THE DIABETIC FOOT

THE DIABETIC FOOT

Edited by

ROBERT J. HINCHLIFFE, MD, FRCS
Senior Lecturer and Honorary Consultant in Vascular Surgery
St George's Vascular Institute
St George's Healthcare NHS Trust
London
UK

NICOLAAS C. SCHAPER, MD, PhD
Professor of Endocrinology
Department of Internal Medicine, Division of Endocrinology
Maastricht University Hospital
Maastricht
The Netherlands

MATT M. THOMPSON, MD, FRCS
Professor of Vascular Surgery
St George's Vascular Institute
St George's Healthcare NHS Trust
London
UK

RAMESH K. TRIPATHI, MD, FRCS, FRACS(Vasc)
Director and Professor of Vascular Surgery
Narayana Institute of Vascular Sciences
Narayana Hrudayalaya Healthcare
Bangalore
India

CARLOS H. TIMARAN, MD
Associate Professor of Surgery
Chief of Endovascular Surgery
Division of Vascular and Endovascular Surgery
Department of Surgery
University of Texas Southwestern Medical Center
Dallas, Texas
USA

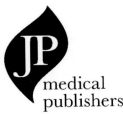

JP medical publishers

London • Philadelphia • Panama City • New Delhi

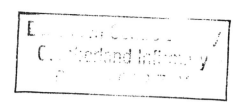

© 2014 JP Medical Ltd.
Published by JP Medical Ltd, 83 Victoria Street, London, SW1H 0HW, UK
Tel: +44 (0)20 3170 8910   Fax: +44 (0)20 3008 6180
Email: info@jpmedpub.com   Web: www.jpmedpub.com

ISBN: 978-1-907816-62-8

British Library Cataloguing in Publication Data
A catalogue record for this book is available from the British Library

Library of Congress Cataloging in Publication Data
A catalog record for this book is available from the Library of Congress

Publisher:	Geoff Greenwood
Development Editor:	Gavin Smith
Design:	Designers Collective Ltd

Typeset, indexed, printed and bound in India.

Preface

Diabetes is reaching epidemic proportions across the globe. It is one of the few diseases that can lay claim to affect multiple organ systems. One of the most feared complications of diabetes for those people who have the misfortune to develop it is lower limb disease, foot ulceration and ultimately, amputation.

Until recently, diabetic foot disease has been a relatively neglected complication of diabetes, but slowly the wheel is turning. Patients, healthcare professionals and politicians have started to realise the quite staggering burden of foot disease for individuals and society. Evidence of this may be seen in the ever increasing numbers of scientific publications on the subject.

Because diabetes is a truly multi-organ disease, it requires input from a variety of healthcare specialists, none of whom should be expected to manage these complications in isolation. Indeed, for many specialists diabetes-related foot disease represents the most challenging aspect of their individual specialty.

If lower limb and specifically foot complications are managed in a timely and expert fashion, ulcers will be healed, limbs preserved and lives saved. Delay, or poor management, including failure to use evidence-based therapies, will result in ulcers that fail to heal, amputations and deaths.

This book was developed with all those who manage patients with diabetes – and specifically, diabetes-related complications of the lower extremity, be they generalists or specialists – in mind. It summarises the current best available evidence on diabetic foot disease for busy clinicians. Bringing together a variety of experts from across the world, it provides a keen insight to the current management of all aspects of diabetic foot disease. Specifically, the experts have amassed and sifted through the wealth of data now emerging on this topic and provided a clear and concise summary that readers will find easy to access rapidly. The book is separated into the main themes of diabetic foot disease, from its epidemiology and natural history, through to the practical organisation of care and the diagnosis and management of neuropathy, peripheral arterial disease, infection and Charcot disease. Each chapter helpfully provides a brief summary, highlights current controversies and focuses the reader on current and future areas of research.

Robert J. Hinchliffe
Nicolaas C. Schaper
Matt M. Thompson
Ramesh K. Tripathi
Carlos H. Timaran
July 2014

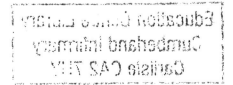

Contents

Preface v

Contributors xi

Introduction xvii
Karel Bakker

SECTION 1: GENERAL ASPECTS

Chapter 1
Epidemiology of diabetic foot disease and etiology of ulceration 3
Jan Apelqvist

Chapter 2
Diabetic foot assessment and classification of risk 11
David G. Armstrong, Nicholas A. Giovinco, Magdiel Trinidad-Hernandez

Chapter 3
Setting up a diabetic foot service 21
Abdul Basit

Chapter 4
Economic aspects of foot care 27
Marion Kerr

Chapter 5
Medical therapy and metabolic control to optimize cardiovascular
risk and reduce overall mortality 33
Jack R. W. Brownrigg, Kausik K. Ray

Chapter 6
Psychological aspects of diabetes-related foot disease 39
George Peach, Robert J. Hinchliffe

Chapter 7
Diabetes self-management education for the preservation of patient
and foot health and the prevention of foot ulcers and amputations 45
Kristien Van Acker, Neil Baker

SECTION 2: INFECTION

Chapter 8
Managing infection in the diabetic foot 57
Edgar J. G. Peters, Benjamin A. Lipsky

Chapter 9
Diabetic foot osteomyelitis: diagnosis and classification 69
Eric M. Senneville

Chapter 10
Osteomyelitis: medical management 75
John M. A. Embil, Elly Trepman

Chapter 11
Osteomyelitis: surgical management 79
F. Javier Aragón Sánchez

SECTION 3: ISCHEMIA

Chapter 12
Peripheral arterial disease in diabetes   95
Carlos H. Timaran, David E. Timaran

Chapter 13
Microvascular disease   101
Sanjeev Sharma, Gerry Rayman

Chapter 14
The diagnosis of peripheral arterial disease   111
Patrick Coughlin

Chapter 15
Imaging of peripheral arterial disease   117
Gerard S. Goh

Chapter 16
Angiosomes   129
Neil C. Wright, Robert Fitridge

Chapter 17
Distal bypass techniques   137
Himanshu Verma, Robbie K. George, Ramesh K. Tripathi

Chapter 18
Angioplasty techniques   153
Ezio Faglia, Giacomo Clerici, Flavio Airoldi

Chapter 19
Outcomes of angioplasty and bypass in diabetes   171
Robert J. Hinchliffe, Keith G. Jones, Rachael O. Forsythe

SECTION 4: NEUROPATHY

Chapter 20
Pathobiology of neuropathy   183
Ketan Dhatariya

Chapter 21
The diagnosis and clinical impact of diabetic distal
symmetrical polyneuropathy   193
Nicolaas C. Schaper, Solomon Tesfaye

Chapter 22
Surgical treatment of diabetic neuropathy   201
A. Lee Dellon

SECTION 5: WOUNDS AND ULCERATION

Chapter 23
Acute and chronic wound healing biology in diabetes   209
Michelle Griffin, Ardeshir Bayat

Chapter 24
Scoring systems and assessment of the ulcerated foot   223
Fran Game

Chapter 25
Wound dressings and debridement   231
Elizabeth J. Mudge, Alastair J. Richards, Keith G. Harding

Chapter 26
Adjuncts to wound healing   243
Magnus Löndahl

Chapter 27
Standardization of outcomes and end points of wound healing
in everyday practice and clinical trials   251
Finn Gottrup

SECTION 6: SURGICAL INTERVENTION

Chapter 28
Surgical anatomy of the foot   259
Adam Ajis

Chapter 29
Surgical debridement   267
Peter Vowden, Soroush Sohrabi

Chapter 30
Skin and local tissue flaps   273
Crystal L. Ramanujam, John J. Stapleton, Thomas Zgonis

Chapter 31
Free tissue transfer   283
Joon Pio Hong

SECTION 7: CHARCOT

Chapter 32
The causes and diagnosis of acute Charcot foot in diabetes   297
William Jeffcoate

Chapter 33
Charcot osteoarthropathy: medical management and off-loading   303
Valeria Ruotolo, Luigi Uccioli

Chapter 34
Charcot osteoarthropathy: surgical management and off-loading   311
Katherine M. Raspovic, Dane K. Wukich

SECTION 8: AMPUTATION

Chapter 35
Minor amputation and major amputation   321
Yiu-Che Chan, Stephen W. Cheng

Chapter 36
Rehabilitation post-amputation   333
S. Sooriakumaran

SECTION 9: BIOMECHANICS AND PREVENTION

Chapter 37
Off-loading   345
Martin C. Berli, Thomas Böni

Chapter 38
Prevention of ulcer recurrence   353
Sicco A. Bus

Chapter 39
Preventive foot care programs   361
Zulfiqarali G. Abbas

Index   369

Contributors

Zulfiqarali G. Abbas, MBBS, MMed, DTM&H(UK)
Consultant Physician, Endocrinologist and Diabetologist
Chair, Pan-African Diabetic Foot Study Group
Abbas Medical Centre and Muhimbili University of Health
and Allied Sciences
Dar es Salaam
Tanzania

Flavio Airoldi, MD
Chief, Endovascular Unit
Cardiovascular Department
IRCCS MultiMedica
Milan
Italy

**Adam Ajis, BMedSc(Hons Physiol), MBChB,
FRCS(Tr & Orth)**
Consultant Trauma and Orthopaedic Surgeon
Specialising in Disorders of the Foot and Ankle
Department of Trauma and Orthopaedic Surgery
Western Sussex NHS Foundation Trust
Worthing
UK

Jan Apelqvist, MD, PhD
Associate Professor, Internal Medicine
Department of Endocrinology, University Hospital of
Skåne, Malmö
Division for Clinical Sciences, University of Lund
Sweden

F. Javier Aragón Sánchez, MD, PhD
Head, Surgery Department
Diabetic Foot and Endoluminal Therapy Unit
La Paloma Hospital
Las Palmas de Gran Canaria
Spain

David G. Armstrong, DPM, MD, PhD
Professor of Surgery
Department of Surgery
University of Arizona College of Medicine
Tucson, Arizona
USA

Neil Baker, BSc, DPod M, FCPod Med, MChS
Principal Diabetes Specialist and Research Podiatrist
Ipswich Diabetic Foot Cente
Ipswich Hospital NHS Trust
Ipswich
UK

Karel Bakker, MD, PhD
Internist/Endocrinologist
Immediate Past –Chair, International Working Group on
the Diabetic Foot
Heemstede
The Netherlands

Abdul Basit, MBBS, FRCP(Lon)
Director, Baqai Institute of Diabetology and Endocrinology
Professor of Medicine, Baqai Medical University
Karachi
Pakistan

Ardeshir Bayat, BSc (Hons) MBBS, MRCS, PhD
Clinical Scientist
Institute of Inflammation and Repair
Manchester Institute of Biotechnology
The University of Manchester
University Hospital of South Manchester NHS Foundation
Trust
Wythenshawe Hospital
Manchester
UK

Martin C. Berli, MD
Deputy Team Leader, Technical Orthopedics
Department of Orthopedic Surgery
University of Zürich
Zürich
Switzerland

Thomas Böni, MD
Team Leader, Technical Orthopedics
Department of Orthopedic Surgery
University of Zürich
Zürich
Switzerland

Jack R. W. Brownrigg, MBChB, MRCS
NIHR Academic Clinical Fellow Vascular Surgery
St George's Vascular Institute
St George's Healthcare NHS Trust
London
UK

Sicco A. Bus, PhD
Senior Investigator and Head, Human Performance
Laboratory
Academic Medical Center
Department of Rehabilitation Medicine
University of Amsterdam
Amsterdam
The Netherlands

Yiu-Che Chan, MB BS, BSc, MD, FRCS,
FRCS(General Surgery)
Division of Vascular and Endovascular Surgery
Department of Surgery
University of Hong Kong Medical Centre
Hong Kong
China

Stephen W. Cheng, MB BS, MS, FRCS
Professor of Surgery
Division of Vascular and Endovascular Surgery
Department of Surgery
University of Hong Kong Medical Centre
Hong Kong
China

Giacomo Clerici, MD
Chief, Diabetic Foot Centre
IRCCS MultiMedica
Milan
Italy

Patrick Coughlin, MB ChB, MD, FRCS
Consultant Vascular and Endovascular Surgeon
Addenbrookes Hospital
Cambridge
UK

A. Lee Dellon, MD, PhD
Professor of Plastic Surgery and Neurosurgery
Johns Hopkins University
Baltimore, Maryland
USA

Ketan Dhatariya, MBBS, MSc, MD, MS, FRCP
Consultant in Diabetes and Endocrinology
Elsie Bertram Diabetes Centre
Norfolk and Norwich University Hospitals NHS
Foundation Trust
Norwich
UK

John M. A. Embil, BSc(Hons), MD, FRCPC, FACP
Consultant, Infectious Diseases
Director, Infection Prevention and Control Program,
Winnipeg Regional Health Authority
Coordinator, Diabetic Foot and Complicated Wound
Clinic, Health Sciences Centre
Professor, Departments of Internal Medicine (Section of
Infectious Diseases) and Medical Microbiology
University of Manitoba
Winnipeg, Manitoba
Canada

Ezio Faglia, MD
Diabetic Foot Centre
IRCCS MultiMedica
Milan
Italy

Robert Fitridge, MB, BS, MS, FRACS
Professor of Vascular Surgery
University of Adelaide
Department of Vascular Surgery
The Queen Elizabeth Hospital
Woodville, South Australia
Australia

Rachael O. Forsythe, MBChB, MRCS
Specialty Registrar in Surgery
St George's Vascular Institute
St George's Healthcare NHS Trust
London
UK

Fran Game, FRCP
Consultant Diabetologist, Honorary Associate Professor
Department of Diabetes and Endocrinology
Derby Hospitals NHS Foundation Trust
Derby
UK

Robbie K. George, MS, DNB, FRCS
Consultant Vascular Surgeon
Narayana Institute of Vascular Sciences
Narayana Hrudayalaya Healthcare
Bangalore
India

Nicholas A. Giovinco, DPM
Assistent Professor of Surgery
Department of Surgery
University of Arizona College of Medicine
Tucson, Arizona
USA

Gerard S. Goh, MBBS, FRANZCR, EBIR
Interventional and Diagnostic Radiologist
Department of Radiology
The Alfred Hospital
Melbourne, Victoria
Australia

Finn Gottrup, MD, DMSci
Professor of Surgery
University of Southern Denmark
Copenhagen Wound Healing Center
Department of Dermatology
Bispebjerg University Hospital
Copenhagen
Denmark

Michelle Griffin, MBChB, MRes, MRCS, MSc
Vascular Research Fellow
St George's Vascular Institute
St George's Hospital Healthcare NHS Trust
London
UK

Keith G. Harding, FRCGP, FRCP, FRCS
Dean of Clinical Innovation
Head of Wound Healing Research Unit
Wound Healing Research Unit
Cardiff University School of Medicine
Cardiff
UK

Robert J. Hinchliffe, MD, FRCS
Senior Lecturer and Honorary Consultant in Vascular
Surgery
St George's Vascular Institute
St George's Healthcare NHS Trust
London
UK

Joon Pio Hong, MD, PhD, MMM
Professor of Plastic Surgery
Department of Plastic surgery
Asan Medical Center
University of Ulsan
Seoul
Korea

William Jeffcoate, MB, MRCP
Consultant Diabetologist
Foot Ulcer Trials Unit
Department of Diabetes and Endocrinology
Nottingham University Hospitals Trust
Nottingham
UK

Keith G. Jones, MS, FRCS
Consultant in Vascular Surgery
St George's Vascular Institute
St George's Healthcare NHS Trust
London
UK

Marion Kerr, MSc
Health Economist
Insight Health Economics Ltd.
London
UK

Benjamin A. Lipsky, MD, FACP, FIDSA, FRCP
Professor of Medicine
Department of Medicine, University of Washington
(Emeritus)
Seattle, USA
University of Geneva (Visiting)
Geneva, Switzerland
Teaching Associate, Green Templeton College
University of Oxford
Oxford
UK

Magnus Löndahl, MD, PhD
Senior Consultant, Endocrinology
Head of Diabetes
Department of Endocrinology
Skåne University Hospital
Department of Clinical Sciences
Lund University
Lund
Sweden

Elizabeth J. Mudge, MSc, BSc, DPodM, SRch, MChS
Research Fellow, Wound Healing
Wound Healing Research Unit
Cardiff University School of Medicine
Cardiff
UK

George Peach, MRCS, MBChB, BSc
Specialist Registrar, Vascular Surgery
St George's Vascular Institute
St George's Healthcare NHS Trust
London
UK

Edgar J. G. Peters, MD, PhD
Internist, Infectious Diseases Specialist, Acute Medicine
Specialist
Department of Internal Medicine
VU University Medical Center
Amsterdam
The Netherlands

Crystal L. Ramanujam, DPM, MSc
Assistant Professor
Division of Podiatric Medicine and Surgery
Department of Orthopaedic Surgery
University of Texas Health Science Center at San Antonio
San Antonio, Texas
USA

Katherine M. Raspovic, DPM
Department of Plastic Surgery
Georgetown University Hospital
Washington, District of Columbia
USA

**Kausik K. Ray, BSc(Hons), MBChB, MD, MPhil(Cantab),
FRCP, FESC, FACC, FAHA**
Professor of CVD Prevention
Cardiovascular Sciences Research Centre
St George's University of London
London
UK

Gerry Rayman, MD, FRCP
Consultant Physician, Diabetes and Endocrinology
Department of Diabetes and Endocrinology
Ipswich Hospital NHS Trust
Ipswich
UK

Alastair J. Richards, MBBCh
Clinical Research Fellow, Wound Healing
Wound Healing Research Unit
Cardiff University School of Medicine
Cardiff
UK

Valeria Ruotolo, MD
Endocrinologist
Department of Internal Medicine
Tor Vergata University
Rome
Italy

Nicolaas C. Schaper, MD, PhD
Professor of Endocrinology
Department of Internal Medicine, Division of
Endocrinology
Maastricht University Hospital
Maastricht
The Netherlands

Eric M. Senneville, MD, PhD
Professor of Infectious Dieases
University Department of Infectious Diseases
Gustave Dron Hospital
Tourcoing
France

Sanjeev Sharma, MD, MRCP
Clinical Research Fellow in Diabetes
Diabetes Research Unit
Ipswich Hospital NHS Trust
Ipswich
UK

Soroush Sohrabi, MD, PhD, MRCS
NIHR Academic Clinical Lecturer in Vascular Surgery
Department of Vascular Surgery
Bradford Teaching Hospitals NHS Foundation Trust
Bradford
UK

Sellaiah Sooriakumaran, FRCP, FRCS
Consultant in Rehabilitation Medicine
Roehampton Rehabilitation Centre
Queen Mary's Hospital
London
UK

John J. Stapleton, DPM, FACFAS
Associate, Foot and Ankle Surgery
VSAS Orthopaedics and Chief of Podiatric Surgery
Lehigh Valley Hospital
Allentown, Pennsylvania
Clinical Assistant Professor of Surgery
Penn State College of Medicine
Hershey, Pennsylvania
USA

Solomon Tesfaye, MB ChB, MD, FRCP
Consultant Physician and Honorary Professor of Diabetic
Medicine
The University of Sheffield
Royal Hallamshire Hospital
Sheffield
UK

Carlos H. Timaran, MD
Associate Professor of Surgery
Chief of Endovascular Surgery
Division of Vascular and Endovascular Surgery
Department of Surgery
University of Texas Southwestern Medical Center
Dallas, Texas
USA

David E. Timaran, MD
Postdoctoral Research Fellow
Division of Vascular and Endovascular Surgery
Department of Surgery
University of Texas Southwestern Medical Center
Dallas, Texas
USA

Elly Trepman, MD
Professional Associate
Department of Medical Microbiology
University of Manitoba
Manitoba
Canada

Magdiel Trinidad-Hernandez, MD
Assistant Professor, Surgery
Department of Surgery
The University of Arizona College of Medicine
Tucson, Arizona
USA

Ramesh K. Tripathi, MD, FRCS, FRACS(Vasc)
Director and Professor of Vascular Surgery
Narayana Institute of Vascular Sciences
Narayana Hrudayalaya Healthcare
Bangalore
India

Luigi Uccioli, MD
Professor of Endocrinology
Department of Internal Medicine
Tor Vergata University
Rome
Italy

Kristien Van Acker, MD, PhD
Chair, IDF Consultative Section Diabetic Foot/
International Working Group on the Diabetic Foot
(IWGDF)
Department of Diabetology
Hospital H. Familie
Rumst (Reet)
Department of Diabetology
Centre de Santé des Fagnes
Chimay
Belgium

Himanshu Verma, MS, FEVS
Vascular Surgeon
Narayana Institute of Vascular Sciences
Narayana Hrudayalaya Healthcare
Bangalore
India

Peter Vowden, MD, FRCS
Consultant Vascular Surgeon
Visiting Professor Wound Healing Research
Department of Vascular Surgery
Bradford Teaching Hospitals NHS Foundation Trust
University of Bradford
Bradford
UK

Neil C. Wright, MBBCh, FCS, FRACS
Vascular Surgeon
Sunninghill Hospital
Johannesburg
South Africa

Dane K. Wukich, MD
Professor of Orthopaedic Surgery
Chief, Division of Foot and Ankle Surgery
Medical Director, UPMC Mercy Center For Healing and
Amputation Prevention
University of Pittsburgh Medical Center
Pittsburgh, Pennsylvania
USA

Thomas Zgonis, DPM, FACFAS
Associate Professor, Director of Externship and
Reconstructive Foot and Ankle Surgery Fellowship
Division of Podiatric Medicine and Surgery
Department of Orthopaedic Surgery
University of Texas Health Science Center at San Antonio
San Antonio, Texas
USA

Introduction

Karel Bakker

BACKGROUND

The 'diabetic foot' defined as 'infection, ulceration and/or destruction of deep tissue associated with neurological abnormalities and various degrees of peripheral vascular disease in the lower limb in people with diabetes' (IWGDF 2011) has for centuries been neglected. It only started to generate serious interest in the 1980s. Diabetic foot complications were rightly feared by patients and clinicians alike because of their association with high rates of lower extremity amputations (LEA). The vast majority, some 85% of these amputations, is preceded by a foot ulcer. The most important factors relating to the development of these ulcers are peripheral neuropathy, foot deformities, minor foot trauma, and peripheral arterial disease (PAD). Once an ulcer has developed, infection and PAD are major causes of amputation. However, with timely and expert care, many amputations may be prevented and most ulcers will heal.

◼ PREVALENCE

It is estimated that in 2013 approximately 382 million – 8.3% of the world's population – people had diabetes, and about 80% of these people live in developing countries. By 2035, the global estimate is expected to rise to >592 million – 9.9% of the adult population. Worryingly, type 2 diabetes is increasing among young people as well as older people around the world (International Diabetes Federation 2013).

The spectrum of foot lesions varies from region to region due to differences in socioeconomic conditions, standards of foot care, and the quality of footwear. It has been calculated that in developed countries, one in six people with diabetes will have an ulcer during their lifetime. In developing countries, diabetes-related foot problems are thought to be even more common. Every year, more than 1 million people with diabetes lose a leg as a consequence of this disease. This means that every 20 seconds a lower limb is lost due to diabetes somewhere in the world.

◼ HISTORY

During the 19th century and for much of the 20th century, disease of the lower limb in patients with diabetes was conceptualized not, as it is now, as 'the diabetic foot' or as 'a diabetic foot ulcer' but as 'gangrene in the diabetic foot' or as 'diabetic gangrene' (Connor 2008). The prognostically and therapeutically important distinction between gangrene due to vascular insufficiency and gangrene due to infection in a limb with a normal or near normal blood supply was not made until about 1893 (Godlee 1893). The advent of aseptic surgery improved the survival of amputation flaps, but surgery remained a hazardous undertaking until the discovery of insulin. The increasing workload attributable to diabetic foot disease after the introduction of insulin is reflected in the publications on diabetes in the 1920s. In some hospitals in North America, this led to initiatives in prophylactic care and patient education, the importance of which were only more widely appreciated some 60 years later. A continuing emphasis on ischemia and infection as the major causes of diabetic foot disease led to a neglect of the role of neuropathy. In consequence, the management of diabetic neuropathic ulceration entered a prolonged period of therapeutic stagnation at a time when significant advances were being made in the management of lepromatous neuropathic ulceration. The association between gangrene and diabetes was recognized by Marchal de Calvi in 1852 (Marchal de Calvi 1852) and also by Thomas Hodgkin in 1854 (Hodgkin 1854). The importance of pressure and callus in the pathogenesis and persistence of ulcers was recognized by Treves in 1884 (Treves 1884). It was understood that foot ulcers could be healed by prolonged bed rest, but that recurrence was likely when the patient mobilized. Amputation of part of the foot was often recommended for persistent or recurrent ulcers, even though the risk of further ulceration in the deformed foot or in the amputation stump was well known.

It was Treves who also described for the first time the use of sharp debridement in the treatment of neuropathic ulceration. He recognized that a reduction in pressure on the foot was required if recurrence was to be prevented. Treves established three principles in the treatment of neuropathic ulceration, namely sharp debridement, off-loading of pressure for both treatment and prevention, and education about foot care and footwear. However, at least as regards diabetic neuropathic ulceration, these three principles were then largely forgotten for the next 40 years.

Whether the arrival of insulin in 1922 improved the survival in patients with gangrene cannot be determined from the literature (Connor 2008). It is likely that many of the patients who are now treated surgically would have been considered unfit for surgery in the preinsulin years. However, the increasing workload attributable to diabetic foot disease is reflected in a fourfold increase in the number of pages that Joslin (1917) devoted to the subject between the second and fourth editions in 1928 of his textbook.

Joslin and others expressed their view that prophylactic care and education were essential and they mentioned virtually all of the points that we would teach our patients today. The teaching of foot care was considered so important that by 1928 the clinic at the Deaconess Hospital in Boston had assigned one graduate nurse and two pupil nurses to this duty; and it was not just theoretical oral teaching and written advice that was provided because 'every diabetic patient receives at least one demonstration and lesson...' (McKittrick & Root 1928) A treatment room for diabetes-related foot problems, staffed by two chiropodists and one nurse, had been opened in the clinic in 1927, an early example of multidisciplinary teamwork and one that extended to the clinic's relationships with chiropodists outside the hospital. Like doctors in other clinics, Joslin had been aware that some diabetic foot problems were the result of uninformed chiropody, but instead of blaming the chiropodists he took steps to bring them on board and by 1934 he could write that: 'Our Boston chiropodists are useful allies. Nowadays we do not see gangrene which has developed at the hands of a chiropodist. At the start of our work with them we consulted with the leaders of their State and National Societies and these excellent men have guided us in our contacts' (Joslin 1934).

Other early converts to the need for education on foot care were the Montreal General Hospital where foot care leaflets were given to all patients by 1927 (Rabinowitch 1927) and the Bellevue Hospital in New

York, which started a diabetic foot room in May 1933 (Brandaleone et al. 1937). It is amazing that it has taken dozens of years for other clinics to embrace these principles and even more amazing that some still do not do so.

Henry Connor wrote 'to those of us who came into the field of diabetic foot disease in the 1970s and early 1980s, it often seemed that the diabetic foot was the forgotten specialty of the chronic complications of diabetes' and there is some evidence to support this belief (Connor 2008). A search of PubMed (www.ncbi.nlm.nih.gov/entrez/query.fcgi 2006) demonstrates that in each decade from 1950 onward there have been fewer papers published on the diabetic foot than on diabetic neuropathy or nephropathy or retinopathy (**Table 0.1**). For example, in the 1950s there were more than twice as many papers on retinopathy as on foot disease. The data show that foot disease lagged further and further behind the other complications until the end of the 1980s. Only in the 1990s did the trend start to reverse. A similar pattern is to be found in the formation of the Study Groups of the European Association for the Study of Diabetes; the Foot Study Group was the last group to be formed, in 1998, some 10 years after the neuropathy, nephropathy, and retinopathy groups.

Why was there this lag period in the study of diabetic foot disease? It is tempting to attribute the deficiency in publications to a lack of technology for investigating foot disease. But this cannot explain the lack of progress in the field of diabetic neuropathic ulceration at a time when significant advances were being made in the management of neuropathic ulcers in leprosy. The use of special footwear to prevent ulcers or their relapse in patients with leprosy was described by Paul Brand already in 1950 (Brand 1950). Brand used clay to obtain standing impressions of his patient's feet and these were used to produce molded rubber insoles. This was 26 years before Holstein's paper on insoles for diabetic shoes (Holstein et al. 1976). By 1963, Brand and his colleagues were using thin transducers in patients with leprosy to make in-shoe pressure measurements that they used to guide their research and shoe manufacturing (Bauman et al. 1963, Ward 1962). He showed that neuropathic ulcers were treatable and preventable. This was 10 years before the earliest diabetic publications on this subject (Barrett & Mooney 1973, Stokes et al. 1975).

Why were those who worked with patients with diabetes in more affluent societies so much slower to learn the same lessons? Connor believes that it was, in large part, due to classification and terminology. The diabetic foot is, of course, a more complex entity than its lepromatous counterpart in that it has a heterogeneous aetiology comprising an important vascular element in addition to the neuropathic component, and also because infection plays a significant role along with hyperglycemia.

The issues over terminology extended beyond neglect of the neuropathic component. The dominance of negative terms such as 'diabetic gangrene' only finally disappeared during in the 1980s–1990s (Kahn & Weir 1994, Oakley 1954). As long as clinicians continued to think of diabetic foot lesions predominantly in negative terms like gangrene and amputation, it was almost inevitable that they would do so in an aura of therapeutic nihilism. When more neutral terms came to the fore, the minds of diabetologists were opened to the possibility of therapeutic advance. The author believes that the number of different specialists involved in diabetic foot care may also have been counterproductive. In essence, no single specialty was able to identify and drive the diabetic foot care agenda. Only after the development of a multi- or interdisciplinary team approach were major steps forward made.

1980 AND ON

An important development following the long lag period was the foundation of diabetic foot clinics in the 1980s in the USA and Europe, notably at the University of Miami, USA; Geneva, Switzerland; San Antonio, USA; Kings College Hospital, London, UK, Manchester Infirmary, UK; Deaconess Hospital, Boston, USA; and the Heemstede Hospital, Heemstede, the Netherlands. The spin-off effect of this was significant throughout the world. Likewise, more awareness was created by the first international diabetic foot meetings. Among the first events of this kind were the University of Texas Health Science Center 1st meeting (1985), the first Malvern Foot meeting (1986) in the UK, the High Risk Diabetic Foot Conference in Boston (1988), and the first International Symposium on the Diabetic Foot (ISDF) in Noordwijkerhout, the Netherlands (May 1991) (**Figure i**).

The foundation of the Diabetic Foot Study Groups (DFSG) was an important development as well. Creating a platform for researchers in the field with the slogan 'together are we stronger' focused on the importance of better management and prevention of diabetic foot ulcers and their consequences.

The American Diabetes Association (ADA) Foot Council had its first meeting in 1987 and, as already mentioned, the DFSG Europe was founded in 1998 in Barcelona. In the meantime, several more study groups were formed elsewhere (e.g., GLEPED [South America] and the Pan African DFSG and the local DFSG in India, Pakistan, Israel, Greece, Egypt, France, Belgium, the Netherlands, Germany, Portugal, Spain, and very recently the Gulf Diabetic Foot Study Group).

Data to underpin the clinical effectiveness of these MDT foot clinics and initiatives started to filter through soon afterward. Edmonds showed for the first time that a multidisciplinary diabetic foot clinic approach could reduce the number of amputations significantly (Edmonds et al. 1986).

A groundbreaking initiative took place in Italy in 1989. At a well-attended international workshop, representatives of government health departments and patient organizations from all European countries met with diabetes experts under the aegis of the regional offices of the World Health Organization (WHO) and the International Diabetes Federation (IDF) in St Vincent, Italy, on 10–12th October, 1989. They unanimously agreed upon the following recommendations and urged that they should be presented in all countries throughout Europe for implementation. The so-called 'St Vincent Declaration' was a result of this important workshop (Saint The Vincent Declaration on diabetes

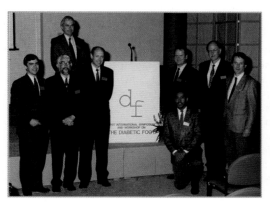

Figure i First International Symposium on the Diabetic Foot (ISDF). Noordwijkerhout, the Netherlands, May 1991: organizing committee. Standing from left to right: Andrew J M Boulton (UK), Karel Bakker (the Netherlands), Jan A Rauwerda (the Netherlands), Per E Holstein (Denmark), Folke Lithner (Sweden), Bob PJ Michels (the Netherlands). Kneeling: Lawrence B Harkless (USA). Standing above: Arie C Nieuwenhuijzen Kruseman (the Netherlands).

care and research in Europe 1989). At the conclusion of the St Vincent meeting, all those attending formally pledged themselves to strong and decisive action in seeking implementation of the recommendations on their return home. One of the 5-year targets was to 'reduce by one half the rate of limb amputations for diabetic gangrene.' Unfortunately this goal, at least for the time being, appears to represent a 'bridge too far.' It is remarkable that there remains a lack of willingness in many countries' ministries of health to invest in preventive measures.

BARRIERS

In recent years, many efforts have been undertaken to teach all healthcare workers involved in the treatment of people with diabetes. Nevertheless, there are numerous barriers to the implementation of universal good care, involving the attitudes and beliefs of doctors, other healthcare professionals, and patients, and the structure of healthcare systems all of which can conspire to prevent patients with diabetes from receiving the appropriate care they desperately need (van Houtum 2012).

Barriers to the implementation of foot care are everywhere. Their presence is often expected in developing countries, but be assured that barriers are easily encountered in the most highly specialized diabetic foot care centers. Sometimes the most glaring barriers are not identified and therefore completely overlooked, preventing patients from receiving the best available foot care. Potential barriers can be grouped together in three distinct categories: availability of healthcare, patient-related factors, and healthcare system (van Houtum 2005).

Availability of healthcare

In some areas of the world, there is a complete lack of dedicated clinics for patients with diabetes-related foot disease. As facilities in certain areas provide care for a large geographical area, patients may be forced to travel enormous distances of up to hundreds of kilometers.

Even when clinics are available, healthcare providers working in those facilities may not be interested in diabetic foot pathology or may not have the appropriate knowledge or training. This will result in delays or even an absence of adequate foot care. Certain doctors may adhere to beliefs that interfere with their willingness to put effort into diabetic foot problems. Patients who seek alternative forms of medicine may be excluded from care as they may be considered unwilling to follow directions (Tripp-Reimer et al. 2001).

The availability of specific tools can differ to a huge extent between different facilities. Even when a strict protocol is implemented and local guidelines have been developed, the care provided is still different. In the Eurodiale study, it was found that among 1232 patients in 14 European centers, 27% of people had a referral delay of >3 months. Casting was performed in only 35% of cases with a plantar ulcer (percentage range: 0–68%). Vascular imaging in severe limb ischemia was performed in 56% of cases, ranging between 14% and 86% in the different centers (Prompers et al. 2008).

Another serious problem is the lack of availability of licensed podiatry education. Podiatry is considered to be the cornerstone of good diabetic foot care. In the >200 countries in the world, there exist only 19 trainings facilities with a course duration of 3 years or more, of which 13 are in Europe. It is estimated that well-trained podiatrists are active in only 35 countries. It is the aim of programs such as the Diabetic Foot Care Assistants education program varying from 2 weeks (basic course) to 10 weeks (advanced course) will help to fill the gap (Tulley et al. 2009), but so far only a very few countries have adopted such programs.

Patient-related factors

The presentation of patients to the appropriate healthcare providers is dependent on many factors. The most recognized barrier is the presence of neuropathy. The absence of the 'gift of pain' creates a patient delay. They do not feel problems with their feet, denying them the ability to act accordingly. The presence of retinopathy in people with diabetes may also prevent them from actually seeing callus, erythema, ulceration, or any other pending foot problem.

Education is therefore pivotal and needs to be provided to patients in a simple, consistent and repetitive manner. Lack of education has proven to be a risk factor for the occurrence of ulceration in >90% of cases in a study from Egypt (El-Nahas et al. 2008). Factors that need to be addressed in providing education are language barriers, illiteracy, availability of educational programs, and documentation. Unfortunately, there remains a lack of funding for preventive measures throughout the world.

A patient's fear of losing a limb may act as another barrier to attending a diabetic foot clinic. In many cultures, there are specific beliefs that prevent patients from getting appropriate care. Alternative healers are present in every corner of the world. This problem is not uniquely encountered in developing countries. In the most modern communities, specific alternative modalities are at hand. Religious habits or lifestyle choices that influence the risk of foot problems include barefoot walking or kneeling while at prayer.

Healthcare system

Differences in the financial organization of care directly influence the possibility of using care facilities. When all care is reimbursed by the government, care may be easily available to patients. However, when care is provided only by private insurance cover or even self-payment, certain types of care may be restricted or simply not obtainable.

On a more macroeconomical level, it is instrumental to realize that the amount of money dedicated to care as a whole and the diabetic foot in particular differs enormously between countries and fluctuates over time (Cavanagh et al. 2012). Ultimately the individual healthcare system at hand determines the availability of specific specialists, multidisciplinary teams, and the presence of protocols.

ACHIEVEMENTS
International Working Group on the Diabetic Foot

Diabetic foot ulcers and their consequences do not only represent a major personal tragedy for the person suffering from an ulcer and his/her family but also place a considerable financial burden on the healthcare system and society in general. Ulcers of the foot in diabetes are the source of major suffering and cost. At least 25% will not heal and up to 28% may result in some form of amputation.

Because of this devastating problem, experts in the field felt the need to do more than organizing and attending meetings to create more awareness to exchange research results and to discuss better management of diabetic foot problems. Internationally acknowledged guidelines were needed. Investing in a diabetic foot care guideline is one of the most cost-effective forms of healthcare expenditure, provided the guideline is goal focused and properly implemented. Therefore, the International Working Group on the Diabetic Foot (IWGDF) was founded in 1996.

Other aims of the IWGDF were to stimulate proper research and to guide scientific meetings, of which the very successful quadrennial ISDF (since 1991 in Noordwijkerhout, the Netherlands) is by far the most striking example.

The IWGDF is instrumental in acting as a consultant for the implementation of programs such as the 'Step-by-Step' (SbS) program, improving diabetic foot care in developing and low income countries, the 'Train-the-Foot-Trainer, how to set up Step-by-Step program' (TtFT) programs, the Diabetic Foot Care education program for Assistants, and postgraduate courses. In 2000, Sir George Alberti, President of the IDF at that time, invited the IWGDF to become a Consultative Section of the IDF.

Development of IWGDF guidelines

The guideline process started with a constituent meeting in Malvern, United Kingdom. A steering committee was installed and gathered in 1997 with the task of designing a first draft on a variety of topics (**Figure ii**). In 1998, 23 representatives from 23 countries met to comment on the concept and to come to an agreement. In 1999, the IWGDF published the *International Consensus on the Diabetic Foot and Practical Guidelines on the Management and the Prevention of the Diabetic Foot to Date* for the first time. This publication has been translated into 26 languages, and more than 80,000 copies were distributed globally. In order to further implement the International Consensus document, the IWGDF recruited local champions as members of the IWDGF and these members now represent >100 countries around the world.

Workings groups of independent experts in the field were asked on a quadrennial basis to revise and update the chapters of the original text, according to current knowledge and standards. Since 2007, the guidelines have been based on evidence in the literature. At a Consensus Day (preceding the ISDF meetings) all representatives of the IWGDF network gather to discuss comments and to give their final approval of and undersign the quadrennial IWGDF Consensus guidelines (**Figures iii** and **iv**). The most recent guidelines were launched in May 2011 (Bakker et al. 2011). This ongoing process is guided by the IWGDF Editorial Board (Bakker & Schaper 2011).

World Diabetes Day 2005

The theme for 2005 was 'Diabetes and Foot Care,' completing the series of themes on diabetes complications that began in 2001. The IWGDF/IDF Consultative Section was asked to lead this project. Unlike previous campaigns, where activity was concentrated on or around World Diabetes Day (WDD) on November 14th, the year marked the beginning of a year-long focus for the campaign. IDF had spread activities over the year in order to extract the maximum benefit from the awareness-raising opportunities that presented themselves. It was that goal that drove the awareness campaign for 2005. Preparation for an annual campaign has allowed the IDF to draw greater attention to the theme of WDD. This has been made possible thanks to the support and collaboration of the IDF's partners in the global diabetes community, the IWGDF country representatives, and its sponsors.

WDD 2005 reached its largest audience ever. The IWGDF/IDF held press conferences, TV interviews, and diabetic foot meetings in all regions. WDD was promoted at 53 important diabetes congresses, exhibitions, and meetings around the world. The Lancet devoted a special issue to diabetic foot disease (**Figure v**). WDD material was translated into 25 different languages. As a result of the 12-month global campaign, it is believed that information on diabetes-related foot problems reached

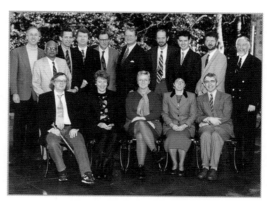

Figure ii International Guidelines on the Management and Prevention of the Diabetic Foot, Tunbridge, UK. June 1997 Steering Committee, sitting from left to right: Jan Apelqvist (Sweden), Gayle Reiber (USA), Lisbeth Vang (Denmark), Jenniffer A Mayfield (USA), Andrew JM Boulton (UK). Standing in front: CV Krishnaswami (USA). Back row: Nicolaas C Schaper (the Netherlands), the late Melcher GK Falkenberg (Sweden), David L Steed (USA), Henry Connor (UK), Per E Holstein (Denmark), Peter R Cavanagh (USA), William H van Houtum (the Netherlands), Lawrence A Lavery (USA), Karel Bakker (the Netherlands).

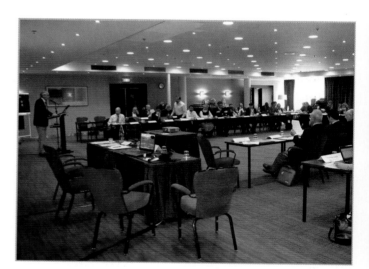

Figure iii International Symposium on the Diabetic Foot (ISDF), Noordwijkerhout, the Netherlands, May 2011 IWGDF Consensus Day.

half a billion people – including people with diabetes, healthcare providers, and, very importantly, healthcare decision makers.

Website

The new IWGDF website was launched in March 2013. The complete 2011 Consensus guidelines (with French and Spanish translations) are on the site, as well as all the IWGDF and IDF Consultative Sections' programs and their implementation processes. In addition, the names and addresses of all of the IWGDF representatives from >100 countries are provided. A news page covering recent developments in 'the foot world' will be updated regularly. This important medium will not only unify the diabetic foot world but will also, without doubt, contribute to more awareness throughout the world (IWGDF 2011).

IMPLEMENTATION

In the new century, several implementation programs have been designed and implemented. The most important ones of these are the

GENERAL ASPECTS

Chapter 1

Epidemiology of diabetic foot disease and etiology of ulceration

Jan Apelqvist

INTRODUCTION

Since diabetes mellitus is growing at epidemic proportions worldwide, the prevalence of diabetes-related complications is bound to increase. Diabetic foot disorders, a major source of disability and morbidity, are a significant burden for the community and a true public health problem. The risk of ulceration and amputation is much higher in those with diabetes compared with those without diabetes. It is estimated that every 20 seconds an amputation is performed for an individual with diabetes somewhere in the world. Foot ulceration is the most common major end point among diabetic complications.

Diabetic foot ulceration represents a major medical, social, and economic problem all over the world. Although >5% of patients with diabetes have a history of foot ulceration, the cumulative lifetime incidence may be as high as 25%. Foot problems in patients with diabetes account for more hospital admissions than any other long-term complications of diabetes and also result in increasing morbidity and mortality.

As reviewed in this chapter, peripheral neuropathy, arterial disease, and foot deformities are the main factors accounting for this increased risk. Age and sex as well as social and cultural status are contributing factors. Knowing these factors is essential to classify every individual with diabetes using a risk grading system and to take preventive measures accordingly.

BACKGROUND

Diabetes is now one of the most common noncommunicable diseases worldwide. It is the fourth or fifth leading cause of death in most of the developed countries and is epidemic in many developing and newly industrialized nations. It is estimated that today approximately 350 million people or 6.6% of the world's population have diabetes. Around 80% of these people live in developing countries. By 2030, the global estimate is expected to rise to some 440 million or 7.8 % of the adult population. Type 1 diabetes accounts for a small percentage of the total burden of diabetes in the population. Type 2 diabetes constitutes about 85–90% of all diabetes in developed countries and accounts for an even higher percentage in developing countries (IDF Atlas). It is increasing in both developed and developing countries.

The diabetic foot defined as infection, ulceration, and/or destruction of deep tissues associated with neurological abnormalities and various degrees of peripheral arterial disease in the lower limb presents a particularly troubling picture and it has been claimed that every 20 seconds, a lower limb is amputated due to diabetes (Int Work Group 2011). It is estimated that 50–70% of all lower extremity amputations are related to diabetes. Of all amputations in patients with diabetes, 85% patients are preceded by a foot ulcer that subsequently deteriorates to a severe infection or gangrene requiring amputation.

Four out of five ulcers are claimed to be preceded by external trauma. Diabetic foot complications result in huge costs for both society and people living with diabetes. Foot problems use 12–15% of the health-care resources for diabetes. In developing countries figures up to 40% have been reported (Boulton 2005, Driver et al. 2010).

FOOT ULCER: PREVALENCE AND INCIDENCE IN INDIVIDUALS WITH DIABETES MELLITUS

A diabetic foot wound is caused by infection, ulceration, and destruction of deep tissues associated with neurological abnormalities and various degrees of peripheral arterial disease in the lower limb. A foot ulcer is the general term to describe a full-thickness wound below the ankle in a patient with diabetes, irrespective of duration (Int Work Group 2011). Active foot disease may be of recent onset or due to a deteriorating chronic situation and refers to anyone with diabetes who presents with a foot lesion.

The major adverse outcomes of diabetic foot problems are foot ulcers and amputations. Up to 85% of all amputations begin with an ulcer; every year, approximately 4 million more people develop a diabetic foot ulcer. More information is available on numbers of amputations than on numbers of ulcers. Until proper population-based registers of people with diabetes are available, reliable data relating to accurate estimates of the prevalence and incidence of these late complications will be limited to community-based studies or studies from dedicated centers or clinics.

As most of the information in the current scientific literature comes from selected populations, and different definitions are used, it is difficult to gauge the extent of foot problems worldwide. It is also likely that the type of ulcer varies around the world: in developed countries, up to 60% of new ulcers are associated with peripheral arterial disease so called neuroischemic and ischemic ulcers; in developing countries, neuropathic ulcers of various origins are more common.

The point prevalence of foot ulcers in developed countries varies between 1.5% and 10% in various populations; a corresponding incidence of 2.2–5.9% has been reported from studies in Western Europe and North America. Foot ulcers occur in both type 1 diabetes and type 2 diabetes. In elderly patients with diabetes type 2 the reported prevalence of foot ulcers has been 5–10%. In studies that focused on younger subjects with type 2 diabetes or individuals with diabetes type 1, the estimated prevalence was 1.7–3.3% (Int Consensus 2011, Richard et al. 2008, Rathur & Boulton 2007, Reiber & LeMaster 2008). In community-based European studies, the prevalence varies between 1.4% and 8.3% and in clinic-based studies from developing countries, a prevalence of 3.6–11.9% is reported especially from Arab countries with a prevalence of diabetes of 19.2–29.2%. In western countries, on average 2 out of 100 individuals with diabetes have a foot ulcer (Richard et al. 2008). The prevalence increases in populations in the presence of predisposing factors.

Box 1.1 Most frequent statements regarding foot ulcers in individuals with diabetes mellitus

- 2.2–5.9% annual cumulative incidence of foot ulcer
- 1.4–8.3% prevalence of foot ulcers
- 7% 1 year incidence of first foot ulcer in neuropathic feet
- 11–25% annual cumulative incidence of re-ulceration or new foot ulcer
- 30–50% new ulcers within 2 years after healed index ulcer
- 10% of ulcers in subjects with previously unknown diabetes

The incidence of diabetic foot ulceration varies with the population studied, the criteria and definitions of foot lesions used, and with differences in study design.

Two studies from Northern European countries reported the annual incidence of foot ulcers in the general population to be just >2% (Abbot et al. 2002, Muller et al. 2002, Richard et al. 2008). However, incidences of 2.5–7.2% have been reported in high risk or selected populations compared with 0.6–2.2% in European community-based studies and 3–6% in clinic-based studies from developing countries (Abbas et al. 2002, Kumar et al. 1994, Ramachandran 2004, Richard et al. 2008). Ulceration is much more common in patients with predisposing risk factors; annual incidence rates in neuropathic individuals vary from 5% to over 7% (Abbot et al. 2002, Manes et al. 2002). It is likely that the cumulative lifetime incidence of foot ulcers may be as high as 25% or even higher in individuals with diabetes, and a previously healed ulcer 30–50% will have a new foot ulcer within 2 years (Abbot et al. 2002, Boulton et al. 2005, Rathur & Boulton 2007).

Studies from the United Kingdom suggest that foot ulcers and amputation are less common in Asian patients of Indian subcontinent origin (Abbot et al. 2005). Possible explanations for the findings in Asian patients relate to differences in limited joint mobility and to better foot care in certain religious groups such as Muslims. North American studies reported that ulceration was more common in Hispanic Americans and in Native Americans than in non-Hispanic whites (Lavery et al. 2003, Resnick et al. 1999). Foot ulceration also appears to be associated with social deprivation (Reiber & LeMaster 2008). In most publications on foot ulcers, there is a male dominance (Gershater 2008, Prompers et al. 2008).

In many reports, prevalence data rely on hospital discharge or claims data (Driver et al. 2010, Payne & Scott 1998, Rathur & Boulton 2007, Reiber & LeMaster 2008). The rate of hospital discharges for patients with diabetes in the United States with leg/foot ulcers for every 1000 patients with diabetes rose from 5.4 in 1980 to 6.9 in 2003. Ulcer prevalence among persons aged >44 years was 6.5/1000 patients with diabetes and it rose progressively to 10.3/ 1000 in individuals aged >75 years (Reiber & LeMaster 2008).

METHODOLOGICAL CONSIDERATIONS WITH REGARD TO INCIDENCE AND PREVALENCE OF FOOT ULCER

Many epidemiological data have been published on the diabetic foot, but they are difficult to interpret because of variability in the methodology and in the definitions used in these studies (Int Work Group 2011, Reiber & LeMaster 2008). Moreover, there is a lack of consistency in population characteristics (ethnicity, social level, accessibility to care) and how results are expressed.

Adequately performed population-based studies regarding the incidence and prevalence of foot ulcer in the lower leg are scarce. Most studies are performed from the perspective of patients attending a dedicated clinic or in a selected study population. The difference in incidence results, in many cases, from differences in the design of the study, demographic factors, and the prevalence of diabetes, as well as variations in registration systems. A major issue is that a foot ulcer is frequently not reported/detected by the patient himself. In one study, 25% of the patients with a full skin foot ulcer denied the presence of the ulcer at an interview followed by a physical examination (Apelqvist & Larsson 2000). In 10% of patients with an ulcer below the ankle, the diagnosis of diabetes was previously unknown. In 50% of patients with diabetes mellitus and a foot ulcer, the treating physician was not aware of the ulcer and the ulcer was not recorded in the medical records. As a consequence, studies tend to underestimate the total number of foot ulcers. The study design and method are essential in that respect. If it is a survey with self-reported questionnaire, interview, analysis of medical records, or cross-sectional clinical study, this will substantially influence the outcome (Apelqvist & Larsson 2000, Reiber & LeMaster 2008). In most countries, the incidence of foot ulcers is underestimated as a continuous registration system is not in place.

Box 1.2 Some pitfalls when evaluating studies regarding incidence and prevalence of foot ulcers

- Foot ulcer definition: etiology type, site
- Study population: hospital, clinic, community- or area based
- Setting: university hospital, referral unit, primary care, home care
- Prevalence of diabetes established or unknown
- Method: clinical investigation, screening, medical records, survey, questionnaire
- Dropout rate: clinical investigation, self-reported survey

ETIOLOGY OF FOOT ULCER IN INDIVIDUALS WITH DIABETES MELLITUS

The most important factors related to development of foot ulcers in individuals with diabetes are peripheral neuropathy, minor foot trauma, foot deformity, and decreased tissue perfusion (Apelqvist & Larsson 2000, Int Work Group 2011). Diabetic foot ulcers are frequently seen in patients with a combination of two or more risk factors occurring together (Gershater 2008, Prompers et al. 2008).

Sensory neuropathy is associated with the loss of pain, awareness of pressure, temperature sensation, and proprioception. Due to the lack of protective sensation, the foot is vulnerable to unattended minor injuries caused by excess pressure or mechanical or thermal injury. Thus, acute injury, ill-fitting shoes, or walking barefoot can precipitate an ulcer. As a consequence, a minor trauma that is not felt by the patient can quickly cause skin damage or ulceration. Prospective studies have shown that sensory neuropathy is a major predictor for the development of foot ulcers.

Motor neuropathy, affecting both the intrinsic foot muscles and leg muscles, results in atrophy and weakness of the intrinsic muscles of the foot, flexion deformities of the toes, and an abnormal walking

CONCEIVABLE PITFALLS IN THE REGISTRATION OF DIABETES-RELATED AMPUTATIONS

Box 1.4 Prevalence/diagnosis of diabetes
- Number of patients, extremities, or number of procedures (e.g. reamputation)
- Under-reporting diabetes status, absence of uniform outpatient data describing major foot problems, and the growing number of minor outpatient surgical procedures
- Amputation level: definition (minor/major), including toe, transmetatarsal, ray, Syme, below knee, through knee, above knee, and hip disarticulations
- Study population: hospital/area based, hospital discharge data, annual estimates of noninstitutionalized, or hospitalized individuals
- Registration: medical records, in-hospital registration, continuous registration, and national records
- Type of study: survey, questionnaire, cross-sectional study, medical records, and physical examination

Indication for amputation

The most common indications for amputation described in the literature are gangrene, infection, and a nonhealing ulcer (Int Work Group 2011). Although frequently reported as such, a nonhealing ulcer should not necessarily be considered an indication for amputation. The indications most commonly cited are gangrene and infection frequently occurring simultaneously. It has to be emphasized that a nonhealing ulcer in itself should not be considered an indication for amputation, since the duration of an ulcer is not an unfavorable factor with regard to amputation (Apelqvist & Larsson 2000). There are very few studies with regard to incidence/prevalence of amputation that report the indication for the surgical procedure as well as the selection of amputation level. The few studies that state the indications for amputation in patients with diabetes suggest the indications are often multifactorial (Larsson & Apelqvist 1995) of which progressive gangrene (50–70%) and infection (25–50%) are most common and frequently in combination (25–50%).

SELECTION OF AMPUTATION LEVEL

Most studies/reports regarding incidence of lower amputations are focused on amputations at or above the ankle than people without diabetes. Studies that focus primarily on above-ankle amputations tend to underestimate the total number of diabetes-related amputations performed. There is still some controversy concerning the benefit of a primary minor amputation versus primary major amputation (below knee) (Apelqvist & Larsson 2000, Schaper et al. 2012). The advantage of primary major amputation is a lower reamputation rate and shorter healing time (Svensson et al. 2011). Minor amputations are associated with higher reamputation rate and as a consequence longer wound healing time. However, in a prospective study the long-term outcome after a healed index amputation in patients with diabetes and foot ulcer was evaluated and it was concluded that those subjects with an index major amputation had a higher mortality rate, an equal rate of new amputations irrespective of level, an increased rate of new contralateral amputations, and a lower potential for rehabilitation than patients with an index minor amputation (Larsson et al. 1998).

Ideally when evaluating diabetes-related amputations, the total amputation rate irrespective of level should be reported as well as indications and rational for level selection.

ADDITIONAL CONFOUNDERS WHEN COMPARING AMPUTATION-RELATED DATA

- Indication for amputation
- Selection of amputation level
- Comorbidity
- Reimbursement
- Resource utilization
- Setting
- Treatment strategies

AMPUTATION AS A MARKER OF QUALITY OF CARE

A considerable number of reports and studies indicate a substantial decrease in amputation rate in people with diabetes. The general conclusion from these studies is that strategies including preventive measures and a multidisciplinary approach to established foot ulcers, strict amputation criteria, and a continuous registration of amputations can bring about a substantial decrease in amputation rate in patients with diabetes (49–85%) (Int Work Group 2011).

Several population-based studies observed a significant reduction in major amputations over time (Krishnan et al. 2008), and after correction for the increasing number of people with diabetes, in some countries a relative decrease was observed over a longer period of time in the number of lower extremity amputations in people with diabetes. However, there are also several countries that report an increase in rates of amputation. The reason for this discrepancy is unclear, but factors such as health-care organization and reimbursement might be, in part, responsible (Apelqvist & Larsson 2000, Reiber & LeMaster 2008).

When assessing the impact of an interventional diabetic foot program, a number of basic underlying factors, such as prevalence of diabetes, the age profile of the population, comorbidity, and smoking habits, must be considered. Such factors may mask the effect of intervention unless compared with a situation where such intervention is not applied and must be considered when assessing future incidence rates (Schaper et al. 2012).

The differences in incidence results, in many cases, are established as a result of differences in the design of the study, demographic factors, and the prevalence of diabetes, as well as variations in registration systems, and differences in reimbursement for a variety of procedures, e.g. minor foot debridements or amputations and revascularizations (Holman et al. 2012, Vamos et al. 2010).

Leg amputations are associated with an increase in mortality in people with diabetes. By the time an amputation is necessary, people have usually had diabetes for many years, and often have severe comorbidity. Death around the time of the amputation (perioperative mortality) occurs in up to 10% of cases. Mortality rates increase over the 5 years following amputation: 30% of patients die within 1 year, 50% die within 3 years, and 70% die within 5 years (Larsson et al. 1998).

In developing countries, these figures tend to be even higher because many people seek medical attention only when their foot problem is so far advanced that their limbs and their lives appear immediately threatened.

Amputation rate should therefore not be used as a sole quality indicator in diabetic foot disease, unless it can be corrected for the relevant characteristics of the patient, the leg and the foot (Schaper et al. 2012). Although there are limitations to clinical research using amputation as an end point, it seems likely to remain the most commonly used way to compare health strategies and to determine the importance of an intervention. The incidence and prevalence figures are helpful in assessing any potential beneficial effect to justify an intervention if they are used and interpreted with caution. Given the limitations explained above, epidemiological research concerning the prevalence and incidence of foot-related complications still forms the backbone of clinical research in the area of the diabetic foot.

■ IMPORTANT FURTHER READING

Abbott CA, Carrington AL, Ashe H, et al. The North-West diabetes foot care study: incidence of, and risk factors for, new diabetic foot ulceration in a community-based cohort. Diabet Med 2002; 20:377–384.

Boulton AJM, Vileikyte L, Ragnarson-Tennvall G, Apelqvist J. The global burden of diabetic foot disease. Lancet 2005; 366:1719–1724.

Holman N, Young RJ, Jeffcoate WJ. Variation in the recorded incidence of amputation of the lower limb in England. Diabetologia. 2012; 55:1919–1925.

Jeffcoate WJ, van Houtum WH. Amputation as a marker of the quality of foot care in diabetes. Diabetologia 2004; 47:2051–2058.

International Working Group on the Diabetic Foot, International consensus on the diabetic foot and practical guidelines on the management and the prevention of the diabetic foot. Amsterdam, the Netherlands (2011). Available on CD-ROM at www.idf. org/bookshop or (www.diabeticfoot.nl).

Krishnan S, Nash F, Baker N, et al. Reduction in diabetic amputations over 11 years in a defined UK population: benefits of multidisciplinary team work and continuous prospective audit. Diabetes Care 2008; 31:99–101.

■ REFERENCES

Abbas ZG, Archibald LK. Epidemiology of the diabetic foot in Africa. Med Sci Monit 2005; 11:RA262–270.

Abbas ZG, Gill GV, Archibald LK. The epidemiology of diabetic limb sepsis: an African perspective. Diabet Med 2002; 19:575–579.

Abbott CA, Carrington AL, Ashe H, et al. The North-West diabetes foot care study: incidence of, and risk factors for, new diabetic foot ulceration in a community-based cohort. Diabet Med 2002; 20:377–384.

Abbott CA, Garrow AP, Carrington AL, et al. Foot ulcer risk is lower in South Asian and African-Caribbean compared to European diabetic patients in the UK. Diabetes Care 2005; 28:1869–1875.

Apelqvist J, Larsson J. What is the most effective way to reduce incidence of amputation in the diabetic foot? Diabetes Metab Res Rev 2000; 16:S75–S83.

Boulton AJM, Vileikyte L, Ragnarson-Tennvall G, Apelqvist J. The global burden of diabetic foot disease. Lancet 2005; 366:1719–1724.

Connelly J, Airey M, Chell S. Variation in clinical decision making is a partial explanation for geographical variation in lower extremity amputation rates. Br J Surg 2001; 88:529–535.

Driver VR, Fabbi M, Lavery LA, Gibbons G. The costs of diabetic foot: the economic case for the limb salvage team. J Am Podiatr Med Assoc 2010; 100(5):335–341.

Gershater MA, Löndahl M, Nyberg P, et al. Complexity of factors related to outcome of neuropathic and neuroischaemic/ischaemic diabetic foot ulcers: a cohort study. Diabetologia 2009; 52:398–407.

Gulliford MC, Mahabir D. Diabetic foot disease and foot care in a Caribbean Community. Diabet Res Clin Pract 2002; 56:35–40.

Holman N, Young RJ, Jeffcoate WJ. Variation in the recorded incidence of amputation of the lower limb in England. Diabetologia Diabetologia 2012; 55:1919–1925.

International Diabetes Federation IDF Diabetes Atlas, 6th edn. International Diabetes Federation, Brussels (2013). http://www.idf.org/diabetesatlas

Jeffcoate WJ, van Houtum WH. Amputation as a marker of the quality of foot care in diabetes. Diabetologia 2004; 47:2051–2058.

Jiminez JT, Palacia SM, Canete F, et al. Prevalence of diabetes mellitus and associated risk factors in an adult urban population in Paraguay. Diabet Med 1998; 15:334–338.

Kidmas AT, Nwadiaso CH, Igun GO. Lower limb amputation in Jos, Nigeria. East Afr Med J 2004; 81:427–429.

Krishnan S, Nash F, Baker N, et al. Reduction in diabetic amputations over 11 years in a defined UK population: benefits of multidisciplinary team work and continuous prospective audit. Diabetes Care 2008; 31:99–101.

Kumar S, Ashe, Ashe H, Fernando DJ, et al. The prevalence of foot ulceration and its correlates in type 2 diabetic patients: a population-based study. Diabet Med 1994; 11:480–483.

Larsson J, Apelqvist J. Towards less amputations in diabetic patients: incidence, causes, cost, treatment and prevention. Acta Ort Scand 1995; 12:56–65.

Larsson J, Agardh CD, Apelqvist J, Stenström A. Long term prognosis after amputation in diabetic patients. Clin Orthop Relat Res 1998; 350:149–158.

Larsson J, Eneroth M, Apelqvist J, Stenström A. Sustained decrease of major amputation in diabetic patients – an analysis of a 20-year period in a defined population (628 amputations in 461 patients). Acta Orth 2008; 79:665–673.

Lavery LA, Armstrong DG, Wunderlich RP, et al. Diabetic foot syndrome: evaluating the prevalence and incidence of foot pathology in Mexican Americans and non-Hispanic whites from a diabetes disease management cohort. Diabetes Care 2003; 26:1435–1438.

LEA Study Group. Epidemiology of lower extremity amputations in centres in Europe, North America and East Asia. Br J Surg 2000; 87:328–337.

Manes C, Papazoglou N, Sassidou E, et al. Prevalence of diabetic neuropathy and foot ulceration: identification of potential risk factors-a population-based study. Wounds 2002; 14:11–15.

Muller IS, DeGraw WJ, van Gerwen WH, et al. Foot ulceration and lower limb amputation in type 2 diabetic patients in Dutch primary care. Diabetes Care 2002; 25:570–574.

Payne CB, Scott RS. Hospital discharges for diabetic foot disease in New Zealand 1980-1993. Diabet Res Clin Pract 1998; 39:69–74.

Pedrosa HC, Leme LAP, Novaes C, et al. The diabetic foot in South America: progress with the Brazilian Save the diabetic foot project. Int Diab Monitor. 2004; 16:10–16.

Peters EJ, Lavery LA. International Working Group on the Diabetic Foot. Effectiveness of the diabetic foot risk classification system of the International Working Group on the Diabetic Foot. Diabetes Care 2001; 24:1442–1447.

Prompers L, Schaper N, Apelqvist J, et al. Prediction of outcome in individuals with diabetic foot ulcers: focus on the differences between individuals with and without peripheral arterial disease. The EURODIALE Study. Diabetologia 2008; 51:747–755.

Ramachandran A. Specific problems of the diabetic foot in developing countries. Diabet Metag Res Rev 2004; 20:S19–S22.

Rathur HM, Boulton AJM. The diabetic foot. Clin Dermatol 2007; 25:109–120.

Reiber GE, LeMaster JW. Epidemiology and economic impact of foot ulcers and amputations in people with diabetes. In: Bowker JH, Pfeifer M (eds.),

Levin and O'Neals the diabetic foot, 7th edn. Philadelphia: Mosby Elsevier, 2008:3-22.

Resnick HE, Valsania P, Philips CL. Diabetes mellitus and nontraumatic lower extremity amputations in black and white Americans: the National Health and Nutrition Examination survey epidemiology follow-up study. Arch Intern Med 1999; 159:2470–2475.

Richard JL, Schuldiner S. Épidémiologie du pied diabétique. Rev Med Interne 2008; 29:S222–30.

Schaper NC, Apelqvist J, Bakker K. Reducing lower leg amputations in diabetes: a challenge for patients, healthcare providers and the healthcare system. Diabetologia. 2012; 55:1869–1872.

Svensson H, Larsson J, Apelqvist J, Eneroth M. Minor amputation in patients with diabetes mellitus and severe foot ulcers achieves good outcomes. J Wound Care 2011; 20:261–262,264–266.

Tapp RJ, Shaw JE, de Courten MP, et al. Foot complications in type 2 diabetes: an Australian population-based study. Diabet Med 2003; 20:105–113.

Tapp RJ, Zimmet PZ, Harper CA, et al. Diabetes care in an Australian population: frequency of screening for eye and foot complications of diabetes. Diabetes Care 2004; 27:688–693.

Tchakonte B, Ndip A, Aubry P, Malvy D, Mbanya JC. The diabetic foot in Cameroon. Bull Soc Pathol Exot 2005; 98:94–98.

Valeri C, Pozzilli P, Leslie D. Glucose control in diabetes. Diabetes Metab Res Rev. 2004; 20:S1–8

Vamos EP, Bottle A, Edmonds ME, et al. Changes in the incidence of lower extremity amputations in individuals with and without diabetes in England between 2004 and 2008. Diabetes Care 2010;33(12):2592–2597.

van Houtum WH, Lavery LA. Methodological issues affect variability in reported incidence of lower extremity amputation due to diabetes. Diabetes Res Clin Pract 1997; 38:177–183.

van Houtum WH, Lavery LA. Regional variation in the incidence of diabetes-related amputations in The Netherlands. Diabetes Res Clin Pract 1996; 31:125–132.

Zhangrong X, Yuzcheng W, Xiancong W, et al. Chronic diabetic complications and treatments in Chinese diabetic patients. Natl Med J China 1997; 77:119–122.

Chapter 2 — Diabetic foot assessment and classification of risk

David G. Armstrong, Nicholas A. Giovinco, Magdiel Trinidad-Hernandez

SUMMARY

- The risk of foot ulceration may be stratified by simple clinical examination
- Always examine the patient standing and walking
- Regular clinical assessment (screening) of the foot is important
- The 10G monofilament is a simple tool to reliably identify neuropathy
- Any patient with diabetes attending hospital requires a clinical foot examination

BACKGROUND AND HISTORY

Despite, and in many ways because of, advances in public health, diabetes has continued to increase over the past 90 years. According to the United States' Centers for Disease Control and Prevention, nearly 8% of the US population alone has some form of diabetes. The rate of new diagnoses tops 1.6 million annually (Centers for Disease Control & Prevention- National Diabetes Fact Sheet 2008, World Health Organization 2009). In 2009, the leading cause of death became, for the first time, noncommunicable disease, of which diabetes is a significant proportion. Diabetes alone accounts for 6.8% of global all-cause mortality in persons between 20 and 79 years of age. It appears that this number is climbing (Unwin et al. 2010).

Many common complications of diabetes manifest in the periphery. This is particularly true of the lower extremity. Indeed, the lifetime risk of developing a wound on the foot may be conservatively placed at 25% (Singh et al. 2005). This is part of what might be considered a 'stairway' to amputation, which begins with development of diabetes, leading to loss of protective sensation (LOPS) (neuropathy), loss of integument (ulcer), loss of ability to protect against infection, frequent loss of sufficient outflow, and loss of limb. This is graphically illustrated in **Figure 2.1**.

PATHOPHYSIOLOGY

Mechanically and functionally, the human foot is a multitissue composite structure. It is remarkably unique and serves a variety of roles, predominantly sensory and locomotory. Because of this complexity of function and potential for pathological dysfunction or imbalance, initial evaluation of the human foot should consist of a thorough, multicomponent examination in order to isolate specific elements of a patient in order to prevent and treat diabetic foot complications. While it is not necessary for this thorough evaluation to be burdensome or extensively time consuming, it should cover a variety of key areas. These include assessment of blood flow, assessment for LOPS, assessment of the integument, and assessment of the musculoskeletal system and, as necessary, shoe gear. Before

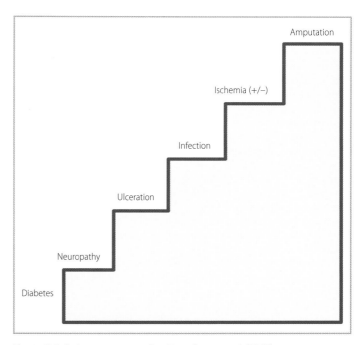

Figure 2.1 Stairway to amputation. From Rogers et al. (2010).

addressing this, we will address frequent patterns of pathology prevalent in people with diabetes that may lead to amputation.

ANGIOPATHY

In combination with the risk factors for ulceration discussed above, the presence of vascular occlusive disease increases the risk of potential amputation. Vascular disease is a common finding in individuals with long-standing diabetes. While vascular insufficiency alone is not usually the primary cause of ulceration, inadequate perfusion can inhibit ulcer healing, leading to further tissue necrosis and the inability to clear infection. **Table 2.1** provides a list of other potential risk factors for amputation. Most cases of vascular disease in individuals with diabetes, interestingly, affect the infrapopliteal vessels with relative sparing of the pedal vessels. In many instances, this allows for a distal bypass to a pedal target artery in order to increase the blood flow to the foot. The vascular examination is addressed in further detail later in this chapter.

NEUROPATHY

Neuropathy, which results in a LOPS of the lower extremity, is the predominant etiology for diabetic foot ulceration. The 'gift of pain' is a natural, nociceptor mediated, defense against tissue trauma

Table 2.1 Risk factors for amputation

Peripheral neuropathy (LOPS)
Vascular insufficiency (PAD)
Infection
Structural foot deformity
Trauma
History of prior foot ulcer or amputation
Charcot foot
Poor glycemic control
Older age
Male gender
Ethnicity (higher in Hispanics and African-Americans)

LOPS, loss of protective sensation; PAD, peripheral arterial disease.

and sensation of a hazardous environment (Yancey & Brand 1997). Without protective sensation, the patient is at a markedly increased risk of serious complications, which may result in loss of limb or life. Peripheral neuropathy can be evaluated as distinct subcategories, such as sensory, motor, and autonomic, but are often witnessed in concert with varying extent of functional compromise. Sensory neuropathy is a symmetric loss of temperature, vibration, pressure, and/or light touch sensation. This often begins distally in the toes and forefoot region, and will progress toward the hindfoot or ankle. More advanced losses will progress toward the proximal lower leg and beyond. The earlier stages of this condition within the foot will resemble a 'stocking and glove' distribution, whereby patients will report numbness or dysthesthesia (abnormal and frequently painful sensations) comparable with a low riding stocking over the foot.

Motor neuropathy is the progressive loss of motor function and control with an eventual imbalance of biomechanical stability and foot posture. Distal, intrinsic foot muscle will lose muscle mass and contractile strength first, which will lead to recruitment and compensation of extrinsic muscles of the leg during ambulation. This, combined with tissue tightness at the joints, will result in several common architectural misalignments such as hammertoe, claw toe, and plantar flexion deformities of the metatarsals. These deformities can cause an increase in focal pressure at the areas of the interphalangeal joints of the digits and beneath the metatarsal heads, respectively, increasing the probability of an ulcer formation from these bony prominences.

Autonomic neuropathy is associated with pathology of the sympathetic nervous system. In the lower extremity, this usually results in the absence of sweat production, inappropriate temperature regulation, and eventual dermatological complications such as drying and scaling of the skin, which increase the likelihood of cracking and fissuring. These cracks or fissures, especially in the heel, may then serve as a portal of entry for bacteria, increasing the chances of developing an infection. Other factors precipitating diabetic foot ulcers have been identified and are listed in (**Table 2.2**) (Boulton et al. 2008).

Table 2.2 Risk factors for ulceration

General or systemic factors	Local factors
Uncontrolled hyperglycemia	Peripheral neuropathy
Duration of diabetes	Structural foot deformity
Peripheral arterial disease	Limited joint range of motion
Older age	Trauma
Chronic renal disease	Improperly fitted shoes
Blindness or visual loss	Callus
	Prolonged elevated focal pressure
	History of previous ulcer or amputation

STRUCTURAL ABNORMALITIES/ GAIT ABNORMALITIES

Through a variety of means, structural derangements of the foot and ankle can be a potential cause of increased pressure and subsequent skin breakdown. The development of foot ulceration is often based on a biomechanical etiology (Frykberg et al. 2000, Lavery et al. 2006). It is important to evaluate both feet and shoe gear, of a patient when possible. As described earlier, motor neuropathy can lead to the loss of functional intrinsic foot musculature causing a deformity (and subsequent overpowering of the intrinsic muscles by the larger extrinsic lower leg muscles). Identification of any of the following contractures will assist in prevention of a potential ulceration: hammertoe (**Figure 2.2**), claw toe, bunion, tailor's bunion (bunionette), hallux limitus/rigidus, flat feet, high arched feet, Charcot deformities, or any postsurgical deformities such as amputations and subsequent further muscular imbalance.

Limited joint and soft tissue mobility should also be evaluated as it can cause an increase in vertical and shear force in certain areas, such as the plantar hallux (**Figure 2.3**), and lead to hypertrophic callosities, preulcerative changes, and tissue breakdown. The Achilles tendon should be evaluated for any type of functional contracture causing equinus deformity (**Figure 2.4**). It is common to find an increase in

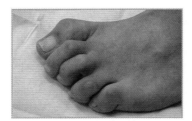

Figure 2.2 Hammertoe.

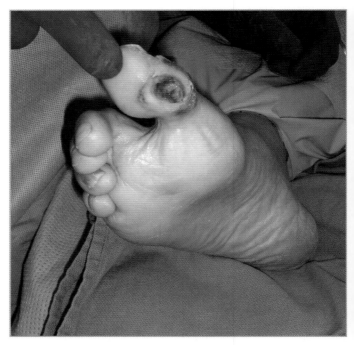

Figure 2.3 Plantar hallux.

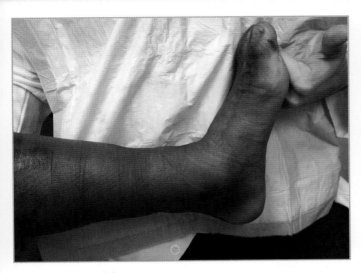

Figure 2.4 Equinus deformity.

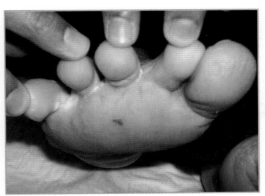

Figure 2.5 An interdigital examination, with significant maceration and secondary infection.

glycosylation of soft tissues and tendons causing contracture of the muscles in the posterior compartment of the leg (Armstrong et al. 1999, Giacomozzi et al. 2005, Grant et al. 2005). This, along with a relatively high body mass index (BMI) will cause an increase in plantar pressures in the forefoot and heel, making these areas more prone to breakdown.

Gait evaluation and muscle testing should also be conducted to evaluate any potential abnormality with ambulation and muscle strength. Thorough evaluation of the muscles in the lower extremity should be done both actively and passively, weight bearing and nonweight bearing in order to gain a more accurate perception of the patient's condition. Plantar foot pressures can also be assessed with the use of a variety of pressure sensitive and pressure recording devices, such as a Harris ink mat. Although these may not always be available, a careful inspection of wear patterns of the inner and outer soles of the patient's footwear can illustrate a great deal of information to the observer.

SCREENING
History and visual screening

A thorough history and physical examination of each patient who presents with a diabetic foot complication are important and should always be obtained at initial patient visit or at the time of a significant change in status. The touchstone datum to consider when obtaining a history includes previous pedal wounds, history of prior amputations, and lower extremity vascular interventions (Boulton et al. 2008, Rogers & Armstrong 2009). A physical examination should always include assessment in at least four of the following categories: biomechanical position and function, neurological status, vascular status, and dermatological presentation.

It is important to remove both shoes and socks for adequate examination. A systematic approach should be taken in order to avoid missing any important aspects of the examination. All surfaces of the foot and ankle should be evaluated including the nails, digits, interdigital webspaces, subdigital sulci, the soles, and the heels, inspecting for cracks, blisters or bullae, hyper/hypopigmentation, fissuring, calluses, macerations, and ulcers. **Figure 2.5** demonstrates an interdigital examination, with significant maceration and secondary infection. The shoe gear should also be inspected for signs

of wear patterns, foreign bodies, and any irregularities. In addition to any gross deformities as described above, malodor, debris, and drainage can be identified during this rapid visual screening (Boulton et al. 2008).

Neurological examination

As stated earlier, peripheral sensory neuropathy and the subsequent LOPS are major risk factors for the development of a diabetic foot complication. Several noninvasive examinations that can be performed to assess the neurological status of a patient, starting with historian, account for neuropathic symptoms such as tingling, burning, numbness, and the feeling of insects crawling on the feet (formication). This may help to identify the onset and progression of neuropathy in those patients at risk of developing foot ulceration (Armstrong & Quebedeaux 1998).

Monofilament testing

One of the most inexpensive and ubiquitous methods used to assess neuropathy is the use of the 10-g Semmes–Weinstein monofilament (Armstrong et al. 1998, Boulton et al. 2008) This technique employs the use of a nylon monofilament, which is placed on 10 different predetermined locations on the foot and pressed down manually until there is a slight bend in the wire. The patient is instructed to say 'yes' if he or she thinks they feel slight pressure or sensation. Loss of accurate sensation to two or more of these 10 locations is clinically positive for neuropathic LOPS.

Vibration testing

Vibratory perception testing can be assessed utilizing several different modalities. The more traditional method of testing is by the use of a 128-Hz tuning fork. The tuning fork is struck and then placed on a prominent bony surface of the foot, such as the great toe or metatarsal head, malleoli or tibial tuberosity. The patient is instructed to identify when the vibration stops. Loss of vibratory sensation at one distal location merits evaluation at the next proximal surface in order to evaluate the locality of compromised sensation.

Alternatively, a vibratory perception threshold monitor (**Figure 2.6**) can be used to test for vibration perception, by means of threshold detection range. The instrument consists of a hand piece with a testing probe on the end, a motor, rheostat, and voltmeter. The probe is held gently on the distal aspect of each hallux, or distal most prominent area. The rheostat is slowly increased until the patient senses the vibration. Once the patient identifies the sensation, the rheostat is then decreased until the sensation is no longer detected. The average value of the two numerical readings is taken and the level of sensation

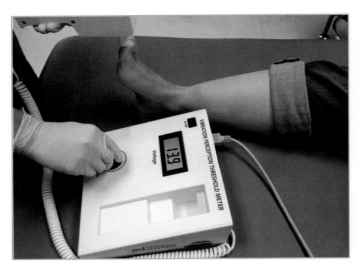

Figure 2.6 Vibratory perception threshold monitor.

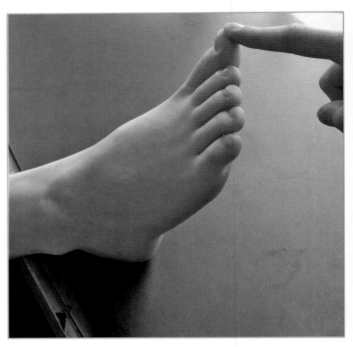

Figure 2.7 Ipswich touch test.

is documented to the location where the numbers were obtained. Average values above 25 Volts are considered positive for neuropathic changes (Boulton et al. 2008).

Neurological examinations traditionally require additional hardware or technology. This is not only costly but requires additional maintenance, electrical power resources, and overhead. Recent study and product designs have made advances in providing reliable and accurate testing modalities for identifying neurological capacity without the expense of burdening carrying capacity (Bowling et al. 2012). This has benefits for underprivileged and underserved regions of the world.

Where no medical instrumentation is present, an Ipswich Touch Test (IpTT) may be utilized. This involves a light touch with the index finger of the examiner for 1–2 seconds to various sites on the patient's foot, as demonstrated by **Figure 2.7** (Rayman et al. 2011). Although not considered as reliable enough to rival standard practices, it does provide care teams a fast and easy means of evaluating a patient's risk of ulceration within a care facility.

Dermatological examination

Following assessment for any loss of sensation, evaluation of the integument is often an important part of the foot screening. The skin can be evaluated for color, texture, turgor, quality, and presence of any areas of moisture, maceration, dryness or fissures, as well as malodor or drainage. This can frequently manifest itself in the interspaces (**Figure 2.5**). Calluses, if present, can be problematic as they indicate areas of increased pressure and an 'at risk' status of preulceration. Wounds can form under the hyperkeratotic lesion, which may cause hemorrhage beneath the callus. **Figure 2.8** shows a hypertrophic rim, encircling the ulceration at the distal aspect of a hammertoe. Debridement of these lesions is recommended in order to increase pressure dispersal (Pataky et al. 2002, Pitei et al. 1999).

Appearance and integrity of the nails should also be noted. If there are nails that are ingrowing, elongated, or there is incurvation of the nails, this could represent a potential area for skin trauma, abscess, and possible infection. Other nail issues to be aware of are onychomycosis (fungal nails), paronychia (ingrown nails with infection and an abscess in the nail fold), dystrophic, atrophic, or hypertrophic growth. Evaluation of any ulceration to the foot or lower leg should be assessed.

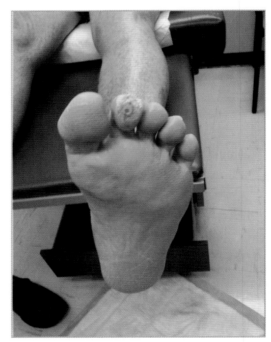

Figure 2.8 Hypertrophic rim encircling ulceration at the distal aspect of a hammertoe.

Important characteristics of ulcers are depth, size, presence of fibrotic or granulation tissue, location, and whether or not the area appears to be infected, malodorous, or draining.

Vascular examination

A complete vascular examination is mandatory in any patient who has symptoms consistent with claudication or ischemic rest pain.

However, due to neuropathy some patients will present with limb-threatening ischemia without the aforementioned complaints. Other patients will present with nonhealing wounds following minor elective or urgent operations. Theses patients may or may not have associated gangrene or infection. The initial physical examination should focus on the pulse examination from the inguinal ligament to the dorsalis pedis and posterior tibial arterial pulses. Nonetheless, perception of the pedal pulses is subjective and there is great variability between examiners who describe its presence and quality (Mowlavi et al. 2002). The ankle-brachial index (ABI) provides an objective measure to screen patients with arterial obstructive disease. Generally, patients with severe ischemia will have an ABI <0.4.

Many patients with diabetes, however, have falsely elevated ankle pressures due to calcification of the arterial wall. This renders some tibial vessels less compressible and others incompressible (pressures >250 mmHg) and the resulting ABI underestimates the severity of the disease (Weitz et al. 1996). In these instances pulse volume recordings (PVR) are helpful to obtain some measure of the degree of arterial occlusive disease involved. PVR are obtained with partially inflated segmental blood pressure cuffs that detect volume changes sequentially down a limb. Volume changes beneath the cuffs during the cardiac cycle cause discrete pressure changes within the cuffs, which can be displayed as arterial waveforms by specific transducers. A normal PVR waveform has a sharp systolic upstroke and peak and a prominent dicrotic notch on the downward portion of the curve. Such a waveform reflects normal arterial inflow to the portion of the extremity under the cuff. With increasing proximal arterial stenosis, the dicrotic notch shrinks and the peak wave becomes rounded with loss of amplitude. With proximal occlusion, the pulse wave may be absent. Pulse volume waveforms are evaluated qualitatively based on the shape of the curve.

Flat and dampened curves are considered severely abnormal. The paucity of reproducible data in PVR limits the utility of air plethysmography (Strandness 1969). An alternative to PVR is the evaluation of digital pressures and waveforms. These noninvasive tests are particularly useful in patients with pedal artery occlusive disease or highly calcified vessels, in whom ankle blood pressures do not accurately reflect real arterial pressure due to incompressibility of the calcified arterial walls. The presence of normal digital waveforms indicates minimal restriction to blood flow despite the calcific arterial disease. In contradistinction, a flat and dampened digital waveform in the presence of normal ankle pulses often indicates pedal artery occlusive disease.

When perfusion cannot be assessed from the indirect noninvasive tests mentioned above, arterial duplex scanning can provide detailed anatomic and hemodynamic information. Duplex scanning combines B-mode ultrasound and pulsed Doppler ultrasound. The combination of color Doppler and B-mode ultrasound can determine anatomical and hemodynamic abnormalities. B-mode imaging alone cannot differentiate hemodynamically significant soft plaque and thrombus from blood. B-mode ultrasound visualizes calcified plaque and enables one to focus on the arterial segment of interest. Doppler ultrasound can demonstrate abnormal flow patterns caused by intra-arterial luminal defects. Blood flow velocities are calculated to determine the degree of stenosis in the artery. Arterial duplex scanning has been compared prospectively with angiography to define standard criteria for normal and diseased arteries. The sensitivity of duplex examination for detecting the presence of a hemodynamically significant lesion (>50% stenosis) ranges from 89% at the iliac artery to 68% at the popliteal artery. Overall sensitivities for predicting interruption of patency are 90% for the anterior tibial, 90% for the posterior tibial, and 82% for the peroneal artery. The sensitivity of arterial duplex ultrasound is not significantly influenced by the severity of atherosclerosis (Moneta et al. 1992).

Intra-arterial digital subtraction angiography continues to be the most accurate method to evaluate arterial circulation of the lower extremity. Nonetheless, it is an invasive procedure that can be associated with complications in up to 2.9% of patients (Balduf et al. 2002). A detailed angiogram must include the inflow vessels and the runoff. Careful selective catheterization of the superficial femoral or popliteal artery allows for detailed visualization of the tibial and pedal vessels with a reduced contrast load. This is important because patients with diabetes despite having a normal creatinine level are at increased risk of contrast-induced nephropathy (Toprak et al. 2007).

■ RISK CLASSIFICATION

■ Diabetes mellitus foot risk classification (risk of ulceration and subsequent amputation)

Based on a thorough history and physical examination, each patient should then be classified and assigned to a specific foot risk category as outlined in **Table 2.3** (Boulton et al. 2008). These categories were designed to direct and expedite the referral process to the necessary specialist and should also serve as a guide for subsequent follow-up visits. Increased categorical levels are associated with increasing risk of ulceration, hospitalization, and amputation.

■ Wound classification systems (risk of nonhealing and subsequent amputation)

Multispecialty teams and hospital facilities employ a variety of specialists and caregivers for the treatment of diabetic foot complications. Wound classification systems are a useful appliance for documentation and peer interaction within a caregiving community. Several wound classification systems have emerged, which are actively in use. Members of the multidisciplinary team should use standard language and descriptions, which include accepted wound classifications. Each of these classifications offers a common descriptor of a clinical scenario, and can be used in addition to the specific details and specific patient evaluation.

Wagner classification for foot ulcers

This classification is primarily based on vascular integrity and depth of involvement within the foot (Wagner 1981). A Grade 0 scenario describes a preulcerative condition overlying an 'at risk' area of skin. A Grade 1 wound describes a partial thickness loss of skin. A Grade 2 wound details a deeper skin or soft tissue involvement, not involving bone. Grade 3 describes a deep wound or abscess involving bone or joint. Grade 4 describes a localized focal gangrenous wound, whereby Grade 5 describes a global foot gangrenous scenario.

University of Texas wound classification system

While many wound classification systems exist, The University of Texas (UT) ulcer classification system was developed to provide a

Table 2.3 American Diabetes Association risk classification for the diabetic foot (Boulton et al. 2008, Lavery et al. 2007)

Risk category	Definition	Yearly ulcer incidence/odds ratio (compared with risk category 0)	Treatment recommendations	Suggested follow-up
0	No LOPS, no PAD, no deformity	2.0%	Patient education including advice on appropriate footwear	Annually (by generalist and/or specialist)
1	LOPS ± deformity	4.5%/2.4	Consider prescriptive or accommodative footwear Consider prophylactic surgery if deformity cannot be safely accommodated in shoes Continue patient education	Every 3–6 months (by generalist and/or specialist)
2	PAD ± LOPS	13.8%/9.3	Consider prescriptive or accommodative footwear Consider vascular consultation for combined follow-up	Every 2–3 months (by specialist)
3	History of ulcer or amputation	32.2%/52.2	Same as category 1 Consider vascular consultation for combined follow-up if PAD present	Every 1–2 months (by specialist)

LOPS, loss of protective sensation; PAD, peripheral arterial disease.

more uniform evaluation of diabetic foot wounds (Armstrong et al. 1998). Like other classification systems, the UT wound classification system builds on the depth-ischemia classification; however, the UT system also considers infection. The presence of infection and ischemia has been found to be more strongly predictive of outcome than the wound depth alone (Oyibo et al. 2001). The UT system uses a 4 by 4 matrix (classes A to D, wound depths 0–3) and evaluates 3 factors of ulceration, which include depth, infection, and peripheral arterial disease (PAD) (Andros 2010). The frequency and level of amputation increases in deeper wounds and in the presence of infection and PAD (Armstrong et al. 1998). Regardless of which specific classification is used, the key factors of depth, infection, and ischemia should generally be communicated in some form. This classification is listed in **Table 2.4**.

PEDIS system

The International Working Group of Diabetic Foot, in an effort to standardize wound classification across research studies, developed and proposed the PEDIS system. Building on previous systems, it also includes wound size and the presence of neuropathy. It also includes these in ordinal variables, which may allow for more precision (Schaper 2004) (**Table 2.5**).

As discussed, classifications are useful to multispecialty care teams for communicating varying descriptions of acuity, benefiting not only clinical dialogue, but also research stratification and investigation. While the use of a specific system is not important, it is important, when patient care involves a number of different specialties and the

treatment of both acute and chronic conditions, to agree a common 'language' of risk and description among members of the team. If a specific classification is preferred, then it is appropriate to define which nomenclature is being applied. Assessment and management of wounds will be discussed in subsequent chapters.

◼ Management of tissue loss, infection, and ischemia: the importance of team

Diabetic foot care demands an interdisciplinary team approach given the multifactorial components and progressive nature of the disease in the foot and the whole patient. If a patient presents with a wound, infection, ischemia, or a combination of these three, then recent evidence as it exists continues to consistently point to a reduction in major amputation rates following the development of an interdisciplinary team (Armstrong et al. 2012, Rogers et al. 2010). The components of a limb salvage team are predicated on the pathology at presentation. The core of the team typically starts with clinicians caring for the structural and surgical aspects of the foot along with clinicians caring for the vascular integrity of the lower extremity. Other specialties of the team, to add a more comprehensive care model, may include Internal Medicine, Diabetology, Infectious Disease, Physical Therapy, Plastic Surgery, Nursing, Emergency Medicine, Endocrinology, Nutrition, and Prosthetics.

Both vasculopathy and neuropathy are two major contributors to diabetic foot disease and subsequent ulceration. In order to reduce amputations, it is proposed that a diabetic rapid response acute foot team would combine the knowledge of certain specialties to promote limb salvage (Fitzgerald et al. 2009). Rather than pointing to specific team members, one may focus on 'skill sets' that transcend borders and specific specialties. We have listed seven important skill sets that can help to define the core of a 'diabetic rapid response foot team (DRRAFT)' (**Box 2.1**) (Rogers et al. 2010). These align well with the National Minimum Skills Framework developed in the UK (Diabetes UK 2011).

Table 2.4 The University of Texas (UT) wound classification system

Grade	Description	Stage
1	Pre- or postulcerative lesion	A–D
2	Superficial	A–D
3	Penetrated to tendon or joint capsule	A–D
4	Penetrates to bone	A–D

Stages: A, no infection or ischemia; B, infection; C, ischemia; D, infection and ischemia.

Table 2.5 PEDIS wound classification

Perfusion	Extent/size	Depth/tissue loss	Infection	Sensation

Grade 1
No symptoms or signs of PAD in the affected foot, in combination with:
Palpable dorsal pedal and posterior tibial artery pulse
or
Ankle-brachial index 0.9 to 1.10
or
Toe-brachial index >0.6
or
Transcutaneous oxygen pressure (tcpO$_2$) >60 mmHg
 	
Grade 2
Symptoms or signs of PAD, but not of critical limb ischemia (CLI):
Presence of intermittent claudication (in case of claudication, additional non-invasive assessment should be performed), as defined in the document of the International Consensus on the Diabetic Foot [8]
or
Ankle-brachial index < 0.9, but with ankle pressure >50 mmHg
or
Toe-brachial index < 0.6, but systolic toe blood pressure >30 mmHg
or
tcpO$_2$ 30–60 mmHg
or
Other abnormalities on non-invasive testing, compatible with PAD (but not with CLI). Note: if tests other than ankle or toe pressure or tcpO$_2$ are performed, they should be specified in each study
 	
Grade 3
CLI, as defined by:
  Systolic ankle blood pressure <50 mmHg
  or
  Systolic toe blood pressure <30 mmHg
  or
  tcpO$_2$ <30 mmHg
	Various means of planimetric analysis have been described in literature from circumference to perpendicular diameter approximations	**Grade 1**
		Superficial full-thickness ulcer, not penetrating any structure deeper than the dermis
		
		Grade 2
		Deep ulcer, penetrating below the dermis to subcutaneous structures, involving fascia, muscle or tendon
		
		Grade 3
		All subsequent layers of the foot involved, including bone and/or joint (exposed bone, probing to bone)
			Grade 1
			No symptoms or signs of infection
			
			Grade 2
			Infection involving the skin and the subcutaneous tissue only (without involvement of deeper tissues and without systemic signs, as described below). At least two of the following items are present:
			  Local swelling or induration
			  Erythema >0.5–2 cm around the ulcer
			  Local tenderness or pain
			  Local warmth
			  Purulent discharge (thick, opaque to white or sanguineous secretion)
			
			Other causes of an inflammatory response of the skin should be excluded (e.g. trauma, gout, acute Charcot neuroarthropathy, fracture, thrombosis, venous stasis)
			
			Grade 3
			Erythema >2 cm plus one of the items described above (swelling, tenderness, warmth, discharge) or infection involving structures deeper than skin and subcutaneous tissues such as abscess, osteomyelitis, septic arthritis, fasciitis. No systemic inflammatory response signs, as described below
			
			Grade 4
			Any foot infection with the following signs of a systemic inflammatory response syndrome. This response is manifested by two or more of the following conditions:
			  Temperature >38 or <36°C
			  Heart rate >90 beats/min
			  Respiratory rate >20 breaths/min
			  $PaCO_2$ <32-mmHg
			  White blood cell count >12.000 or <4.000/cu mm
			  10% immature (band) forms
				Grade 1
				No loss of protective sensation on the affected foot detected, defined as the presence of sensory modalities described below
				
				Grade 2
				Loss of protective sensation on the affected foot is defined as the absence of perception of the one of the following tests in the affected foot:
				  Absent pressure sensation, determined with a 10G monofilament, on two out of three sites on the plantar side of the foot, as described in the International Consensus on the Diabetic Foot
				  Absent vibration sensation (determined with a 128-Hz tuning fork) or vibration threshold >25 V (using semiquantitative techniques), both tested on the hallux

PAD, peripheral arterial disease.

CONCLUSION

Diabetic foot complications are common, complicated, and costly to patients and their communities alike. This makes identification of risk factors through consistent screening and triage very important. Through systematic screening and stratification, patients can be triaged according to risk. Care may thus be standardized with the benefit being a reduction in morbidity and a better quality of life for our patients and their families.

> **Box 2.1 Seven essential skills of a diabetic rapid response acute foot care team**
> - Ability to perform hemodynamic and anatomic vascular assessment with revascularization
> - Ability to perform a neurological assessment
> - Ability to perform site-appropriate culture technique
> - Ability to perform wound assessment and staging/grading of infection and ischemia
> - Ability to perform site-specific bedside and intraoperative incision and debridement
> - Ability to initiate and modify culture-specific and patient-appropriate antibiotic therapy
> - Ability to perform appropriate postoperative monitoring to reduce risks of re-ulceration and infection

IMPORTANT FURTHER READING

Boulton AJ, Armstrong DG, Albert SF, et al. Comprehensive foot examination and risk assessment: a report of the task force of the foot care interest group of the American Diabetes Association, with endorsement by the American Association of Clinical Endocrinologists. Diabetes Care 2008; 31:1679–1685.

Chang CH, Peng YS, Chang CC, Chen MY. Useful screening tools for preventing foot problems of diabetics in rural areas: a cross-sectional study. BMC Public Health 2013; 13:612.

Feng Y, Schlösser FJ, Sumpio BE. The Semmes Weinstein monofilament examination as a screening tool for diabetic peripheral neuropathy. J Vasc Surg 2009; 50:675–682.

National Institute for Health and Care Excellence. Clinical guidelines: type 2 diabetes – footcare (CG10. http://guidance.nice.org.uk/CG10.

Rayman G, Vas PR, Baker N, et al. The Ipswich Touch Test: a simple and novel method to identify inpatients with diabetes at risk of foot ulceration. Diabetes Care 2011; 34:1517–1518.

Singh N, Armstrong DG, Lipsky BA. Preventing foot ulcers in patients with diabetes. JAMA 2005; 293:217–228.

REFERENCES

Andros GL, Lavery LA. Diabetic foot ulcers. In: Cronenwett J, Johnston KW (eds), Rutherford's Vascular Surgery, vol. 2, 7th edn. Saunders Elsevier, 2010:1735–1746.

Armstrong DG, Bharara M, White M, et al. The impact and outcomes of establishing an integrated interdisciplinary surgical team to care for the diabetic foot. Diabetes Metab Res Rev 2012:n/a-n/a.

Armstrong DG, Lavery LA, Harkless LB. Validation of a diabetic wound classification system. The contribution of depth, infection, and ischemia to risk of amputation [see comments]. Diabetes Care 1998; 21:855–859.

Armstrong DG, Lavery LA, Vela SA, et al. Choosing a practical screening instrument to identify patients at risk for diabetic foot ulceration. Arch Intern Med 1998: 289–292.

Armstrong DG, Stacpoole-Shea S, Nguyen HC, Harkless LB. Lengthening of the Achilles tendon in diabetic patients who are at high risk for ulceration of the foot. J Bone Joint Surg (Am) 1999; 81A:535–538.

Balduf LM, Langsfeld M, Marek JM, et al. Complication rates of diagnostic angiography performed by vascular surgeons. Vasc Endovascular Surg 2002; 36:439–445.

Boulton AJ, Armstrong DG, Albert SF, et al. Comprehensive foot examination and risk assessment: a report of the task force of the foot care interest group of the American Diabetes Association, with endorsement by the American Association of Clinical Endocrinologists. Diabetes Care 2008; 31:1679–1685.

Bowling FL, Abbott CA, Harris WE, et al. A pocket-sized disposable device for testing the integrity of sensation in the outpatient setting. Diabet Med 2012; 29:1550–1552.

Centers for Disease Control & Prevention – National Diabetes Fact Sheet: General Information & National Estimates on Diabetes in the United States. Atlanta, GA: Centers for Disease Control & Prevention, 2008.

Diabetes UK. Putting feet first: national minimum skills framework. The national minimum skills framework for commissioning of footcare services for people with diabetes. Revised March 2011. http://www.diabetes.org.uk/About_us/What-we-say/Improving-services--standards/National-Minimum-Skills-Framework-for-commissioning-of-foot-care-services-for-people-with-diabetes-March--2011/

Fitzgerald RH, Mills JL, Joseph W, Armstrong DG. The diabetic rapid response acute foot team: 7 essential skills for targeted limb salvage. Eplasty 2009; 9:15.

Frykberg RG, Armstrong DG, Giurini J, et al. Diabetic foot disorders: a clinical practice guideline. American College of Foot and Ankle Surgeons. J Foot Ankle Surg 2000; 39:S1–60.

Giacomozzi C, D'Ambrogi E, Uccioli L, Macellari V. Does the thickening of Achilles tendon and plantar fascia contribute to the alteration of diabetic foot loading? Clin Biomech (Bristol, Avon) 2005; 20:532–539.

Grant WP, Foreman EJ, Wilson AS, Jacobus DA, Kukla RM. Evaluation of Young's modulus in Achilles tendons with diabetic neuroarthropathy. J Am Podiatr Med Assoc 2005; 95:242–246.

Lavery LA, Armstrong DG, Wunderlich RP, et al. Risk factors for foot infections in individuals with diabetes. Diabetes Care 2006; 29:1288–1293.

Lavery LA, Peters EJ, Williams JR et al., International Working Group on the Diabetic Foot. Reevaluating the way we classify the diabetic foot: restructuring the diabetic foot risk classification system of the International Working Group on the Diabetic Foot. Diabetes Care 2008; 31:154–156.

Moneta GL, Yeager RA, Antonovic R, et al. Accuracy of lower extremity arterial duplex mapping. J Vasc Surg 1992; 15:275–283; discussion 283–274.

Mowlavi A, Whiteman J, Wilhelmi BJ, Neumeister MW, McLafferty R. Dorsalis pedis arterial pulse: palpation using a bony landmark. Postgrad Med J 2002; 78:746–747.

Oyibo SO, Jude EB, Tarawneh I, et al. A comparison of two diabetic foot ulcer classification systems: the Wagner and the University of Texas wound classification systems. Diabetes Care 2001; 24:84–88.

Pataky Z, Golay A, Faravel L, et al. The impact of callosities on the magnitude and duration of plantar pressure in patients with diabetes mellitus. A callus may cause 18,600 kilograms of excess plantar pressure per day. Diabetes Metab 2002; 28:356–361.

Pitei DL, Foster A, Edmonds M. The effect of regular callus removal on foot pressures. J Foot Ankle Surg 1999; 38:251–255; discussion 306.

Rayman G, Vas PR, Baker N, et al. The Ipswich Touch Test: a simple and novel method to identify inpatients with diabetes at risk of foot ulceration. Diabetes Care 2011; 34:1517–1518.

Rogers LC, Andros G, Caporusso J, et al. Toe and flow: essential components and structure of the amputation prevention team. J Vasc Surg 2010; 52:23S–27S.

Rogers LC, Armstrong DG. Diabetic foot ulcers: podiatry care. In: Cronenwitt J (ed.), Rutherford vascular surgery, 7th edn. Amsterdam: Elsevier, 2009.

Schaper NC. Diabetic foot ulcer classification system for research purposes: a progress report on criteria for including patients in research studies. Diabetes Metab Res Rev 2004; 20:S90–95.

Singh N, Armstrong DG, Lipsky BA. Preventing foot ulcers in patients with diabetes. JAMA 2005; 293:217–228.

Strandness DE. Peripheral arterial disease: a physiologic approach. Boston: Little, Brown, 1969.

Toprak O, Cirit M, Yesil M, et al. Impact of diabetic and pre-diabetic state on development of contrast-induced nephropathy in patients with chronic kidney disease. Nephrol Dial Transplant: Official publication of the European Dialysis and Transplant Association – European Renal Association 2007; 22:819–826.

Unwin N, Gan D, Whiting D. The IDF Diabetes Atlas: providing evidence, raising awareness and promoting action. Diabetes Res Clin Pract 2010; 87:2–3.

Wagner FW. The dysvascular foot: a system for diagnosis and treatment. Foot Ankle 1981; 2:64–122.

Weitz JI, Byrne J, Clagett GP, et al. Diagnosis and treatment of chronic arterial insufficiency of the lower extremities: a critical review. Circulation 1996; 94:3026–3049.

World Health Organization Diabetes Fact Sheet, No 312. Geneva: World Health Organization, 2009.

Yancey P, Brand P. The gift of pain. Grand Rapids: Zondervan, 1997.

Chapter 3 Setting up a diabetic foot service

Abdul Basit

SUMMARY

- Diabetic foot amputations can be prevented in most cases
- Significant reduction in amputations can be achieved by well-organized diabetic foot care teams
- Diabetic foot services should focus not only on treatment but also on prevention
- Effective diabetes and diabetic foot care imply an interdisciplinary approach for which a trained interdisciplinary team is indispensable
- Pathways of care should exist between primary and secondary care to ensure timely and expert care
- Any trained health-care professional interested in managing diabetic foot can take the initiative in forming the team
- Minimal model clinics consisting of a physician and a foot care assistant should be part of every primary health-care setting
- High-risk patients and patients with active foot lesions should be referred to an intermediate model foot clinic based in hospital

INTRODUCTION

Foot disease is an enduring complication of diabetes and its effective prevention and management in a particular population is therefore closely dependent on the existence of an efficient diabetic foot service. Developing effective diabetic foot care services within primary and secondary care settings is of paramount importance.

REALIZATION OF DIABETIC FOOT SERVICES: A SHORT HISTORY

Until the mid1990s, a standardized foot care program did not exist in most parts of the world. Foot problems, including those secondary to diabetes, were being treated by general surgeons, orthopedic surgeons, vascular surgeons, physicians, and general practitioners (GPs) in diversified ways. Preventive strategies and swift interventions were seldom offered to avoid foot ulceration and subsequent amputation (Pecoraro et al. 1990).

As the scientific and clinical understanding of etiopathophysiology of foot ulceration and ischemia in diabetes continues, more logical approaches to its prevention and treatment have developed. The natural history of diabetic foot disease is rapidly progressive and as such demands easily accessible specialized multidisciplinary and coordinated care. This is necessary both in the short-term and the long-term. The patients need easy access to systems that are able to provide specialized care under one roof (Rayman et al. 2004).

Such initiatives date back to the 1920s, when Dr E. Joslin established the first foot clinic at New England Deaconess Hospital in Boston.

The clinic specialized in diabetes wound care and developing revascularization approaches in the 1950s. Further techniques for the treatment of ischemic foot ulceration were advocated in 1980s, including extreme distal revascularization (Sanders et al. 2010). Similar clinics were set up in the United Kingdom in the 1980s, with the basic approach of screening and prevention, infection management, and revascularization involving diabetologists, endocrinologists, podiatrists, orthopedic, and vascular surgeons. These measures helped in reducing the amputation rate by 50%.

Experience in various countries has indicated that a nationwide system for the early detection and subsequent referral to a specialized diabetic foot team needs to be implemented to reduce the amputation rate. Clear guidelines have been formulated regarding the identification of at-risk patients, diagnosis of a foot ulcer, classification of disease severity and management (Bakker et al. 2012a) (**Box 3.1**).

> **Box 3.1 Key points in preventing amputation**
> - Early referral to a multidisciplinary team
> - Aggressive (surgical and medical) management of infection
> - Diagnosis of peripheral arterial disease with appropriate investigations
> - Revascularization in cases of impaired tissue perfusion, where possible

MULTIDISCIPLINARY DIABETIC FOOT CARE APPROACH

The diabetic foot cannot be managed by a diabetologist alone. The wide spectrum of diabetic foot problems requires the joint efforts of many allied health-care professionals and a combination of therapeutic methods including revascularization and surgical procedures as well as treatment of infection, pain, metabolic control, comorbidities, meticulous wound care, and biochemical off-loading (Bakker et al. 2011). A number of studies have shown the effectiveness of a unified approach to diabetic foot care (Fusilli et al. 2005, Krishnan et al. 2008, Canavan et al. 2008). If such an approach is instituted, it may be possible to prevent 45–55% of all amputations.

Multidisciplinary approach in the developed world: experience from Europe

The European study group on diabetes and the lower extremity (Eurodiale) is a collaborative network of 14 European centers, consisting of diabetologists, vascular surgeons, and orthopedic surgeons, originally created to initiate multidisciplinary research in the field of diabetic foot disease. The study concluded that many patients with diabetic foot ulcers were severely ill, reflected by the severe underlying pathology and the presence of disabling comorbidities. A high prevalence of infection (58%) in this study and the combination of peripheral arterial disease (PAD) and infection were associated with the poorest outcome. Previous studies have also shown that the combination of infection and ischemia is significantly more likely to lead to a midfoot or higher amputation as compared with less advanced wound stages (Armstrong et al. 1998). Owing to significant comorbidities, a comprehensive, multidisciplinary approach is required. Therefore, a holistic approach by health-care professionals who are familiar with the treatment of patients with diabetes and related complications is essential in order to identify high-risk patients and initiate an appropriate treatment (Prompers et al. 2008).

Traditionally, most people with diabetes in the United Kingdom have had their care supervised by hospital doctors. In the 1970s and 1980s, a number of GPs with a special interest in diabetes care began to develop diabetes clinics within their practices (Moor & Gadsby 1984), whose quality of care was equivalent to hospital clinics. Since then, a shift of routine diabetes care from the secondary (hospital) sector to the primary (general practice) sector has been occurring. This has been encouraged by a number of government initiatives and policy documents and by showing the quality and outcomes framework of the new general practice contract. However, there is still much to be done to ensure that good quality primary foot care screening is performed on everyone on an annual basis, that those with 'at risk feet' get referred and properly managed in foot protection clinics, and that patients presenting with a foot ulcer and/or cellulitis receive appropriate care - from a multidisciplinary foot care team - within 24 hours.

MULTIDISCIPLINARY APPROACH IN THE DEVELOPING WORLD

Singapore

Singapore is a small, developing country that has a large multi-ethnic and multicultural immigrant population. It is a small community with a very good health infrastructure, and the example of its diabetic foot services can be duplicated in other countries as well. In May 2003, the formation of National University Hospital (NUH) multidisciplinary diabetic foot team and the implementation of a precise referral system successfully decreased the major amputation rate from 31% in 2002 to 20% in 2004. In addition, it also reduced the hospital stay and readmission rates of patients with a diabetic foot.

An efficient referral system contributed greatly to this success. In the emergency department, diabetic foot problems are actively sought and patients are classified according to the severity of a foot lesion, particularly taking into account whether the presenting foot problems require a below-knee amputation or above-knee amputation or neither. On this basis, referrals are initiated to the podiatrist and other members of the diabetic foot team, where necessary. The diabetic foot team consists of an endocrinologist, a podiatrist, an orthopedic surgeon, an infectious disease specialist, a specialist wound care nurse, a medico-social worker, and a case manager.

Brazil

In Brazil, the Save the Diabetic Foot Project was initially established in 1991. Nurses were invited to educate patients and perform basic podiatry care that later led to the formal opening of a weekly hospital-based diabetic foot clinic in 1992. With the passage of time, involvement of vascular surgeons, infectious disease specialists, orthopedic surgeons, orthotists, physiotherapists, plastic surgeons, and many more allied health-care professional have led to the development of true interdisciplinary cooperation.

India

India is the country with the maximum number of people with diabetes in the world. There are currently >65.1 million people with diabetes, estimated to rise to >109 million by 2030 (IDF Diabetes Atlas 2013). The situation is made worse by a lack of awareness regarding diabetic foot care as well as a lack of trained personnel to effectively manage these problems. Formulation of the Diabetic Foot Society of India (DFSI) in March 2002 and an amputation prevention initiative were two important steps that helped to improve diabetic foot care in India. The 'Step-by-Step' program (see Introduction and Chapter 7) in India has been very successful in providing foot care to people with diabetes (Bakker et al. 2006) and has shown that the staggering human and economic costs of diabetic foot disease may be reduced by simple measures and preventive foot care practices.

Tanzania

Patients in African communities often present to hospital only after the onset of gangrene or during a stage of sepsis that may be beyond salvage (Abbas et al. 2002). It is not surprising, therefore, that foot infections are especially common where there are no available services for follow-up of the diabetic foot, or lesions are ignored or detected relatively late in the course of infection after unsuccessful home therapy. The importance of delayed presentation to hospital is underscored by the fact that 10% of patients who needed and had agreed to undergo surgery died from advanced sepsis before the planned surgical procedure was actually carried out (Abbas et al. 2002). Thus, education remains the most important preventive tool in Africa and should be an integral part of preventive programs targeted at both health-care workers and patients alike.

In Tanzania, about 1.7 million people have diabetes (IDF Diabetes Atlas 2013). Thirty-three percent of the patients admitted for diabetic foot ulcers undergo amputation with a 54% mortality rate in patients who present late (Abbas et al. 2011). A significant reduction in the incidence of foot ulcer disease and the amputation rate has been documented after the institution of Step-by-Step program (Bakker et al. 2006).

HOW TO START A DIABETIC FOOT SERVICE

Certain factors, such as geographical variations in health-care systems and the local epidemiology of diabetes-related foot disease (incidence and prevalence of the diabetic foot along with amputation rate), should be considered when planning a diabetic foot care service. Treatment focused on ulcer healing should not be the only priority. Diabetic foot disease is a lifelong condition and the patient is at increased risk of developing a new ulcer, requiring amputation and dying prematurely compared with a matched population of people without diabetes. Therefore, a comprehensive management strategy is needed that should focus not only on treatment but also on prevention of ulceration (new and recurrent) and prevention of premature death (**Figure 3.1**).

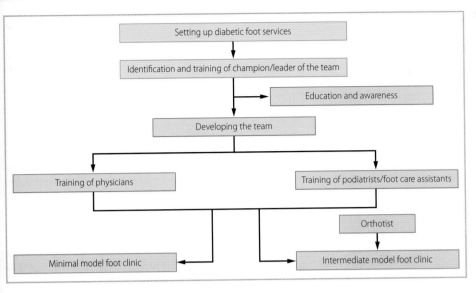

Figure 3.1 Setting up of a diabetic foot care service.

For a national health-care system to be truly efficient both in the developing and developed countries, it would be mandatory to include diabetic foot care at primary, secondary, and tertiary care levels. At primary care level, foot care services would contribute to minimizing the occurrence of neuropathy and PAD. At the secondary care level, these services would aid in the early identification of those feet at increased risk of ulceration or amputation, to minimize the consequences of early peripheral neuropathy, PAD, and foot deformity. Efficient diabetic foot services at tertiary care level would ultimately minimize the number of amputations through complex interventions in those with established foot ulceration.

INTERNATIONAL GUIDELINES ON THE DIABETIC FOOT

In some countries, unfortunately, the diabetic foot is a low priority on the agenda of health-care policy makers. However, in the last decade, an increasing awareness of the need for coordinated diabetic foot care has evolved. Guidelines on prevention and management of the diabetic foot have been formulated and adopted in several countries. However, differences in the specialists involved in developing the guidelines, the aims and scope of the guidelines and the target groups have resulted in documents that vary considerably. The variety of ulcer and risk classification systems has further confused these guidelines.

To narrow the gap and improve coordinated diabetic foot care globally, the international consensus on guidelines of the diabetic foot has been developed. These comprise a group of independent experts, in close association with several international organizations. The International Working Group on the Diabetic Foot (IWGDF), instituted in 1996, coordinates the production of consensus documents and practical guidelines on the management and prevention of diabetic foot, describing the basic principles of prevention and treatment. They summarize strategies for management and prevention and provide a set of definitions of the essential topics in diabetic foot disease (Bakker et al. 2012b).

All health-care workers involved in the care of patients with diabetes may use these guidelines. Depending on the local circumstances, the principles outlined in the document have to be 'translated' to take into account regional socioeconomic differences, accessibility to health care, and cultural factors. These consensus documents have helped to put the diabetic foot on the agenda of policy-makers (commissioners of health care), health-care professionals, and patients by raising awareness not only in the Western world but also in the developing countries.

DIABETIC FOOT SERVICE AT A PRIMARY CARE LEVEL

Minimal model clinic

In the minimal model foot clinic, the foot care team consists of a family practitioner trained in diabetes and a nurse or foot care assistant trained in podiatry. Its aim is prevention and basic curative care and it can be set up in the GP's office or clinic or any other health facility in the primary health-care setting (Diabetes and foot care, 2005).

The foot care assistant plays a pivotal role in these clinics. As a key person, he/she screens out the high-risk group among the patients and treats minor ailments such as calluses and ingrown toenails. They also act as a diabetes educator, teaching the patients proper nail cutting techniques and instructing them how to perform daily self-examination of their feet. High-risk patients identified in such primary clinics should be referred to a specialized multidisciplinary diabetic foot team.

The GPs provide initial and subsequent foot assessment including the neurological and vascular status, skin condition, and level of foot deformity. Neurological evaluation includes vibration sense, proprioception, and monofilament mapping. Screening for PAD includes history of claudication and examination of the pedal pulses. The skin is assessed for integrity, especially between the toes and under the metatarsal heads. Bony deformities and joint stiffness are noted. All patients with active foot problems should be urgently referred to a multidisciplinary foot care team.

DIABETIC FOOT SERVICE AT SECONDARY CARE LEVEL

Intermediate model foot clinic

The intermediate model clinic is staffed by a diabetologist or a general physician with a special interest in diabetes, a podiatrist or nurse trained in podiatry, a surgeon, and possibly an orthotist or someone having knowledge or experience of shoe-making. The intermediate model offers not only preventive care, education, and footwear advice but also detection and treatment of foot problems (Diabetes and foot care, 2005) (**Figure 3.2**). Ideally, such a team should be based in a hospital setting so that patients can be referred here from the primary care setting. There are guidelines as to when to refer these patients. By bringing together relevant expertise and utilizing it without delay, both temporary and permanent disability can be minimized.

The multidisciplinary diabetic foot clinics that were established in the 1980s in the United Kingdom had a significant effect. Evidence demonstrated that their introduction was associated with a reduction in lower extremity amputations as a result of diabetic foot complications (Edmonds et al. 1986, Thomson et al. 1991, Apelquist et al. 1992, McCabe et al. 1998). These models have been adopted in most of the developed world with evidence of benefit. However, the situation is far from satisfactory in the developing world, where there is a lack of health-care infrastructure. Most of the health services are provided by family physicians or GPs at a primary care level. Screening for early or established foot disease and education of patients in the diabetic foot can be performed by these GPs. More severe cases can be referred into a hospital clinic.

Based on the experiences in Brazil, India, Pakistan, and Tanzania, which share the same basic health structure, some common strategies can be developed to initiate diabetic foot clinics in other developing countries. All people with diabetes need to be categorized into a low or high current risk of diabetic foot ulceration on the basis of intact sensation and palpable pulses. Patients at a high risk of ulceration should receive more regular foot examination along with foot care education including the use of proper footwear and good metabolic control (Somannavar et al. 2008).

All these aspects of diabetic foot management can be undertaken at a primary care level. Patients who, in addition to absent sensation, have absent pulses, a history of previous ulceration, or foot deformity are at the highest risk of foot ulceration. These patients should be reviewed more frequently (every 1–3 months) by a podiatrist, and the need for revascularization, as well as specialized orthoses, should be considered in such patients.

PATHWAYS OF CARE

Diabetes and foot complications are managed by a variety of health-care professionals at different stages of the patients' life, including during intercurrent illness and with varying degrees of foot pathology. It is very easy for patients with diabetes to incur treatment delays by 'getting lost in the system' or receiving inadequate advice from nonspecialists. Therefore, it is essential that clear pathways of care are developed or should already exist for any patient with diabetes-related foot problems. This may include both emergency and chronic care. Examples of these pathways include 24-hour emergency hotlines for the referral of new foot lesions. Other examples include the development of 'traffic light' systems to help health-care professionals decide on prioritization and management of patients (developed in England and Scotland). Other health-care systems have empowered patients, for example by issuing them with advice cards about who to contact if they develop foot problems.

ENSURING QUALITY OF DIABETIC FOOT CARE

For many countries, the simple existence of adequate podiatry and a foot care team remains a dream for patients with diabetes. However, some European countries have gone a step further. In Germany, for example, they have been able to formally accredit dedicated diabetic foot clinics. In so doing, they assure the quality of care that patients receive. Peer review and audit against predetermined standards are driving up the quality of care.

In England, national commissioning documents have been issued to health-care commissioners. These identify and lay out the necessary requirements to preserve and manage the foot health of patients with diabetes in large communities. The documents explain the necessary requirements (at all levels) for an integrated foot care service. A further document describes and defines the minimum clinical competencies required for health-care professionals involved at each stage of the care of the diabetic foot.

RESOURCES FOR THE DEVELOPMENT AND SUSTAINABILITY OF DIABETIC FOOT CARE SERVICES

Any health-care professional who has knowledge and understanding of the diabetic foot and is interested in managing these patients may take the initiative in forming the necessary foot care team and pathways of care. A team of professionals interested in the management of diabetic foot needs involvement and commitment by many different experts in the field working in various areas of foot care. These may differ pragmatically according to the local need, geographical variations in foot pathology (e.g. prevalence of PAD), and local expertise. They may include diabetes educators, dieticians, nurses, podiatrists, diabetologists, orthopedic surgeons, vascular surgeons, and plastic surgeons along with physiotherapists. Some

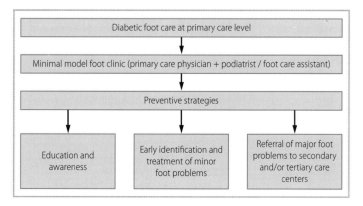

Figure 3.2 Integrated diabetic foot care pathway.

part of the team may be ever-present, whereas others, such as plastic surgeons, may be called upon for specific indications. Primary care physicians have to be trained in diabetes care and diabetic foot care. Short-term postgraduate courses in diabetes care can be introduced, such as the 1 year 'Diploma in Diabetology' being conducted in Pakistan.

Two- to three-day long concise training programs in basic diabetic foot care can provide physicians with an insight into diabetic foot care. Basic and advanced courses being conducted in various countries under the Step-by-Step programs are good example of such training.

Owing to the lack of trained podiatrists in the developing world, foot care assistants can perform the task of wound care and podiatry having been trained locally. The role of a podiatrist or foot care assistant may be multifactorial, including diabetic foot care advice, assessment of feet at risk, examination of pedal pulses, assessment of neuropathy, nail trimming, management of calluses and corns, and assessment of the need for specialized footwear. A precise curriculum of the diabetic foot care assistant course has been developed by IWGDF. A short 6-week foot care assistant course is being successfully conducted in Pakistan and the trained foot care assistants are practically involved in diabetic foot care at foot clinics across the country. Diabetes educators are the key members of a diabetes team. The educators contribute equally to the preventive and management aspects of foot care. Training of diabetes educators is an extremely significant element in the setting up of diabetic foot services. Diabetes educator courses of varying durations have been initiated in various countries in accordance with local circumstances.

As the management of diabetes is consuming an increasingly significant portion of the health budget throughout the world, health-care strategies are shifting, with the main responsibility for prevention and treatment of the diabetic foot moving from secondary to primary care. The primary care setting is required to cope with this increasing pressure of cost-effectiveness along with standardized care.

Ideally, a budget should be allocated and the sustainability of the project planned from the very beginning. Various stakeholders can be involved in initiating the diabetic foot service including the pharmaceutical industry, nongovernmental organizations, government institutions, politicians, and international organizations working on the diabetic foot. Effective diabetes and diabetic foot care implies a multidisciplinary approach for which a trained multidisciplinary team is indispensable. A specialized foot clinic for diabetic patients brings together the skills of podiatrists, orthotists, physicians, and surgeons to manage diabetic foot lesions and reduce the rate of major amputations. However, depending on local circumstances, the diabetic foot care team needs to be modified to achieve the best possible results in preventing and reducing the problems caused by the diabetic foot.

■ IMPORTANT FURTHER READING

Abbas ZG, Lutale JK, Baker K, Baker N, Archibald LK. The 'Step by Step' Diabetic Foot Project in Tanzania: a model for improving patient outcomes in less-developed countries. Int Wound J 2011; 8:169–165.

Bakker K, Apelqvist J, Schaper NC; International Working Group on Diabetic Foot Editorial Board. Practical guidelines on the management and prevention of the diabetic foot 2011. Diabetes Metab Res Rev 2012; 28:225–231.

German Diabetes Society: Working Group on the Diabetic Foot. http://www.ag-fuss-ddg.de/

National Institute for Health and Clinical Excellence. Foot care service for people with diabetes. Commissioning guide: Implementing NICE guidance. October 2006. NICE clinical guideline CG10. http://www.nice.org.uk/media/776/C5/290312_Diabetes_foot_care_service_tool_development_PDF_FINAL.pdf

■ REFERENCES

Abbas ZG, Lutale JK, Baker K, Baker N, Archibald LK. The 'Step by Step' Diabetic Foot Project in Tanzania: a model for improving patient outcomes in less-developed countries. Int Wound J 2011; 8:169–165.

Abbas ZG, Gill GV, Archibald LK. The epidemiology of diabetic limb sepsis: an African perspective. Diabet Med 2002a; 19:895–899.

Abbas ZG, Lutale JK, Morbach S, Archibald LK. Clinical outcome of diabetes patients hospitalised with foot ulcer, Dar es salaam, Tanzania. Diabet Med 2002b; 19:575–557.

Abbas ZG, Lutale JK, Archibald LK, and the Tanzania Diabetic Ulcer Surveillance System (TANDUSS). Epidemiology of foot ulcer in Tanzania: a contrast between African and Asia Diabetes populations. Diabetologia 2002c; 45:1042.

Apelqvist J, Agardh CD. The association between clinical risk factors and outcome of diabetic foot ulcers. Diabetes Res Clin Pract 1992; 18:43–45.

Armstrong DG, Lavery LA, Harkless LB. Validation of a diabetic wound classification system. The contribution of depth, infection, and ischemia to risk of amputation. Diabetes Care 1998; 21:855–859.

Bakker K, Abbas ZG, Pendsey S. Step by Step, improving diabetic foot care in the developing world. A pilot study for India, Bangladesh, Sri Lanka and Tanzania. Practical Diabetes Int 2006; 23:365–369.

Bakker K, Apelqvist J, Schaper NC. Practical guidelines on the management and prevention of the diabetic foot 2011. Diab Metab Res Rev 2012a; 28:225–223.

Bakker K, Apelqvist J, Schaper NC. International Working Group on Diabetic Foot Editorial Board. Practical guidelines on the management and prevention of the Diabetic foot 2011. Diabetes Mateb Res Rev 2012b; 28:225–231.

Canavan RJ, Uniwin NC, Kelly WF, Connolly VM. Diabetes and non-diabetes related lower extremity amputation incidence before and after the introduction of better organized diabetes foot care: continuous longitudinal monitoring using a standard method. Diabetes Care 2008; 31:459–463.

Diabetes and foot care: Time to act. International Diabetes Federation (IDF) and International Working Group of Diabetic foot (IWGDF). 2005. 99 - 01. www.idf.org/webdata/docs/T2A_Introduction.pdf

Edmonds ME, Blundell MP, Morris ME, Cotton LT, Watkins PJ. Improved survival of the diabetic foot: the role of the specialized foot clinic. Q J Med 1986; 60:763–771.

Fusilli D, Alviggi L, Seghieri G, de Bellis A. Improvement of diabetic foot care after the implementation of the International Consensus on the Diabetic Foot (ICDF): result of a 5-year prospective study. Diabetes Res Clin Pract 2005; 75:153–158.

International Diabetes Federation. IDF Diabetes Atlas, 6th edn. Brussels Belgium: International Diabetes Federation, 2013. www.idf.org/diabetesatlas

Krishnan S, Nash F, Baker N, et al. Reduction in diabetic amputations over 11 year in a defined UK population: benefits of multidisciplinary team work and continuous prospective audit. Diabetes Care 2008; 31:99–101.

McCabe CJ, Stevenson RC, Dolan AM. Evaluation of a diabetic foot screening and protection program. Diabet Med 1998; 15:520–523.

Moor MJ, Gadsby R. Non-insulin dependent diabetes mellitus in general practice. Practitioner 1984; 228:675–679.

Pecoraro RE, Reiber GE, Burgess EM. Pathways to diabetic limbs amputation. Basis for prevention. Diabetes Care 1990; 13:513–521.

Prompers L, Schaper N, Apelqvist J, et al. Prediction of outcome in individuals with diabetic foot ulcers: focus on the differences between individuals with and without peripheral arterial disease. The EURODIALE Study. Diabetologia 2008; 51:747–755.

Rayman G, Murali-Kishnan STM, Baker N, Wareham A, Rayman A. Are we underestimating diabetes lower extremity amputation rates? Results and benefits of the first prospective study. Diabetes Care 2004; 27:1892–1896.

Sanders LJ, Robbins JM, Edmonds ME. History of the team approach to amputation prevention: pioneers and milestones. J Vasc Surg 2010; 52:3S–16S.

Somannavar S, Lanthorn H, DeepaM, Pradeepa R, Mohan V. Increase Awareness about Diabetes and its Complications in a Whole City. Effectiveness of the "prevention, Awareness, Counseling and Evaluation" [PACE] Diabetes Project [PACE-6]. JAPI 2008; 56:497–492.

Thomson FJ, Veves A, Ashe H, et al. A team approach to diabetic foot care – the Manchester experience. Foot 1991:1:75-82.

Chapter 4 — Economic aspects of foot care

Marion Kerr

SUMMARY

- It is estimated that 5–7% of people with diabetes have current or past foot ulcers, and 2.5% have current foot ulcers
- Studies suggest that people with diabetic foot ulcers have a lower health-related quality of life than people who have diabetes and macrovascular complications, chronic obstructive pulmonary disease, or end-stage renal disease requiring hemodialysis
- The 5-year mortality rate for people with diabetic foot ulcers has been estimated at 42–44%. For those who undergo major amputation, the rate rises to 68–79%
- The cost of diabetic foot care in England in 2010–2011 is estimated at £580–599 million (US$980–1010 million), which is 0.6% of the National Health Service (NHS) budget. This is higher than the cost of each of the four most common cancers
- There is evidence that diabetic foot care is suboptimal in many areas
- As an example, economic analysis suggests that a multidisciplinary diabetic foot care team (MDT) at The James Cook University Hospital, Middlesbrough, England, was highly cost-effective.
- MDTs reported in the literature vary in composition, cost, and outcomes. The cost-effectiveness of individual interventions will need to be estimated using parameters that reflect local circumstances. As an example, economic analysis suggests that a multidisciplinary diabetic foot care team (MDT) at The James Cook University Hospital, Middlesbrough, England, was highly cost-effective

INTRODUCTION

Health economics is concerned, essentially, with the optimal allocation of scarce health-care resources. There are never sufficient resources in any health-care system for all possible treatments to be provided. Decision makers need to make choices. A key criterion for making such choices is the maximization of health gain. It is not the only criterion: a health-care system may also be concerned with issues such as fairness, or with research objectives or other priorities, but maximizing health gain is generally a key aim.

In order to assess any given proposal against this criterion, it is necessary to make the case in terms that allow for comparison with alternative uses of health-care resources. As a starting point, decision-makers and budget-holders are likely to require the answers to a number of questions, such as:

- How many people have the condition?
- How severe is the effect on their quality of life and survival?
- What impact will a new service have on quality and length of life?
- How will the costs of the new service compare with those for current models of care?

The answers to these questions enable decision makers to determine not only the impacts and costs of a new treatment relative to current care for a given patient group but also – given comparable analysis in other areas and the use of common metrics – to compare the health gain per pound, euro, or dollar of expenditure with that achievable if the money were spent, instead, on treatments for other groups of patients.

In the case of diabetic foot disease, a number of these crucial questions are difficult to answer. In most countries, there is uncertainty over the numbers of people with active ulceration. There have been relatively few studies on the impact of diabetic foot disease on quality of life and survival, and little is known of the true cost of current or improved models of care. Lack of understanding of the human and financial cost of the condition is a key barrier to the provision of high-quality care for people with diabetic foot disease.

In this chapter, we will attempt to address some of these questions in the context of the English NHS, drawing on published studies and on our own economic modeling. We will also identify areas where more clinical or economic evidence is needed. While costs and models of care may differ substantially across health economies, it is hoped that the general approach will provide a starting point for understanding the economic aspects of foot care.

THE HUMAN COST

Incidence and prevalence

Studies suggest that 5–7% of people with diabetes have current or past foot ulcers (Neil et al. 1989, Kumar et al. 1994, Walters et al. 1992). A community-based study in North-West England found that 2.2% of people with diabetes experienced at least one new foot ulcer in a year (Abbott et al. 2002). In Scotland, 2.5% of the diagnosed diabetes population had current foot ulcers at the beginning of December 2010 (Leese et al. 2011).

Approximately, 7 out of every 10,000 people with diabetes underwent a major lower extremity amputation in 2010–2011, and 12 out of 10,000 had a minor amputation (National Diabetes Audit 2012). The risk of a person with diabetes undergoing a lower extremity amputation is around 23 times that of a person without diabetes (Holman et al. 2012).

Quality of life

If quality of life measures are to be used in economic analysis, a generic metric is required, to allow comparison with other clinical conditions. In England, the National Institute for Health and Care Excellence (NICE) has specified that EQ-5D is the preferred measure for cost-effectiveness analysis.

EQ-5D scores are derived from patient questionnaires covering five domains: mobility, pain/discomfort, anxiety/depression, ability to care for oneself, and ability to perform usual tasks. Scores are recorded on a metric in which 0 represents death and 1 represents perfect health. EQ-5D can be used in conjunction with survival data to estimate quality-adjusted life years (QALYs).

Using the EQ-5D instrument, a Swedish study recorded scores for patients treated by a MDT between 1995 and 1998 (Ragnarson Tennvall & Apelqvist 2000). The scores recorded for current ulcers and for major amputation are lower than those recorded in other studies for people with diabetes and macrovascular complications (UKPDS 1999), or with other long-term conditions such as chronic obstructive pulmonary disease (Brazier et al. 2004) or end-stage renal disease requiring hemodialysis (Wasserfallen et al. 2004) (**Figure 4.1**).

Prognosis and mortality

Only two-thirds of diabetic foot ulcers eventually heal without surgery (Apelqvist et al. 1993, Jeffcoate et al. 2006, Pound et al. 2005). Up to 28% may result in some form of amputation (Armstrong et al. 1998). Patients who have had a foot ulcer are at increased risk of further ulceration.

One-year mortality has been estimated at 32.7% for patients who have undergone major amputation in diabetes and 18.3% after minor amputation (Vamos et al. 2010). Five-year cumulative mortality for patients with diabetes undergoing a first major amputation has been estimated at 68–78.7% (Icks et al. 2011, Ikonen et al. 2010).

Even without amputation, diabetic foot ulcers are associated with high levels of mortality. Five-year mortality has been estimated at 42–44% (Apelqvist et al. 1993, Moulik et al. 2003), which is considerably higher than 5-year mortality for high-profile diseases such as breast cancer and prostate cancer. However, available datasets and study evidence do not allow us to determine the discrete impact of diabetic foot disease on mortality risk. In many cases, patients with diabetic foot ulcers have related cardiovascular disease and advanced diabetes complications that contribute to mortality risk.

THE FINANCIAL COST

A number of studies have estimated the cost of care for people with diabetic foot disease, either in absolute or relative terms. For example, a US study found that the cost of care in the year after diagnosis of a foot ulcer was up to 5.4 times as high as the cost of care for people with diabetes who did not have an ulcer (Ramsey et al. 1999). The Eurodiale study compiled data from 14 European centers, and found that costs increased with ulcer severity, with the highest costs recorded for patients with infection and peripheral arterial disease

(Prompers et al. 2008). Comparison across studies is difficult, however, owing to differences in study design, methods, and definitions, and to differences between health-care systems (Matricali et al. 2007). In examining the cost-effectiveness of interventions, it is important to use cost data from the health-care economy in which the interventions will be implemented.

We recently estimated the cost of diabetic foot care in England in 2010–2011 at £580–£599 million (US$980–1010 million), which is 0.6% of the NHS budget (preliminary findings published in Kerr 2012, further analysis in Kerr et al. 2014) (**Figure 4.2**). Of this sum, £262.30 million is for inpatient care related to ulceration or amputation. This portion of expenditure was estimated based on activity recorded

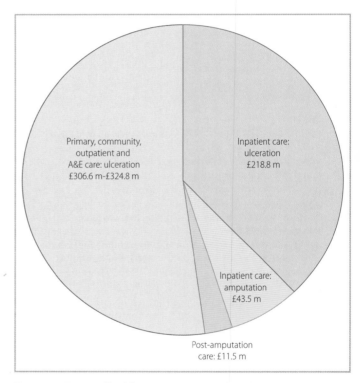

Figure 4.2 Estimated healthcare expenditure on foot ulceration and amputation in diabetes, England, 2010–2011.

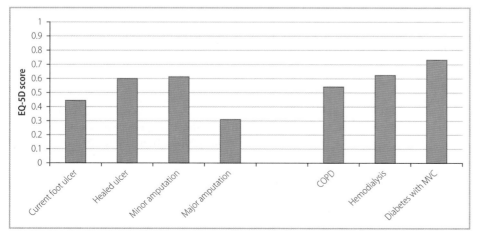

Figure 4.1 EQ-5D scores for ulcer and amputation in diabetes (Ragnarson Tennvall & Apelqvist 2000) and for other conditions (Brazier et al. 2004, UKPDS 1999, Wasserfallen et al. 2004). MVC, macrovascular complications.

Chapter 5

Medical therapy and metabolic control to optimize cardiovascular risk and reduce overall mortality

Jack R. W. Brownrigg, Kausik K. Ray

SUMMARY

- Cardiovascular disease (CVD) risk is approximately twofold higher among individuals with diabetes mellitus (DM) compared with individuals without DM
- Diabetic foot complications are associated with even greater risk of CVD and overall mortality
- Intensive cardiovascular (CV) risk management can reduce CVD and overall mortality in patients with diabetic foot ulcers (DFUs)
- Blood pressure (BP) control and low-density lipoprotein cholesterol (LDL-C) lowering offer the greatest benefits for reduction of CVD events, while intensive glucose control is associated with a reduction in the progression of microvascular disease
- There is likely an unmet potential for CVD prevention among individuals with DFU

INTRODUCTION

During recent decades, the prevention and treatment of diabetic foot complications have received increasing attention from clinicians and investigators as the incidence of DM has surged worldwide. Significant progress has been made with respect to management of diabetic foot ulcers (DFUs); however, many local interventions that may prevent ulceration or enhance healing of existing foot lesions do so without improving long-term survival. DM is associated with a reduction in life expectancy of around 6 years (The Emerging Risk Factors Collaboration 2011), and one half of patients with type 2 diabetes will die prematurely as a result of CVD. Emerging evidence indicates that individuals with DFU carry an even greater risk of premature mortality, attributable in part to a greater burden of CVD (Brownrigg et al. 2012). Against this background, the prevention of CVD should be considered a priority in patients with foot complications of diabetes. The responsibility for prevention falls on individual patients, primary care physicians, and all clinicians who come into contact with patients with DFU in secondary care. This chapter will focus on medical therapies that can reduce excess risk of all-cause and CV mortality seen in patients with DFU.

QUANTIFYING CV RISK IN DFU

CVD is the leading cause of morbidity and mortality among individuals with DM. Data from the large Emerging Risk Factors Collaboration suggests that CVD risk remains approximately twofold higher compared with individuals without DM (Figure 5.1) (The Emerging Risk Factors Collaboration 2010). Current guidelines from the European Society of Cardiology (ESC) (European Guidelines on Cardiovascular Disease Prevention in Clinical Practice 2012) suggest the use of the SCORE risk estimation system that categorizes patients

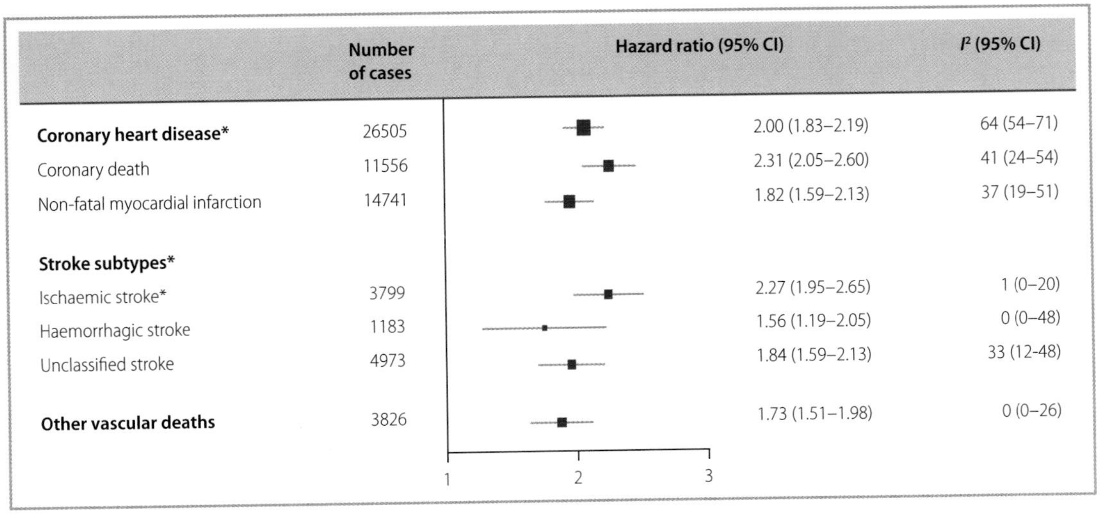

	Number of cases	Hazard ratio (95% CI)		Hazard ratio (95% CI)	I^2 (95% CI)
Coronary heart disease*	26505			2.00 (1.83–2.19)	64 (54–71)
Coronary death	11556			2.31 (2.05–2.60)	41 (24–54)
Non-fatal myocardial infarction	14741			1.82 (1.59–2.13)	37 (19–51)
Stroke subtypes*					
Ischaemic stroke*	3799			2.27 (1.95–2.65)	1 (0–20)
Haemorrhagic stroke	1183			1.56 (1.19–2.05)	0 (0–48)
Unclassified stroke	4973			1.84 (1.59–2.13)	33 (12–48)
Other vascular deaths	3826			1.73 (1.51–1.98)	0 (0–26)

Figure 5.1 Probability of cardiovascular events in people with diabetes versus those without diabetes. Analyses by The Emerging Risk Factors Collaboration were based on 530 083 participants. Hazard ratios were adjusted for age, smoking status, body mass index, and systolic blood pressure, and, where appropriate, stratified by sex and trial arm. With permission from The Emerging Risk Factors Collaboration (2010) with permission from Elsevier. *Includes both fatal and nonfatal events.

into low (<1%), moderate (≥1 and <5%), high (≥5 and <10%), and very high (≥10%) 10-year risk of fatal CVD (**Figure 5.2**) (Conroy et al. 2003). In this system, patients with DM are considered high risk automatically, and very high risk with one or more additional CV risk factors. Given that high BP is reported in over two-thirds of patients with type 2 diabetes, the majority will fall into the very-high risk category. In general, all individuals at risk should be offered lifestyle advice with those with moderate, high, or very high CV risk offered pharmacotherapy to attain specific LDL-C goals, with LDL-C targets being lower among those with the highest absolute risk of CVD. An alternative risk model designed specifically for patients with type 2 diabetes has been generated from the landmark UK Prospective Diabetes Study (UKPDS) data (Stevens et al. 2001); however, this model has demonstrated, at best, moderate discrimination for coronary heart disease (CHD) events in external validation (Guzder et al. 2005, Van Dieren et al. 2000).

While DM is an established risk factor for the development of CVD, there is accumulating evidence that patients with diabetic foot complications may be at even higher risk. A meta-analysis of eight studies reporting comparisons between patients with a history of diabetic foot ulceration and patients with diabetes alone suggests that patients with DFU have an excess risk of CVD events (Brownrigg et al. 2012). In that study, DFU was associated with an increased risk of all-cause mortality [relative risk (RR) 1.89, 95% confidence interval (CI) 1.60–2.23], fatal myocardial infarction (RR 2.22, 95% CI 1.09–4.53), and fatal stroke (RR 1.41, 95% CI 0.61–3.24). Such data suggest there may be an unmet potential to further reduce CV risk in patients with DFU through aggressive risk modification. While the number of CVD deaths is greater in a DFU population, fatal myocardial infarction and cerebrovascular (CV) accounted for 45% of total deaths in both DFU and DM populations. Excess mortality in DFU may, therefore, also reflect the longer duration of DM with a greater burden of disease that is seen in patients with DFU and non-CV complications of DFU, such as sepsis.

EVIDENCE OF CV RISK MODIFICATION IN DFU

The benefits of intensive CV risk modification in a population with diabetes have been demonstrated in an extension of the Steno-2 study

(Gaede et al. 2008). In this study, patients with type 2 diabetes and persistent microalbuminuria were randomized to receive conventional therapy or intensive therapy incorporating tight glucose regulation and the use of renin–angiotensin system blockers, aspirin, and statins. Importantly, this study population was selected for the presence of microalbuminuria, itself a strong predictor of CV events but also associated with microvascular disease, and therefore neuropathy and ulceration. Intensive therapy corresponded to an absolute risk reduction of 20% for all-cause mortality after 7.8 years of intervention and a further 5.5 years of follow-up. At the end of the intervention period, intensive therapy was superior to conventional therapy in controlling the level of glycated hemoglobin, total cholesterol, LDL-C and triglycerides, systolic and diastolic BPs, and the rate of urinary albumin excretion. These observed differences in CV risk factors at completion of the trial period corresponded with a significant difference in CV mortality, with a hazard ratio (HR) of 0.43 (95% CI 0.19–0.94) for death from CV causes in the intensive therapy group.

The direct evidence of CV risk management in patients with DFU is more limited. A single study has evaluated aggressive CV risk management in a foot clinic population (Young et al. 2008). Young et al reported a reduction in 5-year mortality from 48% to 27% following the introduction of a protocol incorporating CVD risk factor screening and modification with an antiplatelet agent, statin, and a angiotensin-converting enzyme (ACE) inhibitor ± beta-blocker in those with hypertension. Ischemic heart disease was the leading cause of death in both cohorts, accounting for 61% and 65% of deaths in the first and second cohorts, respectively.

A recent progress report based on data from the National Health and Nutrition Examination Survey (NHANES) in the United States suggests incremental progress is being made in achieving targets for glycemic control, BP, and lipid levels in diabetes (The Emerging Risk Factors Collaboration 2011). Despite this, important gaps in care remained; notably, smoking rates remained unacceptably high and almost half of US adults with diabetes did not meet the recommended goals for diabetes care. Similar improvements have also been seen in the United Kingdom following the introduction of a pay-for-performance scheme based on meeting targets for the quality of diabetes care in England in 2004 (Campbell et al. 2009). Targets in the scheme include both measurement and intermediate outcomes for BP, cholesterol levels, and glycemic control.

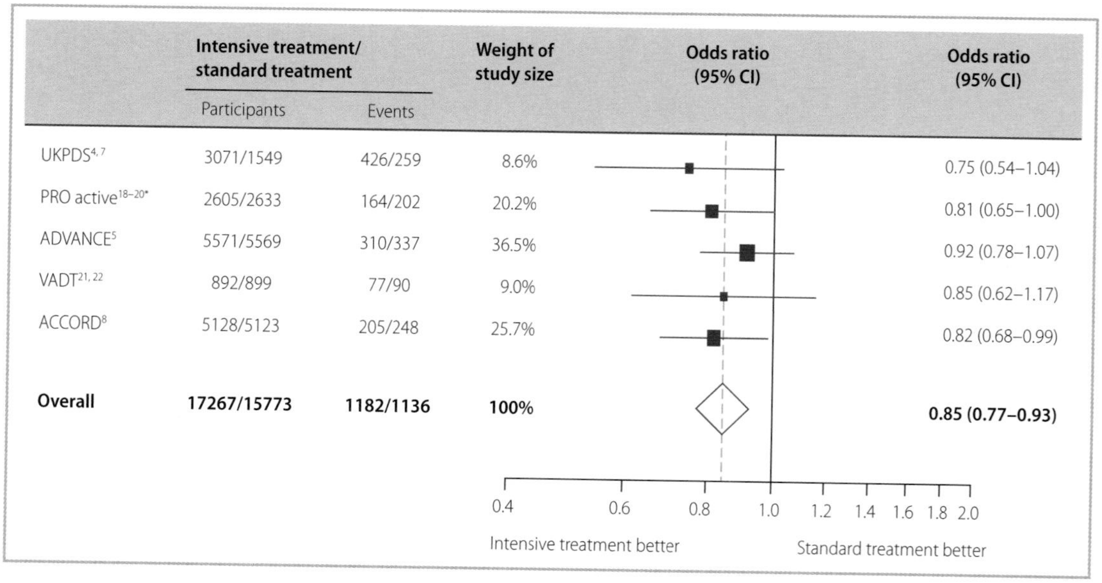

	Intensive treatment/standard treatment		Weight of study size	Odds ratio (95% CI)	Odds ratio (95% CI)
	Participants	Events			
UKPDS[4,7]	3071/1549	426/259	8.6%		0.75 (0.54–1.04)
PRO active[18–20*]	2605/2633	164/202	20.2%		0.81 (0.65–1.00)
ADVANCE[5]	5571/5569	310/337	36.5%		0.92 (0.78–1.07)
VADT[21,22]	892/899	77/90	9.0%		0.85 (0.62–1.17)
ACCORD[8]	5128/5123	205/248	25.7%		0.82 (0.68–0.99)
Overall	**17267/15773**	**1182/1136**	**100%**		**0.85 (0.77–0.93)**

0.4 0.6 0.8 1.0 1.2 1.4 1.6 1.8 2.0

Intensive treatment better   Standard treatment better

Figure 5.2 Probability of events of coronary heart disease with intensive glucose lowering versus standard treatment in people with diabetes. With permission from Ray et al. (2009) with permission from Elsevier. *Included nonfatal myocardial infarction and death from all-cardiac mortality.

BLOOD PRESSURE CONTROL

Hypertension is more prevalent in patients with type 2 diabetes when compared with the general population, and may be even more common in those with DFU (Brownrigg et al. 2012). Much of the evidence of BP reduction in diabetes derives from subgroup analyses of trials conducted in general populations. Treatment effects of antihypertensive regimens have been shown to be greater in patients with diabetes when compared with groups without diabetes in both the Systolic Hypertension in the Elderly Program (SHEP) and Systolic Hypertension in Europe (Syst-Eur) studies (Curb et al. 1996, Birkenhager et al. 2000). In the Hypertension Optimal Study (HOT) (Hansson et al. 1998), which randomly assigned patients to a target diastolic BP, there was a 51% reduction in major CV events in the group with a target of £80 mmHg compared with the target group £90 mmHg. The treatment effect was greater than that observed for equivalent targets in the total study population (28% reduction), emphasizing the need to aggressively treat BP in patients with diabetes. Further evidence of the benefits of tight BP control comes from the UKPDS study (UKPDS Group 1998) in which patients were randomized to tight BP control and less tight BP control, achieving mean BPs of 144/82 mmHg and 154/87 mmHg, respectively. Tight control was associated with a 44% reduction in the risk of stroke and nonsignificant risk reduction of 21% for myocardial infarction. Post-trial monitoring of patients in the UKPDS showed that the benefits of previously improved BP control were not sustained when differences in BP between the groups were lost, indicating a need for continued tight control (Holman et al. 2008). The target BP of 150/85 mmHg in the tight BP control group of UKPDS is less aggressive than a target of <130 mmHg currently advocated for patients with diabetes (Chobanian et al. 2003, Mancia et al. 2007), although this is difficult to achieve in many cases. Certainly, targets of <120 mmHg are both difficult to achieve and potentially harmful for patients, as demonstrated in the ACCORD BP study (Cushman et al. 2010), where this target did not reduce the rate of fatal and nonfatal CV events and increased the risk of serious adverse events associated with antihypertensive treatment. This so-called J-curve effect has also been reported in patients with diabetes and CHD, where reducing systolic BP to lower than 130 mmHg was not associated with reductions in morbidity beyond that achieved with systolic BP <140 mmHg, and was associated with an increase in all-cause mortality (Cooper-DeHoff et al. 2010). However in ACCORD, lowering BP to <120 did significantly reduce stroke that is more closely related to BP than CHD. The recent ESC guidelines recommend a BP target of 140/85 mmHg (ESC Guidelines on Diabetes, pre-diabetes, and Cardiovascular Diseases Developed in Collaboration with the EASD 2013).

While clinical benefits have been shown for all classes of antihypertensives in DM, class-specific effects exist and warrant consideration in this population. A meta-analysis from the Blood Pressure Lowering Treatment Trialists' Collaboration (Turnbull et al. 2005) looked at several placebo-controlled trials of antihypertensives in general populations and in those with DM. They observed no differences in the extent to which CVD events were reduced between patients with and without diabetes, regardless of drug class (antihypertensives regimens included ACE inhibitors, calcium channel blockers, angiotensin receptor blockers, diuretics, and beta-blockers). The ADVANCE trial (Patel et al. 2007), which recruited patients with DM but was not selective for hypertensives, demonstrated reductions in all-cause mortality (14%), CVD mortality (18%), macrovascular events (8%), and microvascular events (9%) in patients treated with combination therapy consisting of an ACE inhibitor and a thiazide-type diuretic. Renin–angiotensin system blockers are attractive in this population by virtue of their renoprotective effects in diabetes. Given that individuals with DM are at risk of end-stage renal disease (ESRD) and dialysis, and renin–angiotensin system blockade reduces the progression to ESRD, it is reasonable for all patients irrespective of BP to be commenced on an ACE inhibitor or an angiotensin receptor blocker (Keane et al. 2003, Mann et al. 2001).

LIPID MODIFICATION

Patterns of dyslipidemia in DM differ from those in populations without diabetes. Individuals with type 2 diabetes typically have lower high-density lipoprotein cholesterol (HDL-C) and higher triglyceride cholesterol (TC) levels than people without diabetes (Wilson et al. 1985, Taskinen 2003), while in patients with type 1 diabetes, triglyceride concentrations tend to be lower than in type 2 diabetes, and HDL-C levels are average or high (Nikkila & Hormila 1978). LDL-C particles are smaller and denser in individuals with diabetes (Feingold et al. 1992); however, total cholesterol and LDL-C concentrations are similar in age- and sex-matched cohorts (Laakso et al. 1985). In this manner, an increased risk associated with atherogenic small and dense LDL particles may be masked by similar overall LDL-C levels. Hence, the European Atherosclerosis Society (EAS) and the ESC recommend using non-HDL-C as a secondary target for those with diabetes (TC-HDL-C).

The Collaborative AtoRvastatin Diabetes Study (CARDS), a randomized-controlled study in patients with type 2 DM without a history of CVD, demonstrated a reduction in CHD and stroke events with atorvastatin 10 mg when compared with placebo (Colhoun et al. 2004). A meta-analysis of 14 randomized trials examining the effect of statins on CV events has confirmed the benefits of lipid reduction (Kearney et al. 2008); a 21% proportional reduction in major CV events was reported for every 1 mmol/L reduction in LDL-C in participants with DM. This reduction was equivalent to that observed in participants without diabetes. Interestingly, the proportional benefit of statin therapy was largely independent of the pretreatment concentration of LDL-C, HDL-C, total cholesterol, and triglycerides. Current guidelines from the National Institute for Health and Care Excellence (NICE) recommend a statin for patients with diabetes and further risk from additional, nonhyperglycemia-related factors (National Institute for Clinical Excellence, 2013). Alternatively, clinicians are advised to utilize the UKPDS risk engine (Stevens et al. 2001), and initiate therapy for those with a projected risk of ≥20% over 10 years. Once lipid-lowering therapy is commenced, patients should undergo repeat assessment of lipid profile between 1 and 3 months after starting treatment and annually thereafter.

Fibrates represent a different class of lipid-lowering therapy with particular efficacy with respect to reducing triglycerides levels, with more modest effects on LDL-C, HDL-C, and total cholesterol (Abourih et al. 2009). The Fenofibrate Intervention and Event Lowering in Diabetes (FIELD) study randomized 9795 patients with type 2 DM to fibrate or placebo therapy (Keech et al. 2005). Investigators observed no significant reduction in the primary outcome measure of coronary events but did report a significant decrease in a composite end point of total CV events, including CHD events; stroke; CV and all-cause mortality; and carotid, peripheral and coronary revascularization procedures. The ACCORD trial suggested that the addition of fenofibrate to statin was not beneficial overall; however, in the prespecified subgroup with a triglyceride ≥204 mg/dL (≥2.30 mmol/L) and an HDL-C ≤34 mg/dL (≤0.88 mmol/L), there was evidence of a statistical benefit but not among those without (The ACCORD Study Group 2010). A meta-analysis of five trials suggested that fibrates only reduce risk of CVD among those with this particular lipid profile but offer no benefit when absent (Sacks et al. 2010). While it is not usual to commence both a statin and fibrate at the same time, it is reasonable to add a fibrate to statin therapy if triglyceride levels remain above 2.30 mmol/L and HDL-C is <0.88 mmol/L. Fenofibrate therapy was also associated with a reduction in microvascular end points in the FIELD study, with less albuminuria progression and less retinopathy needing laser treatment (Keech et al. 2005).

GLYCEMIC CONTROL

Conclusive randomized trial data confirms that intensive blood glucose control results in substantial benefits in microvascular outcomes; however, the evidence of a reduction in macrovascular events has been less convincing. The UKPDS randomized 3867 patients with newly diagnosed type 2 diabetes to conventional treatment or intensive glucose control that resulted in HbA1c levels of 7.9% and 7.0%, respectively, at 10 years of follow-up (UKPDS Group 1998). Intensive therapy was associated with a 25% risk reduction in microvascular end points and a nonsignificant 36% reduction in amputations, but failed to show improvements in CV outcomes, and was likely underpowered to do so. A 10-year postinterventional extension of this study has reported some benefit in CV outcomes despite nonsignificant differences in HbA1c concentration between study arms (Holman et al. 2008). In post-hoc subgroup analyses 10 years postintervention, in patients receiving sulfonylurea-insulin, relative reductions in risk were observed for microvascular disease (24%), myocardial infarction (15%), and all-cause mortality (13%). In the cohort of overweight patients, metformin treatment was associated with risk reductions in myocardial infarction (33%) and all-cause mortality (27%). A similar legacy effect was observed in the Diabetes Control and Complications Trials/Epidemiology of Diabetes Intervention and Complications (DCCT/EDIC) study in patients with type 1 diabetes (DCCT/EDIC Study Research Group 2005). After a mean intervention period of 6.5 years, patients were followed up at 17 years revealing long-term beneficial effects of intensive therapy. The risk of any CVD events was reduced by 42% and remained significant after adjustment for differences in glycosylated hemoglobin and albuminuria.

Microvascular benefits of tight control seen previously were replicated in the ADVANCE study (Patel et al. 2008), which randomized 11,140 patients with type 2 diabetes to standard or intensive glucose control. Intensive control resulted in a significant reduction in the incidence of major microvascular events (HR 0.86; 95% CI 0.77–0.97; P=0.32). A 21% relative reduction in the incidence of nephropathy was observed over a median follow-up of 5 years, although no significant effect on retinopathy was seen. A meta-analysis of five randomized-controlled trials involving 33,040 participants did, however, show a significant reduction in macrovascular events with intensive therapy, including a significant 17% reduction in nonfatal myocardial infarction and a nonsignificant 7% reduction of nonfatal stroke at an average follow-up of 5 years (Ray et al. 2009). No significant effect was observed on events of all-cause mortality, and previous concerns over potential increased risk of all-cause mortality with tight blood glucose control from the ACCORD trial were alleviated (Gerstein et al. 2008). However, the absolute benefits of glucose-lowering therapy are more modest than BP and LDL-C reduction, proportionately 75%, and 60% weaker for a 0.9% lowering of HbA1c versus a 4 mmHg lowering of BP or a 1 mmol/L lowering of LDL-C.

Glucose targets

Observational data from UKPDS suggests that for every 1% reduction achieved in HbA1c concentration, risk of myocardial infarction was reduced by 14%. Accordingly, several guidelines have adopted recommendations for a target glycated hemoglobin of <6.5–7% (European Guidelines on Cardiovascular Disease Prevention in Clinical Practice 2012, National Institute for Clinical Excellence 2013). The major drawback of intensive glucose control is that it carries an increased risk of hypoglycemic events. Pooled data suggest the incidence of severe hypoglycemic events may be twofold that seen with standard treatment (Gerstein et al. 2008). This may be especially important in a population with DFU who tend to be older with longer duration of diabetes and higher HbA1c concentrations than patients with diabetes alone. Less stringent blood glucose targets may be appropriate for such patients, with target blood glucose levels between 6 and 10 mmol/L, although there are no guidelines with specific recommendations for HbA1c concentrations in patients at higher risk of hypoglycemic events.

Glycemic control for ulcer prevention and healing

There is currently no direct evidence to support a role of tight glycemic control in preventing ulceration; however, observational data suggest that optimizing blood glucose levels can prevent peripheral neuropathy and peripheral arterial disease in patients with diabetes. In the UKPDS, a reduction in HbA1c of 1% was associated with a reduction in risk of 43% for amputation or death from peripheral arterial disease (Stratton et al. 2000). Similarly, there are no data to support aggressive glycemic control to aid healing in active ulceration; however, this is also likely to be important, not least because raised blood glucose encourages infection. Data from the EURODIALE study (prospective study of newly presenting patients with DFU to 14 European foot centers) has, however, independently linked poor glycemic control (defined as HbA1c >7.5%) to ulcer recurrence (Dubsky et al. 2013).

MULTIDISCIPLINARY CARE

Several studies have examined the impact of multidisciplinary team (MDT) care on outcomes in DFU, the largest of which involved 341 patients with diabetes who were risk stratified at baseline for risk of developing a DFU (Armstrong & Harkless 1998). Appropriate education and interventions were undertaken in addition to scheduled foot examinations and podiatric care. At 3 years, the incidence of lower-extremity amputations was low (1.1 per 1000 persons per year). Among individuals categorized as high risk for developing a foot lesion, those who missed more than half their follow-up appointments were 54 times more likely to develop an ulcer and 20 times more likely to require an amputation. Multidisciplinary care should occur in both primary and secondary care, although the inclusion of all disciplines involved in caring for this population in secondary care may not be feasible in the community. Reallocating resources toward evidence-based MDT foot clinics may offer a better alternative to primary care-led screening, although this is a subject of debate. The importance of referring all patients presenting with DFU to a MDT involving vascular surgeons, diabetologists, microbiologists, and podiatrists should be emphasized, and it is intuitive that such an approach will achieve good outcomes. Following the introduction of a multidisciplinary foot care team at a single center in the United Kingdom, Krishnan et al observed a 62% reduction in major amputations in a catchment general population (Krishnan et al. 2008).

CONCLUSION

This chapter underlines the importance of managing CV risk in patients with diabetes and foot complications, who are at considerably higher risk of all-cause mortality and CVD morbidity and mortality. There is likely an unmet potential for CVD prevention in this population. Despite a lack of guidelines for managing CVD risk specifically in DFU populations, they should generally be considered as a high-risk group by virtue of frequently coexisting microvascular and macrovascular disease, and will frequently require medical therapy (**Table 5.1**). Optimizing glycemic control will mostly result in benefits in the prevention of microvascular disease, including ulcer recurrence, and will also have a modest effect in reducing CV events. The mainstay of macrovascular event reduction focuses on lifestyle, lipid lowering, and BP control.

AREAS OF CONTROVERSY AND/OR FUTURE RESEARCH

- Future research should focus on quantifying the excess risk associated with foot complications in diabetes, and what measures can be taken to effectively reduce risk in this cohort
- There is a need to identify biomarkers and diagnostic strategies for the early detection of asymptomatic CVD
- The optimal method of reaching the target HbA1c without hypoglycemia or weight gain remains unclear and will likely involve tailored recommendations for specific subgroups
- Reducing HbA1c will translate into microvascular benefits, and microvascular outcomes should be central to trials of novel antihyperglycemic drugs

Table 5.1 European guidelines on cardiovascular disease prevention in diabetes mellitus

Recommendations	Level of evidence
The target HbA1c for the prevention of CVD in diabetes of <7.0% (<53 mmol/mol) is recommended	A
Statins are recommended to reduce cardiovascular risk in diabetes	A
Hypoglycemia and excessive weight gain must be avoided and individual approaches (both targets and drug choices) may be necessary in patients with complex disease	B
Metformin should be used as first-line therapy if tolerated and not contraindicated	B
Further reductions in HbA1c to a target of <6.5% (<48 mmol/mol) (the lowest possible safely reached HbA1c) may be useful at diagnosis. For patients with a long duration of diabetes, this target may reduce risk of microvascular outcomes	B
BP targets in diabetes are recommended to be <140/80 mmHg	A
Target LDL cholesterol is <2.5 mmol/L, for patients without atherosclerotic disease total cholesterol may be <4.5 mmol/L, with a lower LDL cholesterol target of <1.8 mmol/L (using higher doses of statins) for patients with diabetes at very high CVD risk	B
Antiplatelet therapy with aspirin is not recommended for people with diabetes who do not have clinical evidence of atherosclerotic disease	A

Adapted with permission from Perk et al., European guidelines on cardiovascular disease prevention in clinical practice (2012) ©2012 Oxford University Press.

ACS, acute coronary syndrome; BP, blood pressure; CKD, chronic kidney disease; CVD, cardiovascular disease; HbA1c, glycated hemoglobin; LDL, low-density lipoprotein.

IMPORTANT FURTHER READING

Brownrigg JRW, Davey J, Holt PJ, et al. The association of ulceration of the foot with cardiovascular and all-cause mortality in patients with diabetes: a meta-analysis. Diabetologia 2012; 55:2906–2912.

The Emerging Risk Factors Collaboration. Diabetes mellitus, fasting glucose, and risk of cause-specific death. NEJM 2011; 364:829–841.

Gaede P, Lund-Andersen H, Parving HH, Pedersen O. Effect of multifactorial intervention on mortality in type 2 diabetics. N Engl J Med 2008; 358:580–591.

Kearney PM, Blackwell L, Collins R, et al. Efficacy of cholesterol-lowering therapy in 18,686 people with diabetes in 14 randomised trials of statins: a meta-analysis. Lancet 2008; 371:117–125.

Ray KK, Seshasai SRK, Wijesuriya S, et al. Effect of intensive control of glucose on cardiovascular outcomes and death in patients with diabetes mellitus: a meta-analysis of randomized controlled trials. Lancet 2009; 373:1765–1772.

Turnbull F, Neal B, Algert C, et al.; for the Blood Pressure Lowering Treatment Trialists' Collaboration. Effects of different blood-pressure lowering regimens on major cardiovascular events in individuals with and without diabetes mellitus: results of prospectively designed overviews of randomized trials. Arch Intern Med 2005; 165:1410–1419.

Young MJ, McCardle JE, Randall LE, Barclay JI. Improved survival of diabetic foot ulcer patients 1995e2008. Possible impact of aggressive cardiovascular risk management. Diabetes Care 2008; 31:2143–2147.

REFERENCES

Abourih A, Filion KB, Joseph L, et al. Effect of fibrates on lipid profiles and cardiovascular outcomes: a systematic review. Am J Med 2009; 122:962e1–e8.

The ACCORD Study Group. Effects of combination lipid therapy in type 2 diabetes mellitus. NEJM 2010; 362:1563–1574.

Armstrong DG, Harkless LB. Outcomes of preventative care in a diabetic foot specialty clinic. J Foot Ankle Surg 1998; 37:460–466.

Birkenhager WH, Staessen JA, Gasowski J, de Leeuw PW. Effects of antihypertensive treatment on endpoints in the diabetic patients randomized in the Systolic Hypertension in Europe (Syst-Eur) trial. J Nephrol 2000; 13:232–237.

Brownrigg JRW, Davey J, Holt PJ, et al. The association of ulceration of the foot with cardiovascular and all-cause mortality in patients with diabetes: a meta-analysis. Diabetologia 2012; 55:2906e12.

Campbell SM, Reeves D, Kontopantelis E, Sibbald B, Roland M. Effects of pay for performance on the quality of primary care in England. NEJM 2009; 361:368–378.

Chobanian AV, Bakris GI, Black HR, et al. The seventh report of the Joint National Committee on prevention, detection, evaluation, and treatment of high blood pressure (J NC 7). JAMA 2003; 289:2560–2571.

Colhoun HM, Betteridge DJ, Durrington PN, et al. Primary prevention of cardiovascular disease with atorvastatin in type 2 diabetes in the Collaborative Atorvastatin Diabetes Study (CARDS): multicentre randomised placebo-controlled trial. Lancet 2004; 364:685–696.

Conroy RM, Pyö¨ra¨la¨ K, Fitzgerald AP, et al; SCORE project group. Estimation of ten year risk of fatal cardiovascular disease in Europe: the SCORE project. Eur Heart J 2003; 24:987–1003.

Cooper-DeHoff RM, Gong Y, Handberg EM, et al. Tight blood pressure control and cardiovascular outcomes among hypertensive patients with diabetes and coronary artery disease. JAMA 2010; 304:61–68.

Curb JD, Pressel MS, Cutler JA, et al. Effect of diuretic-based antihypertensive treatment on cardiovascular disease risk in older diabetic patients with isolated hypertension. JAMA 1996; 276:1886–1892.

Cushman WC, Evans GW, Byington RP, et al. Effects of intensive blood-pressure control in type 2 diabetes mellitus. N Engl J Med 2010; 362:1575–1585.

Dubsky M, Jirkovska A, Bern R, et al. Risk factors for recurrence of diabetic foot ulcers: prospective follow-up analysis in the Eurodiale subgroup. Int Wound J 2013; 10:555–561.

The Emerging Risk Factors Collaboration. Diabetes mellitus, fasting blood glucose concentration, and risk of vascular disease: a collaborative meta-analysis of 102 prospective studies. Lancet 2010; 375:2215–2222.

The Emerging Risk Factors Collaboration. Diabetes mellitus, fasting glucose, and risk of cause-specific death. NEJM 2011; 364:829–841.

Feingold KR, Grunfeld C, Pang M, et al. LDL subclass phenotypes and triglyceride metabolism in non-insulin dependent diabetes. Arterioscler Thromb 1992; 12:1496–1502.

Gaede P, Lund-Andersen H, Parving HH, Pedersen O. Effect of multifactorial intervention on mortality in type 2 diabetics. N Engl J Med 2008; 358:580e91.

Gerstein HC, Miller ME, Byington RP, et al. Effects of intensive glucose lowering in type 2 diabetes. N Engl J Med 2008; 358:2545–2559.

Guzder RN, Gatling W, Mullee MA, Mehta RL, Byrne CD. Prognostic value of the Framingham cardiovascular risk equation and the UKPDS risk engine for coronary heart disease in newly diagnosed type 2 diabetes: results from a United Kingdom study. Diabet Med 2005; 22:554–562.

Hansson L, Zanchetti A, Carruthers SG, et al. Effects of intensive blood-pressure lowering and low-dose aspirin in patients with hypertension: principal results of the Hypertension Optimal Treatment (HOT) randomised trial. HOT Study Group. Lancet 1998; 351:1755–1762.

Holman RR, Paul SK, Angelyn Bethel M, Neil AB, Matthews DR. Long-term follow-up after tight control of blood pressure in type 2 diabetes. NEJM 2008; 359:1565–1576.

Holman RR, Paul SK, Bethel MA, Matthews DR, Neil HA. 10-year follow-up of intensive glucose control in type 2 diabetes. N Engl J Med 2008; 359:1577–1589.

Keane WF, Brenner BM, De Zeeuw D, et al. The risk of developing end-stage renal disease in patients with type 2 diabetes and nephropathy: The RENAAL Study. Kidney Int 2003; 63:1499–1507.

Kearney PM, Blackwell L, Collins R, et al. Efficacy of cholesterol-lowering therapy in 18,686 people with diabetes in 14 randomised trials of statins: a meta-analysis. Lancet 2008; 371:117–125.

Keech A, Simes RJ, Barter P, et al. Effects of long-term fenofibrate therapy on cardiovascular events in 9795 people with type 2 diabetes mellitus (the FIELD study): randomised controlled trial. Lancet 2005; 366:1849–1861.

Krishnan S, Nash F, Baker N, Fowler D, Rayman G. Reduction in diabetic amputations over 11 years in a defined UK population: benefits of multidisciplinary work and continuous prospective audit. Diabetes Care 2008; 31:99e101.

Laakso M, Voutilainen E, Sarlund H, et al. Serum lipids and lipoproteins in middle aged non-insulin dependent diabetics. Atherosclerosis 1985; 56:271–281.

Mancia G, De Backer G, Dominiczak A, et al. 2007 guidelines for the management of arterial hypertension of the European Society of Hypertension (ESH) and the European Society of Cardiology (ESC). J Hypertens 2007; 25:1105–1187.

Mann JFE, Gerstein HC, Pogue J, et al. Renal insufficiency as a predictor of cardiovascular outcomes and the impact of ramipril: the HOPE randomized trial. Ann Int Med 2001; 134:629–636.

Nathan DM, Cleary PA, Backlund MS, et al. The Diabetes Control and Complications Trial/Epidemiology of Diabetes Interventions and Complications (DCCT/ EDIC) Study Research Group. Intensive diabetes treatment and cardiovascular disease in patients with type 1 diabetes. New Engl J Med 2005; 353:2643–2653.

National Institute for Clinical Excellence. CG 87 – type 2 diabetes: the management of type 2 diabetes. http://www.nice.org.uk/nicemedia/live/12165/44320/44320.pdf. (Last accessed May 1, 2013.)

Nikkila EA, Hormila P. Serum lipids and lipoproteins in insulin-treated diabetes. Demonstration of increased high density lipoprotein concentrations. Diabetes 1978; 27:1078–1086.

Patel A, MacMahon S, Chalmers J, et al. for the ADVANCE Collaborative Group. Effects of a fixed combination of perindopril and indapamide on macrovascular and microvascular outcomes in patients with type 2 diabetes mellitus (the ADVANCE trial): a randomised controlled trial. Lancet 2007; 370:829–840.

Patel A, MacMahon S, Chalmers J, et al. Intensive blood glucose control and vascular outcomes in patients with type 2 diabetes. N Engl J Med 2008; 358:2560–2572.

Perk J, De Backer G, Gohlke H. European guidelines on cardiovascular disease prevention in clinical practice. Eur Heart J 2012; 33:1635–1701.

Ray KK, Seshasai SRK, Wijesuriya S, et al. Effect of intensive control of glucose on cardiovascular outcomes and death in patients with diabetes mellitus: a meta-analysis of randomized controlled trials. Lancet 2009; 373:1765–1772.

Ryden L, Grant PJ, Anker SD, et al. ESC guidelines on diabetes, pre-diabetes, and cardiovascular diseases developed in collaboration with the EASD. Eur Heart J 2013; 34:3035–3087.

Sacks FM, Carey VJ, Fruchart JC. Combination lipid therapy in type 2 diabetes. NEJM 2010; 363:692–694.

Stevens RJ, Kothari V, Adler AI, et al. The UKPDS risk engine: a model for the risk of coronary heart disease in type II diabetes (UKPDS 56). Clin Sci 2001; 101:671–679.

Stevens RJ, Kothari V, Adler AI, Stratton IM, Holman RR. The UKPDS risk engine: a model for the risk of coronary heart disease in type II diabetes (UKPDS 56). Clin Sci 2001; 101:671–679.

Stratton IM, Adler AI, Neil HAW, et al. Association of glycaemia with macrovascular and microvascular complications of type 2 diabetes (UKPDS 35): prospective observational study. Br Med J 2000; 321:405.

Taskinen MR. Diabetic dyslipidaemia: from basic research to clinical practice. Diabetologia 2003; 46:733–749.

Turnbull F, Neal B, Algert C, et al. for the Blood Pressure Lowering Treatment Trialists' Collaboration. Effects of different blood-pressure lowering regimens on major cardiovascular events in individuals with and without diabetes mellitus: results of prospectively designed overviews of randomized trials. Arch Intern Med 2005; 165:1410–1419.

UKPDS Prospective Diabetes Study Group. Tight blood pressure control and risk of macrovascular and microvascular complications in type 2 diabetes: UKPDS 38. BMJ 1998; 317:703–713.

UK Prospective Diabetes Study (UKPDS) Group. Intensive blood-glucose control with sulphonylureas or insulin compared with conventional treatment and risk of complications in patients with type 2 diabetes (UKPDS 33). Lancet 1998; 352:837–853.

Van Dieren S, Peelen LM, Nothlings U, et al. External validation of the UK prospective diabetes study (UKPDS) risk engine in patients with type 2 diabetes. Diabetologia 2011; 54:264–270.

Wilson PWF, Kannel WB, Anderson KM. Lipids, glucose intolerance and vascular disease: the Framingham Study. Monogr Atheroscler 1985; 13:1–11.

Young MJ, McCardle JE, Randall LE, Barclay JI. Improved survival of diabetic foot ulcer patients 1995e2008. Possible impact of aggressive cardiovascular risk management. Diabetes Care 2008; 31:2143e7.

Chapter 6 Psychological aspects of diabetes-related foot disease

George Peach, Robert J. Hinchliffe

SUMMARY

- Diabetes-related foot disease is a common complication of diabetes and can have marked impact on patients' quality of life (QoL)
- Immobility, anxiety, and disruption of social functioning may influence QoL as much as biological factors such as pain and loss of sensation
- Minor amputations may have less adverse effect on QoL than prolonged ulceration
- Although important outcomes in themselves, psychological factors may influence both incidence and severity of diabetes-related foot disease

INTRODUCTION

For many years, it has been recognized that diabetes can have marked psychological impact on patients and cause significant long-term distress. However, with increasingly effective and acceptable ways of controlling blood glucose, living with uncomplicated diabetes has become less of a burden. As a result, it is now the sequelae of the condition, such as visual loss and renal failure that have the greatest impact on patients' QoL. Despite this, relatively little is known about the impact of one of the most common complications – diabetes-related foot disease.

This chapter presents the existing evidence for the psychological impact of diabetes-related foot disease and identifies the tools most suited to assessing it. It also highlights how psychological factors are not only important outcomes in their own right, but may play an important role in determining the course of diabetes-related foot problems.

Diabetes-related foot disease is a chronic, progressive condition that may involve neuropathy, arthropathy, and arteriopathy to varying degrees. In addition to causing significant symptoms in themselves, these pathological processes often lead to debilitating ulceration that may take weeks or even months to resolve. In some cases, ulceration fails to heal despite aggressive medical therapy, resulting in amputation of toes, foot, or even leg. As with many other complications of diabetes, the chronicity and possible severity of diabetes-related foot disease means it has the potential to profoundly affect patients' physical and mental well-being. However, the existence of multiple symptoms with varying etiology has made it difficult to clarify its true impact on QoL.

MEASURING THE IMPACT OF DIABETES-RELATED FOOT DISEASE

The impact that medical conditions have upon QoL is typically assessed using patient-reported outcome measures (PROMs). PROMs usually take the form of patient-completed questionnaires and may be either generic or disease specific, with each type having its merits. Generic PROMs can be used to evaluate outcomes in the general population as well as in groups of patients, whereas disease-specific PROMs cannot. However, disease-specific PROMs allow much more detailed assessment of the issues affecting patients with a particular condition, making them far more useful in clinical practice.

These tools can provide very useful information about health and treatment from the patients' perspective, but their output must be reported appropriately. Many studies that claim to have measured patient QoL have actually used generic health status (HS) tools such as the EuroQol-5D (EQ-5D) (Rabin & de Charro 2001), which measures quality of health (i.e. HS) rather than QoL. In other words, they may identify functional incapacity (e.g. difficulty walking) but they do not assess how this functional incapacity actually affects a patient's QoL.

The tool that has been used most commonly to assess the impact of diabetes-related foot disease is the Medical Outcomes Study 36-item Short Form survey (SF-36) (Ware & Sherbourne 1992). This has been used in a number of randomized-controlled trials of treatments of diabetes-related foot disease (Abetz et al. 2002, Armstrong et al. 2008, Nabuurs-Franssen et al. 2005, Rauck et al. 2007, Rosenstock et al. 2004, Selvarajah et al. 2010, Swislocki et al. 2010) and has been shown to be sensitive to severity of foot ulceration and neuropathy. It has also been shown to be responsive to temporal changes in HS in patients with diabetes-related foot disease (Rosenstock et al. 2004). However, similar to the EQ-5D, this is a generic measure of HS rather than a true measure of QoL. As well as having poor sensitivity, generic tools such as this may also suffer from confounding factors, since it is impossible to establish whether patients are incapacitated by diabetes-related foot disease or other potential complications of diabetes such as retinopathy. Furthermore, since they offer no information about the specific aspects of the condition that are most troubling to patients, they provide little guidance on how clinicians might improve the care they deliver.

In order to address the possible shortcomings of the SF-36 in assessing QoL in this patient population, there are also tools that have been developed specifically for use by patients with diabetes-related foot disease. These are the Diabetic Foot Ulcer Scale (DFS) (Abetz et al. 2002) and the Neuropathy and Foot Ulcer-specific Quality of Life (NeuroQoL) instrument (Vileikyte et al. 2003).

The DFS was developed using semistructured interviews and focus groups of patients with diabetes-related foot ulcers (DFUs) and their caregivers (Abetz et al. 2002). It has been shown to have reliability, validity, and sensitivity to both wound severity and healing (Ribu et al. 2006, Valensi et al. 2005). A shortened version, the Diabetic Foot Ulcer Scale Short Form (DFS-SF), has proven to be similarly robust (Bann et al. 2003). Since the DFS-SF has statistically significant correlation with the DFS and SF-36 and has only 29 questions, it is perhaps a more 'user-friendly' tool for everyday clinical practice. However, while it is indeed disease specific, it may be argued that the DFS is not a true QoL measure, since many of the included items relate to HS rather than QoL – in other words, it gathers much information about physical and mental function (i.e. HS) but does not always require patients to state how much a particular aspect of dysfunction has affected their life (i.e. QoL).

Vileikyte et al. therefore developed the NeuroQoL instrument to assess QoL (rather than HS) in patients with diabetes complicated by peripheral neuropathy and DFUs. It has been validated against the SF-12, to show construct validity and sensitivity to neuropathic symptoms, which the SF-12 (as a generic instrument) was unable to detect. However, while NeuroQoL has demonstrated validity for assessing the impact of neuropathy in these patients, its creators acknowledge that it seems less useful for quantifying the impact of foot ulcer severity on QoL (Vileikyte et al. 2003). This is possibly because the domains of NeuroQoL relate to symptoms of neuropathy rather than ulceration. NeuroQoL's apparent lack of sensitivity to DFUs may also be the result of diminished nociceptive responses in patients with neuropathy, which means those who have ulceration *and* advanced neuropathy have less ulcer-related pain. Poor sensitivity to DFUs may also relate to the fact that NeuoQoL does not assess the impact of ulcer-related therapies such as nonweight bearing regimens, dressing changes, and antibiotic therapy.

While these disease-specific tools have shown sensitivity to symptom severity, their efficacy in assessing how QoL changes over time in these patients remains unproven. Their use in disease monitoring is therefore less valid.

In addition to NeuroQoL and the DFS, which were developed specifically for patients with diabetes-related foot disease, some investigators have suggested using other tools that are partially disease specific, i.e. tools that broadly relate to neuropathy or ulceration but have not been designed specifically to assess the impact of diabetes-related foot disease. The Norfolk Quality of Life for Diabetic Neuropathy instrument (Norfolk QoL-DN) is one such tool devised to evaluate multiple aspects of diabetes-related neuropathic disease including autonomic dysfunction. It is intended for use as a diagnostic aide as well as in disease monitoring and treatment evaluation (Currie et al. 2006, Vinik et al. 2005). However, despite robust validation, the Norfolk QoL-DN lacks specificity to peripheral neuropathy, limiting its use in assessing the specific impact of diabetes-related foot disease (Vinik et al. 2005, 2008). Another tool, The Cardiff Wound Impact Schedule (CWIS), has proven validity in assessing chronic wounds but is not specific to DFUs (Jaksa & Mahoney 2010, Price & Harding 2004). Evaluation alongside the SF-36 showed significant correlations in all domains, but the CWIS did not appear to be sensitive to severity of DFUs, since HS data derived using the CWIS did not correlate with the degree of ulceration (as determined by the University of Texas Wound Classification system) (Jaksa & Mahoney 2010, Price & Harding 2004). However, the CWIS does discriminate between healed and unhealed ulcers (Jeffcoate et al. 2009, Price & Harding 2004).

Combining generic and disease-specific tools may ultimately provide the most useful information on outcomes (Fitzpatrick et al. 1998). Using more than one measure means specific clinical information can be gathered using the disease-specific tool, while a parallel generic measure (such as EQ-5D) (Rabin & de Charro 2001) is used to perform cost–utility analyses and provide comparisons of QoL across different conditions.

THE IMPACT OF DIABETES-RELATED FOOT DISEASE

Neuropathy

Up to 50% of patients with diabetes develop peripheral neuropathy (DPN) (Vinik et al. 2000). Though the most commonly reported symptom is pain, patients may also suffer from poor balance, disturbed sleep, and reduced foot sensation that limits the footwear they can use. These symptoms often coexist and can lead to a marked reduction in physical activity and generally poorer HS (Benbow et al. 1998).

In a well-designed cross-sectional population study using NeuroQoL, Davies et al. found that more severe neuropathy was associated with a higher prevalence of pain and poorer QoL (Davies et al. 2006). However, attempting to study the impact of neuropathic pain in isolation is inherently difficult, particularly in those with mild or moderate neuropathy, since patients will often have painful ulceration as well. The situation is further confounded by the fact that while advanced neuropathy may be associated with an increased risk of *neuropathic* pain it is typically associated with less ulcer-related pain than mild neuropathy. This highlights the importance of using disease-specific QoL measures that are able to differentiate between the various aspects of the condition.

In addition to the impact of physical dysfunction, patients with DPN may also experience fear or anxiety about advancing disease and the possibility of future ulceration or amputation (Jain et al. 2011).

Arthropathy

Few studies have attempted to assess the impact of Charcot arthropathy on QoL/HS in patients with diabetes (Pakarinen et al. 2009, Pinzur & Evans 2003, Sochocki et al. 2008). Of those studies that identified Charcot arthropathy as a separate subgroup, it was suggested [using the American Academy of Orthopaedic Surgeons Diabetic Foot Questionnaire (AAOS-DFQ) and SF-36] that the HS in these patients was comparable with that of patients who had undergone minor lower extremity amputation (Pinzur & Evans 2003). However, these studies were small and a more detailed analysis of a broader spectrum of patients with different stages of Charcot arthropathy is required.

Ulceration

Foot ulceration can cause significant pain over and above that caused by simple neuropathy. Furthermore, prescriptive treatments such as off-loading or casting and the need for frequent dressings may markedly affect patients' mobility and restrict their lifestyle. As such, DFU has been found to have a negative impact on patients' social and emotional well-being (Abetz et al. 2002, Nabuurs-Franssen et al. 2005, Price & Harding 2004, Ribu et al. 2008). In a study of 294 patients with DFU, Nabuurs-Franssen et al. demonstrated (using the SF-36) HS worsened progressively as the duration of ulceration increased (Nabuurs-Franssen et al. 2005). They also demonstrated ulcer healing led to significant improvements in HS. In addition to the impact on patients themselves, this study also assessed the impact of DFU on caregivers. It showed that those providing care for patients with ongoing ulceration had significantly poorer scores for the emotional components of the SF-36 (particularly relating to mood and energy) than those providing care for patients with healed ulcers.

A number of authors have demonstrated that foot ulceration has greater impact on certain subgroups of patients than others. By correlating SF-36 scores with objectively measured clinical parameters (such as ankle-brachial pressure index), Ribu et al. found that those patients with coexisting peripheral arterial disease, large ulcers, or evidence of infection had the poorest HS (Ribu et al. 2007). However, when Valensi et al. explored the same issues (using both SF-36 and DFS), they identified a quite different subgroup of patients with DFU with particularly poor HS (Valensi et al. 2005). In their study, higher age, long-term ulceration, and multiple ulcers were all found to be independent predictors of poorer HS.

These discrepancies may be due to the fact that physiological factors do not necessarily influence QoL directly. During development of the disease-specific NeuroQoL measure, Vileikyte et al. found that there was little correlation between ulcer pain and QoL and that it was the social impact of ulceration (rather than the direct physical impact) that determines QoL in these patients. This is supported by Brod et al., who explored these issues in a series of detailed patient interviews (Brod 1998). They found that it was disruption of daily life, anxiety about future amputation, and the impact of treatment (such as nonweight bearing regimens and prolonged antibiotics) that most affected QoL. Similarly, in the large, cross-sectional 'Eurodiale' study involving 1232 patients with diabetic foot ulcers, Siersma et al. showed that immobility was an important determinant of poor HS (Siersma et al. 2013).

Notably, patients with persistent ulceration have significantly worse HS than patients who have undergone successful minor amputation for DFUs (though definitions of successful amputation are vague) (Carrington et al. 1996, Peters et al. 2001). However, those who undergo major lower extremity amputation have worse HS than those with active DFU (Carrington et al. 1996, Peters et al. 2001).

◼ Amputation

As with other aspects of diabetes-related foot disease, studies of outcome in amputation have generally focused on functional status and mobility rather than QoL. A large cost–utility analysis performed in the USA used three components of the SF-36 to assess HS in patients with diabetes (Eckman et al. 1995). Those with active ulcers had significantly worse scores for 'physical functioning' than those who had undergone successful toe or transmetatarsal amputation. Physical functioning in below knee amputation was no different to that in DFUs, but above-knee amputation scores were worse. Despite the large overall size of this cross-sectional analysis, the subgroups of interest were small and amputation groups poorly represented. Furthermore, only patients who had undergone successful operations were included in this study, with no reference to amputation-related morbidity and mortality, despite the fact that a significant proportion of those who have amputation may require subsequent revision of the stump.

In the United Kingdom, a prospective cohort study used the SF-36 to chart HS outcomes in patients with their first diagnosis of DFU. Eighteen months after diagnosis, those patients who had undergone amputation had no deterioration in SF-36 mental component scores. However, those with persistent or recurrent ulceration had a significant deterioration in mental aspects of HS (Winkley et al. 2009). Similarly, observational studies in Sweden (Ragnarson Tennvall & Apelqvist 2000, Tennvall et al. 2000) and France (Boutoille et al. 2008), using EQ-5D and SF-36 respectively, found that DFU was consistently associated with poorer HS scores than successfully healed minor amputations. Though all patients scored relatively poorly for psychological aspects of HS in these studies, between-group differences were only demonstrated in physical component scores and there was no significant difference in the degree of psychological impact. Furthermore, the majority of studies that have evaluated HS or QoL in patients with diabetes post-amputation have been of poor quality with small, highly selected patient groups (i.e. all patients with well healed rather than amputation stumps with complications).

◼ Demands of care

All patients with diabetes, even those without foot disease, have a poorer QoL than the general nondiabetes population (Abetz et al.

2002, Benbow et al. 1998, Carrington et al. 1996, Davies et al. 2006, Meijer et al. 2001, Price & Harding 2004, Ribu et al. 2007, Valensi et al. 2005, Vinik et al. 2005, 2008). While this may be due to the general lifestyle restrictions and complications of diabetes, it may also reflect the commitment needed to preserve foot health. Indeed, patient focus groups have shown that preventative foot care practices such as regular podiatry and having to wear restrictive footwear can negatively impact QoL (Hjelm et al. 2002, Price & Harding 2004).

Patients who are treated by a supportive multidisciplinary team (MDT) for diabetes care have improved self-management and better health-related outcomes (Davies et al. 2000, Garay-Sevilla et al. 1995, Tang et al. 2008). Using generic and disease-specific PROMs (SF-36 and DFS), a French observational study showed better HS outcomes for patients managed in tertiary centers (Valensi et al. 2005). These patients had less deterioration in physical health scores, less irritation due to ulcer appearance, shorter durations of foot ulcer care, greater closeness with partners and friends, and greater satisfaction with overall medical care. These observations of the efficacy of MDTs have been confirmed in other health-care systems (Rerkasem et al. 2009).

◼ DEPRESSION AND ANXIETY IN DIABETES-RELATED FOOT DISEASE

While it is evident that diabetes-related foot disease may have a profound impact on mental and physical function, the link between diabetes-related foot disease and depression or anxiety is less clear.

It has previously been shown that patients with diabetes have significantly higher rates of depression than the general population (Collins et al. 2009) and this may be particularly true for those with complications of diabetes such as diabetes-related foot disease. Furthermore, anxiety disorders may be even more prevalent than depression among patients with diabetes, with patients experiencing considerable fears about the long-term consequences of their condition.

In a study of 50 patients with DFU, Salomé et al. found that 82% had some evidence of depressive symptoms and 64% had moderate depression, with feelings of self-loathing, negative body image, and grief (Salomé et al. 2011). Though this suggests that there is indeed a link between DFU and depression, other authors have questioned whether it is ulceration that is responsible for low mood in these patients. In a large cross-sectional study, Vileikyte et al. used the Hospital Anxiety and Depression Scale (HADS) to assess the relationship between depressive symptoms and various aspects of diabetes-related foot disease, including pain, poor balance, loss of sensation, and ulceration (Vileikyte 2008). In contrast to the findings of Salomé et al., they found that although unsteadiness and poor sensation were particularly strong predictors of depression, there was no association between foot ulceration and depression. This is perhaps surprising since DFU has been shown to have a significant negative impact on HS, but highlights the importance of separating the concepts of HS, depression, and QoL. While depression does not directly equate to QoL either, the lack of expected association between DFU and depression demonstrates that clinicians should not use HS measures without due consideration when they are actually seeking to assess QoL.

One possible explanation for the apparent lack of association between DFU and depression is that ulcers may cause little pain in those with advanced neuropathy. Chronic pain is a well-recognized cause of depression, but if ulcers are painless they are likely to cause less distress and less disruption to patients' emotional well-being.

Moreover, while ulcers are known to result in poorer physical function, this dysfunction may not be to a degree sufficient to cause depressive symptoms. Indeed, though some patients suffer intractable ulceration, others may have ulcers for a shorter period of time and the ulceration is therefore not sufficiently chronic to induce depression. This situation of potentially curable ulceration contrasts markedly with loss of balance or neuropathic pain, which patients know to be progressive and incurable – again offering a possible explanation for why DPN is more psychologically impactful than DFU.

Whatever the true underlying relationships between diabetes-related foot disease and depression, it is quite clear that these patients are at risk of depressive illness and clinicians should therefore remain vigilant for psychological symptoms and instigate treatment or referral as appropriate.

THE INFLUENCE OF PSYCHOLOGICAL STATE ON OUTCOME IN DIABETES-RELATED FOOT DISEASE

Rather than simply being surrogate markers of outcome, it now seems increasingly clear that psychological factors may have significant impact on the incidence and severity of diabetes-related foot disease.

In a large study of patients with type 2 diabetes, Williams et al. assessed whether the coexistence of depression affected the likelihood of a patient developing ulceration (Williams et al. 2010). They observed 3474 patients with no prior history of DFU over a mean follow-up period of 4 years and showed that although there was no association between minor depression and ulceration, those with major depression had a twofold increased risk of developing DFU.

Gonzalez et al. also examined the influence of depression on ulceration risk (Gonzalez et al. 2010). Their findings supported the suggestion that depression increases the risk of first ulceration, though interestingly they found that this relationship was not mediated by poorer self-care in those patients with depression. Indeed, those patients with depression were actually found to engage in foot care more frequently than those without depression. This suggests that depression may adversely influence ulcer healing by pathways other than simple behavioral change. Though these other pathways require further investigation, it has been proposed that depression may affect healing indirectly via its negative effects on immunological and neuroendocrine responses to injury or infection. Interestingly, this study also found that while depression clearly influences the risk of first ulceration, it seemed to have no effect on the likelihood of ulcer recurrence. However, this lack of apparent association may be because the impact of depression is insufficient to influence ulcer recurrence in a group of patients who are already at extremely high risk of ulceration.

The finding that depression does not lead to poorer foot self-care is perhaps surprising, since poor mental state has been shown to adversely affect many other areas of diabetes self-care, such as glucose monitoring and dietary regulation. However, Altenburg et al. have also suggested that some psychological traits that would normally be considered undesirable may also be protective in diabetes-related foot disease (Altenburg et al. 2011). In their study, anxiety was found to be less common in patients with DFU than in those without ulcers. Though the underlying causes of this association need greater clarification, Altenburg et al. propose that higher levels of anxiety lead to more diligent foot care and therefore reduce the occurrence of ulceration.

Pain may also be influenced by the presence of depression. In a study of >11,000 patients with diabetes, Bair et al. showed that patients with depression reported higher levels of neuropathic pain than those without depression. Furthermore, they found that those with high levels of pain were significantly more likely to have depression, suggesting a synergistic relationship between the two symptoms (Bair et al. 2010).

Beyond its influence on ulcer healing and pain, it seems depression can also have a significant effect on mortality in patients with DFU. In a prospective cohort study of 253 patients, Winkley et al. demonstrated that those patients with DFU who had coexistent depression were twice as likely to have died at 18 months than those who had not had any depressive episodes. They went on to show that this relationship was still observed at 5 years follow-up, demonstrating that the effect seen at 18 months was not simply caused by a peak of depressive symptoms that might be expected following a first diagnosis of DFU, with all its associated restrictions on mobility and lifestyle (Winkley et al. 2012).

SUMMARY

Though the evidence relating to QoL in patients with diabetes-related foot disease remains relatively sparse, it now seems clear that diabetes-related foot disease has the potential to influence – and be influenced by – the psychological well-being of those who suffer with it. The interplay of many factors may result in a self-reinforcing cycle of worsening foot health, as diabetes-related foot disease leads to depression, which in turn causes poorer wound healing and worse pain.

Unfortunately, while the precise factors that underlie this relationship remain unclear, it is inevitably difficult for clinicians to address them. At present there is no single tool that can adequately assess the impact of diabetes-related foot disease on QoL. This is primarily because those tools that do exist are focused on single aspects of the disease. While this is understandable in terms of keeping the questionnaires short enough to be used in clinical practice, it has made it extremely difficult to assess the relative impact of neuropathy, arthropathy, and ulceration on QoL. As clinicians continue to become more aware of the psychological issues that face these patients and their potential to affect the efficacy of treatment, it may be possible to identify increasingly effective strategies to tackle this debilitating condition.

AREAS OF CONTROVERSY AND/OR FUTURE RESEARCH

- The development of new PROMs that are more specifically suited to patients with diabetes-related foot disease may help to clarify the true impact of the condition on QoL
- Further delineation of the relative impact on QoL of amputation versus lower limb revascularization may lead to significant improvements in care
- Determining the true relationship between diabetes-related foot disease and major depressive illness may help clinicians to improve concordance with treatment and minimize the burden of this common complication

■ IMPORTANT FURTHER READING

Hogg FR, Peach G, Price P, Thompson MM, Hinchliffe RJ. Measures of health-related quality of life in diabetes-related foot disease: a systematic review. Diabetologia 2012; 55:552–565.

Nabuurs-Franssen MH, Huijberts MS P, Nieuwenhuijzen Kruseman A C, Willems J, Schaper NC. Health-related quality of life of diabetic foot ulcer patients and their caregivers. Diabetologia 2005; 48:1906–1910.

Ribu L, Hanestad BR, Moum T, Birkeland K, Rustoen T. Health-related quality of life among patients with diabetes and foot ulcers: association with

demographic and clinical characteristics. J Diabetes Complications 2007; 21:227–236.

Siersma V, Thorsen H, Holstein PE, et al. Importance of factors determining the low health-related quality of life in people presenting with a diabetic foot ulcer: the Eurodiale study. Diabet Med 2013; 30:1382–1387.

Vileikyte L. Psychosocial and behavioral aspects of diabetic foot lesions. Curr Diab Rep 2008; 8:119–125.

■ REFERENCES

Abetz L SM, Brady L, McNulty P, Gagnon D. The Diabetic Foot Ulcer Scale (DFS): a quality of life instrument for use in clinical trials. Pract Diabetes Int 2002; 19:167–175.

Altenburg N, Joraschky P, Barthel A, et al. Alcohol consumption and other psycho-social conditions as important factors in the development of diabetic foot ulcers. Diabet Med 2011; 28:168–174.

Armstrong DG, Lavery LA, Wrobel JS, Vileikyte L. Quality of life in healing diabetic wounds: does the end justify the means? J Foot Ankle Surg 2008; 47:278–282.

Bair MJ, Brizendine EJ, Ackermann RT, et al. Prevalence of pain and association with quality of life, depression and glycaemic control in patients with diabetes. Diabet Med 2010; 27:578–584.

Bann CM, Fehnel SE, Gagnon DD. Development and validation of the Diabetic Foot Ulcer Scale-short form (DFS-SF). Pharmacoeconomics 2003; 21:1277–1290.

Benbow SJ, Wallymahmed ME, MacFarlane IA. Diabetic peripheral neuropathy and quality of life. QJM 1998; 91:733–737.

Benbow SJ, Wallymahmed ME, MacFarlane IA. Diabetic peripheral neuropathy and quality of life. QJM 1998; 91:733–737.

Boutoille D, Feraille A, Maulaz D, Krempf M. Quality of life with diabetes-associated foot complications: comparison between lower-limb amputation and chronic foot ulceration. Foot Ankle Int 2008; 29:1074–1078.

Brod M. Quality of life issues in patients with diabetes and lower extremity ulcers: patients and care givers. Qual Life Res 1998; 7:365–372.

Carrington AL, Mawdsley SK, Morley M, et al. Psychological status of diabetic people with or without lower limb disability. Diabetes Res Clin Pract 1996; 32:19–25.

Collins MM, Corcoran P, Perry IJ. Anxiety and depression symptoms in patients with diabetes. Diabet Med 2009; 26:153–161.

Currie CJ, Poole CD, Woehl A, et al. The health-related utility and health-related quality of life of hospital-treated subjects with type 1 or type 2 diabetes with particular reference to differing severity of peripheral neuropathy. Diabetologia 2006; 49:2272–2280.

Davies M, Brophy S, Williams R, Taylor A. The prevalence, severity, and impact of painful diabetic peripheral neuropathy in type 2 diabetes. Diabetes Care 2006; 29:1518–1522.

Davies S, Gibby O, Phillips C, et al. The health status of diabetic patients receiving orthotic therapy. Qual Life Res 2000; 9:233–240.

Eckman MH, Greenfield S, Mackey WC, et al. Foot infections in diabetic patients. Decision and cost-effectiveness analyses. JAMA 1995; 273:712–720.

Fitzpatrick R, Davey C, Buxton MJ, Jones DR. Evaluating patient-based outcome measures for use in clinical trials. Health Technol Assess 1998; 2:i–iv, 1–74.

Garay-Sevilla ME, Nava LE, Malacara JM, et al. Adherence to treatment and social support in patients with non-insulin dependent diabetes mellitus. J Diabetes Complications 1995; 9:81–86.

Gonzalez JS, Vileikyte L, Ulbrecht JS, et al. Depression predicts first but not recurrent diabetic foot ulcers. Diabetologia 2010; 53:2241–2248.

Hjelm K, Nyberg P, Apelqvist J. Gender influences beliefs about health and illness in diabetic subjects with severe foot lesions. J Adv Nurs 2002; 40:673–684.

Jain R, Jain S, Raison CL, Maletic V. Painful diabetic neuropathy is more than pain alone: examining the role of anxiety and depression as mediators and complicators. Curr Diab Rep 2011; 11:275–284.

Jaksa PJ, Mahoney JL. Quality of life in patients with diabetic foot ulcers: validation of the Cardiff Wound Impact Schedule in a Canadian population. Int Wound J 2010; 7:502–507.

Jeffcoate WJ, Price PE, Phillips CJ, et al. Randomised controlled trial of the use of three dressing preparations in the management of chronic ulceration of the foot in diabetes. Health Technol Assess 2009; 13:1–86, iii–iv.

Meijer JW, Trip J, Jaegers SM, et al. Quality of life in patients with diabetic foot ulcers. Disabil Rehabil 2001; 23:336–340.

Nabuurs-Franssen MH, Huijberts MS, Nieuwenhuijzen Kruseman AC, et al. Health-related quality of life of diabetic foot ulcer patients and their caregivers. Diabetologia 2005; 48:1906–1910.

Pakarinen TK, Laine HJ, Maenpaa H, et al. Long-term outcome and quality of life in patients with Charcot foot. Foot Ankle Surg 2009; 15:187–191.

Peters EJ, Childs MR, Wunderlich RP, et al. Functional status of persons with diabetes-related lower-extremity amputations. Diabetes Care 2001; 24:1799–1804.

Pinzur MS, Evans A. Health-related quality of life in patients with Charcot foot. Am J Orthop (Belle Mead NJ) 2003; 32:492–496.

Price P, Harding K. Cardiff Wound Impact Schedule: the development of a condition-specific questionnaire to assess health-related quality of life in patients with chronic wounds of the lower limb. Int Wound J 2004; 1:10–17.

Rabin R, de Charro F. EQ-5D: a measure of health status from the EuroQol Group. Ann Med 2001; 33:337–343.

Ragnarson Tennvall G, Apelqvist J. Health-related quality of life in patients with diabetes mellitus and foot ulcers. J Diabetes Complications 2000; 14:235–241.

Rauck RL, Shaibani A, Biton V, et al. Lacosamide in painful diabetic peripheral neuropathy: a phase 2 double-blind placebo-controlled study. Clin J Pain 2007; 23:150–158.

Rerkasem K, Kosachunhanun N, Tongprasert S, Guntawongwan K. A multidisciplinary diabetic foot protocol at Chiang Mai University Hospital: cost and quality of life. Int J Low Extrem Wounds 2009; 8:153–156.

Ribu L, Birkeland K, Hanestad BR, et al. A longitudinal study of patients with diabetes and foot ulcers and their health-related quality of life: wound healing and quality-of-life changes. J Diabetes Complications 2008; 22:400–407.

Ribu L, Hanestad BR, Moum T, et al. A comparison of the health-related quality of life in patients with diabetic foot ulcers, with a diabetes group and a nondiabetes group from the general population. Qual Life Res 2007; 16:179–189.

Ribu L, Hanestad BR, Moum T, et al. Health-related quality of life among patients with diabetes and foot ulcers: association with demographic and clinical characteristics. J Diabetes Complications 2007; 21:227–236.

Ribu L, Rustoen T, Birkeland K, et al. The prevalence and occurrence of diabetic foot ulcer pain and its impact on health-related quality of life. J Pain 2006; 7:290–299.

Rosenstock J, Tuchman M, LaMoreaux L, Sharma U. Pregabalin for the treatment of painful diabetic peripheral neuropathy: a double-blind, placebo-controlled trial. Pain 2004; 110:628–638.

Salomé GM, Blanes L, Ferreira LM. Assessment of depressive symptoms in people with diabetes mellitus and foot ulcers. Rev Col Bras Cir 2011; 38:327–333.

Selvarajah D, Gandhi R, Emery CJ, Tesfaye S. Randomized placebo-controlled double-blind clinical trial of cannabis-based medicinal product (Sativex) in painful diabetic neuropathy: depression is a major confounding factor. Diabetes Care 2010; 33:128–130.

Siersma V, Thorsen H, Holstein PE, et al. Importance of factors determining the low health-related quality of life in people presenting with a diabetic foot ulcer: the Eurodiale study. Diabet Med 2013. Diabet Med 2013; 30 1382–1387.

Sochocki MP, Verity S, Atherton PJ, et al. Health related quality of life in patients with Charcot arthropathy of the foot and ankle. Foot Ankle Surg 2008; 14:11–15.

Swislocki A, Orth M, Bales M, et al. A randomized clinical trial of the effectiveness of photon stimulation on pain, sensation, and quality of life in patients with diabetic peripheral neuropathy. J Pain Symptom Manage 2010; 39:88–99.

Tang TS, Brown MB, Funnell MM, Anderson RM. Social support, quality of life, and self-care behaviors among African Americans with type 2 diabetes. Diabetes Educ 2008; 34:266–276.

Tennvall GR, Apelqvist J, Eneroth M. Costs of deep foot infections in patients with diabetes mellitus. Pharmacoeconomics 2000; 18:225–238.

Valensi P, Girod I, Baron F, et al. Quality of life and clinical correlates in patients with diabetic foot ulcers. Diabetes Metab 2005; 31:263–271.

Vileikyte L. Psychosocial and behavioral aspects of diabetic foot lesions. Curr Diab Rep 2008; 8:119–125.

Vileikyte L, Peyrot M, Bundy C, et al. The development and validation of a neuropathy- and foot ulcer-specific quality of life instrument. Diabetes Care 2003; 26:2549–2555.

Vinik EJ, Hayes RP, Oglesby A, et al. The development and validation of the Norfolk QOL-DN, a new measure of patients' perception of the effects of diabetes and diabetic neuropathy. Diabetes Technol Ther 2005; 7:497–508.

Vinik AI, Park TS, Stansberry KB, Pittenger GL. Diabetic neuropathies. Diabetologia 2000; 43:957–973.

Vinik EJ, Paulson JF, Ford-Molvik SL, Vinik AI. German-translated Norfolk quality of life (QOL-DN) identifies the same factors as the English version of the tool and discriminates different levels of neuropathy severity. J Diabetes Sci Technol 2008; 2:1075–1086.

Ware JE, Sherbourne CD. The MOS 36-item short-form health survey (SF-36). I. Conceptual framework and item selection. Med Care 1992; 30:473–483.

Williams LH, Rutter CM, Katon WJ, et al. Depression and incident diabetic foot ulcers: a prospective cohort study. Am J Med 2010; 123:748–754.e3.

Winkley K, Sallis H, Kariyawasam D, et al. Five-year follow-up of a cohort of people with their first diabetic foot ulcer: the persistent effect of depression on mortality. Diabetologia 2012; 55:303–310.

Winkley K, Stahl D, Chalder T, et al. Quality of life in people with their first diabetic foot ulcer: a prospective cohort study. J Am Podiatr Med Assoc 2009; 99:406–414.

shoes should be fabricated according to these same guidelines. Patients, particularly those at risk due to prior infection, ulceration, or amputation, must be educated that a program of lifelong surveillance is essential in order to prevent repeated episodes of these complications.

Recurrence of foot ulcers is very common, with 70% of patients developing new foot ulcers within 5 years of healing. It might be expected that these patients would benefit the most from education. However, in a randomized trial this was found not to be the case (Lincoln et al. 2008). Even though the educational intervention was associated with improved foot care behavior, there was no evidence that this program of targeted education was associated with clinical benefit in this population, when compared with 'normal' care. They concluded that the usefulness and optimum delivery of education to such a high-risk group required further evaluation (Lincoln et al. 2008). It is perhaps noteworthy that the incidence of new foot disease is dominated by established physical factors and that educational input and surveillance may have only limited impact (Gershater et al. 2011, Jeffcoate 2011, McInnes et al. 2011).

Is preventive patient education regarding diabetic foot conditions evidence-based?

Dorresteijn has performed a Cochrane review on the effect of patient education on the diabetic foot (Dorresteijn et al. 2012), One of the randomized-controlled trials (RCTs) recorded a reduced incidence of foot ulceration and amputation during an annual follow-up in patients at high risk of foot ulceration, who had undergone a 1-hour group education session. However, a similar study, with a lower risk bias, did not confirm this finding, and three other studies also failed to demonstrate any effect of education on the primary outcomes; these studies may have lacked sufficient power. Patient knowledge regarding foot care was improved, in the short term, in five of the eight RCTs in which this outcome was assessed, as was the patients' self-reported short-term self-care behavior in seven of nine RCTs. Callus, nail problems and fungal infections improved in only one of five RCTs. Only one of the RCTs included was at low risk of bias. The authors came to the conclusion that foot care knowledge and self-reported patient behavior seemed to be positively influenced by education in the short term. However, based on only two sufficiently detailed studies to report the effect of patient education on primary outcomes, they concluded that there was insufficiently robust evidence to show that patient education alone was effective in achieving clinically relevant reductions in ulcer and amputation incidence (Dorresteijn et al. 2012).

It is startling to see that the published evidence seems to suggest that education appears to be a totally ineffective intervention. However, this factor should be interpreted with caution. There may be a lack of evidence, rather than a lack of effect. A future direction of research and practice may be to concentrate preventive effort on those patients who appear to be at highest risk of foot ulceration after careful screening, and selection. Larger randomized clinical trials are needed to assess which patient education formats are the most effective, how often periodic reinforcement is required, and the overall long-term effectiveness of various program.

Improving access to quality of patient education and foot care

Health-care organizations have used various strategies to improve clinicians' performance regarding patient education. In one strategy,

a computerized registry reminded doctors to enter the patient's risk status for lower-extremity amputation (Khoury 1998). After 28 months, the percentage of patients who had received foot screening and risk assessment increased from 15% to 76%. Project LEAP (Lower-Extremity Amputation Prevention), developed by the US Department of Health and Human Services, is a 1-day workshop on diabetic foot care (Wheatley 2001). When this was delivered to 560 clinicians from 85 organizations, it improved the rate of documenting foot care education from a baseline of 38% to 62% after 9 months. More importantly, appropriate foot care self-management increased from 32% to 48%, and a trend toward reduced lower-extremity amputations was recorded. Another approach is to implement foot care clinical practice guidelines. An Indian Health Service diabetes program observed 669 patients during three periods: a standard care period (1986–1989) with routine foot screening, a public health period (1990–1993) with an annual foot examination and initial risk stratification to give those at high-risk special interventions, and a staged diabetes management period (1994–1996) during which clinicians used clinical practice guidelines (Rith-Najarian et al. 1998). The average lower-extremity amputation incidence per 1,000 diabetes person-years was 29 during the standard care period, 21 during the public health period, and 15 during staged management. The overall reduction in lower-extremity amputation was 48% ($P = 0.02$), and the incidence of first amputation decreased from 21 per 1000 to 6 per 1000, from the first to the third period ($P<0.001$). These considerations demonstrate that the effectiveness of patient education must be assessed in the context of a holistic approach to a diabetic foot prevention program.

PATIENT DIABETIC FOOT EDUCATION AS PART OF A DIABETIC FOOT PREVENTION PROGRAM

When considering education, it is best viewed as an integrated part of a diabetic foot prevention program. The important attributes of a diabetic foot prevention program undertaken within the framework of the multidisciplinary team are as follows (Frykberg et al. 2006).

1. Podiatric care: regular visits, examinations, foot care, risk assessment, as well as early detection and aggressive treatment of new lesions
2. Protective shoes: adequate room to protect from injury; well-cushioned walking shoes, extra depth, custom-molded shoes with special modifications, as necessary
3. Pressure reduction: cushioned insoles, custom orthoses, padded hosiery, pressure measurements (computerized or Harris mat)
4. Prophylactic surgery: correct structural deformities (hammertoes, bunions, Charcot). Prevent recurrent ulcers over deformities, intervene at opportune time
5. Preventive education:
   a. Patient education: need for daily inspection and intervention
   b. Practitioner education: significance of foot lesions, importance of regular foot examination, and current concepts of diabetic foot management

When there is interest in implementing programs to prevent diabetic foot ulcers and the number of amputations, it becomes more evident that patient education cannot be considered an isolated activity, either in research or in the development of programs. The next step is to overcome the barriers – especially the barriers of hospital managers and policy makers – which require an understanding of the health economic outcomes.

■ COST-EFFECTIVENESS OF PREVENTIVE MEASURES

Health-care policy makers and financiers, faced with considerable resource constraints, increasingly focus on interventions that work well and do so at a reasonable cost. Glycemic control among those with diabetes is a cost-effective strategy, and health management programs that empower people with chronic illnesses to self-manage their condition are of interest in the workplace.

Diabetes education is effective in helping people with diabetes control their illness and maximize their health status, and is generally accepted as a cost-effective strategy (Boren et al. 2009). There is, however, a lack of available published information regarding the economic evaluation of the costs and benefits of diabetes education, and the value that may be added by a diabetes educator. Even among those providing DSME and training, the studies demonstrating these facts are not well understood (see Chapter 4).

A different approach is therefore required to convince policy makers to support a National Diabetic Foot Prevention Program. Is it possible to state that the cost of prevention will be lower than the combined cost of foot ulcer care and amputations?

Several studies have examined the cost-effectiveness of interventions for the prevention of diabetic foot ulceration. In a cost–utility analysis performed by Tennvall and Apelqvist, preventive measures to decrease the incidence of ulceration (including podiatric foot examinations, specialist footwear, and patient education) were found to be cost-effective, showing a decrease in the ulceration and amputation rate of 25% (Matricali et al. 2007, Ragnarson-Tenvall & Apelqvist 2001). Another study by Ortegon also concluded that preventive measures of intensive glycemic control and optimum foot care were cost-effective, showing a 40% risk reduction (Ortegon et al. 2004).

A recent 'cost of illness' model, based on published data from numerous sources regarding diabetic complications and the value of health resources, found that the mean annual cost of treatment in 2001 was $9306 for an uninfected diabetic foot ulcer, $24,582 for an infected foot ulcer, and $45,579 for a foot ulcer with osteomyelitis. Another review compiled cost data from 1990 to 1997 from seven studies; four conducted in the United States, and three in other countries. After adjustment for inflation and currency conversion, the cost of treating foot ulcers not requiring amputation ranged from $993 to $17,519, and approached $30,724 in one study that spanned 2 years following diagnosis.

A few groups have modeled cost–utility analyses for strategies to prevent foot ulcers. A Markov model from Sweden of intensive prevention (patient education, use of appropriate footwear, and access to therapeutic foot care) for high-risk patients was found to be cost-effective, and the incidence of foot ulcers and lower-extremity amputations was reduced by 25%. A similar model for patients with newly diagnosed type 2 diabetes found that implementing a guideline-based foot care program that included intensive glycemic control, regular foot examinations, risk stratification, patient education, clinician education, and multidisciplinary foot care increased life expectancy and quality-adjusted life, and reduced the incidence of foot complications. The cost of achieving a 10% reduction in the incidence of foot lesions was <$25,000 per quality-adjusted life-year gained (Gordois et al. 2003, Matricali et al. 2007, Ortegon et al. 2004, Ragnarson-Tenvall & Apelqvist 2001, 2004).

■ SPECIAL CONSIDERATIONS FOR DEVELOPING COUNTRIES

■ Are we accomplishing the actions that we are advocating in Europe?

A Maltese report stated: 'research suggests that the complications of diabetes, including foot ulceration, could be prevented or ameliorated by good, long-term glycemic control. However, optimum long-term glycemic control requires appropriate self-management and [with] less than one-third of people suffering with diabetes in Europe achieving good glycemic control' (HbA$_{1c}$ level ≤6.5% [≤48 mmol/mol]) (Liebl et al. 2002). Thus, it has been suggested that people with diabetes are not being educated and supported effectively, in order to achieve good self-management.

Strine et al. (2005) reported that 50–80% of people with diabetes worldwide have significant knowledge deficiencies in relation to the management of their condition. The data suggest that individuals are either not receiving diabetes education or that the education offered is not effective.

■ What can be learnt from the IDF and IWGDF?

In the International Diabetes Federation (IDF) Atlas, updated in December 2011, there is a considerable amount of information regarding diabetes care on a global basis. In developing countries, financial and human resources are limited, despite serious needs and multiple health challenges. More than three-quarters of people suffering from diabetes globally live in developing countries. Between 2000 and 2025, the forecast increase in the number of people with diabetes mellitus in these countries will be approximately 170%. In the developing world, diabetes, in common with other chronic diseases, is often ignored in terms of health-care priorities; the focus remains largely on immediate and acute care, rather than on prevention. The challenges involved in providing education to enable people to self-manage their chronic condition exist at three levels: patients, health-care providers, and health-care systems.

A recent report in *Diabetes Voice* analyzed the challenges to diabetes self-management in developing countries. The various interactions and influences in a person's environment, at social, cultural, and material levels, make the relationship between knowledge, attitudes, and behaviors complex (Debussche et al. 2009).

Despite the problems relating to insufficient numbers of health-care providers and minimal access to treatment and screening, several potential solutions could be explored: peers and health-care providers other than doctors can be used in follow-up, prevention, and education. If these individuals received adequate training, and were supported by the medical expertise required to treat diabetes and its complications, they could take responsibility for follow-up. This approach potentially allows doctors to spend time in their field of expertise. Patient organizations play a major role in this context, and perhaps the Western countries can learn from them, in order to reintegrate patient and peer involvement.

In those countries, decentralization has enabled simultaneous access to treatment and basic diabetes education. The structure of care is complementary to the establishment of education. The 'Step-by-Step' approach, which has been piloted in India and Tanzania, optimized the prevention and management of foot lesions, with spectacular results in Tanzania.

Foot complications cause substantial morbidity in Tanzania, in which 70% of leg amputations occur in patients with diabetes. The Step-by-Step Foot Project was initiated to train health-care personnel in diabetic foot management, facilitate transfer of knowledge and expertise, and improve patient education. The project comprised a 3-day basic course with an interim 1-year period for screening, followed by an advanced course, and evaluation of activities. Fifteen centers from across Tanzania participated during 2004–2006, and 12 during 2004–2007. Of the 11,714 patients screened in 2005, 4335 (37%) had high-risk feet and, of 461 (11%) with ulcers, 45 (9·8%) underwent major amputation. The 3860 patients screened during 2006–2007, demonstrated a significant increase in the proportion with ulcers and amputations, compared with 2005 ($P < 0.001$), probably a result of enhanced case findings. During 2005–2008, there was a fall in the incidence of foot ulcers, in patient referrals to the main tertiary care center in Dar es Salaam, and a parallel fall in amputation among these referrals. In conclusion, the Step-by-Step Foot Project in Tanzania improved foot ulcer management for individuals with diabetes and resulted in permanent, operational foot clinics across the country. This program is an effective model for improving outcomes in other less-developed countries (Abbas 2011, Bakker et al. 2006, Pendsey & Abbas et al. 2007). Many other 'Step-by-Step' courses were organized, as in the Caribbean, where the Rotary clubs acted as as fascilitators (**Figures 7.1–7.4**).

The International Faculty of the International Working Group, formed in December 2012 started a new initiative, called the Train the

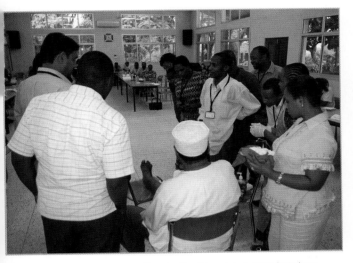

Figure 7.1 Education program: 'Step-by Step' from International Working Group on the Diabetic Foot (IWGDF). A live case presentation during the course in Dominica, 2013.

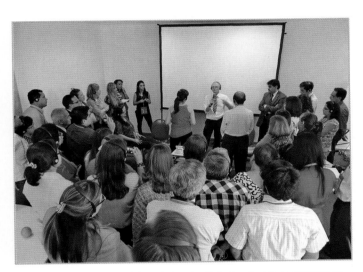

Figure 7.2 Interactive workshop during the 'Train-the-Foot-Trainer' course to implement the 'Step-by-Step' courses in a region. This course was held with the cooperation of International Diabetes Federation (IDF) and International Working Group on the Diabetic Foot (IWGDF). Region: South and Central America; Brasilia, December 2012.

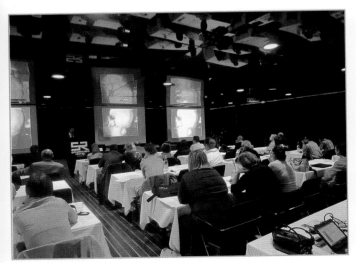

Figure 7.3 The international course for specialists working in reference diabetic foot clinics. Pisa course organized by Professor Dr Alberto Piagesi with the cooperation of International Working Group on the Diabetic Foot (IWGDF). Pisa, 2012.

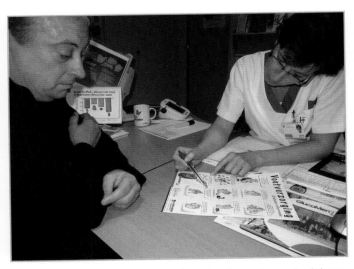

Figure 7.4 The importance of diabetic foot education on the regular diabetes outpatient clinic by dedicated diabetes nurses.

Foot Trainer courses, so as to implement the Step-by-Step programs. This unique initiative integrates the three levels of education necessary: the trainers/experts, the staff on the daily working platform, and the patients and their relatives. In addition to that, the course is focused on the implementation of national and regional foot care provisions, from a structural, educational, clinical, and research perspective. The first region involved is the entire South and Central American region, in which 14 counties within Brazil were reached. Only two and a half months after the course, 13 out of the 14 had initiated and developed a supportive plan for implementation. The question remains as to whether it is possible to reduce the amputations by 50%, the target outlined in the Saint Vincent Declaration in 1989.

Marketing aspects of patient education

Despite all that has been written about the prevention of diabetic foot ulcers and amputation and the education of patients, why is success in their prevention so limited? One of the most recent study by Waaijman et al. (2013) shows that adherence to wearing custom-made footwear is insufficient, particularly at home, where patients exhibit their largest walking activity. This low adherence is a major threat for reulceration. These objective findings provide directions for improvement in adherence, which could include prescribing specific off-loading footwear for indoors, and set a reference for future comparative research on footwear adherence in diabetes. By the end of this chapter, it will be evident that prevention needs to be a combination of systemic disease control and foot care self-management. As health-care professionals, we find it challenging to devise effective methods to influence behaviors in our patients, especially because behaviors are difficult to address in the short period of time we have with them.

In Robbins' study, some of the methods used to influence behaviors were examined, as well as their relative effectiveness (Robbins et al. 2010). The authors explored the concept of marketing the risks associated with diabetes, as a potential strategy to consider in the quest to motivate patients to adopt and maintain healthy behaviors. In 1999, Rothschild was one of the first to proffer the notion of social marketing in order to affect change in human health behaviors. He lamented that social marketing had been co-opted by education and that insufficient marketing strategies were utilized. In his article, he suggested that individuals who are not motivated or able to change on their own could be convinced to do so through a marketing approach based on incentives (for desired behavior) and consequences (for unwanted behavior) (Rothschild 1999). Andreasen examined Rothschild's concept further and investigated the barriers that have prevented social marketing strategies from being utilized more fully. Although the growth of social marketing has not been expansive, Andreasen cited its use by the CDC and UNAIDS, as a tool in fighting AIDS.

The authors defined four barriers to the growth of social marketing (Andreasen 2002):
- Lack of appreciation of social marketing at top management levels
- Poor brand positioning, and the perception that social marketing is manipulative and not community based
- Inadequate documentation and publicity of successes
- Lack of academic stature

Another potential approach is to learn from the advertising industry, and to begin to market risk as a strategy in order to motivate behavioral change. There are many examples of informational 'sound bites' that have marketed risk to various cohorts, which include 'The Silent Killer' for hypertension. Social marketing techniques may help with the clinical application of behavioral change interventions particularly when the target audience involves larger communities or populations, as is the case for patients with diabetes and with a high risk of developing a diabetic foot ulcer. Robbins et al. believed that a similar approach would be effective for patients who have diabetes and present with a foot ulcer. In order to communicate the risk to mortality associated with this foot ulcer, we may wish to use the term 'Diabetic Foot Attack' as suggested by specialists within the United Kingdom.

Diabetes is rarely described as a fatal disease, nor does it have the same implications as a cancer diagnosis. However, when we look at the 5-year mortality rates, we find that they are significantly higher for those with diabetes-related foot ulceration (46%) than for Hodgkin's disease (18%) or for breast cancer (18%). It is time for the multidisciplinary team that provides care for patients with diabetes and foot ulcers to properly communicate that mortality risk to patients, in order to provide more urgent motivation to comply with self-care practices. In this context, we hope that using such social marketing techniques will reduce the delay of referral at the level of the patient and the health-care provider, taking into account that the lack of pain sensation due to neuropathy has a very negative and completely opposite effect.

AREAS OF CONTROVERSY AND/OR FUTURE RESEARCH

- To date, the evidence that patient education has a beneficial outcome in preventing foot ulcers is poor
- The role of expert patients in facilitating health-care education and life skills should be explored
- The ways in which people learn rather than the content of what they should learn needs to be examined
- The role of new information technologies in delivering patient interactive education should be investigated
- Instruments to benchmark the quality of diabetic patient education should be developed

IMPORTANT FURTHER READING

Dorresteijn JA, Kriegsman DM, Assendelft WJ, Valk GD. Patient education for preventing diabetic foot ulceration. Cochrane Database Syst Rev 2012; 17:10.

Funnell MM, Brown TL, Childs BP, et al. National Standards for Diabetes Self-management Education. Diabetes Care 2011; 34:S89–96.

Inzucchi SE, Bergenstal RM, Buse JB, et al. Management of hyperglycemia in type 2 diabetes: a patient-centered approach: position statement of the American Diabetes Association (ADA) and the European Association for the Study of Diabetes (EASD). Diabetes Care 2012; 35:1364–1379.

Lincoln N, Radford K, Game F, Jeffcoate WJ. Education for secondary prevention of foot ulcers in people with diabetes: a randomised controlled trial. Diabetologia 2008; 51:1954–1961.

McInnes A, Jeffcoate W, Vileikyte L, et al. Foot care education in patients with diabetes at low risk of complications: a consensus statement. Diabetic Med 2011; 28:162–167.

Milenkoviæ T, Gavriloviæ S, Percan V, Petrov G. Influence of diabetic education on patient well-being and metabolic control. Diabetologia 2004; 33:91–96.

REFERENCES

Abbas ZG, Lutale JK, Bakker K, Baker N, Archibald LK. The 'Step by Step' Diabetic Foot Project in Tanzania: a model for improving patient outcomes in less-developed countries. Int Wound J 2011; 8:169–175.

Andreasen AR. Marketing social marketing in the social change marketplace. J Publ Pol Market 2002; 21:3–13.

Assal JP. Revisiting the approach to treatment of long-term illness: from the acute to the chronic state. A need for educational and managerial skills for long-term follow-up. Patient Edu Couns 1999; 37:99–111. http://www.ncbi.nlm.nih.gov/pubmed/14528538

Bakker K, Abbas ZG, Pendsey S. Step by Step, improving diabetic foot care in the developing world. A pilot study for India, Bangladesh, Sri Lanka and Tanzania. Pract Diab Int 2006; 23:1–6.

Boren S, Fitzner K, Panhalkar PS, Specker JE. Costs and benefits associated with diabetes education: a review of the literature. Diabetes Educ 2009; 35:72–96.

Bradley C, Gamsu DS. Guidelines for encouraging psychological well-being; report of a working group of WHO Regional Office for Europe and IDF European Region St. Vincent Declaration Action Program for Diabetes. Diab Med 1994; 11:510–516.

Campbell EM, Redman S, Moffitt PS, Sanson-Fisher RW. The relative effectiveness of educational and behavioral instruction programs for patients with NIDDM: a randomized trial. Diabetes Educ 1996; 22:379–386.

Connor H. Some historical aspects of diabetic foot disease. Diabetes Metab Res Rev 2008; 24:S7–S13.

Debussche X, Balcou-debussche M, Besançon S, Traoré S A. Challenges to diabetes self-management in developing countries. Diabetes Voice 2009; 54:12–14.

Dorresteijn JA, Kriegsman DM, Assendelft WJ, Valk GD. Patient education for preventing diabetic foot ulceration. Cochrane Database Syst Rev. 2012; 17:10.

Duprez V, De Pover M, De Spiegelaere M, Beeckman D. The development and psychometrical evaluation of a set of instruments to evaluate the effectiveness of diabetes patient education. J Clin Nursing 2014 23:42P–3S. doi: 10.1111/jocn.12044. [Epub ahead of print]

Edmonds M. Improved survival of the diabetic foot: the role of a specialized foot clinic. Q J Med 1986; 232:763–771.

Frykberg RG, Zgonis T, Armstrong DG, et al. Diabetic foot disorders: a clinical practice guideline. J Foot Ankle Surg 2006; 45:S2–S66.

Funnell MM, Brown TL, Childs BP, et al. "National Standards for Diabetes Self-management Education." Diabetes Care 2011; 34:S89–96.

Gershater MA, Pilhammar E, Apelqvist J, Alm-Roijer C. Patient education for the prevention of diabetic foot ulcers; Interim analysis of a randomised controlled trial due to morbidity and mortality of participants. EDN Autumn 2011; 8:102–107b.

Gordois A, Scuffham P, Shearer A, Oglesby A, Tobian JA. The health care costs of diabetic peripheral neuropathy in the US. Diabetes Care 2003; 26:1790–1795.

Grimshaw JM, Shirran L, Thomas R, et al. Changing provider behaviour: an overview of systematic reviews of interventions. Medical Care 2001; 39:II2–II45.

Haas L, Maryniuk M, Beck J, et al. National Standards for Diabetes Self-management Education and Support. Diabetes Educ 2012; 38:619–629.

International Working Group on the Diabetic Foot. International Consensus on the Diabetic Foot & Practical Guidelines and Management and Prevention of the Diabetic Foot, 2007, 2011–www.iwgdt.org.

Inzucchi SE, Bergenstal RM, Buse JB, et al. Management of hyperglycemia in type 2 diabetes: a patient-centered approach: position statement of the American Diabetes Association (ADA) and the European Association for the Study of Diabetes (EASD). Diabetes Care 2012; 35:1364–1379.

Iversen MM, Tell GS, Riise T, et al. History of foot ulcer increases mortality among individuals with diabetes. Diabetes Care 2009; 32:2193–2199.

Jeffcoate W. Stratification of foot risk predicts the incidence of new foot disease, but do we yet know that the adoption of routine screening reduces it? Diabetologia 2011; 54:991–993.

Joslin EP. The treatment of diabetes mellitus, 4th edn. Lea and Febiger: Philadelphia, PA, 1928:785–802.

Khoury A, Landers P, Roth M, et al. Computer-supported identification and intervention for diabetic patients at risk for amputation. MD Comput. 1998; 15:307–310.

Liebl A, Mata M, Eschwège E, ODE-2 Advisory Board. Evaluation of risk factors for development of complications in type II diabetes in Europe. Diabetologia 2002; 45:S23–S28.

Lincoln N, Radford K, Game F, Jeffcoate WJ. Education for secondary prevention of foot ulcers in people with diabetes: a randomised controlled trial. Diabetologia 2008; 51:1954–1961.

Matricali GA, Dereymaeker G, Muls E, Flour M, Mathieu C. Economic aspects of diabetic foot care in a multidisciplinary setting: a review, diabetes/metabolism research and reviews, review article. Diabetes Metab Res Rev 2007; 23:339–347.

McInnes A, Jeffcoate W, Vileikyte L, et al. Foot care education in patients with diabetes at low risk of complications: a consensus statement. Diabetic Med 2011; 28:162–167.

Milenkoviæ T, Gavriloviæ S, Percan V, Petrov G. Influence of diabetic education on patient well-being and metabolic control. Diabetologia 2004; 33:91–96.

Mühlhauser I, Bruckner I, Berger M, et al. Evaluation of an intensified insulin treatment and teaching programme as routine management of type 1 (insulin-dependent) diabetes. Diabetologia 1987; 30:681–690.

NICE Clinical guideline CG10– type 2 diabetes: prevention and management of foot problems. 2004. www.nice.org.uk/CG10

Norris SL, Lau J, Smith SJ, Schmid CH, Engelgau MM. Self-management education for adults with type 2 diabetes: a meta-analysis of the effect on glycemic control. Diabetes Care 2002; 25:1159–1171.

Ortegon MM, Redekop WK, Niessen LW. Cost-effectiveness of prevention and treatment of the diabetic foot: a Markov analysis. Diabetes Care 2004; 27:901–907.

Peters EJ, Lavery LA. Effectiveness of the diabetic foot risk classification system of the International Working Group on the Diabetic Foot. Diabetes Care. 2001; 24:1442–1447.

Pendsey S, Abbas ZG. The step-by-step program for reducing diabetic foot problems: a model for the developing world. Curr Diabetes Reports 2007; 7:425–428.

Ragnarson Tennvall G, Apelqvist J. Health-economic consequences of diabetic foot lesions. Clin Infect Dis 2004; 39:S132–S139.

Ragnarson-Tennvall G, Apelqvist J. Prevention of diabetes-related foot ulcers and amputations: a cost-utility analysis based on Markov model simulations. Diabetologia 2001; 44:2077–2087.

Rith-Najarian S, Branchaud C, Beaulieu O, et al. Reducing lower-extremity amputations due to diabetes: application of the staged diabetes management approach in a primary care setting. J Fam Pract 1998; 47:127–132.

Robbins JM, Strauss G, Regler J. Marketing risk: beyond diabetic foot education. 2010. http://lowerextremityreview.com/article/marketing-risk-beyond-diabetic-foot-education.

Rothschild ML. Carrots, sticks, and promises: a conceptual framework for the management of public health and social issue behaviors. J Market. 1999; 63:24–37.

Singh N, Armstrong DG, Lipsky BA. Preventing foot ulcers in patients with diabetes. JAMA 2005; 293:217–228.

Strine TW, Okoro CA, Chapman DP, et al. The impact of formal diabetes education on the preventive health practices and behaviors of persons with type 2 diabetes. Prev Med 2005; 41:79–84.

Van Acker K. The diabetic foot: a challenge for policymakers and health care professionals. PhD thesis. University of Antwerp.

Van Acker K. Lavery, Peters, and Bush (Editors). Impact of Specialized Foot Clinics in High Risk Diabetic Foot: Treatment and Prevention (published by Informa Healthcare USA, Inc.), 2010.

Van Acker K. Employing interdisciplinary team working to improve patient outcomes in diabetic foot ulceration – our experience. EWMA J 2012; 12:31–35.

Waaijman R, Keukenkamp R de Haart M, et al. Adherence to wearing prescription custom-made footwear in patients with diabetes at high risk for plantar foot ulceration. Diabetes Care 2013; 12:31–35.

Wheatley C. Audit protocol: part one: prevention of diabetic foot ulcers—the non-complicated foot. J Clin Govern 2001; 9:3–100.

Section 2

INFECTION

Chapter 8

Managing infection in the diabetic foot

Edgar J. G. Peters, Benjamin A. Lipsky

SUMMARY

- The incidence of infections of the foot in patients with diabetes mellitus is high, and increases with the duration of diabetes
- Diabetes influences the immune system in several ways, making patients prone to infection
- The risk of infection increases if chronic, recurrent, traumatic, or deep ulcers are present, especially in the case of peripheral arterial disease, peripheral neuropathy, or a previous partial foot amputation
- The main classification systems for infection are as follows:
  - Infectious Diseases Society of America (IDSA)
  - International Working Group on the Diabetic Foot (IWGDF)
- The predominant organisms involved in mild infections are gram-positive cocci, but deeper and more severe infections are more often caused by mixed gram-positive cocci and gram-negative rods, sometimes including nonfermentative gram-negative rods and obligate anaerobes
- Treating and culturing noninfected wounds is not recommended
- Empiric antibiotic treatment of mild, previously untreated infections should be aimed at gram-positive cocci, while empiric antibiotic coverage of more severe infections should include gram-negative organisms and anaerobes as well
- Recommended duration of antibiotic treatment of soft tissue infection ranges from 1 to 2 weeks in mild infections to up to 4 weeks in moderate infections, usually combined with adequate surgical debridement and other treatment modalities such as arterial revascularization

INTRODUCTION

The incidence of infections of the foot in patients with diabetes mellitus is high, and increases with the duration of diabetes and the onset of its attendant complications. Estimates of the incidence of foot infections range from a lifetime risk of 4% in the general population to 3.7% annually in patients treated in a specialized diabetic foot center (Lavery et al. 2003). Persons with diabetes have a 10-fold greater risk of being hospitalized for a lower-extremity infection compared with persons without diabetes. Most of these hospitalizations occur in patients with poor glycemic control or who have infections classified as moderate or severe (Kosinski & Lipsky 2010). There is a variety of infectious syndromes of the diabetic foot, as summarized in **Table 8.1**.

The most common sequence leading to foot infection is a foot ulcer (usually neuropathic in origin) serves as *port d'entrée* for pathogenic organisms. Infections in a patient with concomitant foot ischemia are especially liable to lead to soft tissue necrosis. About half of all patients with a foot infection will undergo some form of lower-extremity amputation, 10% of which are major (proximal to the ankle) (Eneroth et al. 1997). A foot infection, therefore, often constitutes the pivotal event

leading to an amputation. Not surprisingly, in most risk classification schemes patients with foot infections are considered at highest risk of amputation. Thus, prompt and appropriate treatment of infections is required to halt the cascade toward amputation.

Treating diabetic foot infections is financially costly. A study from Sweden published in 2000 found that the cost of treatment of a diabetic foot infection without need for an amputation (corrected for inflation in 2007, calculated from Swedish krona) was EUR 22,000 and if amputation was required up to EUR 43,000 (Ragnarson Tennvall et al. 2000). Overall, 95% of these costs were related to the prolonged time until healing of the wound and surgical procedures, 51% to bandages and topical treatments, and only 4% to antibiotics. In another study published in 2008, the costs of a diabetic foot-related major amputation averaged EUR 25,200 in both low- and high-income European countries (Prompers et al. 2008). Studies have suggested that optimizing antibiotic protocols based on published recommendations lead to a reduction in health care expenditure for diabetic foot wounds (Sotto et al. 2010).

PATHOPHYSIOLOGY OF INFECTIONS IN DIABETES MELLITUS

Data to support the assertion that patients with diabetes are more prone to infections are less robust than many believe. A retrospective study matched insurance claims for a cohort of over 500,000 subjects with diabetes against those without diabetes (Shah & Hux 2003). Almost 50% of patients with diabetes were hospitalized or had a physician claim for an infection, compared with 38% in the cohort without diabetes (risk ratio of 1.2). The relative risks were 2.2 for hospitalization overall, 2.0 hospitalization for infection, 4.0 for osteomyelitis, 2.0 for sepsis, and 1.8 for death due to an infection. Patients with diabetes had an 80% increased risk of cellulitis compared with those without diabetes. Another 1-year cohort study in 7417 Dutch patients in general practice with diabetes suggested that compared with persons without diabetes, they had a higher incidence of pneumonia, urinary tract infection, and skin infections (Muller et al. 2005).

The changes related to diabetes at a physiological level that increase the risk of infection are not well understood. The influence of diabetes seems to be multifactorial and affects various elements of the immune system, as summarized in **Box 8.1**.

Cellular innate immune system

The major component of the cellular immune system is the polymorphonuclear (PMN) cell or phagocyte. This cell works to destroy micro-organisms by a variety of methods, including chemotaxis, adherence, phagocytosis, and intracellular killing, each of which is impaired in patients with diabetes. Insulin treatment improves these functions, presumably through better metabolic control but also by a more direct effect independent of metabolic control (Walrand et al. 2004). Advanced glycation end products lead to impaired PMN

Table 8.1 Definitions

Diabetic foot	Deformity, ulceration, or destruction of superficial or deep tissues of the foot associated with neuropathy and/or peripheral arterial disease, often associated with infection, below the malleoli of a person with diabetes (International Working Group on the Diabetic Foot 2011)
Colonization	New bacteria introduced into ulcer replicate and establish a physiological state of coexistence without overt tissue damage or host response (International Working Group on the Diabetic Foot 2011)
Contamination	External introduction of nonresident bacteria into host tissue. The number and virulence of the organisms and the robustness of the host's immune system determine the next steps (International Working Group on the Diabetic Foot 2011). Can also mean contamination of a culture sample after obtaining it from the patient
Infection	A pathologic state caused by invasion and multiplication of micro-organisms in tissues accompanied by tissue destruction and/or a host inflammatory response (International Working Group on the Diabetic Foot 2011)
Soft tissue	
Superficial infection	An infection of the skin and soft tissues that does not extend to any structure below the dermis (International Working Group on the Diabetic Foot 2011)
Deep infection	An infection involving tissues deeper than the dermis, including abscess, septic arthritis, osteomyelitis, septic tenosynovitis, and necrotizing fasciitis (International Working Group on the Diabetic Foot 2011)
Bone	
Osteitis	Infection of bone cortex, without the involvement of bone marrow
Acute osteomyelitis	Infection involving the marrow that is usually of recent onset and characterized by polymorphonuclear infiltrate but without necrosis (Mader et al. 1997)
Chronic osteomyelitis	Infection involving the marrow that has usually been present for at least several weeks and is characterized by round cell infiltrates and necrosis (Mader et al. 1997)

Adapted from International Working Group on the Diabetic Foot (2011) and Mader et al. (1997).

Box 8.1 Immune systems affected by diabetes mellitus

Cellular innate system
- Phagocyte function impairment
  - Decreased chemotaxis
  - Decreased adherence
  - Decreased phagocytosis
  - Decreased superoxide formation, leading to diminished intracellular killing capacity

Humoral innate system
- Dysfunction of eNOS/NO system leading to vasoconstriction
  - Ischemia
  - Impaired influx of phagocytes
- Complement disturbances
  - General complement cascade activation
  - Inhibition of specific complement response
  - Decrease in complement-mediated phagocytosis
- Increased production of proinflammatory cytokines
  - General increase in inflammation
  - Decreased insulin sensitivity

Adaptive immune system
- T and B cell function
  - Possibly impaired vaccination response
  - Glycation of immunoglobulins

---

transendothelial migration (Collison et al. 2002). Studies on the effect of diabetes on chemotaxis of PMNs suggest that hyperglycemia impairs phagocyte chemotaxis, but that it can be restored by insulin therapy (Geerlings & Hoepelman 1999). Other studies have suggested that PMN chemotaxis is reduced in diabetes independent of metabolic control (Delamaire et al. 1997). Other cells besides PMNs, such as monocytes, that act as phagocytes have also been found to function less well in patients with diabetes.

Superoxide, a key antimicrobial agent in phagocytes, is produced by the activity of the enzymes myeloperoxidase and nicotinamide

adenine dinucleotide phosphate (NADPH) oxidase. The activity of myeloperoxidase seems unaffected by hyperglycemia (Sato et al. 1993). However, high glucose levels inhibit the enzyme glucose-6-phosphate dehydrogenase (G6PD), which catalyzes the formation of NADPH (Perner et al. 2003). In this way, high glucose concentrations impair the production of superoxide formation. NADPH is an integrated part of the polyol pathway. Increased utilization of this pathway and NADPH leads to reduced levels of superoxide production (Sato et al. 1993).

Some research has been done on ways to overcome the loss of innate cellular immune functions in diabetes. There are conflicting data on the effectiveness of agents that might improve leukocyte function in diabetic foot infections, such as granulocyte colony-stimulating factor (G-CSF) (Cruciani et al. 2009). In meta-analyses of randomized controlled trials in 2005 and 2009, G-CSF did not seem to have any significant beneficial effect on cure of infection or on healing of pedal ulcers. However, patients receiving G-CSF did have significantly lower rates of lower-extremity surgery, including amputations (Cruciani et al. 2009).

■ Humoral innate immune system

The humoral innate immune response consists of the proinflammatory cytokines: local vasoactive cytokines and the complement system. Normally, the release of local vasoactive cytokines, such as bradykinin, leads to vasodilatation through a nitric oxide (NO) response. In hyperglycemia, however, the dysregulation of the endothelial nitric oxide synthase (eNOS) /NO system can lead to vasoconstriction instead, which in turn may both inhibit phagocytes reaching a location of infection and lead to hypoxia (Santilli et al. 2004). In an older study, generalized complement activation appeared to be more common in patients with type 2 diabetes on insulin therapy (Bergamaschini et al. 1991). More recent studies have suggested that elevated glucose concentrations inhibit complement-mediated immune responses. In normal human neutrophils, activation of protein kinases C α and β leads to a decrease in complement receptor-3 and Fc-γ receptor-mediated phagocytosis (Saiepour et al. 2006). Hyperglycemia is associated with an increase in levels of proinflammatory cytokines, including tumor necrosis factor (TNF)-α, interleukin (IL) 1β, IL6, and IL18. These cytokines lead to more insulin resistance through several pathways, such as decreased mRNA expression of glucose transporter, augmented lipolysis, and activation of stress hormones. The increased insulin resistance leads to a cycle of hyperglycemia, further elevated proinflammatory cytokines, and insulin resistance (Turina et al. 2005).

Adaptive immune system

The influence of diabetes on the adaptive immune system with T cells and immunoglobulin-producing B cells is less well characterized. Some specific cellular adaptive immune system defects have been identified in vaccination studies in patients with both poorly and adequately controlled type 1 diabetes (Eibl et al. 2002). In another study, however, among patients with adequately metabolically controlled type 1 and 2 diabetes the immune response appeared to be intact, suggesting normal T memory cell and CD4 positive lymphocyte function (Pozzilli et al. 1987). This suggests that better metabolic control might help to optimize the adaptive immune system.

The level of glycated hemoglobin (HbA1c) is correlated with glycation of immunoglobulin (IgG). Glycation of the antigen-binding fragment (Fab) of IgG might lead to a reduced molecular antibody-antigen recognition capacity (Lapolla et al. 2002). However, protection after (polysaccharide) vaccination against influenza, *Streptococcus pneumoniae*, and hepatitis B has been found to be adequate in clinical studies (el-Madhun et al. 1998). Therefore, the likelihood of clinical relevance of the findings from in vitro studies to glycation of immunoglobulins seems low.

RISK FACTORS FOR DIABETIC FOOT INFECTION

Only a few published studies have examined specific risk factors for diabetic foot infection. One prospective, multicenter study compared 150 patients with a diabetic foot infection (of whom 20% had osteomyelitis) with 97 controls with diabetes but no foot infection (Lavery et al. 2006). Factors significantly associated with the development of a foot infection included a positive probe to bone test [a wound extending to bone, odds ratio (OR) of 6.7], a chronic foot ulcer [present for >30 days (OR 4.7)], a history of recurrent foot ulcers (OR 2.4), a traumatic etiology of the foot ulcer (OR 2.4), and the presence of peripheral arterial disease [absent peripheral pulsation or an ankle–brachial index (ABI) < 0.9 (OR 1.9)]. Only one infection occurred in a patient without a foot ulcer. The second study was a retrospective review of 112 patients with severe diabetic foot infection, possibly requiring an amputation (Peters et al. 2005). Factors associated with an infection in a multivariate analysis were a previous lower-extremity amputation (OR 19.9), peripheral arterial disease (OR 5.5), and peripheral sensory neuropathy (OR 3.4). Other noncontrolled studies have identified renal insufficiency and renal transplantation (George et al. 2004) and walking barefoot as risk factors for diabetic foot infection (Jayasinghe et al. 2007). Risk factors for diabetic foot infection are summarized in **Box 8.2**.

> **Box 8.2 Risk factors for diabetic foot infection**
> - Positive probe-to-bone test
> - Ulcer present for >30 days
> - History of recurrent ulcers
> - Traumatic etiology of the ulcer
> - Previous lower-extremity amputation
> - Sensory peripheral neuropathy
> - Peripheral arterial disease
> - Renal insufficiency or renal transplantation

CLINICAL SIGNS AND SYMPTOMS

Three recently published national and international guidelines affirmed the viewpoint that the diagnosis of diabetic foot infection should be made on clinical (rather than microbiological) parameters (Lipsky et al. 2012a and 2012b, National Institute for Health and Clinical Excellence 2011). Classical clinical signs and symptoms of inflammation such as redness, warmth, swelling, pain/tenderness, and loss of function are subjective by nature, but there is consensus on their use (**Table 8.2**) (Lipsky et al. 2012a, Schaper 2004). Other 'secondary' signs suggesting infection are the presence

Table 8.2 IDSA and PEDIS classification on diabetic foot infection (Lipsky et al. 2012a, Schaper 2004)

Clinical manifestation of infection	IDSA infection severity	PEDIS grade
No symptoms or signs of infection	Uninfected	1
Infection involving the skin and subcutaneous tissue only (not deeper tissues) and without systemic signs (as described below). At least two of the following items are present: Local swelling or induration Erythema >0.5–2 cm around the ulcer Local tenderness or pain Local warmth Purulent discharge (thick, opaque to white or sanguineous secretion) Other causes of skin inflammation excluded (e.g. trauma, gout, acute neuro-osteoarthropathy, fracture, thrombosis, venous stasis)	Mild	2
Erythema >2 cm plus one of the items described above (swelling, tenderness, warmth, discharge) or Infection involving structures deeper than skin and subcutaneous tissues as abscess, osteomyelitis, septic arthritis, fasciitis No systemic inflammatory response signs, as described below	Moderate	3
Any foot infection with signs of the systemic inflammatory response syndrome (SIRS), manifested by ≥2 of the following: Temperature >38 or < 36°C Heart rate >90 beats/min Respiratory rate >20 breaths/min or $PaCO_2$< 32 mmHg White blood cell count >12,000 or < 4000 cu/mm or 10% immature (band) forms	Severe	4

IDSA, Infectious Diseases Society of America; PEDIS, Perfusion, Extent (size), Depth (tissue loss), Infection, Sensation (neuropathy)

of necrosis, lack of wound healing, purulent or nonpurulent discharge, a fetid odor, undermining of wound edges, and the lack of healthy granulation tissue (Richard et al. 2012). In patients with diabetes, signs and symptoms of inflammation are usually less obvious than in patients without diabetes (Lavery et al. 1995). This is partly because pain sensation and tenderness are often diminished due to neuropathy. Additional signs, such as erythema and induration, might be less visible due to peripheral arterial disease. Blood influx to the wound may also be decreased due to autonomous neuropathy and subsequent diminished dermal blood flow. The improper functioning of leukocytes (see above) can also contribute to the absence of signs of inflammation. Systemic signs such as fever, malaise, hypotension, and laboratory tests such as an elevation of white blood cell count, erythrocyte sedimentation rate, and C-reactive protein are usually not present in diabetic foot infections. If present, however, several of these findings would lead to the infection being classified as severe (see below) (Lipsky et al. 2012a and 2012b). Microbiological data do not contribute to the diagnosis of infection, but are important to optimize antimicrobial therapy (see below).

CLASSIFICATION

Several classification schemes are available to assess infection severity, with the hope of predicting outcome and helping determine appropriate empirical therapy. There is no consensus on which classification to use in various situations, largely because these classifications often have different purposes. Most of the available schemes are subsections of ulcer classifications and many were originally devised for patients in clinical trials. A classification for research purposes should be selective and exclusive to allow comparison of different study populations. A clinical classification, however, should be simple, descriptive, and fit any patient.

Examples of diabetic foot wound classification systems are the Meggit–Wagner (Meggitt 1976) PEDIS (see below) (Schaper 2004) S(AD) (Size [Area and Depth])/SAD (Sepsis, Arthropathy, Denervation) and SINBAD (Site, Ischemia, Neuropathy, Bacterial infection, Depth) (Jeffcoate et al. 2006), and the University of Texas (UT) (Armstrong et al. 1998). All are originally diabetic foot ulcer classifications, but have a separate section to assess infection severity. Other schemes were specifically developed as wound scores, such as the Ulcer Severity Index (USI) (Knighton et al. 1986), the DUSS (Diabetic Ulcer Severity Score) and MAID (Multiple ulcers, Area, Ischemia, Duration) (Beckert et al. 2006 and 2009), and the DFI (Diabetic Foot Infection) (Lipsky et al. 2009). The Meggit–Wagner, SINBAD classifications are not useful to describe infection because they provide only a dichotomous description of infection (present or absent) without further definitions of infection. The UT classification uses a dichotomous description for infection as well, but infection is better defined in stages and there is evidence that the system adequately predicts outcome. The USI is complex and there are no data available on the predictive qualities for infection. The DUSS and DFI are less complex, and are wounds scores that have been successfully tested in large clinical trials. The DFI has the advantage that it helps demonstrating improvement in signs of infection and wound healing during treatment, and may help compare the severity of foot wounds in patients in different studies (Lipsky et al. 2009). Only the IDSA and the similar subcategory of the IWGDF and PEDIS scheme are specifically designed to classify severity of a foot infection. Both of these, and the S(AD)/SAD, provide a semiquantitative four point scale to describe infection and may help predict the outcome

of a diabetic foot infection (Lipsky et al. 2012a, Schaper 2004). There is no evidence that one classification or wound score is better than any other.

PEDIS and IDSA

The PEDIS ulcer classification, an acronym for perfusion, extent (size), depth (tissue loss), infection, sensation (neuropathy), was originally developed by the IWGDF for research purposes, but can be used for clinical practice as well (Schaper 2004). It offers a semiquantitative gradation of ulcer severity. The infection part of the classification is almost the same as the one by IDSA (see **Table 8.2**) (Lipsky et al. 2012a). The IDSA classification describes a moderate infection as having more extensive cellulitis or deeper invasion than a mild infection, possibly with the presence of lymphangitic streaks, deep soft tissue, or bone infection or gangrene (Lipsky et al. 2012a). The IWGDF defines moderate infection as cellulitis of >2 cm diameter plus at least one other sign of inflammation or a deep infection, such as septic arthritis, osteomyelitis, or an abscess (Schaper 2004). Severe foot infection in the IDSA classification is defined as being associated with systemic toxicity or metabolic disturbance, while in the PEDIS classification this is more strictly defined as a patient with a foot infection-related sepsis, i.e. two or more criteria of the systemic inflammatory response syndrome (SIRS). In clinical practice, however, these classifications are unlikely to differ. A major advantage of both classifications is that they are analogous to other infection classifications, e.g. those for pneumonia or sepsis, making them easier to work with for clinicians less experienced in diabetic foot management. The IDSA/IWGDF system has been validated in prospective studies in patients with diabetes (Lavery et al. 2007). In these studies, it predicted the need for hospitalization and for limb amputation to a statistically significant level. In a recent study, the system was not used for prospective research, but for a comparative audit between 14 European diabetic foot centers (Prompers et al. 2007).

MICROBIOLOGY

Microbiological data should be interpreted with knowledge of the clinical situation. All wounds are colonized with bacteria, making findings of cultures or Gram-stained smears potentially misleading as the identified organisms may only be colonizers or contaminants. Because clinically noninfected wounds should not be treated with systemic antibiotics, there is no value in obtaining cultures, unless they are being used for epidemiological studies. For clinically infected wounds, however, collecting specimens for microbiological processing is certainly useful for selecting the most appropriate antibiotic therapy. Using the proper sampling technique is essential (International Working Group on the Diabetic Foot 2011). In general, colonizing organisms are not found within vital tissue, making a sample of deep tissue taken through noncolonized surroundings, or of pus, less likely to produce a false positive culture. For example, in one study of previously untreated patients with osteomyelitis and a foot ulcer, culture of bone matched results of superficial wound swabs in only 22.5% of patients (Senneville et al. 2006). Blood cultures are rarely positive except in patients with severe infection, especially those with fever or rigors.

The predominant pathogens in diabetic foot infections are aerobic gram-positive cocci, particularly *Staphylococcus aureus* and β-hemolytic streptococci, especially of Lancefield group B, and occasionally A and G, as well as coagulase-negative staphylococci. These are usually the only organisms causing mild infections in patients not previously treated with antibiotics (Lipsky et al. 2012b, Ge et al. 2002). Outside the developed world, *S. aureus* is somewhat less predominant as a cause of diabetic foot infections (approximately 30% compared with 75% in developed world) (Gadepalli et al. 2006). In warm climates in less developed countries, infections with aerobic gram-negative rods (especially *Pseudomonas*) are more frequent. Deeper or more severe infections are more often caused by mixed gram-positive cocci and gram-negative rods (*Escherichia coli, Proteus,*

Klebsiella), sometimes including nonfermentative gram-negative rods (e.g. *Pseudomonas*) and obligate anaerobes (e.g. *Peptostreptococcus, Bacteroides*) (Lipsky et al. 2012a and 2012b). *Pseudomonas aeruginosa* has been associated especially with deep puncture wounds and with patients exposed to water (Lavery et al. 1995). Anaerobes are usually found in wounds with necrosis or severe ischemia (Lipsky et al. 2012a). The most likely infecting micro-organisms according to local circumstances are summarized in **Table 8.3**.

Table 8.3 Suggestions for empiric antibiotic regimens based on the Infectious Diseases Society of America's (IDSA) guidelines on diabetic foot infection (Lipsky et al. 2012a)

Infection severity	Likely pathogen(s)	Antibiotic agent(s)	Comments
Mild (usually treated with oral antibiotics)	*Staphylococcus aureus* (MSSA), *Streptococcus* spp.	Dicloxacillin or flucloxacillin	QID dosing, narrow spectrum, inexpensive
		Clindamycin	Usually, but not always, active against community acquired MRSA. Inhibits protein synthesis of some toxins
		Cephalexin	QID dosing, inexpensive
		Levofloxacin	Once-daily dosing, suboptimal coverage of *S. aureus*
		Amoxicillin/clavulanate	Relatively broad-spectrum oral agent, includes anaerobic coverage
	MRSA	Doxycycline	Active against many MRSA and some gram-negative organisms, uncertain activity against *Streptococcus* spp.
		Trimethoprim/ sulfamethoxazole (co-trimoxazole)	Active against MRSA and some gram-negative spp. Uncertain activity against *Streptococcus* spp.
Moderate (oral or initial parenteral, followed by oral antibiotics) or Severe (usually treated with parenteral antibiotics)	MSSA, *Streptococcus* spp., *Enterobacteriaceae*, obligate anaerobes	Levofloxacin	Suboptimal against *S. aureus*
		Cefoxitin	Second-generation cephalosporin with anaerobic coverage
		Ceftriaxone	Third-generation cephalosporin, once-daily dosing
		Ampicillin/sulbactam	Adequate if low suspicion of *Pseudomonas aeruginosa*. Anaerobic coverage
		Moxifloxacin	Once-daily oral dosing. Relatively broad-spectrum, including most obligate anaerobic organisms
		Ertapenem	Once-daily dosing. Relatively broad-spectrum including anaerobes, but not active against *P. aeruginosa*
		Tigecycline	Active against MRSA. Spectrum may be excessively broad. High rates of nausea and vomiting and increased mortality warning
		Levofloxacin or ciprofloxacin with clindamycin	Limited evidence supporting clindamycin for severe *S. aureus* infections; PO and IV formulations for both drugs
		Imipenem/cilastatin	Very broad-spectrum (but not against MRSA); use only when this is required. Consider when ESBL-producing pathogens suspected
	MRSA	Linezolid	Expensive; increased risk of toxicities when used >2 weeks
		Daptomycin	Once-daily dosing. Requires serial monitoring of CPK
		Vancomycin	Vancomycin MICs for MRSA are gradually increasing
	Pseudomonas aeruginosa	Piperacillin/tazobactam	TID/QID dosing. Useful for broad-spectrum coverage. *P. aeruginosa* is an uncommon pathogen in diabetic foot infections except in special circumstances
	MRSA, *Enterobacteriaceae*, *Pseudomonas*, and obligate anaerobes	Vancomycin* with ceftazidime, cefepime, piperacillin/tazobactam aztreonam, or a carbapenem	Very broad-spectrum coverage; usually only used for empiric therapy of severe infection. Consider addition of obligate anaerobe coverage if ceftazidime, cefepime, or aztreonam selected

Narrow-spectrum agents (e.g. vancomycin, linezolid, daptomycin) should be combined with other agents (e.g. a fluoroquinolone) in case of a polymicrobial infection (especially moderate or severe) is suspected

Use an agent active against MRSA for patients who have a severe infection, evidence of infection or colonization with this organism elsewhere, and when there are epidemiological risk factors for MRSA infection

Select definitive regimens after considering the results of culture and susceptibility tests from wound specimens, as well as the clinical response to the empiric regimen

Similar agents of the same drug class can probably be substituted for suggested agents

CPK, creatine phosphokinase; ESBL, extended-spectrum β-lactamase; FDA, US Food and Drug Administration; IV, intravenous; MIC, minimum inhibitory concentration; MRSA, methicillin-resistant *S. aureus*; MSSA, methicillin-sensitive *S. aureus*; PO, oral; QID, 4 times a day; TID, 3 times a day

*Vancomycin may be substituted for daptomycin or linezolid or teicoplanin

Chronic wounds that are infected (and, inappropriately, sometime uninfected) have often recently been unsuccessfully treated with antibiotics, a situation that can lead to the selection of unusual and resistant bacterial flora (Hartemann-Heurtier et al. 2004, Mendes et al. 2012). In cases caused by multidrug-resistant organisms (MDROs), antimicrobial therapy is often inappropriate (Mendes et al. 2012). Studies of the outcome of diabetic foot ulcers infected with resistant organisms, such as methicillin-resistant *S. aureus* (MRSA), vancomycin-resistant *Enterococcus* (VRE), or extended-spectrum β-lactamase (ESBL) producing gram-negative rods, have produced conflicting data. In one, where 25% of patients had osteomyelitis, patients whose ulcer cultures grew MDROs did not seem to have a worse outcome than patients without resistant bacteria (Hartemann-Heurtier et al. 2004). However, other studies have suggested that patients with MRSA did do worse (Wagner et al. 2001). A possible confounder in these studies might be that patients colonized with MRSA had been subjected to previous unsuccessful treatments or hospitalizations that led to the colonization. Another issue that makes generalization of the results of this latter study difficult is that most specimens were cultured from superficial swabs. This might also explain why most of the patients from whom MDROs were cultured healed without antimicrobial drugs specifically targeting these bacteria (Lipsky et al. 2004). The prevalence of MRSA, both hospital and community acquired, and ESBL producing organisms in diabetic foot infections is rising (Tentolouris et al. 2006). Identified risk factors for resistant bacteria in foot infections include previous antibiotic therapy, especially of long duration; frequent hospitalization for the same ulcer, especially of long duration; and presence of underlying osteomyelitis (Hartemann-Heurtier et al. 2004, Kandemir et al. 2007).

Molecular microbiology

Standard techniques for culture of wounds have been used for over 150 years. While they are relatively easy to do and well standardized, they are designed to isolate the organisms currently known to cause infections. Culture-based techniques select for species that flourish under the typical nutritional and physiological conditions of the diagnostic microbiology laboratory, not necessarily the most abundant or clinically important organisms (Lipsky et al. 2013). Furthermore, they depend on taking appropriately collected specimens and take at least 2–3 days to provide results. In the past decade, studies with molecular microbiological techniques have raised doubts about the accuracy of wound culture results. In light of these deficiencies, newer molecular methods have been explored for detecting micro-organisms in infected wounds.

Using amplification and sequence analysis of 16S rRNA has revealed vastly more complex bacterial communities than those identified by culture, particularly in chronic wounds. One study of diabetic foot chronic wounds that used by polymerase chain reaction-based methods and standard cultures found that the wounds generally harbored greater eubacterial diversity than healthy skin on the contralateral foot, but the isolation of known pathogens was not associated with qualitatively distinct consortial profiles or otherwise altered diversity (Oates et al. 2012). These data suggest that there may be utility of both culture and molecular techniques for the microbial characterization of chronic wounds. Another study of patients with diabetic foot wounds found that cultures, when compared with molecular techniques, greatly underestimated the microbial load, overestimated the relative abundance of staphylococci, and underrepresented the prevalence of obligate anaerobes (Gardner et al. 2013). Molecular sequencing demonstrated great heterogeneity in the colonizing flora, but they could generally be divided into those with a high relative abundance either *Staphylococcus* spp., *Streptococcus* spp., or anaerobes and proteobacteria (gram-negatives). One other study that included patients with chronic diabetic foot wounds found that using comprehensive molecular diagnostic techniques, fungi (mostly *Candida* species, but many others as well) were more important wound pathogens than suspected and opportunistic pathogens than previously reported (Dowd et al. 2011).

While molecular techniques have demonstrated that there are many more micro-organisms of greater variety than we were able to appreciate with standard culture techniques, we do not currently know the clinical significance of these findings. It is likely, however, that molecular techniques, both for identifying causative pathogens and also demonstrating whether or not virulence factors and antibiotic resistance genes are present, will become the standard in the near future.

■ TREATMENT
■ Uninfected wounds

Some argue for using systemic antibiotic treatment of clinically uninfected wounds, believing that high levels of surface colonization may inhibit healing or that overt signs of infection are obscured in diabetes (Edmonds & Foster 2004). In one small nonrandomized study, only published as an abstract, patients with an uninfected wound who were prescribed antibiotics underwent fewer amputations (Foster et al. 1999). Most authorities argue against this approach, as it has not been found to be effective for either improving ulcer healing or reducing the likelihood of clinical infection (Chantelau et al. 1996) and it exposes the patient to the expense, potential for adverse effects, and the possibility of infection with antibiotic-resistant pathogens.

Published trials reporting on treatment of a colonized wound without clinical infection (PEDIS grade 1/IDSA uninfected) found that antibiotics were ineffective in the healing of ulcers or as prophylaxis against infections (Peters et al. 2012). Prescribing antibiotics for clinically uninfected wounds is discouraged in virtually all currently published diabetic foot guidelines (Lipsky et al. 2012a and 2012b). Potential adverse effects can range from mild side effects, such as upset stomach or diarrhoea, to fatal reactions or severe bacteriological complications such as *Clostridium difficile*-associated disease. On a population level, prescribing antibiotics to patients needs to be weighed against the spread of antibiotic resistance. More studies are needed to determine the efficacy of treating uninfected wounds with various types of antimicrobials. Of course, clinically uninfected wounds do need other forms of treatment to ensure healing, such as proper off-loading, dressing and, if necessary, improvement in arterial supply (International Working Group on the Diabetic Foot 2011, Schaper et al. 2012).

■ Infected wounds
General measurements

A combination of several different interventions is required to treat a diabetic foot infection. Antibiotic therapy alone will not heal a severe infection; it should be combined with appropriate debridement, proper off-loading, and often surgical procedures. Surgical management encompasses cleansing, removal of callus and necrotic material, and drainage of pus collections. Edema is usually treated with limb elevation and compression. Furthermore, vascular interventions to optimize supply of both nutrients and immune cells are crucial in cases of peripheral arterial disease.

Systemic antimicrobial therapy

Assessing the severity, e.g. with the IWGDF/IDSA classification, is useful in determining appropriate empirical antimicrobial therapy (Lipsky et al. 2012a and 2012b, Vardakas et al. 2008). Empirical therapy is usually based on local epidemiological data and clinical findings. Then, culture and antibiogram results, as well as the clinical response, can be used to tailor definitive therapy. Suggested empirical therapies are summarized in **Table 8.3** (Lipsky et al. 2012a). Most of these recommendations are based on expert opinion. In 2008, a meta-analysis on factors associated with treatment failure in diabetic foot infection found 18 randomized clinical trials (Vardakas et al. 2008). Two factors were associated with treatment failure in the 1715 subjects: use of an antibiotic other than a carbapenem and the presence of MRSA or streptococci. However, the reported studies were likely to suffer from bias and the outcomes of these studies were dependent on local antimicrobial resistance. In another systematic review published in 2006, 23 trials were identified with 19 unique comparisons among interventions (Nelson et al. 2006). In 2011, a critical review of randomized controlled trials on the antibiotic treatment of diabetic foot infections between 1999 and 2009 concluded that it is difficult to compare the available trials, or to determine which regimen may be the most appropriate (Crouzet et al. 2011). Reasons for this difficulty are discrepancies in study design, inclusion criteria, statistical methodology, and the varying definitions of both clinical and microbiological end points among the studies.

In 2012, the IWGDF, a consultative section of the International Diabetes Federation IDF, published a systematic review on treatment of diabetic foot infections (Peters et al. 2012). The literature search of papers published prior to August 2010 conducted for this study identified 7517 articles, 33 of which fulfilled predefined criteria for detailed data extraction. Of these studies, 29 were randomized controlled trials, and 4 were cohort studies. Among 12 studies comparing different antibiotic regimens in the management of skin and soft-tissue infection, none reported a better response with any particular regimen. Of 7 studies that compared antibiotic regimens in patients with infection involving both soft tissue and bone, one reported a better clinical outcome in those treated with cefoxitin compared with ampicillin/sulbactam, but the others reported no differences between treatment regimens. In two health economic analyses, there was a small saving using one regimen (ertapenem in one, ceftriaxone + metronidazole in the another) versus the more expensive other (piperacillin/tazobactam or ticarcillin/clavulanate). No published data clarify the optimal duration of antibiotic therapy in either soft-tissue infection or osteomyelitis or support the superiority of any particular route of delivery of systemic antibiotics. In one nonrandomized cohort study, the outcome of treatment of osteomyelitis was better when the antibiotic choice was based on culture of bone specimens as opposed to wound swabs (Senneville et al. 2006). This study, however, was not randomized, and the results may have been affected by confounding factors such as the use of rifampicin in patients receiving bone biopsy-guided therapy. Results from two studies suggested that early surgical intervention was associated with a significant reduction in major amputation, but the methodological quality of both studies was low (Peters et al. 2012).

All of the systematic reviews concluded that no single antibiotic regimen has been proven superior over other regimens for diabetic foot infections (Crouzet et al. 2011, Nelson et al. 2006, Peters et al. 2012, Vardakas et al. 2008) Unfortunately, there have not been many trials performed and the methodological quality of the available studies was poor. The sample sizes in most studies were insufficient to identify differences between antimicrobial regimes in part because they used a variety of definitions and outcomes. Based on the available data, there is no strong evidence of recommending any particular antimicrobial agent to prevent amputation, aid the resolution of infection, or hasten ulcer healing.

There is some debate on the importance of the diffusion of antibiotics into infected tissue of the foot. One literature review of studies of the serum and tissue levels of antibiotics (Lipsky 1999) found that levels in viable tissues of gentamicin and clindamycin adjacent to the surgical site were low, while tissue concentrations of penicillin derivatives were generally higher. It also appeared that most β-lactam antibiotics achieved relatively high serum levels, but lower tissue levels, possibly with the exception of ceftazidime (Storm et al. 1994). In contrast, in other small studies it has been suggested that clindamycin and quinolones achieve adequate levels in bone, biofilm and necrotic tissue (Duckworth et al. 1993, Mueller-Buehl et al. 1991). For oral therapy, it is important to demonstrate that the oral absorption (or bioavailability) is high enough to ensure adequate serum levels. A direct relationship, however, between serum or tissue antibiotic levels and clinical outcome is as yet unproven.

A crucial issue currently is the development of resistance among many pathogens to antimicrobial agents. Some newer drugs have shown efficacy in cases of drug resistance including:

- Linezolid (intravenously (IV) or orally (PO)) for gram-positive and anaerobic organisms
- Daptomycin once-daily IV for gram-positive organisms
- Dalbavancin IV once-weekly for gram-positive organisms
- Telavancin once-daily IV for gram-positive organisms, including glycopeptides-resistant strains
- Tigecycline IV twice daily for gram-positive and gram-negative bacteria including anaerobes, VRE and ESBL producers, but not *Pseudomonas*
- Ceftardin IV twice daily for gram-positive organisms, including MRSA moxifloxacin IV or PO once daily, broad spectrum but not for MDROs
- Ertapenem IV once daily for gram-positive and negative organisms including ESBL producing organisms, but not for *Pseudomonas*

Mild infections

Mild infections (PEDIS grade 2) in patients who have not been recently treated with antimicrobials are usually caused by streptococci and staphylococci. Outpatient treatment is safe in mild infection provided that the clinical and social circumstances allow this (Lipsky et al. 2012a and 2012b). Although gram-negative rods are sometimes cultured, these are usually thought to be colonizing rather than infecting organisms. In areas where the prevalence of MRSA is low, a semisynthetic penicillin with antistaphylococcal activity such as flucloxacillin, or a first-generation cephalosporin such as cephalexin for 2 weeks is appropriate. An alternative is clindamycin, although the susceptibility of staphylococci can vary (Lipsky et al. 2012a, de Vries et al. 2014). In areas of endemic MRSA, wound cultures are advisable to prevent prescription of an inadequate antibiotic regime (Lipsky 1999). For MRSA, potentially appropriate agents include trimethoprim–sulfamethoxazole (cotrimoxazole, which has weak antistreptococcal activity), doxycycline (also weak antistreptococcal activity), or linezolid (expensive) (Lipsky et al. 2012a).

Moderate infections

Patients with a moderate infection (PEDIS grade 3) often require broader spectrum coverage than those with mild infections, including gram-positive cocci and gram-negative rods. The combination of the two is more often present in chronic wounds and in patients who have been previously treated with antibiotics. Obligate anaerobes are not encountered frequently except in the presence of necrosis or ischemia (Lipsky et al. 2012a and 2012b). In the IDSA and IWGDF guidelines, the empirical treatment for the group with moderate infection is the same as for severe infection (PEDIS grade 4) (Lipsky et al. 2012a and 2012b). Options for empirical therapy are combinations of a fluoroquinolone with clindamycin or a β-lactam antibiotic with anti-β-lactamase activity (e.g. amoxicillin–clavulanate) (Lipsky et al. 2012). In cases where colonization with multiresistant organisms may be anticipated, a carbapenem, such as imipenem or meropenem, might be an option (Lipsky et al. 2012a). For PEDIS grade 3 infection hospitalization is often necessary for surgical or diagnostic procedures or for initial parenteral administration of antibiotics. Inappropriate management of the patients with PEDIS 3 infections resulted in more proximal amputations in up to 10% of cases (Lipsky 1999). Antimicrobial regimens should be as narrow spectrum as possible and adjusted based on the results of cultures (and Gram-stains) and clinical response. The duration of therapy depends on infection severity, clinical response, the need for surgical intervention such as vascular reconstruction or debridement and the presence of osteomyelitis, but is usually not longer than 2–3 weeks (Lipsky et al. 2012a, Johnson et al. 2013).

Severe infections

The treatment of severe or grade 4 PEDIS infections is essentially the same as for moderate infections. The main difference is that the patients are systemically ill, and obligate anaerobe organisms and bacteria resistant to antibiotics are more likely to play a role (Lipsky 1999, Lipsky et al. 2012a and 2012b) Given the serious nature of the infection, the anticipated high bacterial load, and uncertain gastrointestinal absorption in systemic illness, antibiotics prescribed in these patients should generally be broad spectrum and IV administered (Lipsky et al. 2012 and 2012b).

Switch to oral antibiotics and duration of antibiotic therapy

Initial treatment of moderate and severe infections is often parenteral, as the pathogen load is high, the margins for error are small, and adequate serum levels need to be attained. After the first phase of treatment, when the local and systemic inflammatory signs are responding, a switch to oral antibiotics is often possible. Oral treatment is cheaper, safer, and easier for patients and medical staff. As mentioned earlier, the oral absorption and effectiveness of selected antibiotics is excellent (Embil & Trepman 2006). In one study in osteomyelitis, long-term oral antibiotic treatment seemed an effective alternative to prolonged IV treatment and surgery (Vardakas et al. 2008). No studies are available to the most optimal timing of switch to oral antibiotics (**Table 8.4**).

■ ADJUNCTIVE THERAPY

■ Topical treatment

Most studies of the effectiveness of topical antimicrobial treatment in patients with infected diabetic foot ulcers have used topical agents (e.g. hypochlorite, peroxide, zinc oxide, mafenide acetate, silver dressings, povidone- and cadexomer-iodine solutions, honey) as adjuncts to systemic antimicrobial treatment. No single agent has been proven superior to other agents (Game et al. 2012). Some agents might have nonantimicrobial effects on the process of wound healing itself. Although topical silver is widely used, two recent systematic reviews could not confirm its effectiveness (Bergin & Wraight 2006, Game et al. 2012). Two studies have examined the effect of larvae in diabetic foot ulcers (Game et al. 2012). In one study, conducted in patients with vascular disease, application of larvae seemed to decrease the need for systemic antibiotics and the occurrence of amputations, suggesting both an antibacterial effect and an effect on ulcer healing (Game et al. 2012). Other preclinical studies have suggested both direct antimicrobial and antibiofilm effects of larval application (Game et al. 2012). Although there have been some studies published on negative pressure wound therapy and wound healing, none could be identified on its effectiveness on diabetic foot infections (Game et al. 2012).

■ Hyperbaric oxygen treatment

There is much debate about hyperbaric oxygen treatment of diabetic foot infections. Severe infections with obligate anaerobic bacteria might benefit from this treatment modality, especially in the presence of necrosis or ischemia. In a Cochrane analysis in 2012, it was

Table 8.4 Expert opinion on route, setting, and duration of antibiotic therapy in diabetic foot infection (Lipsky et al. 2012a)

Site and extent of infection	Route of administration	Outpatient or hospitalization	Duration of antibiotic therapy
Soft tissue only			
Mild	Oral	Outpatient	1–2 Weeks (up to 4 weeks if slowly resolving)
Moderate	Oral, or initially parenteral	Outpatient/inpatient	1–3 Weeks (up to 4 weeks if slowly resolving)
Severe	Parenteral, switch to oral when possible	Inpatient, then outpatient	2–4 Weeks
Bone or joint			
No residual infected tissue, e.g. after amputation	Parenteral or oral	-	2–5 Days
Residual infected soft tissue, but not bone	Parenteral or oral	-	1–3 Weeks
Residual infected, but viable bone	Initial parenteral, then consider oral switch	-	4–6 Weeks
No surgery or residual dead bone after surgery	Initial parenteral, then consider oral switch	-	≥3 Months

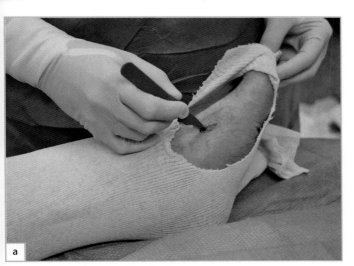

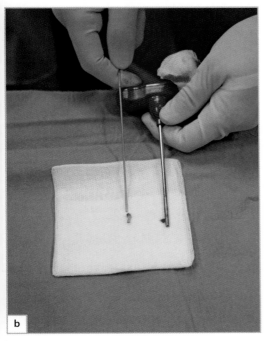

Figure 9.1 (a) Skin incision via a noninfected area prior to the insertion of the bone-cutting needle. (b) Bone fragment obtained by transcutaneous biopsy.

histological examination of the bone samples can be helpful. A study comparing culture to histopathology on 44 surgically obtained bone specimens from patients with DFO found that histological and microbiological examinations performed similarly (Weiner et al. 2011). Given the available data regarding bone biopsy in the management of DFO, it appears that this diagnostic procedure is,overall, a valuable tool for reliably identifying the bacteria involved in the bone infection.

When the severity of the foot infection requires surgical intervention, a bone biopsy should be performed with sterile surgical instruments that have not been used during the debridement in order to reduce the risk of contamination of the samples.

■ Imaging studies

Plain X-rays of the foot are first-line diagnostic tools when DFO is suspected, as they are widely available, repeatable, and relatively inexpensive. Bone abnormalities, especially cortical erosion, periostal reaction, and sometimes fractures (or even bone fragmentation and complete disappearance of osteoarticular structures underlying a soft tissue ulcer) should lead physicians to consider a diagnosis of DFO (**Box 9.1**, **Figure 9.2**). However, a recent meta-analysis reported a pooled sensitivity of 0.54 and pooled specificity of 0.68 of plain X-rays in patients with DFO (Dinh et al. 2008). In addition, it may take 2–4 weeks after the onset of bone disease for osteomyelitis to become evident on plain radiographs (Newman et al. 1991, Sella & Grosser 2003, Shults et al. 1989). Progressive changes seen on serial plain radiographs repeated after 2–4 weeks may have greater sensitivity and specificity but this has never been established in cases of diabetic foot osteomyelitis (Hartemann-Heurtier & Senneville 2008). The continued absence of any bony abnormalities on repeated radiographs probably excludes osteomyelitis. Another limitation of plain X-rays (as with other current imaging techniques) is the similarity of bone abnormalities seen on both neuro-osteoarthropathy and osteomyelitis.

Radioisotope scans (leukocyte or antigranulocyte scan) are more sensitive than radiographs for detecting early osteomyelitis but unfortunately they are rather nonspecific (Sella & Grosser 2003) and have been shown to be less specific than MRI (Kapoor et al. 2007). The best techniques are either labeled leukocyte (with ^{99m}Tc or ^{111}In) or antigranulocyte Fab fragment (e.g. sulesomab). They are limited by their availability, complexity (may take >2 days to be completed), need for blood manipulation, and costs (Schweitzer et al. 2008).

MRI is currently considered the most accurate imaging study for defining bone infection (Chatha et al. 2005, Kapoor et al. 2007,

free period appear to be optimal in avoiding false-negative cultures but must be weighed against the risk of progressive infection in the absence of treatment. While not always necessary, percutaneous bone biopsy should preferably be done under fluoroscopic or CT guidance by traversing uninfected skin if possible, taking at least two specimens, one for culture and another for histological analysis (White et al. 1995). When undertaken by trained physicians, percutaneous bone biopsy appears to be a safe procedure (Senneville et al. 2008, 2009).

Even when performed using the results of previous imaging studies and real-time fluoroscopic guidance, percutaneous bone biopsy may miss the area of active osteomyelitis, giving a potentially false-negative result. In a recent retrospective study, it was shown, however, that of patients with diabetes with the suspicion of osteomyelitis and a negative percutaneous bone biopsy, only one in four developed osteomyelitis within 2 years of the biopsy (Senneville et al. 2012). However, preventive antiseptic measures may not always prevent contamination of the bone samples during the biopsy procedure, giving a potentially false-positive result. In light of these deficiencies,

---

Box 9.1 Features of osteomyelitis on plain radiography

- Periosteal reaction or elevation
- Loss of cortex with bony erosion
- Focal loss of trabecular pattern or marrow radiolucency
- New bone formation
- Bone sclerosis with or without erosion
- Sequestrum
  - Devitalized bone with radiodense appearance that has become separated from normal bone
- Involucrum
  - A layer of new bone growth outside existing bone resulting from the elevation of the periosteum from the cortex and new bone growing beneath
- Cloaca
  - Opening in involucrum or cortex through which sequestra or granulation tissue may be discharged

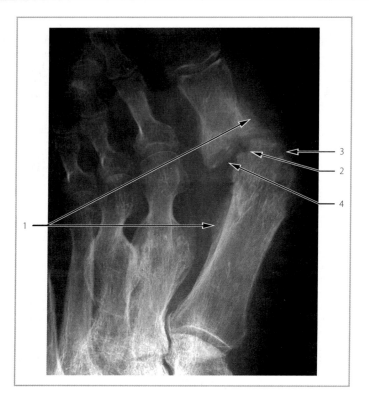

Figure 9.2 Plain X-ray of the left foot in a patient with diabetes with a chronic ulcer of the plantar surface showing (1) periosteal reaction, (2) disappearance of the distal part of the 1st metatarsal bone, (3) cortical erosion, and (4) joint dislocation.

Schweitzer et al. 2008), but it requires well-trained and experienced 'readers' to interpret the scans obtained. When compared with other imaging techniques, MRI provides the best sensitivity and specificity for the detection of DFO with values established in two recent meta-analyses as high as respectively 90% and 79–82.5% (Dinh et al. 2008, Kapoor et al. 2007).

The UK NICE guidelines recommend that when DFO is suspected but not confirmed by initial plain radiographs, clinicians should use MRI or, if unavailable or contraindicated, white blood cell scanning (Tan et al. 2011). MRI has an advantage over other imaging techniques in that it provides data on soft tissue infection, including sinus tracts and tissue necrosis (Kapoor et al. 2007). There is no specificity of DFO in the bone changes except for the difficulties in distinguishing DFO from the neuroarthropathic foot (Charcot foot) (Berendt & Lipsky 2004). MRI may provide information that is useful when selecting the most appropriate surgical option (Tomas et al. 2000). Its use may, however, be limited by its low availability in some centers and difficulties in interpreting the findings.

The distinction between osteomyelitis and diabetic neuro-osteoarthropathy (Charcot foot) may be particularly difficult, and requires consideration of the overall clinical and imaging information (Schweitzer & Morrison 2004). Clinical clues supporting neuro-osteoarthropathy in this context include a midfoot location and the absence of a soft tissue wound, while those favoring osteomyelitis include the presence of an overlying ulcer (Tan & Teh 2007). Consultation with an experienced musculoskeletal radiologist to distinguish between these entities is of major importance (Berendt et al. 2008).

In preliminary studies, fluorodeoxyglucose positron emission tomography has a better accuracy for confirming or excluding a diagnosis of chronic osteomyelitis than MRI, but its role in patients with diabetes is not yet established (Termaat et al. 2005) (**Box 9.2**).

Box 9.2 Features of osteomyelitis on magnetic resonance imaging (MRI)

- Low focal signal intensity on T1-weighted images
- High focal signal on T2-weighted images
- High short tau inversion recovery (STIR) sequences in bone marrow
- Less specific or secondary changes:
  - Cortical disruption
  - Adjacent cutaneous ulcer
  - Soft tissue mass
  - Sinus tract
  - Adjacent soft tissue inflammation or edema

■ Classification

Osteomyelitis is defined as an inflammatory process in bone that is caused by microorganism infection and causes osseous fragmentation and overall destruction of the skeletal architecture (Berendt et al. 2008, Jeffcoate & Lipsky 2004, Jeffcoate et al. 2008, Lew & Waldvogel 1997, 2004). According to the Waldvogel classification (Waldvogel et al. 1970), DFO appears to be both an osteomyelitis associated with a contiguous focus and a chronic osteomyelitis. The Cierny-Mader classification is based on both the anatomy of bone infection and the physiology of the host (Cierny & Mader 1987, Cierny et al. 2003). It has been suggested that this classification may be less helpful in classifying DFO, especially in cases where there is involvement of the small bones in the foot (Lew & Waldvogel 2004).

According to recent studies reported by Aragon-Sanchez, three types of osteomyelitis can be found in the diabetic foot: acute, chronic, and acute exacerbation of chronic osteomyelitis (Aragon-Sanchez et al. 2008). In their report, the different histopathological types of osteomyelitis were related to the white blood cell count, successful conservative surgery, and minor amputations. Histopathological findings have been correlated to the MRI results (Craig et al. 1997). In a multivariate analysis, the histopathological type of osteomyelitis was not an independent risk factor for the risk of failure of conservative surgery.

There is currently no classification of DFO that would help to select the most appropriate therapeutic approach to the patient or predict the outcome regarding the risk of amputation of the limb or recurrence of DFO. The sensitivity/specificity, diagnostic odds ratio and likelihood ratio of some clinical, biological and imaging tests for DFO are reported in **Table 9.2**.

More recently, Aragon Sanchez (2012) has proposed a separation of DFO into four classes:

- Class I: without ischemia and soft tissue involvement
- Class II: with ischemia and without soft tissue involvement
- Class III: with soft tissue involvement
- Class IV: with ischemia and soft tissue involvement

This study showed a statistically significant trend toward increased severity (i.e. from class I to class IV) and increased amputation rate and mortality (**Table 9.3**). However, as stated by the author, the diagnosis of deep tissue infection associated with DFO may be difficult to achieve before surgery, which makes this classification more useful for conducting clinical research studies than for helping a physician to choose the most appropriate treatment strategy for a given patient prior to surgery.

Table 9.2 Accuracy of diagnostic tests for diabetic foot osteomyelitis

Diagnostic test	Sensitivity (%)	Specificity (%)	Diagnostic odds ratio	Likelihood ratio
Exposed bone or probe-to-bone test	60	91	49	6.4*
Ulcer area >2 cm²	NA	NA	NA	7.2
Erythrocyte sedimentation rate >70 mm/h	NA	NA	NA	11
Plain radiography	54	68	2.8	2.3
Magnetic resonance imaging	90	79	24	3.8
Bone scan	81	28	2.1	NA
Leukocyte scan	74	68	10	NA

Data derived from Dinh et al. (2008).

Sensitivity: total number of infected patients divided by the number of patients with true positive test results

Specificity: total number of uninfected persons divided by the number of persons with negative test results

Diagnostic test ratio: ratio of the odds of the test being positive if the subject has the disease relative to the odds of the test being positive if the subject does not have the disease.

Likelihood ratio of predicting presence of osteomyelitis, based on test abnormality; data from Butalia et al. (2008).

*Probe-to-bone test only.

NA, not available.

Table 9.3 Classification of diabetic foot osteomyelitis. Increased class level is associated with significantly increased severity of infection and risk of amputation and mortality.

Class	Osteomyelitis	Ischemia	Soft tissue involvement
I	Yes	No	No
II	Yes	Yes	No
III	Yes	No	Yes
IV	Yes	Yes	Yes

Adapted from Aragón-Sánchez (2012).

CONCLUSIONS

Bone involvement secondary to the spread of infection of a foot ulcer in a person with diabetes is rarely a situation that needs urgent surgery or antibiotic therapy. However, data issued from the clinical experience and the current literature show that this complication is clearly associated with a high risk of failure, relapses, and limb amputation even in the absence of impaired limb perfusion. Additional studies are needed to clarify the place of the different imaging techniques and to what extent they can impact the management of patients with DFO.

AREAS OF CONTROVERSY AND/OR FUTURE RESEARCH

- The best combination of clinical factors and imaging to most reliably diagnose osteomyelitis needs to be confirmed
- The role of bone biopsy in everyday clinical practice should be more clearly defined
- The reliability of bone histology in the diagnosis of osteomyelitis requires further investigation
- Research is need to confirm whether bone biopsy-directed antibiotic regimens improve outcomes compared with empirical or deep wound culture regimens
- Will fluorodeoxyglucose positron emission tomography prove more accurate than MRI in confirming or excluding chronic osteomyelitis?
- Are current classification schemes helpful in the prognosis and management of osteomyelitis in everyday clinical practice?

IMPORTANT FURTHER READING

Aragón-Sánchez FJ. Pathological characterization of diabetic foot infections: grading the severity of osteomyelitis. Lower extremity wounds. Int J Clinical 2012; 11:107–112.

Berendt AR, Peters EJ, Bakker K, et al. Diabetic foot osteomyelitis: a progress report on diagnosis and a systematic review of treatment. Diabetes Metab Res Rev 2008; 24:S145–161.

Butalia S, Palda VA, Sargeant RJ, et al. Does this patient with diabetes have osteomyelitis of the lower extremity? JAMA 2008; 299:806–813.

Dinh MT, Abad CL, Safdar N. Diagnostic accuracy of the physical examination and imaging tests for osteomyelitis underlying diabetic foot ulcers: meta-analysis. Clin Infect Dis 2008; 47:519–527.

Senneville E, Gaworowska D, Topolinski H, et al. Outcome of patients with diabetes with negative percutaneous bone biopsy performed for suspicion of osteomyelitis of the foot. Diabet Med 2012; 29:56–61.

Senneville E, Melliez H, Beltrand E, et al. Culture of percutaneous bone biopsy specimens for diagnosis of diabetic foot osteomyelitis: concordance with ulcer swab cultures. Clin Infect Dis 2006; 42:57–62.

REFERENCES

Aragón-Sánchez FJ. Pathological characterization of diabetic foot infections: grading the severity of osteomyelitis. Lower extremity wounds. Int J Clinical 2012; 11:107–112.

Aragón-Sánchez FJ, Cabrera-Galván JJ, Quintana-Marrero Y, et al. Outcomes of surgical treatment of diabetic foot osteomyelitis: a series of 185 patients with histopathological confirmation of bone involvement. Diabetologia 2008; 51:1962–1970.

Aragon-Sanchez J, Lipsky BA, Lazaro-Martinez JL. Diagnosing diabetic foot osteomyelitis: is the combination of probe-to-bone test and plain radiography sufficient for high-risk inpatients? Diabet Med 2011; 28:191–194.

Armstrong DG, Harkless LB. Outcomes of preventative care in a diabetic foot specialty clinic. J Foot Ankle Surg 1998; 37:460–466.

Berendt AR, Peters EJ, Bakker K, et al. Specific guidelines for treatment of diabetic foot osteomyelitis. Diabetes Metab Res Rev 2008; 24:S190–191.

Berendt AR, Lipsky B. Is this bone infected or not? Differentiating neuro-osteoarthropathy from osteomyelitis in the diabetic foot. Curr Diab Rep 2004; 4:424–429.

Berendt AR, Peters EJ, Bakker K, et al. Diabetic foot osteomyelitis: a progress report on diagnosis and a systematic review of treatment. Diabetes Metab Res Rev 2008; 24:S145–161.

Chantelau E, Wolf A, Ozdemir S, Hachmoller A, Ramp U. Bone histomorphology may be unremarkable in diabetes mellitus. Med Klin (Munich) 2007; 102:429–433.

Chatha DS, Cunningham PM, Schweitzer ME. MR imaging of the diabetic foot: diagnostic challenges. Radiol Clin North Am 2005; 43:747–759.

Cierny G 3rd, Mader JT, Penninck JJ. A clinical staging system for adult osteomyelitis. Clin Orthop Relat Res 2003; 414:7–24.

Cierny G 3rd, Mader JT. Approach to adult osteomyelitis. Orthop Rev 1987; 16:259–270.

Craig JG, Amin MB, Wu K, et al. Osteomyelitis of the diabetic foot: MR imaging--pathologic correlation. Radiology 1997; 203:849–855.

Dinh MT, Abad CL, Safdar N. Diagnostic accuracy of the physical examination and imaging tests for osteomyelitis underlying diabetic foot ulcers: meta-analysis. Clin Infect Dis 2008; 47:519–527.

Eckman MH, Greenfield S, Mackey WC, et al. Foot infections in diabetic patients. Decision and cost-effectiveness analyses. JAMA 1995; 273:712–720.

Elamurugan TP, Jaqdish S, Kate V, Chandra Parija S et al. Role of bone biopsy specimen culture in the management of diabetic foot osteomyelitis. Int J Surg 2011; 9:214–216.

Embil JM. The management of diabetic foot osteomyelitis. The Diabetic Foot 2000; 3:76–84.

Fleischer AE, Didyk AA, Woods JB, et al. Combined clinical and laboratory testing improves diagnostic accuracy for osteomyelitis in the diabetic foot. J Foot Ankle Surg 2009; 48:39–46.

Grayson ML, Gibbons GW, Balogh K, Levin E, Karchmer AW. Probing to bone in infected pedal ulcers. A clinical sign of underlying osteomyelitis in diabetic patients. JAMA 1995; 273:721–723.

Hartemann-Heurtier A, Senneville E. Diabetic foot osteomyelitis. Diabetes Metab 2008; 3:87–95.

Howard CB, Einhorn M, Dagan R, Yagupski P, Porat S. Fine-needle bone biopsy to diagnose osteomyelitis. J Bone Joint Surg Br 1994; 76:311–314.

Jeffcoate WJ, Lipsky BA, Berendt AR, et al. Unresolved issues in the management of ulcers of the foot in diabetes. Diabet Med 2008; 25:1380–1389.

Jeffcoate WJ, Lipsky BA. Controversies in diagnosing and managing osteomyelitis of the foot in diabetes. Clin Infect Dis 2004; 39:S115–S122.

Jeffcoate WJ, Lipsky BA. Controversies in diagnosing and managing osteomyelitis of the foot in diabetes. Clin Infect Dis 2004; 39:S115–122.

Kapoor A, Page S, Lavalley M, Gale DR, Felson DT. Magnetic resonance imaging for diagnosing foot osteomyelitis: a meta-analysis. Arch Intern Med 2007; 167:125–132.

Kessler L, Piemont Y, Ortega F, et al. Comparison of microbiological results of needle puncture vs. superficial swab in infected diabetic foot ulcer with osteomyelitis. Diabet Med 2006; 23:99–102.

Khatri G, Wagner DK, Sohnle PG. Effect of bone biopsy in guiding antimicrobial therapy for osteomyelitis complicating open wounds. Am J Med Sci 2001; 321:367–371.

Lavery LA, Sariaya M, Ashry H, Harkless LB. Microbiology of osteomyelitis in diabetic foot infections. J Foot Ankle Surg 1995; 34:61–64.

Lavery LA, Armstrong DG, Peters EJ, Lipsky BA. Probe-to-bone test for diagnosing diabetic foot osteomyelitis: reliable or relic? Diabetes Care 2007; 30:270–274.

Lavery LA, Peters EJ, Armstrong DG, et al. Risk factors for developing osteomyelitis in patients with diabetic foot wounds. Diabetes Res Clin Pract 2009; 83:347–352.

Ledermann HP, Schweitzer ME, Morrison WB. Nonenhancing tissue on MR imaging of pedal infection: characterization of necrotic tissue and associated limitations for diagnosis of osteomyelitis and abscess. AJR Am J Roentgenol 2002; 178:215–222.

Lesens O, Desbiez F, Vidal M, et al. Culture of per-wound bone specimens: a simplified approach for the medical management of diabetic foot osteomyelitis. Clin Microbiol Infect 2011; 17:285–291.

Lew DP, Waldvogel FA. Osteomyelitis. Lancet 2004; 364:369–379.

Lew DP, Waldvogel FA. Osteomyelitis. N Engl J Med 1997; 336:999–1007.

Lipsky BA, Peters EJ, Berendt AR, et al. International Working Group on Diabetic Foot. Specific guidelines for the treatment of diabetic foot infections 2011. Diabetes Metab Res Rev 2012; 28:234–235.

Lipsky BA. A report from the international consensus on diagnosing and treating the infected diabetic foot. Diabetes Metab Res Rev 2004; 20:S68–77.

Lipsky BA. Osteomyelitis of the foot in diabetic patients. Clin Infect Dis 1997; 25:1318–1326.

Mader JT, Ortiz M, Calhoun JH. Update on the diagnosis and management of osteomyelitis. Clin Podiatr Med Surg 1996; 13:701–724.

Morales Lozano R, González Fernández ML, Martinez Hernández D. Validating the probe-to-bone and other tests for diagnosing chronic osteomyelitis in the diabetic foot. Diabetes Care 2010; 33:2140–2145.

Newman LG, Waller J, Palestro CJ, et al. Unsuspected osteomyelitis in diabetic foot ulcers. Diagnosis and monitoring by leukocyte scanning with indium in 111 oxyquinoline. JAMA 1991; 266:1246–1251.

Rajbhandari SM, Sutton M, Davies C, Tesfaye S, Ward JD. 'Sausage toe': a reliable sign of underlying osteomyelitis. Diabet Med 2000; 17:74–77.

Schweitzer ME, Morrison WB. MR imaging of the diabetic foot. Radiol Clin North Am 2004; 42:61–71.

Schweitzer ME, Daffner RH, Weissman BN, et al. ACR Appropriateness Criteria on suspected osteomyelitis in patients with diabetes mellitus. J Am Coll Radiol 2008; 5:881–886.

Sella EJ, Grosser DM. Imaging modalities of the diabetic foot. Clin Podiatr Med Surg 2003; 20:729–740.

Senneville E, Gaworowska D, Topolinski H, et al. Outcome of patients with diabetes with negative percutaneous bone biopsy performed for suspicion of osteomyelitis of the foot. Diabet Med 2012; 29:56–61.

Senneville E, Melliez H, Beltrand E, et al. Culture of percutaneous bone biopsy specimens for diagnosis of diabetic foot osteomyelitis: concordance with ulcer swab cultures. Clin Infect Dis 2006; 42: 57–62.

Senneville E, Morant H, Descamps D, et al. Needle puncture and transcutaneous bone biopsy cultures are inconsistent in patients with diabetes and suspected osteomyelitis of the foot. Clin Infect Dis 2009; 48:888–893.

Senneville E, Lombart A, Beltrand E, et al. Outcome of diabetic foot osteomyelitis treated nonsurgically: a retrospective cohort study. Diabetes Care 2008; 31:637–642.

Shone A, Burnside J, Chipchase S, Game F, Jeffcoate W. Probing the validity of the probe-to-bone test in the diagnosis of osteomyelitis of the foot in diabetes. Diabetes Care 2006; 29:945.

Shults DW, Hunter GC, McIntyre KE, et al. Value of radiographs and bone scans in determining the need for therapy in diabetic patients with foot ulcers. Am J Surg 1989; 158:525–529.

Slater RA, Lazarovitch T, Boldur I, et al. Swab cultures accurately identify bacterial pathogens in diabetic foot wounds not involving bone. Diabet Med 2004; 21:705–709.

Snyder RJ, Cohen MM, Sun C, Livingston J. Osteomyelitis in the diabetic patient: diagnosis and treatment. Part 2: Medical, surgical, and alternative treatments. Ostomy Wound Manage 2001; 47:24–30.

Tan T, Shaw EJ, Siddiqui F, et al. Guideline Development Group. Inpatient management of diabetic foot problems: summary of NICE guidance. BMJ 2011; 23:342.

Tan JS, File TM Jr. Diagnosis and treatment of diabetic foot infections. Baillieres Best Pract Res Clin Rheumatol 1999; 13:149–161.

Tan PL, Teh J. MRI of the diabetic foot: differentiation of infection from neuropathic change. Br J Radiol 2007; 80:939–948.

Termaat MF, Raijmakers PG, Scholten HJ, et al. The accuracy of diagnostic imaging for the assessment of chronic osteomyelitis: a systematic review and meta-analysis. J Bone Joint Surg Am 2005; 87:2464–2471.

Tomas MB, Patel M, Marwin SE, Palestro CJ. The diabetic foot. Br J Radiol 2000; 73:443–450.

Waldvogel FA, Medoff G, Swartz MN. Osteomyelitis: a review of clinical features, therapeutic considerations and unusual aspects. 3. Osteomyelitis associated with vascular insufficiency. N Engl J Med 1970; 282:316–322.

Weiner RD, Viselli SJ, Fulkert KA, Accetta P. Histology versus microbiology for accuracy in identification of osteomyelitis in the diabetic foot. J Foot Ankle Surg 2011; 50:197–200.

Wheat J. Diagnostic strategies in osteomyelitis. Am J Med 1985; 78:218–224.

White LM, Schweitzer ME, Deely DM, Gannon F. Study of osteomyelitis: utility of combined histologic and microbiologic evaluation of percutaneous biopsy samples. Radiology 1995; 197:840–842.

Zuluaga AF, Galvis W, Jaimes F, Vesga O. Lack of microbiological concordance between bone and non-bone specimens in chronic osteomyelitis: an observational study. BMC Infect Dis 2002; 2:8.

Chapter 10   Osteomyelitis: medical management

John M. A. Embil, Elly Trepman

SUMMARY

- Some patients with diabetes and foot osteomyelitis may respond to medical therapy without surgery. Osteomyelitis can be controlled successfully in 60% cases with antibiotic treatment, alone or in combination with surgery
- The probe-to-bone test for any diabetic foot infection with an open wound can help diagnose or exclude osteomyelitis
- Plain radiographs have low sensitivity and specificity for osteomyelitis, but serial radiographs may be helpful for diagnosis and monitoring. Magnetic resonance imaging (MRI) is the study of choice when diagnosis of osteomyelitis is equivocal from plain radiographs
- Empiric antimicrobial treatment regimens should include agents with activity against the staphylococci. The decision to target methicillin-resistant *Staphylococcus aureus* (MRSA) is based upon knowledge of the local epidemiology and whenever possible, antibiotic treatment should be based upon the results of a bone culture
- There are currently insufficient data to favor either intravenous or oral route for antibiotics, or to provide guidance for duration of antibiotic treatment
- The route of therapy may be determined by the severity of the patient's condition and extent of the infection
- Surgical debridement of necrotic bone may facilitate resolution of infection

INTRODUCTION

Historically, osteomyelitis was considered primarily a surgical disease. Antimicrobials were associated with poor bone penetration and poor outcomes when used as the only treatment modality for osteomyelitis. However, more recent reports have been published that have caused physicians to challenge the assumption that osteomyelitis may be treated successfully only by removal or extensive debridement of infected bones. Authors of these reports have challenged the apparently successful outcomes of surgery. They have suggested that successful antibiotic therapy may be the result of improved antimicrobial agents and regimens, better patient selection, improved bioavailability of antimicrobials, and longer duration of therapy.

INDICATIONS FOR MEDICAL THERAPY

Antimicrobial therapy is indicated for patients with established or suspected diabetic foot infection including osteomyelitis. Optimal treatment may include antibiotics selected to cover pathogenic organisms identified on cultures from infected overlying soft tissue, bone, or blood. However, in the absence of culture results, empiric antibiotics are indicated in patients who have clinical signs of infection, such as fever, chills, rigors, erythema, swelling, ulcer wound drainage, or imaging signs of infection, including infected bone or abscess. Whenever possible, a specimen should be obtained for culture to help guide antimicrobial therapy.

PATIENT SELECTION

Some patients with diabetes and foot osteomyelitis may respond to medical therapy without surgery. However, no specific rules are available to guide the clinician to identify patients who may be treated successfully without surgery. Intuitively, medical therapy alone is less likely to be successful in the presence of necrotic tissue or sequestrum, foul smelling tissue, purulent drainage, or abscess. In addition, patient factors may help guide which therapeutic options can be pursued, including the ability of the patient to adhere to therapeutic regimens and tolerate oral or parenteral therapy, antimicrobial susceptibility profiles for pathogens recovered from the affected area, vascular status of the patient, and magnitude of the affected area (Lipsky et al. 2004a, Lipsky et al. 2012a). However, antibiotics are important even in those patients with osteomyelitis who are managed primarily with surgery (debridement or removal of infected bone).

DIAGNOSIS

Sinus tract or surface wound swab cultures are unreliable and do not provide accurate information about the pathogen involved in the underlying bone infection (Mackowiak et al. 1978, Elamurugan et al. 2011). The bone pathogen is identified from a superficial swab culture in only 38% patients with diabetes and foot osteomyelitis (Elamurugan et al. 2011), and therefore using these data on which to base antimicrobial therapy is unreliable.

The most definitive approach to make the diagnosis of osteomyelitis is to use the combination of bone culture and histology (Lipsky et al. 2012a). Bone culture and histology are equally effective at confirming the presence of diabetic foot osteomyelitis (Weiner et al. 2011). However, bone histology is dependent on the accuracy of interpretation by the pathologist; a difference in interpretation of histologic specimens by different pathologists, with two pathologists differing between presence or absence of osteomyelitis, may occur in 41% patients who have undergone bone biopsy for suspected diabetic foot osteomyelitis (Meyr et al. 2011).

When bone debridement is not performed, a diagnostic bone biopsy may be done to address diagnostic uncertainty, inadequate culture information, or failure to respond to empiric therapy (Lipsky et al. 2012a). This may be done percutaneously through a small incision or at the time of surgical debridement. In some patients who have persistent clinical signs of infection despite a negative percutaneous bone biopsy, repeat biopsy may confirm the presence of osteomyelitis (Senneville et al. 2012).

TREATMENT REGIMENS

Dilemmas in treating diabetic foot osteomyelitis include (1) optimal route of antibiotic treatment (oral or intravenous) and (2) duration of antibiotic therapy. Limited reliable data are available on which to assess the efficacy of local antimicrobial administration such as installation of antibiotics into wound beds or the use of antibiotic impregnated beads. Empiric therapy may depend on multiple factors including severity of infection, local antimicrobial epidemiology, renal function, and clinical response (**Table 10.1**).

Diabetic foot infections frequently are polymicrobial (Wheat et al. 1986). Chronic or previously treated diabetic foot infections typically are polymicrobial and may include aerobic gram-positive cocci and aerobic gram-negative bacilli or anaerobes (Lipsky et al. 1990). In diabetic foot osteomyelitis, the most common organisms isolated are *Staphylococcus aureus* followed by other aerobic gram-positive

cocci (Lipsky 1997). Most cases of diabetic foot osteomyelitis are polymicrobial and may include *S. aureus* (50%), *S. epidermidis* (25%), streptococci (30%), and enterobacteriaceae (40%) (Lipsky 1997, Lipsky et al. 2012b). In addition, microorganisms that frequently are not considered pathogenic in other circumstances may cause diabetic foot osteomyelitis (Hunt 1992).

Treatment regimens for diabetic foot osteomyelitis vary widely. Some centers use intravenous antibiotics for 2 to 6 weeks followed by a long course of oral antibiotics, and others use shorter courses of parenteral therapy or oral antibiotics alone (Embil et al. 2006, Byren et al. 2009).

There is a lack of data from clinical trials about the most appropriate antimicrobial agents, and no specific antimicrobial regimen is most effective for diabetic foot osteomyelitis (Berendt et al. 2008a, 2008b). However, empiric antimicrobial therapy initially may target the most likely pathogens, and subsequent therapy may be modified after culture results become available. Empiric regimens include coverage against staphylococci, with or without coverage for MRSA, depending on local prevalence of MRSA (Berendt et al. 2008a, 2008b, Lagacé-Wiens et al. 2009, Lipsky et al. 2012b).

Adequate antimicrobial bone levels can be achieved with intravenous antibiotics or highly bioavailable oral agents; no data support an advantage of either intravenous or oral route for the treatment of diabetic foot osteomyelitis, or provide guidelines for duration of antimicrobial treatment (Berendt et al. 2008a, 2008b). However, bone concentrations and adverse reactions of antibiotics vary (Rao et al. 2011), and treatment with highly bioavailable oral antibiotics may be as effective as parenteral therapy (Spellberg & Lipsky 2012).

It is currently recommended that antibiotic treatment for diabetic foot osteomyelitis be based, if possible, on results of a bone culture. Approximately, two thirds of cases of diabetic foot osteomyelitis can be arrested or cured with antibiotics alone (without surgery) and antibiotics given at doses higher than usual for 2 to 6 months. However, many patients can be switched to oral therapy after 1 week of intravenous antibiotics, and a short course of antibiotics (2–14 days) may be considered in patients who have had complete surgical debridement of all infected tissue (Embil et al. 2006, Lipsky et al. 2012b).

A review of > 90 clinical trials performed over 30 years showed that the available literature does not provide adequate validated information about optimal antibiotic agent, route, or duration (Lazzarini et al. 2005). This review suggested that the outcomes were better for acute than chronic osteomyelitis, but there was no evidence in favor of intravenous or oral antibiotics (Lazzarini et al. 2005). In a review of > 7500 published articles about the treatment of foot infection in diabetes, there were seven studies that compared different antibiotic regimens for infections of soft tissue and bone; however, there were no published data that confirmed the superiority of any particular route of antibiotic delivery or duration of therapy (Peters et al. 2012). One study reported better clinical outcome with cefoxitin than with ampicillin/sulbactam (Erstad & McIntyre 1997), but other studies did not demonstrate a difference between antibiotic regimens (Peters et al. 2012). There has been only one randomized trial available that compared oral and intravenous antibiotics, and this showed comparable cure rates with oral and intravenous antibiotics (Lipsky et al. 2004b, Berendt et al. 2008a). Oral therapy with fluoroquinolones for chronic osteomyelitis may be curative in 60% to 80% patients, and treatment outcome may be better with combination therapy that includes oral rifampin (Spellberg & Lipsky 2012). However, further study is needed about rifampin in

Table 10.1 Empiric therapy for osteomyelitis in the diabetic foot*

Osteomyelitis	Antimicrobial agent†
• Treated with intravenous therapy or long-term oral antimicrobial therapy with agents that are well absorbed from the gastrointestinal tract and have good distribution to bone and tissue • Surgical debridement is indicated for the removal of necrotic debris, abscess, or sequestrum • If MRSA is present or suspected, addition of vancomycin, or linezolid, may be considered	Oral options • Cloxacillin • Cephalexin • TMP-SMX • Clindamycin • Amoxicillin-clavulanic acid • Linezolid • Doxycycline • TMP-SMX and metronidazole or clindamycin • Levofloxacin or ciprofloxacin and metronidazole or clindamycin Parenteral options • Combination of β-lactam antibiotic and β-lactamase inhibitor (piperacillin and tazobactam) • Clindamycin and third-generation cephalosporin (i.e. cefotaxime, ceftriaxone, or ceftazidime) • Carbapenem (i.e. imipenem/cilastatin, meropenem, ertapenem, or doripenem) • Tigecycline

MRSA, methicillin-resistant *Staphylococcus aureus*; TMP-SMX, trimethoprim-sulfamethoxazole.

*Adapted with permission from Embil and Trepman (2012). Antibacterial therapy should always be guided by available culture results. If in doubt about the most appropriate antimicrobial regimen, discussion with an infectious diseases consultant may be prudent.

†Dosage may depend on renal function and drug levels. Prior to initiating antimicrobial therapy, verify creatinine clearance and modify dose and interval accordingly.

The agents suggested in this section are for empiric therapy prior to the availability of final culture and susceptibility results. Knowledge of local epidemiology must also guide therapeutic choices, and some agents (β-lactams) are ineffective against methicillin-resistant *Staphylococcus aureus* (MRSA).

Many of the agents identified in this table do not have a specific Food and Drug Administration (FDA) indication for the management of diabetic foot infections including osteomyelitis but may have an indication for the management of skin and soft tissue infections or may have antimicrobial activity effective against the typical pathogens encountered in osteomyelitis of the diabetic foot. Therapy must be refined on the basis of the final culture and susceptibility profiles for the pathogens recovered.

Duration of therapy is based on clinical response. However, typical treatment courses for skin and soft tissue infections range from 7 (mild) to 21 (severe) days, and the treatment of osteomyelitis may require 4–6 weeks of parenteral or several months of oral antimicrobial therapy. Whenever possible it is desirable to switch to oral antimicrobial therapy to avoid complications from parenteral administration.

treating diabetic foot osteomyelitis because rifampin may interact with multiple drugs. Rifampin should usually not be used as the only antimicrobial agent, because it is associated with the development of marked frequency of resistance.

Surgical debridement may not be necessary routinely in treating diabetic foot osteomyelitis, but debridement of necrotic bone may facilitate resolution of infection (Berendt et al. 2008a). After radical surgical debridement, antibiotics may be used for a short period (2-5 days); when there is persistent infected or necrotic bone, a prolonged course of antibiotics (≥4 week) may be used (Lipsky et al. 2004a, Byren et al. 2009, Lipsky et al. 2012a). However, residual osteomyelitis at the margin of debridement of diabetic foot osteomyelitis may be associated with a significantly increased risk of treatment failure and amputation (Kowalski et al. 2011). Furthermore, revascularization may be considered when ischemia is present (Berendt et al. 2008a, 2008b).

Response to antibiotic therapy is monitored by clinical examination, laboratory tests [erythrocyte sedimentation rate (ESR) and C-reactive protein (CRP)], and radiographic studies. Satisfactory response to treatment is evidenced by resolution of clinical findings (swelling, erythema, and wound drainage), wound healing, and improvement of the elevated white blood cell count, ESR, and CRP. Serial plain radiographs may show improvement of soft tissue swelling and bone remodeling. Further investigation, including repeat MRI, is indicated when the clinical course is prolonged or exacerbated.

Currently, there is insufficient evidence to support the use of adjunctive treatments such as hyperbaric oxygen, growth factors, larval therapy, granulocyte colony stimulating factor, or vacuum-assisted closure in the treatment of diabetic foot osteomyelitis (Berendt et al. 2008a, 2008b, Lipsky et al. 2012a).

OUTCOMES OF MEDICAL THERAPY

Diabetic foot osteomyelitis can be successfully controlled in 60% cases with antibiotic treatment, alone or in combination with surgery (Berendt et al. 2008a). Amputation may be required in 5% to 10% cases treated with antibiotics alone (Berendt et al. 2008a).

A meta-analysis of eight small clinical trials (228 patients) about treatment of chronic osteomyelitis (nondiabetic) showed that there was no significant difference in frequency of remission of osteomyelitis between patients treated with oral or parenteral antibiotics; however, trials of diabetic osteomyelitis were excluded from this meta-analysis, and the results may not be applicable to diabetic foot osteomyelitis (Conterno & da Silva Filho 2009).

Failure of treatment of diabetic foot infections is significantly more likely when there is growth of resistant organisms (Ertugrul et al. 2012). Presence of ischemia may also worsen the prognosis (Edmonds 2009).

AREAS OF CONTROVERSY AND/OR FUTURE RESEARCH

- The duration of therapy and route of antibiotic administration for osteomyelitis should be confirmed
- The optimum antimicrobial regimens for osteomyelitis require further investigation
- The utility of local administration of antimicrobial therapy (e.g. antibiotic beads) should be studied
- The selection of patients who will respond favorably to primarily nonsurgical management of osteomyelitis is important
- The indications for and timing of surgical intervention in patients with osteomyelitis are important

IMPORTANT FURTHER READING

Embil JM, Trepman E. Diabetic foot infections. In: McKean SC, Ross JJ, Dressler DD, et al. (eds), Principles and practice of hospital medicine. New York: American College of Physicians and McGraw-Hill; 2012:1162–1169, Chapter 145.

Game FL, Jeffcoate WJ. Primarily non-surgical management of osteomyelitis of the foot in diabetes. Diabetologia 2008; 51:962–967.

Lipsky BA, Berendt AR, Cornia PB, et al. Executive summary: 2012 Infectious Diseases Society of America clinical practice guideline for the diagnosis and treatment of diabetic foot infections. Clin Infect Dis 2012; 54:e132-e173.

Lipsky BA, Peters EJ, Senneville E, et al. Expert opinion on the management of infections in the diabetic foot. Diabetes Metab Res Rev 2012; 28(suppl 1):163–178.

Senneville E, Lombart A, Beltrand E, et al. Outcome of diabetic foot osteomyelitis treated nonsurgically: a retrospective cohort study. Diabetes Care 2008; 31:637–642.

Spellberg B, Lipsky BA. Systemic antibiotic therapy for chronic osteomyelitis in adults. Clin Infect Dis 2012; 54:393–407.

Valabhji J, Oliver N, Samarasinghe D, et al. Conservative management of diabetic forefoot ulceration complicated by underlying osteomyelitis: the benefits of magnetic resonance imaging. Diabet Med 2009; 26:1127–1134.

REFERENCES

Berendt AR, Peters EJ, Bakker K, et al. Diabetic foot osteomyelitis: a progress report on diagnosis and a systematic review of treatment. Diabetes Metab Res Rev 2008a; 24(suppl 1):S145–S161.

Berendt AR, Peters EJ, Bakker K, et al. Specific guidelines for treatment of diabetic foot osteomyelitis. Diabetes Metab Res Rev 2008b; 24(suppl 1):S190–S191.

Byren I, Peters EJ, Hoey C, Berendt A, Lipsky BA. Pharmacotherapy of diabetic foot osteomyelitis. Expert Opin Pharmacother 2009; 10:3033–3047.

Conterno LO, da Silva Filho CR. Antibiotics for treating chronic osteomyelitis in adults. Cochrane Database Syst Rev 2009:CD004439.

Edmonds M. Double trouble: infection and ischemia in the diabetic foot. Int J Low Extrem Wounds 2009; 8:62–63.

Elamurugan TP, Jagdish S, Kate V, Chandra Parija S. Role of bone biopsy specimen culture in the management of diabetic foot osteomyelitis. Int J Surg 2011; 9:214–216.

Embil JM, Rose G, Trepman E, et al. Oral antimicrobial therapy for diabetic foot osteomyelitis. Foot Ankle Int 2006; 27:771–779.

Embil JM, Trepman E. Diabetic foot infections. In: McKean SC, Ross JJ, Dressler DD, et al. (eds), Principles and practice of hospital medicine. New York: American College of Physicians and McGraw-Hill; 2012:1162–1169, Chapter 145.

Erstad BL, McIntyre KE Jr. Prospective, randomized comparison of ampicillin/sulbactam and cefoxitin for diabetic foot infections. Vasc Endovasc Surg 1997; 31:419–426.

Ertugrul BM, Oncul O, Tulek N, et al. A prospective, multi-center study: factors related to the management of diabetic foot infections. Eur J Clin Microbiol Infect Dis 2012; 31:2345–2352.

Hunt JA. Foot infections in diabetes are rarely due to a single microorganism. Diabet Med 1992; 9:749–752.

Kowalski TJ, Matsuda M, Sorenson MD, Gundrum JD, Agger WA. The effect of residual osteomyelitis at the resection margin in patients with surgically treated diabetic foot infection. J Foot Ankle Surg 2011; 50:171–175.

Lagacé-Wiens PR, Ormiston D, Nicolle LE, Hilderman T, Embil J. The diabetic foot clinic: not a significant source for acquisition of methicillin-resistant Staphylococcus aureus. Am J Infect Control 2009; 37:587–589.

Lazzarini L, Lipsky BA, Mader JT. Antibiotic treatment of osteomyelitis: what have we learned from 30 years of clinical trials? Int J Infect Dis 2005; 9:127–38.

Lipsky BA. Osteomyelitis of the foot in diabetic patients. Clin Infect Dis 1997; 25:1318–1326.

Lipsky BA, Berendt AR, Cornia PB, et al. Executive summary: 2012 Infectious Diseases Society of America clinical practice guideline for the diagnosis and treatment of diabetic foot infections. Clin Infect Dis 2012a; 54:e132-e173.

Lipsky BA, Berendt AR, Deery HG, et al. Diagnosis and treatment of diabetic foot infections. Clin Infect Dis 2004a; 39:885–910.

Lipsky BA, Itani K, Norden C, Linezolid Diabetic Foot Infections Study Group. Treating foot infections in diabetic patients: a randomized, multicenter, open-label trial of linezolid versus ampicillin-sulbactam/amoxicillin-clavulanate. Clin Infect Dis 2004b; 38:17–24.

Lipsky BA, Pecoraro RE, Wheat LJ. The diabetic foot. Soft tissue and bone infection. Infect Dis Clin North Am 1990; 4:409–432.

Lipsky BA, Peters EJ, Senneville E, et al. Expert opinion on the management of infections in the diabetic foot. Diabetes Metab Res Rev 2012b; 28(suppl 1):163–178.

Mackowiak PA, Jones SR, Smith JW. Diagnostic value of sinus-tract cultures in chronic osteomyelitis. JAMA 1978; 239:2772–2775.

Meyr AJ, Singh S, Zhang X, et al. Statistical reliability of bone biopsy for the diagnosis of diabetic foot osteomyelitis. J Foot Ankle Surg 2011; 50:663–667.

Peters EJ, Lipsky BA, Berendt AR, et al. A systematic review of the effectiveness of interventions in the management of infection in the diabetic foot. Diabetes Metab Res Rev 2012; 28(suppl 1):142–162.

Rao N, Ziran BH, Lipsky BA. Treating osteomyelitis: antibiotics and surgery. Plast Reconstr Surg 2011; 127(suppl 1):177S–187S.

Senneville E, Gaworowska D, Topolinski H, et al. Outcome of patients with diabetes with negative percutaneous bone biopsy performed for suspicion of osteomyelitis of the foot. Diabet Med 2012; 29:56–61.

Spellberg B, Lipsky BA. Systemic antibiotic therapy for chronic osteomyelitis in adults. Clin Infect Dis 2012; 54:393–407.

Weiner RD, Viselli SJ, Fulkert KA, Accetta P. Histology versus microbiology for accuracy in identification of osteomyelitis in the diabetic foot. J Foot Ankle Surg 2011; 50:197–200.

Wheat LJ, Allen SD, Henry M, et al. Diabetic foot infections. Bacteriologic analysis. Arch Intern Med 1986; 146:1935–1940.

Chapter 11 Osteomyelitis: surgical management

F. Javier Aragón Sánchez

SUMMARY

- Surgery plays a pivotal role in the management of diabetic foot osteomyelitis
- A variety of surgical techniques may be employed from conservative to more radical approaches, depending on the site and extent of infection, along with soft tissue involvement
- Medical therapy with antibiotics alone is unlikely to be successful when osteomyelitis is associated with severe soft tissue sepsis, abscess, or necrosis
- The outcome from forefoot osteomyelitis is better than that from midfoot or hindfoot osteomyelitis (which are frequently the complications of Charcot deformity)
- Residual bone infection (margin involvement), soft tissue infection, and ischemia are associated with worse outcomes after surgery for osteomyelitis

INTRODUCTION

Osteomyelitis is a common diabetic foot infection. Some authors have reported higher rates of osteomyelitis among patients with diabetic foot infections requiring admission (Eneroth et al. 1999, Aragon-Sanchez et al. 2008, Aragon-Sanchez et al. 2012c).

Despite the importance of diabetic foot osteomyelitis, the best approach for treating patients with a high risk of amputation remains debatable. Traditionally, the type of contiguous, chronic osteomyelitis that occurs in the diabetic foot required all or most of the necrotic bone to be surgically removed. Emerging data suggest newer antibiotic regimens alone may be effective in treating diabetic foot osteomyelitis. However, it remains difficult to predict which patients will benefit from antibiotic therapy alone.

Although osteomyelitis is highly prevalent in patients with diabetic foot infections and surgery has been widely accepted as the main treatment of diabetic foot osteomyelitis, there is some confusion regarding the types of surgical procedures that can be carried out and the outcomes in patients with diabetes and surgically treated foot osteomyelitis.

ANATOMICAL BASIS OF SURGERY FOR DIABETIC FOOT OSTEOMYELITIS

Hematogenous osteomyelitis is rare in adults. Diabetic foot osteomyelitis is invariably associated with ulceration due to polyneuropathy, peripheral arterial disease, or both, and/or penetrating injury inoculating the infection in the bone. Bacteria gain access to bone by contiguous spread, entering from overlying soft tissue and penetrating the cortex before reaching the marrow. The first layer affected by the infection is the periostium (periostitis). Subsequently, the cortical bone may be affected (i.e. osteitis) and if the infection progresses into the bone marrow, osteomyelitis is established. This sequence is very important because soft tissues around the bone may be affected by the infection, and the clinical picture will become very complicated. It is very important to evaluate the point of entry of the infection into the bone to ascertain the anatomical structures involved (Aragon-Sanchez 2010). Before reaching the bone, the infection may involve subcutaneous tissue, aponeurosis, tendons, and the joint. For example, ulcers located on the tip of the toe easily reach bone because only a thin layer of subcutaneous tissue separates the skin and periosteum. Ulcers located in the interphalangeal joint on the dorsum of the toes may easily involve the joint. This is frequently found in cases of digital deformity, such as claw or hammertoes, subject to foot wear related trauma. Another typical location in which the ulcers can easily reach the joint and the bone is the space located between the toes. These ulcers appear on the lateral side of the toes due to high pressure from the adjacent condyle as a result of wearing tight shoes. Lateral deformities such as bunions are high-risk locations for osteomyelitis. Plantar ulcers with osteomyelitis may become especially difficult to treat due to the complex anatomy of this region, which is divided into compartments occupied by structures that may be affected by the infection (see Chapter 28) (Aragon-Sanchez 2011, Aragon-Sanchez et al. 2012d). Before reaching the bone, the infection may involve the tendons inside the compartments and can spread both proximally and distally from the point of entry. The floor of the compartments is the rigid plantar aponeurosis, which is attached to the calcaneus and spreads distally to the toes. The plantar aponeurosis is the outermost fascia and is located beneath the subcutaneous tissue. The medial and central compartments are separated by the medial intermuscular septum, which extends from the medial calcaneal tuberosity to the first metatarsal head. The central and lateral compartments are separated by the lateral intermuscular septum, which extends from the calcaneus to the fifth metatarsal head. The medial compartment contains the flexor hallucis brevis, abductor hallucis, and flexor hallucis longus tendons. The flexor hallucis longus tendon is located between the sesamoid bones below the first metatarsal head. When a plantar ulcer beneath the first metatarsal head is complicated by sesamoid osteomyelitis, it is easy to see inflammatory changes in the tendons. The central compartment contains the flexor digitorus brevis, lumbrical muscles, flexor digitorum longus tendons, and quadratus plantae muscle. The lateral compartment consists of the flexor digiti minimi brevis and abductor digiti minimi. The interosseus compartment is located between the metatarsal bones and contains the interossei muscles. Osteomyelitis of the first ray may spread through the medial compartment; osteomyelitis of the second to fourth ray may spread through the central compartment, whereas those of the fifth ray can move through the lateral compartment (Aragon-Sanchez 2011).

CLINICAL PRESENTATION OF DIABETIC FOOT OSTEOMYELITIS REQUIRING SURGERY

There is general agreement that when the infection is potentially life threatening (severe or PEDIS 4), immediate surgery after appropriate patient resuscitation is indicated (Frykberg et al. 2007). Deep tissue infections generally speaking rarely respond to antimicrobial therapy alone and frequently require surgery. Recently, osteomyelitis was reported to be a severe infection in only 8.6% of a prospective series that included 81 patients with diabetic foot osteomyelitis (Aragon-Sanchez 2012a). The clinical presentation of osteomyelitis varies considerably and is frequently associated with soft tissue infection. In another earlier series, 72.2% of the infected patients had osteomyelitis, of which 21.8% had both osteomyelitis and soft tissue infection (Aragon-Sanchez et al. 2008). Eneroth et al. 1999 found osteomyelitis in 79.3% of a series of 223 consecutive patients with deep foot infections, where it was the most frequent type of infection. In this same group of patients, 50.2% presented only with osteomyelitis and 29.1% both osteomyelitis and deep soft tissue infection. Of those with osteomyelitis only, 73% underwent a surgical procedure, compared with 96% with a deep soft tissue infection and 100% with a combined infection (Eneroth et al. 1999). The presence of bone or joint infection in association with deep foot infection in a patient with diabetes frequently necessitates local aggressive debridement, resection, or partial foot amputation. The types of deep soft tissue infections have been previously reported (Eneroth et al. 1999, Aragon-Sanchez 2012a) and are shown in **Table 11.1**. The presence (and severity) or absence of deep soft tissue infection should be taken into account when dealing with osteomyelitis. Two different clinical presentations of diabetic foot osteomyelitis can be seen in **Figure 11.1**. **Figure 11.1a** – osteomyelitis of the phalanx without soft tissue involvement that could be resolved with surgery without amputation. **Figure 11.1b** demonstrates diabetic foot osteomyelitis accompanied by necrotizing tenosynovitis that required hallux amputation.

Guidelines for treating diabetic foot osteomyelitis suggest urgent surgery for necrotizing fasciitis, deep soft tissue abscesses, or gangrene accompanying osteomyelitis. Nonurgent surgery may be necessary if there is a significant compromise of the soft tissue envelope (Berendt et al. 2008b). When osteomyelitis is not linked to such complicating factors, some researchers advocate antibiotic treatment and others surgery or combined approaches. Currently, there are no studies directly comparing primarily surgical and primarily medical strategies.

Infectious Diseases Society of America guidelines state that there are four situations in which nonsurgical management of osteomyelitis might be considered (Lipsky et al. 2012).

Table 11.1 Soft tissue infections accompanying osteomyelitis

Superficial soft tissue infections	Deep soft tissue infections
• Cellulitis: Inflammation involving subcutaneous tissues around the point of entry of the infection without necrosis • Subepidermal abscess: bullae filled by purulent collection • Subcutaneous abscess: purulent collection in the subcutaneous tissue • Necrotizing cellulitis: infection spreading along subcutaneous tissue causing progressive necrosis of the skin and/or subcutaneous tissue	• Deep abscess: purulent collection below the fascia • Acute tenosynovitis: inflammation of the tendons and their sheaths without necrosis • Necrotizing tenosynovitis/fasciitis: infection spreading along fascial planes and/or tendons causing necrosis • Myonecrosis: infection spreading along muscle causing necrosis

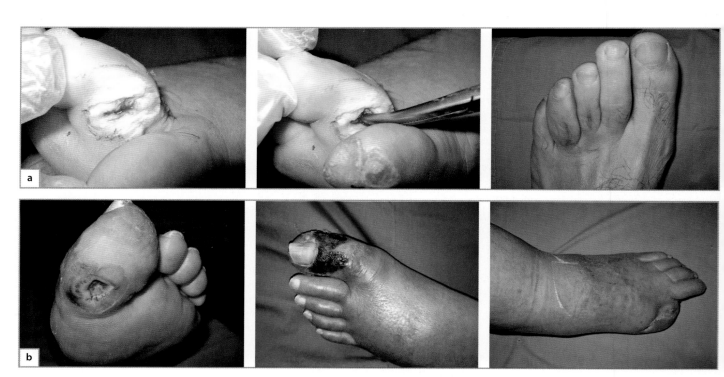

Figure 11.1 (a) Osteomyelitis without soft tissue infection resolved by conservative surgery. (b) Osteomyelitis with necrotizing tenosynovitis resolved by hallux amputation.

1. There is no acceptable surgical target (i.e. radical cure of the infection would cause unacceptable loss of function)
2. The patient has ischemia caused by unreconstructable vascular disease but wishes to avoid amputation
3. Infection is confined to the forefoot, and there is minimal soft tissue loss
4. The patient and health care professionals agree that surgical management carries excessive risk or is otherwise not appropriate or desirable

REMOVING THE INFECTED BONE: TYPES OF SURGERY

Operative removal of most, all, or part of an infected bone may potentially decrease the duration of antimicrobial therapy by removing devitalized tissue and reducing bacterial load. Surgical treatment of diabetic foot osteomyelitis belongs to class 3 or 4 of a previously described and validated diabetic foot surgery classification system (Armstrong et al. 2006). In this classification system, there are four classes: class 1 (elective), class 2 (prophylactic), class 3 (curative), and class 4 (emergency). Curative surgery (class 3) is performed on people with open wounds, and the goal is to heal and prevent subsequent recurrence. Emergency surgery (class 4) is performed on people with severe infections. The goal is to limit the spread of a potentially limb- or life-threatening infection. The most frequent method of achieving this goal is to perform several types of foot amputation; however, conservative surgeries, which deal satisfactorily with the source of life- and limb-threatening infection and prevent its spread, are an attractive and may prevent subsequent amputation.

Amputation

The most frequent location of osteomyelitis in the feet of patients with diabetes is the forefoot: phalanges and metatarsal heads (Aragon-Sanchez, et al. 2008, Game & Jeffcoate 2008; Valabhji et al. 2009, Lesens et al. 2011, Aragon-Sanchez et al. 2012c).

Several types of amputation have been classically used to remove infected bone in patients with diabetic forefoot osteomyelitis. Toe, ray, and transmetatarsal amputations are the most frequent procedures reported in the literature. Prompt toe amputation has been advocated in cases of toe osteomyelitis as a cost-saving procedure when compared with long-term antibiotic therapy (Kerstein et al. 1997); however, the data to support either approach over the other are weak.

The goals of minor amputation for osteomyelitis are to remove the infected bone and conserve as much of the foot as possible, make the foot stable and restore its function, and prevent or reduce the risk of reulceration. Toe and ray resections allow the patient to use footwear with no or minimal alterations. However, these amputations may also produce biomechanical disturbances. This, in turn, may result in new high-pressure points and predispose patients to subsequent reulceration. In a retrospective study of 90 patients undergoing amputation of the big toe, 60% underwent a second amputation and 17% subsequently required a below-the-knee amputation (Murdoch et al. 1997). However, the number of reulcerations and reamputations could probably be reduced with a specialized multidisciplinary postoperative treatment based on custom-made shoes and foot care. Dalla Paola et al. 2003 reported that only 15 out of 89 patients (16.8%) presented with reulceration and 8 (8.9%) required further surgical treatment. No patients in the group with reulceration underwent a major amputation (Dalla Paola et al. 2003).

In cases of phalanx involvement, the toe can be amputated through the phalanx, the interphalangeal joint, the metatarsophalangeal joint or the metatarsal bone (**Figure 11.2**). Several considerations should be taken into account when performing amputations for osteomyelitis in patients with diabetes. One of the most important is whether to close the surgical wound or leave it open to heal by secondary intention or to be closed secondarily. The decision to close a surgical wound will depend on whether the surgeon is sure that no infected bone and/ or infected soft tissue remain in the surgical wound. A dehiscence

Figure 11.2 Levels of toe amputation.

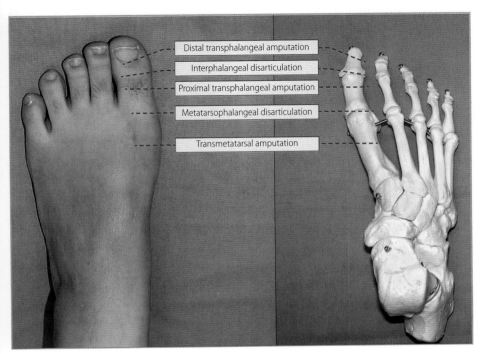

Distal transphalangeal amputation

Interphalangeal disarticulation

Proximal transphalangeal amputation

Metatarsophalangeal disarticulation

Transmetatarsal amputation

rate of surgical wounds of 10.3% (10/97) has been reported when the indication for surgery is osteomyelitis. In that study, the authors used at least 4 weeks of antibiotic therapy and local dressings before performing the amputation (Faglia et al. 2012a).

Other authors have systematically undertaken alternative approaches. In a series of 185 patients, minor amputations consisted of 70 partial or total amputations of toes and 9 open transmetatarsal amputations combined with healing by secondary intention (Aragon-Sanchez et al. 2008). Healing was achieved in 120 days (range 21–365) where minor amputations were performed and the wound was left open to heal by secondary intention. However, this series included a significant proportion of patients 30.2% (56/185) with deep abscess and necrotizing soft tissue infections accompanying osteomyelitis, and therefore, the results have to be extrapolated accordingly (because of the different behaviors of osteomyelitis associated with deep soft tissue infections, as already highlighted in the literature) (Eneroth et al. 1999, Aragon-Sanchez et al. 2009b, Aragon-Sanchez 2010, 2012a, Faglia et al. 2012b). Open transmetatarsal amputation is a useful technique when the surgeon is not certain that residual infection remains in the stump in cases of advanced forefoot infections. **Figure 11.3** demonstrates an open transmetatarsal amputation with opening of the plantar central compartment.

◼ Conservative surgery without amputation in cases of forefoot osteomyelitis

Surgical treatment of diabetic foot osteomyelitis without amputation is an attractive option to remove infected bone while conserving the soft tissue envelope and maintaining the external appearance of the foot. This option may be a good option for a patient with diabetes, because it is aesthetically acceptable (Faglia et al. 2012a). However, the impact of this type of conservative surgery on function and quality of life compared with minor (or major) amputations has not been fully assessed. Furthermore, amputation is frequently seen as an admission of failure of treatment and yet there is a paucity of data to suggest whether patients function better after conservative or amputation surgery.

The surgical approach to osteomyelitis is a balance of the removal of as much infected bone as possible against the need to preserve foot function (Frykberg et al. 2007). In theory, a conservative surgical approach also changes the foot biomechanics, although the risk of reulceration may be lower than that with traditional surgery, where more bone segments are removed. Additional advantage of the procedure would be the removal of bone prominences to eliminate areas of high pressure in the foot. The aims of the surgeon are both curative (osteomyelitis with/without soft tissue infection) and prophylactic (recurrent osteomyelitis and ulceration). In any case of conservative forefoot osteomyelitis surgery, when the wound has healed, the patient will need regular podiatric care, customized insoles, and adequate footwear to minimize the risk of reulceration.

Some disagreement exists around the term that should be used when surgery without amputation is carried out. The term 'internal pedal amputation' has been used by some authors (Koller 2008, Faglia et al. 2012a). This describes the procedures of resecting the metatarsals, midtarsal bones, or talus while preserving the toes and soft tissue envelope (Koller 2008). The term amputation means surgical removal of all or part of a limb, and for this reason, the term in the authors opinion is imprecise and unhelpful and should not be used for these operations (many of which already have a precise name) including arthroplasties (some of these procedures have a proper name), external and internal fixations, or antibiotic-loaded bone cement (Schweinberger et al. 2008, Aragon-Sanchez 2010, 2012b, Melamed et al., 2012).

Some authors have used the term 'bone incision and drainage' (Diamantopoulos et al. 1998) or 'bone debridement.' The problem is that the term 'debridement' is often used in an imprecise way in the literature dealing with diabetic foot problems. Debridement is currently understood to mean, for example, the elimination of the surrounding hyperkeratosis in plantar ulcers, removal of necrotic soft tissues from any wound or 'limited bone debridement.' The term 'debridement'

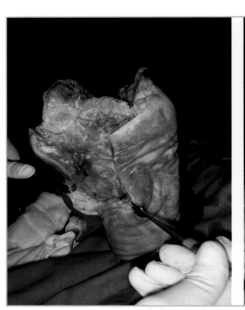
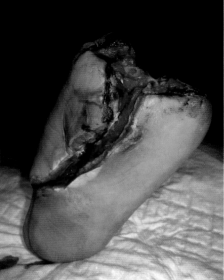
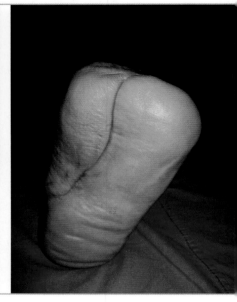

Figure 11.3 Open transmetatarsal amputation with opening of the plantar central compartment.

should be used when referring to the removal of infected, devitalized, or necrotic skin or soft tissue, but when referring to surgery performed on infected bones, more precise terms should be used to permit valid comparisons between the results of different studies.

The term 'conservative surgery' could be more appropriate for defining this type of foot surgery without amputation. The contribution of conservative surgery in treating patients with diabetic foot osteomyelitis was reported in 1996 (Ha Van et al. 1996). Conservative surgical treatment was initially defined as a limited resection of the infected part of the phalanx or the metatarsal bone under the wound, with no other resection associated with the removal of the ulcer site. Other authors later defined this type of surgery as any procedure in which only the infected bone and nonviable soft tissues are removed, but no amputation of any part of the foot is undertaken. Conservative surgery preserves the soft tissue envelope and more distal tissues, in effect resecting the infected bone while preserving the soft tissue envelope (Aragon-Sanchez et al. 2008). **Figure 11.4** demonstrates a typical case of conservative surgery of osteomyelitis of the interphalangeal joint of the hallux. Only ostectomy of infected and soft bone was carried out through a minimal incision.

A classification of the common types of conservative surgery for treating diabetic foot osteomyelitis is shown in **Table 11.2**.

Removing the distal phalanx can be successfully carried out to treat osteomyelitis of the distal phalanx of any toe. Percutaneous tenotomy can be performed in an outpatient clinic in cases of claw toe deformities with distal phalanx osteomyelitis. A research group treated 34 toes in 14 patients, of whom three had osteomyelitis of the distal phalanx. Toes without osteomyelitis healed within an average of 3 weeks, whereas those with osteomyelitis healed within an average of 8 weeks (Tamir et al. 2008). They did not report on whether infected bones on the tip of the toes were removed in addition to tenotomy or were treated exclusively with antibiotics. In cases of involvement of the interphalangeal joint, a resection arthroplasty can be carried out (Aragon-Sanchez et al. 2008, Kim et al. 2008, Aragon-Sanchez 2010, Melamed & Peled 2012). Other authors have reported using modified arthroplasty to treat osteomyelitis of the proximal and distal interphalangeal joint and the tip of the second, third, fourth, and fifth toes. In one such study, no great toe (hallux) osteomyelitis was included in a group of 52 patients (57 feet and 72 toes). The bone was removed through a dorsal wound, the wound was irrigated and a Kirschner wire 1.2 mm in diameter was placed (Kim et al. 2008). The authors performed closure of the wound only when the interphalangeal joint was free of symptomatic infection. However, the term 'symptomatic infection' was not defined, and the authors did

Table 11.2 Description of procedures of conservative surgery used in cases of diabetic foot osteomyelitis

Ostectomy	Any removal of bone tissue without formal anatomic limits; possibly, the 'limited debridements' described in some publications matches with this type of surgery
Metatarsal head resection	Removal of metatarsal head
Metatarsophalangeal joint resection	Removal of metatarsophalangeal joint. It includes metatarsal head and base of the proximal phalanx
Metatarsal resection	Removal of any part of the metatarsal bone excluding the head of the metatarsal
Distal phalangectomy	Removal of any part (or all) of the distal phalanx
Interphalangeal joint resection	Removal of any interphalangeal joint. Arthroplasty or modified arthroplasty may include the joint resection or the head of the phalanx resection
Sesamoidectomy	Removal of one or both sesamoid bones
Partial calcanectomy	Removal of a partial amount of calcaneus bone
Total calcanectomy	Removal of calcaneus bone
Exostectomy	Totally or partial removing of exostoses. Frequently used in cases of Charcot deformity with plantar bony prominences

not report how the joint evaluation was made. Eight cases underwent vascular intervention: angioplasty and stenting in six cases and bypass surgery in two. Surgery was carried out ≥3 weeks after vascular intervention. Twelve toes (30.5%) required reoperation to remove soft tissue and/or residual infected bone and three toes underwent amputation. Healing was achieved in 25.6 ± 6.2 days. The authors concluded that modified resection arthroplasty was an excellent treatment option for managing toe deformities with nonhealing ulcers, including patients with osteomyelitis (Kim et al. 2008). Additional conclusions were extracted from this study. First, putting a Kirschner wire in small bones that had had infections was a safe procedure, including wounds that were left open to heal by secondary intention. Second, although 30.5% of the cases required reoperations, these additional surgeries were successful in saving the toe. This is consistent with the experience of other authors (Aragon-Sanchez et al. 2008, 2012c). An example of arthroplasty for osteomyelitis of the proximal interphalangeal joint is shown in **Figure 11.5**. The probe-to-bone test was positive (**Figure 11.5a**) and X-ray showed signs of bone destruction of the interphalangeal joint (**Figure 11.5b**). Arthroplasty was carried out, as seen in the postoperative X-ray (**Figure 11.5c**). Healing was

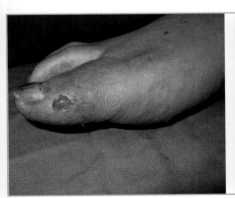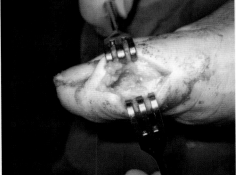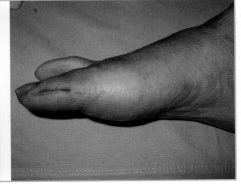

Figure 11.4 Conservative surgery of osteomyelitis of the interphalangeal joint of the hallux.

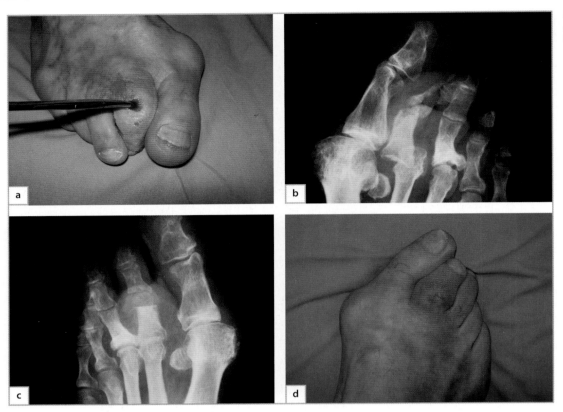

Figure 11.5 Arthroplasty for osteomyelitis of the proximal interphalangeal joint.

achieved 3 weeks after surgery (**Figure 11.5d**), and no recurrence has been found 7 years after surgery.

A common location of osteomyelitis in the foot of patients with diabetes is the metatarsal head. Metatarsal head resection is a very useful procedure employed by different study groups in cases with or without osteomyelitis (Wieman et al. 1998, Armstrong et al. 2005, Freeman et al. 2007, Aragon-Sanchez et al. 2008, 2012c, Faglia et al. 2012a). Two techniques may be used to remove the infected metatarsal head: the dorsal or plantar approach. After removing the infected bone, the surgical wound must be properly managed. Healing either by a secondary intention or primary closure approach is possible. A typical case of osteomyelitis of the second metatarsal head is shown in **Figure 11.6**. A dorsal approach was chosen in this case for removing the second metatarsophalangeal joint. A drain communicating plantar ulcer and dorsal wound was placed.

Antibiotic-impregnated cement spacer to fill the cavity resulting from the elimination of the infected bone and debriding soft tissues has also been reported. Only 2 out of 23 cases included in a retrospective study underwent a subsequent amputation using this management approach. Patients who did not have ischemia, gangrene, or necrotizing fasciitis were selected and included in the study. Of the 20 cases, 11 had one operation, 10 needed two operations, and 2 required three operations, averaging 1.6 operations per patient/site of infection, including the two amputation operations (Melamed & Peled 2012).

The location of forefoot osteomyelitis that is the most difficult to treat is the first metatarsophalangeal joint, which is the largest joint and the most complex. Hallux or first ray amputations are associated with the development of new plantar ulcers due to biomechanical changes and increased plantar pressures. Maintenance of the first ray is likely to reduce rates of recurrent reulceration and amputation (Schweinberger & Roukis 2008). However, published reports dealing

with surgery of osteomyelitis of the first metatarsophalangeal joint are few, retrospective, and frequently fail to demonstrate an advantage over amputation. Different authors have reported conservative surgery in small patient groups to avoid first ray or hallux amputations. One-stage resection and pin stabilization were reported in a retrospective series consisting of 15 patients (18 feet) with an average follow-up of 48.8 months (Johnson & Anderson 2010). The authors reported that only one patient required a transmetatarsal amputation after the procedure for worsening infection and wound complications. Although the procedure was successful, 50% of the feet developed a new ulcer. However, after secondary procedures, the new ulcers did not lead to subsequent amputation. Another option is to use external fixation after removing the infected bone, as reported in a group of six patients. Five of these had involvement of the first metatarsophalangeal joint, whereas the remaining one exhibited involvement of the interphalangeal joint of the hallux (Schweinberger & Roukis 2008). The authors used staged surgical procedures consisting of ulcer excision, removal of all necrotic soft tissue and bone, followed by pulse lavage irrigation, culturing, and polymethylmethacrylate antibiotic cement administration. After that, a miniexternal fixator was placed in four out of six cases. When the infection was cleared according to clinical and laboratory data, they carried out the deformity correction and wound closure. They subsequently used allogenic bone graft, iliac crest bone graft, or arthroplasty without bone grafting with the external fixator. One of the patients died from pulmonary embolus >2 months after the index procedure, and none of the surviving subjects developed recurrent ulceration or required amputation after 14 months of follow-up (Schweinberger & Roukis 2008). Using antibiotic-impregnated cement spacer to fill the cavity resulting from the removal of the infected bone is another option. The author describing this therapy treated 7 patients out of 20 patients who

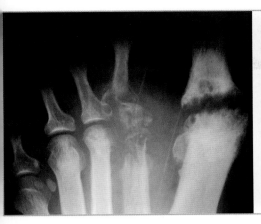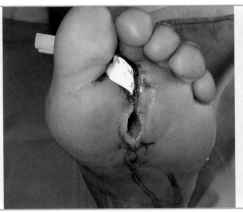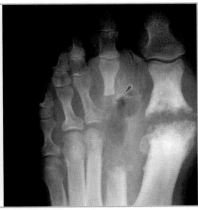

Figure 11.6 Osteomyelitis of the second metatarsal head was removed through dorsal approach. A drain communicating plantar ulcer and dorsal wound was placed.

presented with osteomyelitis of the first metatarsophalangeal joint. Bone debridement and antibiotic-impregnated cement spacer were used in every patient, and Kirschner wire was used in three patients. Five patients required further operations including cement removal and metatarsophalangeal arthrodesis (Melamed & Peled 2012). The outcomes in this subgroup of patients were good. One patient required a below-the-knee amputation due to complications arising from a new ulcer under the fifth metatarsal head. A postoperative radiograph showing a gentamicin-impregnated cement spacer and Kirschner wire is demonstrated in **Figure 11.7**.

◼ Conservative surgery in midfoot osteomyelitis

Osteomyelitis of the mid- and hindfoot is associated with a higher rate of major amputations than that of the forefoot (Karchmer & Gibbons 1994). Fortunately, osteomyelitis is less common in the mid- and hindfoot compared with the forefoot. In one surgical series, osteomyelitis was located in the forefoot in 90% of cases, in the midfoot in 5%, and in the hindfoot in another 5% of the cases (Aragon-Sanchez et al. 2008). Others have reported higher figures of hindfoot osteomyelitis at 21.8% of patients in one study (Karchmer & Gibbons 1994). Unfortunately, the data on mid- and hindfoot osteomyelitis in diabetes are relatively sparse owing to a paucity of published data. Most published studies are case reports, and it is very difficult to extract conclusions from them.

Cases involving midfoot osteomyelitis are frequently associated with underlying Charcot deformity. It has been suggested that repeat bone resection followed by the insertion of antibiotic cement spacers or antibiotic beads may be helpful therapeutic approaches (Capobianco et al. 2010). As a consequence of bone resection, the foot becomes destabilized and immobilization has to be enforced. Several ways of immobilizing an unstable foot have been reported, including internal fixation, external fixation, or both. Internal fixation is contraindicated in an area of previous osteomyelitis (Capobianco et al. 2010). Circular fixation based on Ilizarov principles provides stabilization following correction of deformities (Pinzur 2010). Complex procedures of flapping can be used together with external fixation to achieve limb salvage (Capobianco et al. 2010, Ramanujam et al. 2011). A group of authors have reported two cases of extensive midfoot osteomyelitis and an unstable foot successfully treated by a different approach. The radiograph of one of these two cases can be seen in **Figure 11.8**. Limb salvage was achieved and the following

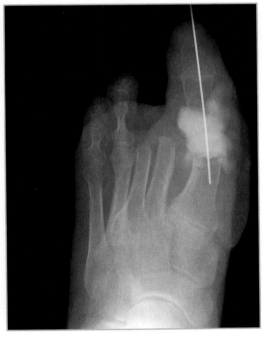

Figure 11.7 Postoperative X-ray showing a gentamicin-impregnated cement spacer and Kirschner wire after removing the first metatarsophalangeal joint.

three points were proposed for the success of this method: (1) the most part of the infected bone was removed, (2) culture-guided antibiotic treatment was administered, and (3) the infected foot was stabilized using a total contact cast (Aragon-Sanchez et al. 2012b). The use of total contact cast was controversial in these two cases, because evidence in the medical literature supports the use of a total contact cast for off-loading neuropathic plantar ulcers, but it is contraindicated in cases of infection and/or ischemia. The authors made two decisions to provide safe management of the patients. First, an opening was left in the cast for performing wound care and to check the healing course. Second, changes of the total contact cast were made weekly to evaluate the foot and monitor complications such as spreading infection, necrosis, or pressure ulcers. Total contact casts were used to stabilize extensive bone destruction in the midfoot and achieve a stable foot after surgery that produced additional instability because of the partial removal of the infected bones (Aragon-Sanchez et al. 2012b). Immobilization of the foot was critical, because it decreased

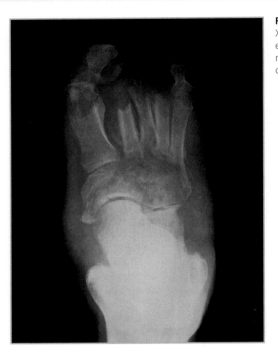

Figure 11.8
X-ray showing extensive midfoot bone destruction.

inflammation, in agreement with the results observed in cases of Charcot neuroarthropathy. Patients maintained their preoperative ambulatory status, and long-term follow-up demonstrated neither reulceration nor recurrence.

Conservative surgery in hindfoot osteomyelitis

Saving the foot in cases of heel ulceration and calcaneal osteomyelitis is a challenge because failure frequently leads to a major amputation. Subtotal and total calcanectomy has been suggested as an option to achieve limb salvage in patients, including those with diabetes (Perez et al. 1994, Baravarian et al. 1999, Fleischli & Laughlin 1999, Lehmann et al. 2001, Bollinger & Thordarson 2002, Randall et al. 2005).

A systematic review of partial or total calcanectomy as an alternative to below-the-knee amputation was recently reported (Schade 2012). The author reviewed 31 publications, and only 16 met the inclusion criteria, which were patients 18 years and older with a diagnosis of calcaneal osteomyelitis, who had undergone partial or total calcanectomy without adjunctive free tissue transfer, were ambulatory pre- and postoperatively, and had follow-up for at least 12 months. The combined data represented 100 patients who had undergone 76 partial and 28 total calcanectomy, giving a total of 104 calcanectomies. From the articles reviewed, only eight publications reported the number of patients with diabetes; there were a total of 45 patients with this condition. Forty-nine out of 76 partial calcanectomies (64.4%) did not have complications. Total calcanectomy was carried out without complications in 14 out of 28 (50%) cases. Minor complications were breakdown, subcutaneous abscess, papilloma, postoperative hematoma, and delayed healing. The risk of minor complications based on the number of total procedures performed after partial versus total calcanectomy was similar for partial and total calcanectomies at 23.7% and 21.4%, respectively. Regarding major complications, the rate was 36.1% after total calcanectomy and 15.8% after a partial one. Seven cases of partial calcanectomy (9.2%) and four cases of total calcanectomy (14.3%) subsequently required a major amputation. Patients with diabetes

had a fivefold greater risk of undergoing a major amputation (Schade 2012). Another review also reported that patients with diabetes and those with peripheral arterial disease are at high risk of failure after undergoing partial calcanectomy (Randall et al. 2005). Seventy-five per cent of patients maintained their preoperative ambulatory status postoperatively after either partial or total calcanectomy. Orthotic devices, custom shoes, ankle–foot orthoses, and Charcot restraint orthotic walkers were used to assist the patients to maintain their ambulatory status (Schade 2012).

A group of authors reported a series that was not included in the aforementioned review, which consisted of 24 patients who had undergone a partial calcanectomy (Van Riet et al. 2012). Eighteen had the procedure as a consequence of a large heel ulcer complicated by calcaneal osteomyelitis and six as a consequence of complications from internal fixation after surgery due to calcaneal fracture. Eight patients had diabetes mellitus: seven in the group with ulcers and another one in the group with calcaneal fracture. Using a midline incision, the authors removed the necrotic soft tissue and bone. Resection of the insertion of the Achilles tendon was sometimes required when it was involved in the infection. If primary closure was possible, they closed the wound in a single layer with 2/0 nylon. If not possible, the wound was left open and repeat debridement with secondary closure was planned. Only 1 patient out of 24 underwent a below-the-knee amputation. And in one out of the eight patients with diabetes, the infection was not controlled and required further resection. Four patients with diabetes required secondary suture. Mean hospital stay in patients with diabetes was 56.7 days, and healing was achieved in 118 days. Six patients with diabetes did not have a recurrence, and the other two could not be evaluated at the time the study was reported. There was no major difference in the failure rate between patients with and without diabetes. All patients were able to walk with or without external support (Van Riet et al. 2012).

Charcot neuropathy of the ankle is a severe complication that becomes limb threatening when it is complicated by osteomyelitis. A group of authors reported a prospective cohort of 45 patients with Charcot foot and ankle osteomyelitis (Dalla Paola et al. 2009). The location of the ulcer complicated by osteomyelitis was plantar at the rear of the foot in 13 cases, 18 in the medial malleolus, and 13 in the lateral malleolus. The authors used extensive debridement of infected bone, and the foot was subsequently stabilized with external fixation. The authors reported the key elements of their successful experience: complete debridement of the infected tissue, application of an external fixator with pins and wires not interfering with the infection site, use of only tensioned thin wires on the foot, 6–8 weeks of parenteral antibiotics in the postoperative period and use of negative pressure wound therapy for the postoperative treatment of open wounds. Fifteen patients had critical limb ischemia and underwent percutaneous transluminal angioplasty (PTA) ($n = 12$) or bypass ($n = 3$) before orthopedic surgery. Only four high-risk patients (8.8%) required a major amputation (Dalla Paola et al. 2009).

WHEN SHOULD SURGERY BE PERFORMED?

There is no evidence about the best time for performing surgery to treat osteomyelitis. Some working groups believe that osteomyelitis in the feet of patients with diabetes should undergo surgery as soon as osteomyelitis is diagnosed (Henke et al. 2005, Frykberg et al. 2007). Patients included in one series underwent surgical treatment during the first 12 hours after admission to hospital, although it was not possible to extract from the report when the diagnosis was made

(Aragon-Sanchez et al. 2008). The authors argued that early surgical treatment aided a quick stabilization of the condition of the patient, reducing costs and shortening the hospital stay, but this option needed to be investigated in a prospective trial and was not addressed in the study. Another approach was reported by Hartemann-Heurtier et al. They gave their patients a preoperative course of antibiotics for a period of 10–15 days and argued that in this way, surgery may be limited to the site of bone infection (Hartemann-Heurtier et al. 2002). A similar approach was reported by another group of authors (Faglia et al. 2012a). They operated on patients after administering antibiotics for at least 4 weeks. The authors argued that although this therapy might not have ensured complete resolution of the bone infection, it allowed the eradication of the infection from soft tissues and a reduction in the ulcer size (Faglia et al. 2012a). Other authors believe that early surgery minimizes the chance of bacteria spreading to soft tissues, and that any residual infection can be treated postoperatively by culture-guided antibiotics (Aragon-Sanchez et al. 2008, Aragon-Sanchez 2010, 2012b). However, it should be noted that patients with deep soft tissue infections accompanying osteomyelitis were included in this study (Aragon-Sanchez et al. 2008). This type of patient may benefit from early surgery. There is evidence that aggressive surgical treatment in the first 72 hours can reduce the need for below-the-knee amputations in diabetic foot infections (Tan et al. 1996) and that failure to remove necrotic tissue and purulent cavities by debridement increases the risk of amputation (Karchmer & Gibbons 1994).

HOW MUCH BONE SHOULD BE REMOVED?

Recent publications have highlighted the fact that patients with bone margins affected by infection after undergoing amputation for osteomyelitis have a poor prognosis. A group of researchers reported a retrospective series of 111 patients, evaluating the impact of residual osteomyelitis on surgical margins after surgical resection of infected bone (Kowalski et al. 2011). Forty-seven patients underwent digital amputation, 21 partial ray (metatarsal) resections, 38 ray resections, and 5 other procedures. Of the 111 patients included in the study, 39 (35.14%) had pathologically confirmed margins positive for residual osteomyelitis. Patients with positive margins had significantly higher rates of proximal amputations, as well as skin and soft tissue infections. The authors concluded that residual osteomyelitis at the pathologic margin was associated with a higher rate of treatment failure, despite the longer duration of antibiotic therapy (Kowalski et al. 2011). Another retrospective observational study involving 27 patients with diabetes showed that the overall rate of residual osteomyelitis was 40.7% (11/27). Nine out of eleven patients (81.8%) with positive margins had poor outcomes, including three reamputations, three wound dehiscences, one reulceration, one death, and one chronic wound that required skin grafting (Atway et al. 2012).

FACTORS RELATED TO SURGERY OUTCOME

The location of the bone infection is related to the outcome of treatment. Karchmer and Gibbons reported the outcomes of the surgical treatment of diabetic foot osteomyelitis in 110 patients, with bone infection proven by biopsy in 96% of the cases. In this group, 88% of minor and 12% of major amputations were performed in 86 cases of forefoot osteomyelitis (Karchmer & Gibbons 1994). Another study reported that 48.5% of 167 patients with forefoot osteomyelitis underwent conservative surgery, 45.5% minor amputations, and 6% major amputations (Aragon-Sanchez et al. 2008). Faglia et al. (2012b) stated that toe or ray amputation was performed in 198 out of 234 patients with forefoot osteomyelitis (84.6%), whereas the rest underwent 25 transmetatarsal and 1 Lisfranc amputation. Mid- and hindfoot osteomyelitis are associated with worse prognosis than forefoot osteomyelitis (Karchmer & Gibbons 1994, Aragon-Sanchez et al. 2008, Aragon-Sanchez 2010).

The outcome of conservative surgery treating diabetic foot osteomyelitis is not well defined. One report investigated a group of 185 patients, including those with severe soft tissue infections accompanying osteomyelitis. After excluding the patients for whom conservative surgery was found to be impossible on admission, 111 patients underwent conservative surgery as the first choice. Of those, only 20 (18%) required subsequent amputations: 13 minor (11.7%) and 7 major amputations (6.3%). Conservative surgery was successful in 82% of the cases (Aragon-Sanchez et al. 2008). The same working group reported a new cohort of 81 patients with the same characteristics. Forty-eight patients (59.3%) had conservative surgery, 32 (39.5%) minor amputations, and 1 (1.2%) major amputation (Aragon-Sanchez et al. 2012c). The factors associated with amputation in the logistic regression model were previous ulceration [$p = 0.03$, odds ratio (OR) 0.23, 95% confidence interval (CI) 0.06–0.9], soft-tissue infection accompanying osteomyelitis ($p = 0.02$, OR 4.9, 95% CI 1.2–20), capillary glucose monitoring in quartiles 2–4 ($p = 0.04$, OR 5.9, 95% CI 1.6–24.7), peripheral arterial disease ($p < 0.01$, OR 6.2, 95% CI 1.6–24.7), and skin necrosis ($p < 0.01$, OR 12.2, 95% CI 2.9–50.9). The authors also found that the bone changes seen in simple X-rays in osteomyelitis cases did not have any prognostic value when surgical treatment was undertaken. The outcomes were more related to soft tissue involvement than any bone destruction viewed on simple X-rays (Aragón-Sánchez et al. 2012a).

Careful vascular status determination must be made before performing amputation. The combination of peripheral arterial disease and infection has a major impact on healing rates. Ischemia has long been recognized as a factor contributing to prolonged hospitalization, the spread of infection, and avoidable amputation in patients with diabetes and foot ulcers. Peripheral arterial disease should always be excluded. Minor amputation in a foot without adequate foot perfusion may be complicated by nonhealing wounds, the spread of infection, and necrosis, with major amputation subsequently being required. Failure of treatment was linked to values of ankle systolic blood pressure < 50 mmHg, toe systolic blood pressure < 30mmHg, ankle/brachial index < 0.5, and transcutaneous oxygen pressure < 20 mmHg in a prospective series of diabetic foot infections, including 58% of patients with osteomyelitis (Diamantopoulos et al. 1998). Other authors also reported peripheral arterial disease as a risk factor for the failure of conservative surgery and amputation (Aragon-Sanchez et al. 2008, Aragon-Sanchez & Lazaro-Martinez 2011, Aragon-Sanchez 2012a). Hartemann-Heurtier et al. showed that an increase in the time to heal correlated with the existence of peripheral arterial disease and end-stage renal disease treated with hemodialysis. In this study, the authors did not show the outcomes of six patients with osteomyelitis and ischemia, because these patients were included in the group of 30 patients with severe peripheral arterial disease. In this ischemic group, 24 had undergone bypass surgery. The authors showed a limb-salvage rate of 97.5% with this aggressive approach (Hartemann-Heurtier et al. 2002). Henke et al. demonstrated that peripheral arterial disease was associated with a lower rate of wound healing and limb salvage. In their sample, bypass surgery was linked to wound healing and limb salvage. Aggressive surgical debridement accompanied by early revascularization can achieve a high rate of limb salvage (Hartemann-Heurtier et al. 2002, Henke et al. 2005).

The optimum timing for vascular surgery in patients with diabetes, ischemia, and foot osteomyelitis has not yet been identified. In cases of severe infections, it is important to proceed with surgical debridement as soon as possible with the intention of performing revascularization after debridement. For a patient with a severely infected ischemic foot, it is preferable to perform revascularization within 1 to 2 days of the initial surgical debridement (Zgonis et al. 2008). When the patient is metabolically stable and osteomyelitis is not accompanied by necrotizing changes, deep abscesses, or systemic response to infection, it is preferable to continue antibiotic treatment and perform revascularization as soon as possible. Thus, increased distal flow can be attained to promote wound healing after a surgical procedure on the infected bone. A team in Rome monitored transcutaneous oxygen tension ($TcPO_2$) after PTA in patients with ischaemic foot ulcers and diabetes (Caselli et al. 2005). They found that in the group of patients with successful revascularization, the percentage of patients with a $TcPO_2 \geq 30$ mmHg was 38.5% 1 week after PTA, but this increased to 75% after 3 weeks. They concluded that when it is possible to delay surgery, the best time to perform a more aggressive debridement or minor amputations is 3 to 4 weeks after successful revascularization (Caselli et al. 2005). There is a lack of evidence related to the optimum time for performing bone surgery after a revascularization. The decision to offer open bypass surgery rather than endovascular revascularization rests primarily with the pattern of arterial occlusion, the experience of the team and is best made in a multidisciplinary meeting of surgeons and interventionists.

A group of authors (Ha Van et al. 1996) retrospectively compared the results of the treatment of osteomyelitis without ischemia over two different periods. Thirty-two patients belonged to a historical group (1986 to 1993) of patients treated with antibiotic therapy, off-loading, and local wound care. The second group consisted of 32 patients who underwent conservative surgery followed by the same regime of care (September 1993 to March 1995). Healing rates were 57% for the former group and 78% for the latter ($p < 0.008$); there was also a significant difference in healing time: 462 ± 98 days and 181 ± 30 days ($p < 0.008$), respectively. In the group who underwent conservative surgery, only two patients (6.25%) required a minor amputation. In the antibiotic group, failure of the medical management resulted in 40% of patients undergoing amputations: nine toe, three transmetatarsal, and two below the knee. These authors concluded that in the case of osteomyelitis of the foot in patients with diabetes, conservative surgery reduced healing time, the duration of antibiotic therapy, and the number of secondary surgical procedures. Healing was achieved in 181 +/- 30 days (Ha Van et al. 1996). Aragón-Sánchez et al. reported that open wounds healed by secondary intention over a median period of 90 days. The median wound healing times in patients with successful conservative surgery was 80 days (12 to 365) compared with 120 days (21–365) for those who had minor amputations ($p = 0.003$). Median wound healing times were longer in cases where there was associated soft tissue infection ($p = 0.0005$) and limb ischemia ($p = 0.001$) (Aragon-Sanchez et al. 2008).

Another investigation assessed 157 patients with complicated foot ulcers and 51 patients had osteomyelitis. Forty-five patients had osteomyelitis without foot ischemia and 41 of these (91%) underwent surgical treatment: 28 conservative surgery (68%) and 13 minor amputations (32%) (Hartemann-Heurtier et al. 2002). Another group reported 51 patients without ischemia or soft tissue infection. They performed 44 conservative surgical procedures (86.3%) and 7 minor

amputations (13.7%). In this selected population, no patients required major amputation or died (Aragon-Sanchez et al. 2008).

The presence of deep soft tissue infections accompanying osteomyelitis has an influence on the outcome of surgery. Game (2010) reviewed and compared two modern series. Conservative surgery (Aragon-Sanchez et al. 2008) was compared with primarily nonsurgical management of diabetic foot osteomyelitis (Game & Jeffcoate 2008). The review stated that the minor amputation rate in the former series was much higher than that in the latter one (48% versus 23%, respectively). The major amputation rate was similar (8.8% versus 8.1%) (Aragon-Sanchez et al. 2008, Game & Jeffcoate 2008). It is important to highlight the fact that 55 out of 185 patients included in the surgical series (29.7%) were admitted with osteomyelitis accompanied by abscesses or necrotizing soft tissue infections (Aragon-Sanchez et al. 2008). It is reasonable to postulate that the type of infections treated by Game and Jeffcoate differed from those treated by Aragon-Sanchez et al. As previously mentioned, soft tissue infections accompanying osteomyelitis were a risk factor for amputation in this surgical group (Aragon-Sanchez et al. 2008, Aragón-Sánchez et al. 2012a). Moreover, patients with osteomyelitis and deep tissue infections have worse prognosis than those with isolated bone infections (Eneroth et al. 1999). This has also been recently highlighted; patients with osteomyelitis have better prognosis than those with deep tissue abscesses (Faglia et al. 2012b). The former group has a higher rate of major amputations and a much more proximal level of minor amputations. These outcomes highlight the need for defining the type of osteomyelitis present. An attempt to characterize the grading of the severity of osteomyelitis was recently made. Osteomyelitis was classified as follows: osteomyelitis without ischemia and without soft tissue involvement (class 1), osteomyelitis with ischemia without soft tissue involvement (class 2), osteomyelitis with soft tissue involvement (class 3), and osteomyelitis with ischemia and soft tissue involvement (class 4). No amputation was required in a subgroup of 25 out of 81 patients without ischemia and soft tissue infections. The characterization of osteomyelitis into four classes showed a statistically significant trend toward increased severity and increased amputation rate and mortality (Aragon-Sanchez 2012a).

Conservative management based only on antibiotics prior to admission worsened the lower extremity salvage rate in adults with osteomyelitis of the foot and toe in a group of patients who did not exclusively have diabetes (Henke et al. 2005). The authors reported on a sample of 237 patients who were treated for osteomyelitis at the University of Michigan over a period of 7 years. In this dataset, the patients were treated using one of two forms of treatment: medical or surgical. The criteria used to select treatment were not discussed. Of the 237 patients, 13 were excluded because they could not be followed up and another 14 because they had undergone an immediate major amputation. Thus, the sample contained 210 patients of whom 80% had diabetes. Fifty-two per cent of the patients had previously been given antibiotics: 19% intravenous and 33% oral with a mean treatment time of 5 ± 2 months. On admission, 95 patients were treated surgically and 115 were given only antibiotics. In the surgical group, 77% underwent conservative surgery and 23% a minor amputation. Subsequently, 18% of the patients in this group underwent a major amputation so the rate of limb salvage was 82% after 31 months of follow-up. In the 115 patients receiving medical treatment, the limb salvage rate was 81%. Thus, there was no statistically significant difference between the two groups. Unfortunately, however, without knowing the criteria used to select treatment, it is impossible to assess the significance of this finding. It is often the case that patients with the most severe infections receive an operation. The initial debridement and bypass surgery

for women. In 1984, in Australia, Welborn et al. described the prevalence of occlusive PAD in 1084 patients with either type 1 or type 2 diabetes mellitus (Welborn et al. 1984). They used IC and pulse deficit as diagnostic criteria of PAD. The prevalence was 38%. Both the Rochester study and Welborn study had to deal with the great difficulty of diagnosing PAD in those with diabetes using claudication as the exclusive diagnostic criterion. Pure clinical criteria may underestimate the prevalence of PAD in patients with diabetes (Jude 2010, Melton et al. 1980, Welborn et al. 1984). Those limitations are related to the high rate of asymptomatic PAD among those with diabetes and the frequent occurrence of neuropathy, which may delay the onset of claudication symptoms. In most cases, vascular dysfunction and autonomous deregulation develop simultaneously with neuropathy. In those patients, ulcers may develop earlier and more advanced disease may be evident at the time of diagnosis (Lepantalo et al. 2011).

Claudication may be present in only one-third of patients with diabetes and PAD. Trying to overcome these limitations, Becks et al. and Walters et al. in the Netherlands and England, respectively, used as the diagnostic criterion of PAD an ABI <0.9 (Beks et al. 1995, Walters et al. 1992). Becks, in the Hoorn study, found that the prevalence of ABI <0.9 in individuals with normal glucose tolerance was 7%, increasing to 20.9% in patients with diabetes (Beks et al. 1995). Walters described a 23.5% prevalence of PAD among 864 patients with type 2 and type 1 diabetes mellitus. This study showed that the prevalence of PAD was much higher in patients with type 2 diabetes than in patients with type 1 diabetes mellitus (23.5% vs. 8.7%, respectively) (Walters et al. 1992). The Framingham study reported that diabetes, hypertension, and coronary artery disease were all associated with the development of IC. Diabetes and hypertension conferred a greater than twofold increased risk, whereas coronary artery disease almost tripled the risk for claudication (Kannel 1985, Jude 2010).

The duration and severity of diabetes correlate with the incidence and extent of PAD. In a prospective cohort study, Al-Delaimy et al. found a strong positive association between the duration of diabetes and the risk of developing PAD (Al-Delaimy et al. 2004). The association was stronger among men with hypertension or who were current smokers. The prevalence of PAD was higher in those patients with a longer duration of diabetes. The degree of diabetes control was also an independent risk factor for PAD. With every 1% increase in glycated hemoglobin, the risk of PAD was shown to increase by 18% (Selvin et al. 2004). In people with diabetes, the risk of PAD is increased by age, duration of diabetes, and the presence of peripheral neuropathy. Due to the delay in diagnosis of PAD in patients with diabetes, a substantially higher risk of mortality exists, primarily from cardiovascular disease, compared with the general population. Selvin and Erlinger found that the crude OR for patients with diabetes to develop PAD was 3.2, decreasing to 2.1 when adjusting for age, gender, and comorbidities (Selvin & Erlinger 2004). Both findings were statistically significant.

In the Framingham study, 26% of the participants had a history of diabetes mellitus (Kannel 1985). Among people with diabetes, a 3.5- and 8.6-fold excess risk of developing PAD was reported for men and women, respectively. In this study, an incidence of PAD in patients with diabetes of 12.6/1000 in males and 8.4/1000 in females was reported (Kannel 1985, Jude et al. 2001). In the Rochester study, the cumulative incidence of PAD was 15% 10 years after the diagnosis of diabetes, increasing to 45% 20 years later (Melton et al. 1980).

Patients with diabetes and PAD are more likely to present with an ischemic ulcer or gangrene than patients without diabetes, increasing the risk of lower-extremity amputation. Faglia et al. (1998) observed a positive trend between PAD severity and amputation rates in patients with diabetes. People with diabetes are 25 times more likely to have an amputation than those without diabetes (Bild et al. 1989).

NATURAL HISTORY OF PERIPHERAL ARTERIAL DISEASE IN THE GENERAL POPULATION

The clinical manifestations of PAD depend on the location and severity of arterial disease and range from mild claudication to limb-threatening ischemia (**Table 12.1**). Approximately 75% of all patients with claudication experience clinical stabilization or improvement in their condition and symptoms over their lifetime without the need for intervention; however, patients who contine to smoke or those with concomitant diabetes or renal insufficiency tend to have a more rapid deterioration of their symptoms (Norgren et al. 2007).

Aboyans et al. studied the factors that predict progression of PAD in a longitudinal study involving 403 patients using a standard questionnaire, clinical examination, ABI, and TBI over a mean follow-up of 4.6 years (Aboyans et al. 2006). The authors defined significant PAD progression as a decline of 0.3 or more in the ABI. Significant risk factors after adjustment included current cigarette smoking [hazard ratio (HR), 3.2; 95% CI, 1.5–6.8], ratio of total cholesterol to HDL cholesterol (HR, 1.4; 95% CI, 1.1–1.7), elevated high sensitivity C-reactive protein (HR, 1.4; 95% CI, 1.0–1.9), and elevated lipoprotein (HR, 1.4; 95% CI, 1.0-1.8). Diabetes, hypertension, homocysteine, and body mass index were not significant for large-vessel disease progression as measured by ABI changes. However, among patients with TBI decrement, diabetes was the only significant predictor of

Table 12.1 Fontaine and Rutherford classifications of peripheral arterial disease

Fontaine		Rutherford		
Stage	Clinical presentation	Grade	Category	Clinical presentation
I	Asymptomatic	0	0	Asymptomatic
IIa	Mild claudication	I	1	Mild claudication
IIb	Moderate-to-severe claudication	I	2	Moderate claudication
		I	3	Severe claudication
III	Ischemic rest pain	II	4	Ischemic rest pain
		III	5	Minor tissue loss
IV	Ulceration or gangrene	III	6	Major tissue loss

progression (Aboyans et al. 2006). Both NHANES and MESA confirmed that current smoking status, diabetes, hyperlipidemia, and black race are significant predictors of progression of PAD (Aboyans et al. 2006, Allison et al. 2009).

Asymptomatic PAD

Most patients with PAD are unaware of their disease. Fewer than 50% of patients with PAD and about 30% of their physicians are aware of their disease, which is remarkable considering that PAD is a major predictor of cardiovascular outcomes (Novo 2002). Overall, the annual cardiovascular event rate is 5–7% for patients with PAD (**Figure 12.1**) (Norgren et al. 2007). Fowkes et al. in the AGATHA study demonstrated that patients with PAD in one vascular bed had a 35% chance of having disease in at least one other territory (Fowkes et al. 2006). Patients with asymptomatic PAD had a threefold increase in the occurrence of angina compared with the control group. Diehm et al. and Nicoloff et al. found that asymptomatic PAD is a risk factor for increased mortality, with no difference in mortality between patients with symptomatic and asymptomatic PAD (Diehm et al. 2009, Nicoloff et al. 2002). Nicoloff found that patients with a low initial ABI tended to develop a more rapid decline in the ABI during follow-up (Nicoloff et al. 2002). The progression of the disease from an asymptomatic stage to claudication, as shown in the Framingham study, may be related to the presence of elevated serum cholesterol, cigarette smoking, moderate hypertension, and diabetes (Kannel 1985).

Intermittent claudication

IC is characterized by slow symptom progression. Critical limb ischemia seldom occurs. Only 1–2% of patients with claudication are estimated to develop critical limb ischemia within 5 years, whereas 70–80% will continue with stable claudication (Hirsch et al. 2006). Claudication is a marker for generalized atherosclerosis and for other cardiovascular and cerebrovascular morbidity and mortality. Muluk and collaborators in a series of 2777 patients with IC found that the mortality rate per year during a 47-month period was 12% (Muluk et al. 2001). This rate was much higher than the age-adjusted US male population in 2001. In addition, the rate of progression from claudication to either minor or major amputation was <10%. Significant predictors for either mortality or amputation were older age (RR = 1.3), lower ABI (RR = 1.2), diabetes requiring medication (RR = 1.4), and stroke (RR = 1.4). Revascularization procedures occurred with a 10-year cumulative rate of 18%. Aquino et al. in a long-term study with a cohort of 1244 patients with IC found that low ABI and diabetes were the most important predictors for the evolution of IC to ischemic rest pain and ischemic ulceration (Aquino et al. 2001). According to McDermott et al. (2003) and the PARTNERS study (Hirsch et al. 2001), patients with IC have a poor quality of life and high rates of depression. It seems that IC and emotional well-being affect walking ability.

Critical limb ischemia

Critical limb ischemia is a late and fatal manifestation of PAD with a prevalence in the European and North American population estimated at between 500 and 1000/million. Both Aboyans (Aboyans et al. 2006) and Aquino (Aquino et al. 2001) in their respective studies found that the rate of progression from IC to chronic limb ischemia (CLI) was related to diabetes (fourfold), smoking (threefold risk), and hypercholesterolemia (twofold risk). Amputation rates in patients with CLI remained high at 25%, and long-term survival was poor. The course of CLI depended to some extent on the treatment center, although it was estimated that 50–90% of affected patients would undergo some form of revascularization (Norgren et al. 2007). According to Wolf and collaborators, the mortality rate for cardiovascular causes in patients with CLI was 25% after 1 year of the initial presentation (Wolfe & Wyatt 1997). The TASC II document revealed that 40% of patients with CLI and nonreconstructible disease underwent amputation within 6 months, and 20% died within the same period (Norgren et al. 2007, Wolfe & Wyatt 1997).

NATURAL HISTORY OF PERIPHERAL ARTERIAL DISEASE IN DIABETES

Diabetes and PAD individually increase the risk of adverse cardiovascular events and mortality, disability, amputation, and poor outcome after revascularization. Diabetes is a common cause of mortality and morbidity, associated with a fourfold increased risk of cardiovascular disease. In a large meta-analysis of 13 prospective cohort studies published by Selvin et al. (2004), for every 1% increase in glycated hemoglobin, the RR for any cardiovascular event was 1.18 (95% CI, 1.1–1.3).

Diabetes is associated with a higher prevalence of PAD and increased risk of adverse outcomes. In the Prevention of Progression of Arterial Disease and Diabetes (POPADAD) trial (Belch et al. 2008), 16% of 1276 asymptomatic patients with diabetes and PAD progressed to IC, 3% to critical limb ischemia, and 1.6% to a major amputation at 6 years. The findings were consistent with the Framingham study, in which diabetes was considered an important predictor of IC (OR, 2.6) (Kannel 1985).

Among individuals in the general population, diabetes has also been associated with increased disability and poorer physical functioning. Currently, it is not clear if the excess risk of disability associated with diabetes is exacerbated in subjects with PAD. In a cross-sectional study that included 460 patients, Dolan et al. assessed ABI, neuropathy score, 6-min walk distance, and 4-m walking velocity (Dolan et al. 2002). Patients with concomitant PAD and diabetes walked shorter distances in the 6-min walk test (1,040.2 vs. 1,168.2 feet), had lower 4-m walking velocity (0.83 vs. 0.90 m/s) and lower completed full tandem stand (41.4% vs. 61.6%), and required more time to complete the five chair rises (12.7 vs. 11.7 s).

Patients with diabetes have more severe PAD at the time of diagnosis. In a retrospective study with 403 patients assessed over a 10-year period, Aboyans et al. found that patients with ABI >1.4 and evidence of arterial occlusive disease (according to Doppler waveform patterns) have poorer prognosis in terms of death and cardiovascular events than patients with normal ABI after adjusting for comorbidities and smoking status (HR, 2.2; 95%IC, 1.2–4.2, P<0.01) (Aboyans et al. 2006).

Jude et al. assessed the severity and distribution of PAD in patients with and without diabetes using angiography findings (Jude et al. 2001). The study included 136 patients, of whom 58 (43%) had diabetes with duration of 13.0 +/- 11.1 years. Patients with diabetes were found to have higher severity scores in below the knee vasculature. The posterior tibial artery was the vessel with higher score severity. No statistically significant difference was found among vessels above the knee vascular system. Other studies such as one published by Strandness et al. supported the idea that patients with diabetes had more infrapopliteal disease (Strandness et al. 1964), whereas King et al. (1984) found greater involvement of the profunda femoris artery in those with diabetes. Patients with diabetes are more susceptible to developing more heavily calcified atherosclerotic arteries and tibial artery occlusive disease. Patients with diabetes may have lower technical success rates after revascularization procedures compared with patients without diabetes due to the morphological distribution of PAD and calcified vessels.

Although the results of revascularization among patients with diabetes will be discussed in detail in Chapter 19, it is worth mentioning that patients with diabetes and PAD have poor outcomes in terms of technical success, limb salvage, and patient survival. Melliere et al. (1999) in a retrospective study over a 5-year period of fully computerized data of 1003 patients in France found that the mortality rate for patients with diabetes following aortic or lower-extremity revascularization was 9.6% compared with 2.2% in patients without diabetes. Lazaris et al. (2004) performed a retrospective review on 99 patients suffering from CLI who underwent primary infrainguinal subintimal angioplasty in 112 limbs within a 6-month period. In this cohort, 33 patients had diabetes. The overall technical success was 89%, although the technical success rate in patients with diabetes was 81% compared with 93% in those without diabetes ($P = 0.05$). The rate of complications was significantly higher in patients with diabetes [16.7% vs. 3.9% ($P = 0.03$)]. Dick et al. compared both surgical and endovascular interventions for iliac, femoropopliteal, and tibial artery occlusive disease and found lower rates of Rutherford classification improvement and a shorter term of amputation-free survival in patients with diabetes (**Table 12.1**) (Dick et al. 2007).

Most nontraumatic lower-limb amputations in the Western world are performed on patients with diabetes, whose RR of major amputation is 12- to 24-fold compared with those without diabetes (American Diabetes 2003). Diabetes and PAD are both frequently complicated by neuropathy and foot ulceration, and each condition is associated with an increased risk of gangrene and amputations. In patients with concomitant diabetes and CLI, the probability of major amputation is 30% and of death 20% within 6 months (Dormandy & Rutherford 2000).

Malmstedt et al. in a population-based cohort study identified 1840 patients who had their first leg bypass procedure for critical lower-limb ischemia in a 1-year period, of which 742 patients had diabetes (Malmstedt et al. 2008). The rate of ipsilateral amputation or death per 100 person-years was higher in patients with diabetes (30.2; 95% CI, 26.6–34.2) than in patients without diabetes (22.0; 95% IC, 19.4–24.9). Almost one-half of the patients with diabetes and one-third of those without diabetes had undergone a major amputation or died 2 years after the procedure. The median time of death and/or amputation was 2.3 years in patients with diabetes and 3.4 years in those without it. The effect of diabetes on amputation-free survival was more pronounced in male patients (age-adjusted HR, 1.8; 95% CI, 1.5–2.1) than in female patients (1.4; 95% CI, 1.1–1.6). Patients with PAD and diabetes present later with more severe disease and have a greater risk of amputation. Patients with diabetes undergoing amputation have a 3-year survival rate lower than 50% and a higher risk of a second amputation; patient survival is lower among those with diabetes than in those without diabetes undergoing successful revascularization (Jude et al. 2001).

AREAS OF CONTROVERSY AND/OR FUTURE RESEARCH

- A multidisciplinary approach is needed for early diagnosis of PAD in patients with diabetes
- The timing for screening and follow-up of PAD in patients with diabetes needs to be established
- Noninvasive vascular methods for the screening of PAD in patients with diabetes need to be investigated more fully
- Practitioners should consider early and aggressive intervention of atherosclerotic risk factors in addition to opportune revascularization to improve the outcomes of PAD in diabetic patients
- It is important to establish therapeutic goals in the management of diabetes to prevent the onset of PAD and/or to slow its progression

IMPORTANT FURTHER READING

Criqui MH, Allison MA, McDermott MM, et al. Ethnic differences and risk factors for peripheral arterial disease (PAD) in the multi-ethnic study of atherosclerosis (MESA). Circulation 2004; 109:E78.

Hirsch AT, Haskal ZJ, Hertzer NR, et al. ACC/AHA 2005 Practice Guidelines for the management of patients with peripheral arterial disease (lower extremity, renal, mesenteric, and abdominal aortic): a collaborative report from the American Association for Vascular Surgery/Society for Vascular Surgery, Society for Cardiovascular Angiography and Interventions, Society for Vascular Medicine and Biology, Society of Interventional Radiology, and the ACC/AHA Task Force on Practice Guidelines (Writing Committee to Develop Guidelines for the Management of Patients With Peripheral Arterial Disease): endorsed by the American Association of Cardiovascular and Pulmonary Rehabilitation; National Heart, Lung, and Blood Institute; Society for Vascular Nursing; TransAtlantic Inter-Society Consensus; and Vascular Disease Foundation. Circulation 2006; 113:e463–e654.

Jude EB, Oyibo SO, Chalmers N, Boulton AJ. Peripheral arterial disease in diabetic and nondiabetic patients: a comparison of severity and outcome. Diabetes Care 2001; 24:1433–1437.

Kannel WB, McGee DL. Update on some epidemiologic features of intermittent claudication: the Framingham Study. J Am Geriatr Soc 1985; 33:13–18.

Norgren L, Hiatt WR, Dormandy JA, et al. Inter-Society Consensus for the Management of Peripheral Arterial Disease (TASC II). J Vasc Surg 2007; 45:S5–67.

Selvin E, Erlinger TP. Prevalence of and risk factors for peripheral arterial disease in the United States: results from the National Health and Nutrition Examination Survey, 1999-2000. Circulation 2004; 110:738–743.

REFERENCES

Aboyans V, Criqui MH, Denenberg JO, et al. Risk factors for progression of peripheral arterial disease in large and small vessels. Circulation 2006; 113:2623–2629.

Al-Delaimy WK, Merchant AT, Rimm EB, et al. Effect of type 2 diabetes and its duration on the risk of peripheral arterial disease among men. Am J Med 2004; 116:236–240.

Allison MA, Cushman M, Solomon C, et al. Ethnicity and risk factors for change in the ankle-brachial index: the Multi-Ethnic Study of Atherosclerosis. J Vasc Surg 2009; 50:1049–1056.

American Diabetes A. Peripheral arterial disease in people with diabetes. Diabetes Care 2003; 26:3333–3341.

Aquino R, Johnnides C, Makaroun M, et al. Natural history of claudication: long-term serial follow-up study of 1244 claudicants. J Vasc Surg 2001; 34:962–970.

Beks PJ, Mackaay AJ, de Neeling JN, et al. Peripheral arterial disease in relation to glycaemic level in an elderly Caucasian population: the Hoorn study. Diabetologia. 1995; 38:86–96.

Belch J, MacCuish A, Campbell I, et al. The prevention of progression of arterial disease and diabetes (POPADAD) trial: factorial randomised placebo controlled trial of aspirin and antioxidants in patients with diabetes and asymptomatic peripheral arterial disease. BMJ 2008; 337:a1840.

Bild DE Selby JV, Sinnock P, et al. Lower extremity amputation in people with diabetes: epidemiology and prevention. Diabetes Care 1989; 12:24–31.

Criqui MH, Allison MA, McDermott MM, et al. Ethnic differences and risk factors for peripheral arterial disease (PAD) in the multi-ethnic study of atherosclerosis (MESA). Circulation 2004; 109:E78–E78.

Criqui MH, Fronek A, Barrett-Connor E, et al. The prevalence of peripheral arterial disease in a defined population. Circulation 1985; 71:510–515.

Dick F, Diehm N, Galimanis A, et al. Surgical or endovascular revascularization in patients with critical limb ischemia: influence of diabetes mellitus on clinical outcome. J Vasc Surg 2007; 45:751–761.

Diehm C, Allenberg JR, Pittrow D, et al. Mortality and vascular morbidity in older adults with asymptomatic versus symptomatic peripheral artery disease. Circulation 2009; 120:2053.

Dolan NC, Liu K, Criqui MH, et al. Peripheral artery disease, diabetes, and reduced lower extremity functioning. Diabetes Care 2002; 25:113–120.

Dormandy JA, Rutherford RB. Management of peripheral arterial disease (PAD). TASC Working Group. TransAtlantic Inter-Society Consensus (TASC). J Vasc Surg 2000; 31:S1–S296.

Faglia E, Favales F, Quarantiello A, et al. Angiographic evaluation of peripheral arterial occlusive disease and its role as a prognostic determinant for major amputation in diabetic subjects with foot ulcers. Diabetes Care 1998; 21:625–630.

Fowkes FG, Housley E, Cawood EH, et al. Edinburgh Artery Study: prevalence of asymptomatic and symptomatic peripheral arterial disease in the general population. Int J Epidemiol 1991; 20:384–392.

Fowkes FG, Low LP, Tuta S, Kozak J, Investigators A. Ankle-brachial index and extent of atherothrombosis in 8891 patients with or at risk of vascular disease: results of the international AGATHA study. Eur Heart J 2006; 27:1861–1867.

Hirsch AT, Criqui MH, Treat-Jacobson D, et al. Peripheral arterial disease detection, awareness, and treatment in primary care. JAMA 2001; 286:1317–1324.

Hirsch AT, Haskal ZJ, Hertzer NR, et al. ACC/AHA 2005 Practice Guidelines for the management of patients with peripheral arterial disease (lower extremity, renal, mesenteric, and abdominal aortic): a collaborative report from the American Association for Vascular Surgery/Society for Vascular Surgery, Society for Cardiovascular Angiography and Interventions, Society for Vascular Medicine and Biology, Society of Interventional Radiology, and the ACC/AHA Task Force on Practice Guidelines (Writing Committee to Develop Guidelines for the Management of Patients With Peripheral Arterial Disease): endorsed by the American Association of Cardiovascular and Pulmonary Rehabilitation; National Heart, Lung, and Blood Institute; Society for Vascular Nursing; TransAtlantic Inter-Society Consensus; and Vascular Disease Foundation. Circulation 2006; 113:e463–e654.

Jude EB, Oyibo SO, Chalmers N, Boulton AJ. Peripheral arterial disease in diabetic and nondiabetic patients: a comparison of severity and outcome. Diabetes Care 2001; 24:1433–1437.

Jude EB. Peripheral arterial disease in diabetes—a review. Diabet Med 2010; 27:4–14.

Kannel WB, McGee DL. Update on some epidemiologic features of intermittent claudication: the Framingham Study. J Am Geriatr Soc 1985; 33:13–18.

King TA, DePalma RG, Rhodes RS. Diabetes mellitus and atherosclerotic involvement of the profunda femoris artery. Gynecol Obstet 1984; 159:553–556.

Kullo IJ, Turner ST, Kardia SL, et al. A genome-wide linkage scan for ankle-brachial index in African American and non-Hispanic white subjects participating in the GENOA study. Atherosclerosis 2006; 187:433–438.

Lazaris AM, Tsiamis AC, Fishwick G, Bolia A, Bell PR. Clinical outcome of primary infrainguinal subintimal angioplasty in diabetic patients with critical lower limb ischemia. J Endovasc Ther 2004; 11:447–453.

Lepantalo M, Apelqvist J, Setacci C, et al. Chapter V: Diabetic foot. Eur J Vasc Endovasc Surg 2011; 42:S60–S74.

Malmstedt J, Leander K, Wahlberg E, et al. Outcome after leg bypass surgery for critical limb ischemia is poor in patients with diabetes: a population-based cohort study. Diabetes Care 2008; 31:887–892.

Marso SP, Hiatt WR. Peripheral arterial disease in patients with diabetes. J Am Coll Cardiol 2006; 47:921–929.

McDermott MM, Greenland P, Guralnik JM, et al. Depressive symptoms and lower extremity functioning in men and women with peripheral arterial disease. J Gen Intern Med 2003; 18:461–467.

Melliere D, Berrahal D, Desgranges P, et al. Influence of diabetes on revascularisation procedures of the aorta and lower limb arteries: early results. Eur J Vasc Endovasc Surg 1999; 17:438–441.

Melton LJ III, Macken KM, Palumbo PJ, Elveback LR. Incidence and prevalence of clinical peripheral vascular disease in a population based cohort of diabetic patients. Diabetes Care 1980; 3:650–654.

Muluk SC, Muluk VS, Kelley ME, et al. Outcome events in patients with claudication: a 15-year study in 2777 patients. J Vasc Surg 2001; 33:251–257; discussion 257–258.

Nicoloff AD, Taylor LM Jr, Sexton GJ, et al. Relationship between site of initial symptoms and subsequent progression of disease in a prospective study of atherosclerosis progression in patients receiving long-term treatment for symptomatic peripheral arterial disease. J Vasc Surg 2002; 35:38.

Norgren L, Hiatt WR, Dormandy JA, et al. Inter-Society Consensus for the Management of Peripheral Arterial Disease (TASC II). J Vasc Surg 2007; 45:S5–67.

Novo S. Classification, epidemiology, risk factors, and natural history of peripheral arterial disease. Diabetes Obes Metab 2002; 4:S1–S6.

Pahlsson HI, Lund K, Jorneskog G, Gush R, Wahlberg E. The validity and reliability of automated and manually measured toe blood pressure in ischemic legs of diabetic patients. Eur J Vasc Endovasc Surg 2008; 36:576–581.

Potier L Abi Khalil C, Mohammedi K, Roussel R. Use and utility of ankle brachial index in patients with diabetes. Eur J Vasc Endovasc Surg 2011; 41:110–116.

Selvin E, Erlinger TP. Prevalence of and risk factors for peripheral arterial disease in the United States: results from the National Health and Nutrition Examination Survey, 1999-2000. Circulation 2004; 110:738–743.

Selvin E, Marinopoulos S, Berkenblit G, et al. Meta-analysis: glycosylated hemoglobin and cardiovascular disease in diabetes mellitus. Ann Intern Med 2004; 141:421–431.

Strandness DE, Priest RE, Gibbons GE. Combined clinical and pathological study of diabetic and non-diabetic peripheral arterial disease. Diabetes Care 1964; 13:366–372.

Walters DP GW, Mullee MA, Hill RD. The prevalence, detection, and epidemiological correlates of peripheral vascular disease: a comparison of diabetic and non-diabetic subjects in an English community. Diabet Med 1992; 9:710–715.

Welborn TA, Knuiman M, McCann V, Stanton K, Constable IJ. Clinical macrovascular disease in Caucasoid diabetic subjects: logistic regression analysis of risk variables. Diabetologia 1984; 27:568–573.

Wolfe JH, Wyatt MG. Critical and subcritical ischaemia. Eur J Vasc Endovasc Surg 1997; 13:578–582.

Chapter 13 | Microvascular disease

Sanjeev Sharma, Gerry Rayman

SUMMARY

- The microvasculature of the skin is composed of a complex network of capillary loops, arteriovenous shunts, arterioles, and venules, which play a key role in maintaining skin nutrition
- The diabetic foot demonstrates a number of structural and functional changes in these microvessels, which alter microvascular blood flow and potentially impair skin nutrition
- There are various methods for assessing skin blood flow, each having individual advantages and limitations. These factors need to be considered when interpreting their results
- The endothelium is postulated to play an important role in the pathogenesis of diabetic microangiopathy, with disturbance of the nitric oxide (nitrergic) pathways being central
- Critical limb ischemia (CLI) denotes an advanced stage of peripheral arterial disease where capillary blood flow is severely compromised, leading to diminished tissue viability

INTRODUCTION

Diabetic foot disease is a major cause of morbidity and mortality. The key pathologies leading to ulceration and amputation are neuropathy and peripheral vascular disease, with trauma, foot infection, or a combination of the two often tipping the balance. This chapter describes the normal anatomy and physiology of the skin's microcirculation and the methods that can be used to assess this in human skin. It describes the functional and structural microvascular abnormalities seen in the foot skin of people with diabetes and discusses their potential role in the development of foot ulceration and in contributing to impaired ulcer healing and ultimately amputation.

Diabetes, whether type 1 or type 2, is associated with a variety of complications affecting both micro- and macrocirculations. Previous chapters have addressed macrovascular (peripheral arterial) disease, its relationship to poor glycemic control, hypercholesterolemia, hypertension, smoking as well as its associated two- to fourfold increase in stroke and myocardial infarction. The propensity for macrovascular disease of the lower limb arteries particularly those below the knee in people with diabetes has also been discussed.

Although the susceptibility of people with diabetes to macrovascular disease is a major cause of morbidity and mortality, it is microvascular disease that is unique to the diabetic state. Microangiopathy is classically viewed as important in the retina, nerves, and kidneys. Retinopathy can lead to loss of sight and nephropathy to renal failure. The relationship of microangiopathy to long-term glycemic control has been well established in both the Diabetes Control and Complications Trial (1993) and United Kingdom Prospective Diabetes Study (UKPDS) (1998) studies. Although microangiopathy of the skin was identified decades ago, with abnormal nail fold capillary structure having being described more than 50 years ago (Landau & Davis 1960), the extent to which it contributes to skin ulceration and impaired wound healing in humans is still to be fully determined. It is not yet established whether microangiopathy is of greater significance in the neuropathic or the ischemic foot. Furthermore, it remains to be established whether microvascular disease compromises the outcomes of people with diabetes and CLI and further influences wound healing after successful revascularization.

A detailed understanding of the microvascular impairments afflicting the diabetic foot is fundamental in consolidating the concepts involved in the pathogenesis of diabetic foot disease.

▉ THE ANATOMY AND PHYSIOLOGY OF THE SKIN MICROCIRCULATION

▉ Microvascular structure of the skin

The skin of the foot comprises an outer epidermis predominantly composed of keratin and devoid of any intrinsic blood supply and an inner dermis consisting of papillary and reticular layers of collagen and elastic fibers. The skin is supplied by a dense network of cutaneous arterioles in the dermis. These resistance vessels control flow through two horizontal plexuses, one situated 1–1.5 mm below the epidermis and the other at the dermal–subcutaneous junction. From the arterioles in the upper plexus, arise smaller meta-arterioles with their precapillary sphincters, which function as high resistance conduits to a network of nutritional capillaries loops. The nutritional capillaries are organized into functional units with each dermal papilla supplied by one to three capillary loops (**Figure 13.1**).

The venous end of the capillary loop leaves the dermal papilla and enters into the subpapillary venous plexus. Areas subserving thermoregulation such as the skin of the hands and feet are additionally supplied by numerous arteriovenous anastomoses. These low resistance vessels directly connect the meta-arterioles to the venous plexus, which when open shunt large volumes of blood to the skin to aid heat dissipation. Both the precapillary sphincters and the arteriovenous anastomoses are innervated by vasoconstrictor sympathetic small nerve fibers (**Figure 13.2**).

Each capillary is composed of a single layer of endothelial cells lying on a basement membrane, which is thicker in the foot than in other tissues because of increased hydrostatic pressure associated with the bipedal stance (Williamson et al. 1971). The endothelium serves a variety of functions including regulation of blood flow through the synthesis of vasoactive substances, lipoprotein metabolism, nutrient transport, and angiogenesis as well as contributing to tissue defense and homeostasis.

The principle function of the microcirculation is the exchange of nutrients and metabolites between blood and tissues, which occurs at the capillary level, and hence any abnormalities of the microcirculation will have an adverse impact on the health of the entire skin.

▉ The regulation of skin blood flow

There are numerous regulatory mechanisms that control skin blood flow, and the key ones are as follows:

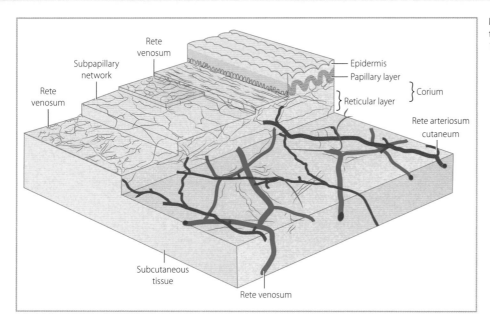

Figure 13.1 The distribution of the blood vessels in the skin of the sole of the foot. Adapted from Gray 1918.

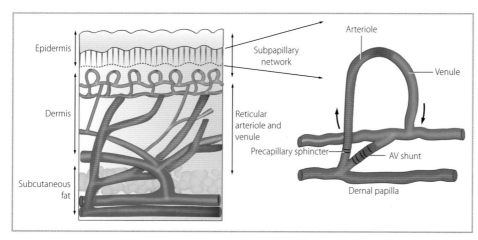

Figure 13.2 Diagrammatic representation of skin microvasculature depicting the dermal capillary network. A single capillary loop comprising a dermal arteriovenous anastomosis is shown on the right.

Central regulation of skin blood flow

Total blood flow to the skin can be considered to have two components: the nutritive component, which comprises flow through the capillary network, and the thermoregulatory component, which comprises flow through the arteriovenous anastomoses. In a comfortable environment, skin blood flow is normally subjected to a high degree of sympathetic vasoconstrictor tone balanced by a sympathetic active vasodilator system. With whole body heat stress, the former is released and sympathetic vasodilation activated, resulting in a substantial increase in skin blood flow (Charkoudian 2003).

Local reflexes
Vasodilation due to nerve axon reflex
Also known as the Lewis triple response, this mechanism is neurally mediated by nociceptive C-fibers, which are stimulated by noxious stimuli, including mechanical, chemical, and thermal injury.

Direct injury to the skin and the underlying microvessels results in a reduction in precapillary sphincter tone, which increases local blood flow limited at site of injury. Significant injury such as heating the skin to above 42°C will result in the maximum blood flow at that site. In addition to this direct vasodilator response, nociceptive C nerve fibers at the injury site are stimulated, resulting in orthodromic neural conduction to the spinal cord and onward to the sensory cortex to alert the subject of the painful stimulus. There is also antidromic conduction to the neural network adjacent to the site of injury. The latter results in the release of vasoactive substances including substance P, histamine, and calcitonin gene-related peptide into the surrounding skin beyond the injury site; this causes vasodilation in the vessels surrounding the injury site and is seen as the 'red flare' described by Thomas Lewis (**Figure 13.3**). Both direct and reflex vasodilation responses are of relevance to the diabetic skin as later described.

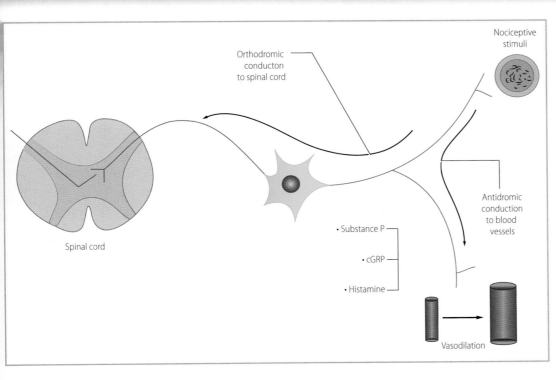

Figure 13.3 Schematic representation of the nerve axon reflex. Stimulation of the C-nociceptive nerve fibers leads to antidromic stimulation of the adjacent C fibers and mediated by substance P, calcitonin gene related peptide, and histamine.

Local autoregulation and the venoarteriolar axon reflex

Changes in vascular transmural pressure can alter skin blood flow. Two principal mechanisms are involved, autoregulation and the venoarteriolar reflex. Autoregulation is the tendency to maintain constant blood flow during changes of arteriolar perfusion pressure (Johnson et al. 1986). It is present in various tissues, including the brain, skeletal muscle, adipose, and cutaneous tissue. It is a myogenic response in the resistance arterioles, unrelated to neural control mechanisms but influenced by the endothelium as described later. Autoregulation is over-ridden when the limb is lowered >40 cm below the heart by a vasoconstrictor reflex mediated by a local sympathetic axon reflex involving the venules and the arterioles. Activation of this reflex in response to the gravitational increase in venous pressure in venules of the dependent limb causes a reduction in microvascular blood flow by as much as 90%. The physiological purpose of this reflex is to limit the excessive and potentially damaging rise in capillary pressure that would otherwise occur on dependency, and also to prevent the resulting interstitial edema. The degree of vasoconstriction is proportional to the change in the height of the column of the blood between the heart and the limb (Rayman et al. 1986).

■ Endothelium-dependent regulation

In recent decades, the role of the endothelium in the control of blood flow at both the macro- and microvascular levels has received considerable attention. It has become evident that the endothelium is by no means a passive inner lining of blood vessels but has an essential role in the regulation of perfusion, fluid and solute exchange, hemostasis and coagulation, inflammatory responses, vasculogenesis, and angiogenesis (**Figure 13.4**). The endothelium generates nitric oxide endogenously from L-arginine, oxygen, and nicotinamide

adenine dinucleotide phosphate by various nitric oxide synthase enzymes in response to shear stress and agonists such as acetylcholine. Nitric oxide is a powerful smooth muscle relaxant, resulting in vasodilation and increasing perfusion to the downstream vascular bed.

■ STRUCTURAL MICROVASCULAR ABNORMALITIES IN THE DIABETIC FOOT

The most prominent structural changes in the diabetic microcirculation are thickening of the capillary basement membrane (CBM), diminished capillary size, and pericyte (contractile cells that wrap around the endothelial cells of capillaries and venules throughout the body and are found in the basement membrane) degeneration. These changes are more pronounced in lower extremities due to gravity-induced hydrostatic pressure.

It is believed that CBM thickening is related to an increase in capillary pressure and shear stress as a result of the loss of control of precapillary sphincter vasoconstriction. This is greatest in the feet, because this capillary bed is not protected from the additional hydrostatic pressure due to the loss of postural regulation of capillary pressure (see later). This increases fluid filtration and induces an inflammatory response in the microvascular endothelium that leads to CBM thickening and hyalinosis of the arterioles.

Observational studies have shown that the degree of CBM thickening correlates with the level of glycemic control – with poorly controlled patients with diabetes having a greater degree of thickening when compared with well-controlled patients (Raskin et al. 1983). CBM thickening and increased stiffness of the precapillary vessel wall have also been linked to increased glycosylation and formation of nonenzymatic advanced glycosylation end products (Mullarkey et al. 1994).

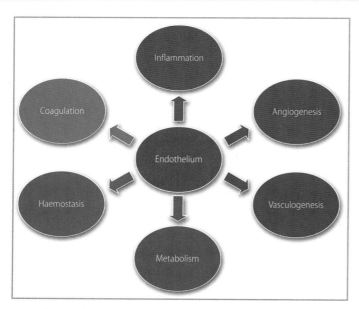

Figure 13.4 Multiple functions of the endothelium.

ASSESSMENT OF MICROVASCULAR FUNCTION AND ABNORMALITIES OBSERVED IN THE DIABETIC FOOT

In the last two decades, there have been significant improvements in existing methodologies and techniques for assessing the functional microcirculation of the skin as well as the development of new technologies. The concept of measuring skin microcirculation is based on quantifying the optical and thermal properties of the skin with particular relevance to blood flow, blood volume, intracellular oxygenation, and cellular respiration. The most commonly used techniques include laser Doppler flowmetry (LDF), laser Doppler imaging (LDI), transcutaneous oxygen tension (TcPO$_2$) measurements, capillary video-microscopy, and cannulation to measure capillary flow and pressure. Hyperspectral imaging (HSI) is a relatively new technique and is briefly mentioned as this may have a future role in assessing nutritive perfusion of the skin. The relative merits and limitations of each technique as well as the findings in people with diabetes are discussed in this section.

Laser Doppler flowmetry

The LDF is the most widely used technique for evaluating microvascular blood flow in the skin as it is easy to use and under controlled conditions gives reproducible results. The principle governing LDF is the noninvasive continuous measurement of skin blood flow based on the scattering of light by moving particles, principally red blood cells. All LDF instruments use monochromatic low-powered lasers with the light being delivered to the skin though a fiber optic cable. Light backscattered by moving red cells undergoes a frequency shift related to the speed and volume of moving cells. The backscattered light is returned to the instrument by the fiber optic cable. Through a mathematical algorithm, a voltage output related to the velocity and number of moving cells is calculated, which through further modeling generates an output expressed as units of perfusion flux. This reflects particle movement in the upper 1–1.5 mm of the skin,

which will include capillaries, very superficial meta-arterioles, venous plexuses, and arteriovenous anastomoses. In the pulps of the fingers and toes in a warm environment, its output is largely dominated by flow in the arteriovenous anastomoses unlike when used in the dorsum of these appendages, which are largely devoid of arteriovenous anastomoses. The method is well validated but limited by uncertainty of its penetration depth and its restriction to single-point measurement, which will result in point-to-point variation related to difference in skin thickness, microvascular density, and microvascular architecture. Moreover, it cannot directly measure the absolute flow but only provides an index of perfusion proportional to the skin blood flow (Fagrell 1990).

A variety of functional defects have been detected in the microcirculation of the diabetic foot using the LDF techniques. Impairment of the maximum hyperemic response to skin heating is well described, and the degree of impairment has been shown to relate to the duration of diabetes and the presence of other microvascular complications in both type 1 (Rayman et al. 1986) and type 2 diabetes (Krishnan et al. 2004).

The LDF has also been used in diabetes to assess the postocclusive hyperemic response of the microcirculation to ischemia induced by arterial occlusion. Time to peak is delayed in those without large vessel disease (Jaffer et al. 2008), indicating a microvascular defect; however, this was not the case in those with proximal disease who actually had a shorter time to peak probably reflecting the rigid nature of their vessels (Wahlberg et al. 1990).

Laser Doppler imaging

The principles governing the LDI are the same as the LDF, but it differs in being a noncontact method and can be adapted to scan tissue areas of various sizes instead of just measuring a single point as in LDF. Like LDF it can be used to measure the maximal hyperemic response to skin heating or other forms of injury but has the advantage of being able to do this on a wider area thus reducing the problem of point-to-point variations seen with the LDF. It also has the advantage of being able to measure the integrity of the nerve–axon related hyperemic response to injury. The resultant hyperemic flare (called LDIflare) has been shown to be a sensitive and well-validated method of assessing C-fiber nerve function (**Figure 13.5**). Like the LDF, it is subject to depth limitation and is unable to differentiate nutritive blood flow because of the inclusion of a variety of microvascular tissues in its measurement volume.

As with the LDF method, studies in diabetes using LDI have confirmed reduced skin maximum hyperemia but additionally have found impaired neurogenic flare responses in early type 2 diabetes before maximum blood flow is impaired (Krishnan et al. 2004). This suggests that small fiber neuropathy may be an early abnormality and has an important impact on the control of microvascular blood flow to skin in people with diabetes. The integrity of the neurovascular response may have an important role in wound healing, and its loss in neuropathy may, in part, explain delayed healing of neuropathic ulcers.

Assessment of endothelial function using iontophoresis and laser Doppler

Endothelial function was initially studied using venous occlusion plethysmography, but later with ultrasonography, most commonly in the brachial artery. The latter measures increase in arterial diameter after arterial occlusion to determine endothelial function. More recently, it has become possible to directly assess endothelial function in the microcirculation using iontophoresis of acetylcholine combined with either LDF or LDI. A transdermal current is used to drive positively charged acetylcholine into the skin leading to the generation of nitric oxide from the endothelium resulting in microvascular vasodilation. The increase in blood flow can be measured using either of the two laser Doppler techniques. Endothelial dysfunction or injury is seen as a relative smaller increase in perfusion in comparison with normative data derived from healthy volunteers.

The technique though relatively quick is operator dependent and influenced by the duration and amplitude of the current, which in itself may generate vasodilation. Importantly, in conditions such as diabetes where the skin structure is altered, it has been suggested that the diffusion of acetylcholine may be impaired, giving rise to a smaller stimulus, resulting in what may be falsely interpreted as reduced endothelial function. Impaired endothelial function has been demonstrated by a number of investigators in a variety of different diabetes states; however, the relationship to tissue ischemia and skin healing has not been established (Veves et al. 1996).

Transcutaneous oxygen tension measurement

The TcPO$_2$ is a noninvasive method that measures the partial pressure of oxygen molecules diffusing through the skin. The oxygen is derived from the superficial microvasculature. The TcPO$_2$ in the skin surface is relatively low; however, heating the skin to above 42°C greatly increases the measured level. The normal TcPO$_2$ level under these circumstances is in the region of 60 mmHg. Early studies demonstrated reduced TcPO$_2$ in the skin of people with diabetes without peripheral arterial disease and were thought to indicate abnormalities of oxygen diffusion and skin metabolism. However, it is now recognized that in the absence of large vessel disease, the measurement is influenced by the ability to maximize microvascular blood flow in response to heating; indeed the measurement correlates well with maximum microvascular blood flow measured by the LDF when both are used at the 44°C (Ray et al. 1997). TcPO$_2$ method is used in many vascular laboratories to help confirm CLI and by some to help determine the amputation level in patients with peripheral arterial disease (Faglia et al. 2007). In patients without diabetes patients, a TcPO$_2$ outcome of <30 mmHg confirms CLI. However, in patients with diabetes, the presence of microvascular disease will also influence the TcPO$_2$, but in the absence of macrovascular disease, lower results can also be seen in children with diabetes (Ewald et al. 1981). The TcPO$_2$ being influenced by both macro- and microvascular disease may, therefore, be of unique benefit in diabetes and, indeed, has been used to predict ulcer healing (Kalani et al. 1999).

Unfortunately, there is no standardization of the technique, and results vary from laboratory to laboratory. The technique has also the disadvantage of being time consuming, less reliable in the presence of tissue edema, operator dependent, and influenced by skin and room temperature.

Photoplethysmography

Photoplethysmography involves the measurement of both pulsatile arterial and venous blood flow by recording the changes in optical intensity of the moving blood column using an infrared light source and a photodetector. The light source is scattered, reflected, refracted, and absorbed in varying proportions by the blood column before reaching the photodetector, and these changes are represented as an electronic signal. It is a relatively cheap and easy to use method, but it is limited by restricted spatial resolution, and varying density of tissues since skin and underlying muscle absorb light in different proportions. It is an index of total blood flow to the area under the photodetector rather than flow in the superficial microvessels. Studies in patients with diabetes have shown good correlation with toe blood pressure and toe brachial index (Danescu et al. 2013). However, there is a lack of evidence to demonstrate its utility following revascularization of the diabetic foot.

Capillaroscopy

This is a useful experimental technique that allows visualization of the density, morphology, and rheology of capillaries using a sensitive real-time two-dimensional video technique. It has good spatial resolution and can be directed to the visualization of single capillaries. It has the advantage of being the only technique that measures nutritive blood flow. However, its use is limited to peripheral areas like the finger nail bed where the capillary loops run parallel to the epidermis allowing the whole capillary loop to be visualized. Its use in the toe nail fold is technically more difficult. The method is complex and time consuming, but it provides high-quality images of capillary diameter, length, and density in the specified areas and real-time capillary red blood cell velocity. To date, its use has been limited to research purposes. As discussed later, the technique has demonstrated reduced capillary flow during reactive hyperemia in people with diabetes despite there being an increase in total blood flow suggesting the blood is being shunted through the arteriovenous anastomoses (Jörneskog et al. 1995a, 1995b).

Hyperspectral imaging

The HSI is a novel method that assesses nutritive skin blood flow noninvasively. It is based on the hypothesis that ischemic ulceration is associated with hypovascular tissue as opposed to inflamed tissues that are usually hyperemic. Ischemia alters the ratio of oxyhemoglobin to deoxyhemoglobin concentrations at the affected site when compared with nearby unaffected tissues. With the aid of imaging algorithms this difference is measured to give information regarding the vascularity of tissues. The technique shows promise and may be important in monitoring healing of and the development of diabetic foot ulcers and in predicting the risk of ulceration. To date, this remains an experimental technique (Yudovsky et al. 2010).

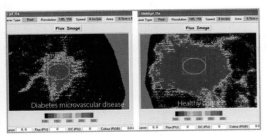

Figure 13.5
Nerve axon-mediated flare response by laser Doppler imaging method in response to heat stimulus in diabetes microvascular disease in comparison with healthy controls.

PATHOGENESIS OF MICROANGIOPATHY AND IMPAIRED NUTRITION IN DIABETIC FOOT SKIN

Although the pathogenesis of diabetic microvascular disease is clearly multifactorial and complex, hyperglycemia is considered to be the single most important risk factor. However, the nature of the metabolic imbalances induced by hyperglycemia in vascular cells and the interactions that result in vascular dysfunction remain unclear. The temporal evolution of diabetic microangiopathy has been suggested by several authors (Azzam et al. 1995) to develop over two stages, namely, an initial 'functional' stage that is largely reversible with normalization of the blood glucose levels and a latter 'remodeling' stage, which involves structural adaptation as mentioned above. Two mechanisms for microvascular dysfunction in the diabetic foot have been proposed, although neither is mutually exclusive, and the evidence suggests that both may be involved (**Table 13.1**).

The hemodynamic hypothesis

The hemodynamic hypothesis was first proposed by Parving et al. 1983, this hypothesis suggests that loss of regulation of microvascular blood flow results in increased capillary pressure causing endothelial injury and later CBM thickening, arteriolar hyalinosis, and diminished vasodilatory capacity. CBM thickening and arteriolar hyalinosis have been suggested to structurally 'lock' the microcirculation such that it can neither autoregulate nor respond to central and local reflexes and cannot maximize microvascular blood flow in response to vasogenic stimuli. This dysfunction has an anatomical preponderance with the most severe dysfunction demonstrated in the distal lower extremity. It is proposed that this results from the loss of protective postural regulation of microvascular blood flow in the dependent diabetic limb such that considerably greater and damaging pressures are generated in the capillaries of the foot accelerating the structural changes (Chao et al. 2009).

The capillary steal syndrome

Capillary steal syndrome mediated by opening of arteriovenous shunts has also been proposed to explain microvascular dysfunction. The initial events are heralded by loss of vasoconstriction due to autonomic sympathetic denervation, which leads to increased blood flow through arteriovenous shunts (**Figure 13.6**).

As a result, there is relatively reduced blood flow and nutrition of the upper dermis and epidermis, impairing ulcer healing. Studies by several authors, including Boulton et al. 1982 and Uccioli et al. 1992, have shown that arteriovenous blood flow is, indeed, increased in patients with diabetes and foot ulceration and neuropathy when compared with diabetic subjects with or without neuropathy alone.

However, these findings have been questioned by other investigators, including Rendell et al. 1989, who found that the arteriovenous shunt flow was reduced in patients with type 1 diabetes as compared with healthy control subjects, which is contradictory to other findings and would not support the 'capillary steal syndrome' hypothesis. Jörneskog et al. 1995b have reported the capillary circulation to be markedly reduced in patients with diabetes without complications, whereas total skin circulation was similar in patients with type 1 diabetes and control subjects. Furthermore, in another study Jörneskog et al. 1995a reported a reduction in capillary blood flow but not in arteriovenous shunt flow in patients with diabetes and peripheral arterial disease, indicating that sufficient blood reaches the area but does not enter the capillaries.

Irrespective of the individual relevance of either the hemodynamic or capillary steal syndrome in the development of diabetic foot microangiopathy, glycemic burden remains the most important factor in the causation of diabetic microvascular disease.

THE ROLE OF ENDOTHELIAL DYSFUNCTION IN DIABETIC MICROANGIOPATHY

The role of the endothelium in the regulation of blood flow has been described earlier. Our understanding of the mechanisms of endothelial dysfunction and the effects on diabetic microangiopathy have increased manifold in the past two decades. Both hyperglycemia and hyperinsulinemia have been suggested as aggravating factors leading to endothelial dysfunction on type 1 and type 2 diabetes (Johnstone et al. 1993, Williams et al. 1996).

At the cellular level, the main mechanisms involve the nitric acid pathway and increased vascular permeability. Although it is beyond the scope of this chapter to examine and understand these mechanisms and their evidences in detail, the broad cellular changes are outlined in **Figure 13.7**.

Although a substantial number of vasoactive substances have been shown to be increased in response to endothelial injury, the following biomarkers have been shown to consistently reflect the quantum of endothelial injury:

- von Willebrand factor (vWF): in both type 1 and type 2 diabetes, increased plasma levels of vWF have been demonstrated, and

Table 13.1 Proposed mechanisms leading to microvascular dysfunction and impaired skin nutrition

	Hemodynamic hypothesis	Capillary steal syndrome
Initial trigger	Disordered endothelial and smooth muscle function secondary to hyperglycemia resulting in loss of control of precapillary vasoconstriction	Loss of the regulation of the partitioning of skin blood flow resulting from sympathetic dysfunction
Vascular effects	• Increase in microvascular flow and capillary pressure • Increase in vascular endothelial permeability • Capillary basement membrane thickening and microvascular sclerosis leading to reduced vascular elasticity • Loss of reactive hyperemia • Loss of hyperemia response to injury	• Shunting of blood through arteriovenous anastomoses bypassing the capillary network • Increased total peripheral blood flow but reduced nutritive blood flow
Consequence	Impaired skin nutrition – reduced nutritive and regenerative blood flow after injury	

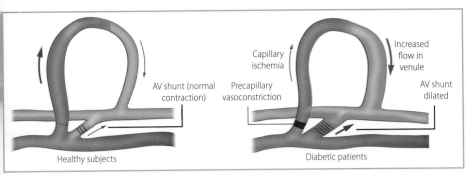

Figure 13.6 Capillary steal syndrome in patients with diabetes showing increased flow through the arteriovenous shunts.

these elevations have been found to precede the development of microvascular complications (Verrotti et al. 2003)

- Cellular adhesion molecules (CAMs): Ferri et al. 1998 have reported that CAMs are higher in both patients with diabetes and patients with impaired glucose tolerance

Studies in both type 1 and type 2 diabetes have demonstrated the temporal relationship between changes in the endothelial function and vascular dysfunction. However, this is better defined in type 2 diabetes where it has been shown that endothelial dysfunction precedes the development of diabetes; being present in the prediabetic stage (Su et al. 2008). However, in type 1 diabetes, Elhadd et al. 1999 have shown that endothelium-dependent vasodilation is impaired in the absence of microvascular complications, suggesting that endothelium dysfunction may be involved in the later development of microvascular disease.

DIABETIC MICROANGIOPATHY AND CLI

The mechanisms governing the etiopathogenesis of the diabetic microcirculatory state have been described as has the important role of the endothelium and its effects in those with diabetes. Traditionally, the role of vascular insufficiency in the lower limbs has been related to large vessel atherosclerosis that is associated with glycemic burden, smoking, hypertension, and hyperlipidemia. The UKPDS has shown that 11% of patients with type 2 diabetes developed peripheral arterial disease 6 years after diagnosis (Adler et al. 2002) and for each 1% increase in HbA1c, the risk increased by 25–28% (Adler et al. 2010).

In addition to the atherosclerotic process, Monckeberg's medial sclerosis and the resulting vascular calcification are more common in the lower limbs of patients with diabetes. Hence, traditional methods of measuring vascular insufficiency including ankle systolic pressure, ankle-brachial index (ABI), and Doppler estimations may give falsely reassuring results on a background of microvascular dysfunction. The above changes of medial sclerosis are less apparent in digital arteries, and hence measurement of toe blood pressure and calculation of toe:brachial ratio have been suggested as a more reliable alternative to ABI. Nevertheless, it must be recognized that calcification of the digital arteries is not unknown in diabetes, and therefore, even toe pressures can be misleading.

The concept of CLI is derived from an advanced stage of peripheral arterial disease where capillary blood flow is severely compromised leading to diminished tissue viability. The atherosclerotic changes of the larger conduit vessels lead to an increased resistance to blood flow

Figure 13.7 Mechanisms of endothelial dysfunction.

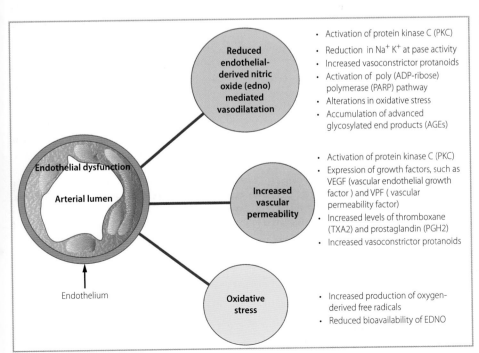

with a critical reduction in perfusion pressure and blood supply to the tissues. The reduced blood supply may lead to tissue ischemia causing rest pain, tissue necrosis, nonhealing foot ulcers, and gangrene. Rest pain in the supine position is a classic symptom of CLI, which improves in the standing or sitting position due to improvement of perfusion as a result of the additional gravitational hydrostatic pressure. It is important to recognize that people with diabetes and neuropathy may not complain of claudication or rest pain.

Norgren et al. 2007 from the Trans-Atlantic Inter-Society Consensus on Management of Peripheral Arterial Disease (TASC II) have reported that 1–3% of patients with diabetes have evidence of CLI on first investigation, whereas > a 5-year duration, 5–10% progress from peripheral arterial disease to CLI. The same committee has recommended that in view of significant underlying microangiopathy in patients with diabetic foot ulcer, tests of microcirculation are very pertinent to evaluate capillary ischemia.

In the face of overwhelming evidence of significant structural and functional damage to the microcirculation of the foot skin in type 1 and 2 diabetes, the key question is how important are these to the development of diabetic foot ulceration in the neuropathic and ischemic limb? In addition, do they contribute to the outcome of the critically ischemic limb and to wound healing in ulcerated and postsurgical wounds? There are considerable difficulties in answering these questions as patients with diabetes have multiple comorbidities, which in themselves influence wound healing. These include cardiac failure, renal disease, and anemia. Cardiac failure is associated with reduced cardiac output and edema of peripheral tissues both of which influence healing. End-stage renal disease is common in these patients as is renal anemia, both of which may significantly impair wound healing. Primary healing rates of foot ulcers in such patients are only 65% and following a major amputation 40% of stumps are still unhealed at the time of the patient's death (Lavery et al. 2010, Ndip et al. 2010).

In the absence of peripheral arterial disease, foot ulceration is almost always associated with peripheral neuropathy. Here, loss of sensation, neuropathy-related foot deformity, and resulting high pressure in focal areas combine to cause pressure ulceration – the typical neuropathic ulcer. Similarly, loss of the benefit of protective sensation is a recipe for unrecognized traumatic skin injury. Furthermore, a breach in the skin defenses due to sensory loss opens the tissue to infection with can rapidly spread without being recognized because of the same sensory loss. Whether microvascular disease in the skin increases the propensity to pressure-induced skin ulceration or impaired tissue defense, the spread of infection is still unknown.

Intuitively, it seems very likely that in the presence of significant peripheral arterial disease, reduced hyperemic responses to injury, reduced capillary blood flow, and impaired neurogenic vasodilation could tip the balance to further compromise skin nutrition. This must be considered when assessing a patient with poor wound healing in whom traditional noninvasive tests such as ABI and toe pressures would otherwise suggest a degree of large vessel disease that in an individual without diabetes would not be considered severe enough to benefit from intervention. Early vascular imaging should be considered in all patients with diabetes in whom healing is delayed beyond 6 weeks irrespective of the results of such noninvasive tests. As previously discussed, TcPO2 may be helpful in this situation as it is influenced by both large vessel disease and the ability of the microcirculation to maximally vasodilate.

Following revascularization and re-establishment of adequate flow by either distal bypass or endovascular procedures, wound healing may be delayed or fail in people with diabetes. It has been suggested that this is the result of persistent 'functional capillary ischemia.'

These areas show persistent lactic acidosis and are believed to result from microangiopathy, with the inability of the microvasculature to dilate and to proliferate in response to ischemia and inflammation accounting for the lack of formation of granulation tissue and healing despite successful revascularization.

It is important to recognize that despite the multiple defects in the microcirculation, on their own, these are unlikely to sufficiently impair the skin's nutrition to cause ulceration or impair wound healing as all such abnormalities have been demonstrated in the skin of children with diabetes (Khan et al. 2000), in people with impaired glucose tolerance (Jaap et al. 1994), and in newly diagnosed type 2 diabetes (Sandeman et al. 1991); groups in whom the absence of neuropathy and/or ischemia do not suffer critical skin ischemia or impaired wound healing.

Of relevance, one study failed to demonstrate impairment in the rate of wound closure after skin biopsy in patients with diabetes, despite gross reduction in maximal skin hyperemic response to heating, impaired neurovascular function, reduced vascular endothelial growth factor, and reduced small nerve fiber density (Krishnan et al. 2007).

CONCLUSION

Over the last few decades, a vast number of studies have provided substantial evidence of structural and functional microvascular abnormalities in the skin of people with diabetes. In the absence of large vessel disease, there is evidence of maldistribution of microvascular blood flow, resulting in reduced capillary blood flow; loss of postural regulation of blood flow, resulting in damaging capillary hypertension; disordered endothelial regulation of blood flow, impaired maximum blood flow, and impaired neurovascular response to injury. In the meantime, it is important that all clinicians assessing diabetic foot problems are aware that dysfunction in the microcirculation, the final vascular pathway to healing, is almost certainly present in every patient with diabetic foot disease and that they need to factor this into the equation, thus lowering their thresholds for intervention.

AREAS OF CONTROVERSY AND/OR FUTURE RESEARCH

- The shunting of skin blood flow through arteriovenous anastomoses in the diabetic state has been postulated to result in reduced nutrient capillary blood flow; however, not all studies support this concept
- There is difference of opinion as to which plays the predominant role in the pathogenesis of diabetic microangiopathy – the hemodynamic hypotheses and/or the capillary steal syndrome
- The extent to which diabetic microangiopathy impacts on the critically ischemic diabetic foot, neuropathic foot ulceration, and wound healing is still unknown
- The exact role of microvascular disease in the pathogenesis of the diabetic foot disease remains to be fully defined; further research is needed to fully understand which, if any, of these microvascular abnormalities are implicated in the genesis of skin ulceration and their influence on healing
- Research is needed to develop techniques that can be used at the bedside or in a vascular laboratory to determine nutrient capillary blood flow, and the effectiveness of the microcirculation in delivering nutrients and factors involved in defense to the tissues

IMPORTANT FURTHER READING

Adler AI, Erqou S, Lima TA, Robinson AH. Association between glycated haemoglobin and the risk of lower extremity amputation in patients with diabetes mellitus-review and meta-analysis. Diabetologia 2010; 53:840–849.

Chao C, Cheing G. Microvascular dysfunction in diabetic foot disease and ulceration. Diabetes Metab Res Rev 2009; 25:604–614.

Jörneskog G, Brismar K, Fagrell B. Skin capillary circulation severely impaired in toes of patients with IDDM, with and without late diabetic complications. Diabetologia 1995a; 38:474–480.

Krishnan ST, Quattrini C, Jeziorska M, et al. Neurovascular factors in wound healing in the foot skin of type 2 diabetic subjects. Diabetes Care 2007; 30:3058–3062.

Rayman G, Williams SA, Spencer PD, et al. Impaired microvascular hyperaemic response to minor skin trauma in type I diabetes. Br Med J (Clin Res Ed) 1986; 292:1295–1298.

Su Y, Liu XM, Sun YM, et al. The relationship between endothelial dysfunction and oxidative stress in diabetes and prediabetes. Int J Clin Pract 2008; 62:877–882.

REFERENCES

Adler AI, Erqou S, Lima TA, Robinson AH. Association between glycated haemoglobin and the risk of lower extremity amputation in patients with diabetes mellitus-review and meta-analysis. Diabetologia 2010; 53:840–849.

Adler AI, Stevens RJ, Neil A, et al. UKPDS 59: hyperglycemia and other potentially modifiable risk factors for peripheral vascular disease in type 2 diabetes. Diabetes Care 2002; 25:894–899.

Azzam ZS, Barton S, Corbett M, et al. Quantitative evaluation of the dermal vasculature of diabetics. Q J Med 1995; 54:229–239.

Boulton AJ, Scarpello JH, Ward JD. Venous oxygenation in the diabetic neuropathic foot: evidence of arteriovenous shunting? Diabetologia 1982; 22:6–8.

Chao C, Cheing G. Microvascular dysfunction in diabetic foot disease and ulceration. Diabetes Metab Res Rev 2009; 25:604–614.

Charkoudian N. Skin blood flow in adult human thermoregulation: how it works, when it does not, and why. Mayo Clin Proc 2003; 78:603–612.

Danescu LG, Roe CA, Johnson LW. Photoplethysmography: a simplified method for the office measurement of ankle brachial index in individuals with diabetes. Endocr Pract 2013; 19:439–443.

Diabetes Control and Complications Trial Research Group. The effect of intensive treatment of diabetes on the development and progression of long-term complications in insulin-dependent diabetes mellitus. N Engl J Med 1993; 329:977–986.

Elhadd TA, Kennedy G, Hill A, et al. Abnormal markers of endothelial cell activation and oxidative stress in children, adolescents and young adults with type 1 diabetes with no clinical vascular disease. Diabetes Metab Res Rev 1999; 15:405–411.

Ewald U, Tuvemo T, Rooth G. Early reduction of vascular reactivity in diabetic children detected by transcutaneous oxygen electrode. Lancet 1981; 1:1287–1288.

Faglia E, Clerici G, Caminiti M, et al. Predictive values of transcutaneous oxygen tension for above-the-ankle amputation in diabetic patients with critical limb ischemia. Eur J Vasc Endovasc Surg 2007; 33:731–736.

Fagrell B. Peripheral vascular disease. In: Shepherd AP, Öberg AA (eds), Laser: Doppler flowmetry. Boston, MA: Kluwer Academic Publishers; 1990:201–214.

Fagrell B, Hermansson IL, Karlander SG, et al. Vital capillary microscopy for assessment of skin viability and microangiopathy in patients with diabetes mellitus. Acta Med Scand Suppl 1984; 687:25–28.

Ferri C, Desideri G, Baldoncini R. Early activation of vascular endothelium in nonobese, nondiabetic essential hypertensive patients with multiple metabolic abnormalities. Diabetes 1998; 47:660–667.

Gray H. Anatomy of the human body. Philadelphia, PA: Lea & Febiger; 1918. Bartleby.com, 2000. www.bartleby.com/107/ (accessed 05 March, 2104).

Jaap AJ, Hammersley MS, Shore AC, Tooke JE. Reduced microvascular hyperaemia in subjects at risk of developing type 2 (non-insulin-dependent) diabetes mellitus. Diabetologia 1994; 37:214–216.

Jaffer U, Aslam M, Standfield N. Impaired hyperaemic and rhythmic vasomotor response in type 1 diabetes mellitus patients: a predictor of early peripheral vascular disease. Eur J Vasc Endovasc Surg 2008; 35:603–606.

Johnson JM, Brengelmann GL, Hales JR, et al. Regulation of the cutaneous circulation. Fed Proc 1986; 45:2841–2850.

Johnstone MT, Creager SJ, Scales KM. Impaired endothelium-dependent vasodilation in patients with insulin-dependent diabetes mellitus. Circulation 1993; 88:2510–2516.

Jörneskog G, Brismar K, Fagrell B. Skin capillary circulation severely impaired in toes of patients with IDDM, with and without late diabetic complications. Diabetologia 1995a; 38:474–480.

Jörneskog G, Brismar K, Fagrell B. Skin capillary circulation is more impaired in the toes of diabetic than non-diabetic patients with peripheral vascular disease. Diabet Med 1995b; 12:36–41.

Kalani M, Brismar K, Fagrell B, et al. Transcutaneous oxygen tension and toe blood pressure as predictors for outcome of diabetic foot ulcers. Diabetes Care 1999; 22:147–151.

Khan F, Elhadd TA, Greene SA, et al. Impaired skin microvascular function in children, adolescents, and young adults with type 1 diabetes. Diabetes Care. 2000; 23:215–220.

Krishnan ST, Quattrini C, Jeziorska M. Neurovascular factors in wound healing in the foot skin of type 2 diabetic subjects. Diabetes Care 2007; 30:3058–3062.

Krishnan ST, Rayman G. The LDIflare: a novel test of C-fiber function demonstrates early neuropathy in type 2 diabetes. Diabetes Care 2004; 27:2930–2935.

Landau J, Davis E. The small blood-vessels of the conjunctiva and nailbed in diabetes mellitus. Lancet 1960; 2:731–734.

Lavery L, Hunt N, Ndip A, et al. Impact of chronic kidney disease on survival after amputation in individuals with diabetes. Diabetes Care 2010; 33:2365–2369.

Mullarkey CJ, Brownlee M. Biochemical basis of microvascular disease. In: Pickup JC, Williams G (eds), Chronic complications of diabetes. Oxford, United Kingdom: Blackwell Scientific Publications; 1994:20–29.

Ndip A, Lavery L, Boulton AJM. Diabetic foot disease in people with advanced nephropathy and those on renal dialysis. Curr Diab Rep 2010; 10:283–290.

Norgren L, Hiatt Wr, Dormandy JA, et al. Inter-society consensus for the management of peripheral arterial disease (TASC II). Eur J Vasc Endovasc Surg 2007; 33:S1–75.

Parving HH, Viberti GC, Keen H, et al. Hemodynamic factors in the genesis of diabetic microangiopathy. Metabolism 1983; 32:943–949.

Raskin P, Pietri AO, Unger R, et al. The effect of diabetic control on the width of skeletal muscle capillary basement membrane in patients with type 1 diabetes mellitus. N Engl J Med 1983; 309:1546–1550.

Ray SA, Buckenham TM, Belli AM, et al. The predictive value of laser Doppler fluxmetry and transcutaneous oximetry for clinical outcome in patients undergoing revascularisation for severe leg ischaemia. Eur J Vasc Endovasc Surg 1997; 13:54–59.

Rayman G, Williams SA, Spencer PD, et al. Impaired microvascular hyperaemic response to minor skin trauma in type I diabetes. Br Med J (Clin Res Ed) 1986; 292:1295–1298.

Rendell M, Bergman T, O' Donnell G, et al. Microvascular blood flow, volume, and velocity measured by laser Doppler techniques in IDDM. Diabetes 1989; 38:819–824.

Sandeman DD, Pym CA, Green EM, et al. Microvascular vasodilatation in feet of newly diagnosed non-insulin dependent diabetic patients. BMJ 1991; 302:1122–1123.

Su Y, Liu XM, Sun YM, et al. The relationship between endothelial dysfunction and oxidative stress in diabetes and prediabetes. Int J Clin Pract 2008; 62:877–882.

Uccioli L, Mancini L, Giordano A, et al. Lower limb arteriovenous shunts, autonomic neuropathy and diabetic foot. Diabetes Res Clin Pract 1992; 16:123–130.

UK Prospective Diabetes Study (UKPDS) Group. Intensive blood-glucose control with sulphonylureas or insulin compared with conventional treatment and risk of complications in patients with type 2 diabetes (UKPDS 33). Lancet 1998; 352:837–853.

Verrotti A, Greco R, Basciani F, et al. Von Willebrand factor and its propeptide in children with diabetes. Relation between endothelial dysfunction and microalbuminuria. Pediatr Res 2003; 53:382–6.

Veves A, Donaghue VM, Sarnow MR, et al. The impact of reversal of hypoxia by revascularization on the peripheral nerve function of diabetic patients. Diabetologia 1996; 39:344–348.

Wahlberg E, Jörneskog G, Olofsson P, et al. The influence of reactive hyperaemia and leg dependency on skin microcirculation in patients with peripheral arterial occlusive disease (PAOD), with and without diabetes. Vasa 1990; 19:301–306.

Williams SB, Cusco JA, Roddy M et al. Impaired nitric oxide-mediated vasodilation in patients with noninsulin-dependent diabetes mellitus. J Am Coll Cardiol 1996; 27:567–574.

Williamson JR, Vogler NJ, Kilo C. Regional variations in the width of the basement membrane of muscle capillaries in man and giraffe. Am J Pathol 1971; 63:359–370.

Yudovsky D, Nouvong A, Pilon L. Hyperspectral imaging in diabetic foot wound care. J Diabetes Sci Technol 2010; 4:1099–1113.

Chapter 14

The diagnosis of peripheral arterial disease

Patrick Coughlin

SUMMARY

- The diagnosis of peripheral arterial disease (PAD) can be challenging within the population of patients with diabetes as they may have a significant burden of PAD yet be asymptomatic

- PAD may be due to significant neuropathy or a more sedentary lifestyle on the back of significant cardiovascular comorbidity

- The first manifestation of PAD may be a nonhealing ulcer caused by a trivial injury. It is therefore essential that as part of screening of patients with diabetes that close scrutiny is placed on determining the state of the lower limb arterial circulation

- A major cause of high amputation rates in this cohort of 'at risk' patients is the delayed recognition of PAD and thus referral on to vascular surgeons is often too late as the tissue loss burden can be too great to heal even with successful revascularization

- Although, no treatment is required for asymptomatic patients, the determination of PAD allows aggressive cardiovascular risk management to be initiated, which may halt or slow the progress of atherosclerotic burden

- An accurate history and in-depth examination will often give a diagnosis of PAD in patients with diabetes. However, this can often be challenging

- There are a number of complimentary noninvasive examination techniques that are available to aid diagnosis. These are often relatively straightforward to perform, meaning that there is the potential for them to be delivered within a primary care setting. At present, however, they are often limited to vascular studies units

INTRODUCTION

Diabetes mellitus is a strong risk factor for the development of atherosclerosis as a whole and specifically PAD (Eraso et al.). Insulin resistance, a precursor to the development of diabetes is also associated with the presence of PAD in an older population, increasing the risk of PAD by approximately 50–60% (Britton et al. 2012, Muntner et al. 2005). Intermittent claudication is twice as common in people with diabetes compared with those without diabetes and its prevalence is associated with the glycemic control, with a 1% increase in Hb1Ac levels being associated with a 26% increase in risk of PAD (Selvin et al. 2004).

Lower limb PAD is a relatively common condition. It is caused by the development of atherosclerosis that leads to arterial stenosis or occlusion in the major vessels within the lower limb. Diabetes, however, is also associated with microvascular disease that further hinders blood supply to the lower limb and specifically the foot, which is not easily amenable to any form of treatment. In the population as a whole, the prevalence of PAD is based on objective testing [an ankle brachial pressure index (ABPI)] (Criqui et al. 1985, Hiatt et al. 1995, Selvin & Erlinger 2004). Diabetes mellitus will accelerate the atherosclerotic process, with earlier presentation of complications associated with lower limb ischemia especially when combined with other risk factors, specifically cigarette smoking.

This chapter will focus on the diagnosis of PAD, which may often be challenging within the diabetes population, focusing specifically on the history, clinical examination, and noninvasive assessments of blood flow.

SYMPTOMS OF PERIPHERAL ARTERIAL DISEASE

A large proportion of patients with PAD will be asymptomatic (Bozkurt et al. 2011) (**Table 14.1**). This is in part either due to a limited exercise requirement thus not subjecting the lower limb muscle to an ischemic condition or the development of sufficient collateral supply. This is in itself significant in patients with diabetes as the presence of lower limb arterial disease (be it symptomatic or asymptomatic) increases the risk of longer-term cardiovascular morbidity/mortality. Furthermore, it places any patient's foot 'at risk' from developing ulceration/gangrenous changes. Based on these observations, a consensus statement from the American Diabetes Association recommends PAD screening with an ABI every 5 years in patients with diabetes (http://www.diabetes.org/living-with-diabetes/complications/peripheral-arterial-disease.html).

Intermittent claudication

The classical presentation of patients with PAD is that of intermittent claudication – the onset of muscular cramp like pain brought on by walking and relieved with rest. The symptoms commonly affect the calf muscle but can also affect the thigh and buttock. Patients with intermittent claudication have enough blood flow at rest not to develop symptoms. At the onset of exercise, often walking, the atherosclerotic disease within the arteries supplying the lower limb limit the increase in blood required to adequately perfuse the muscle groups of the lower limb thus causing a mismatch between oxygen supply and muscle metabolic demand. This mismatch ultimately results in anaerobic metabolism and the subsequent onset of pain. Resting (i.e. cessation of walking) eventually re-establishes the equilibrium between resting blood flow and the reducing metabolic needs of the muscle. The onset of pain is often accelerated when patients walk up an incline due to the increasing metabolic needs of the muscles. Furthermore, following resting and the associated relieving of pain, the patient is often able to then walk the same distance again before developing the pain.

Although the symptoms of claudication are quite typical, there are a number of other conditions that cause leg pain on exertion. The differential diagnosis of claudication includes chronic compartment syndrome, popliteal entrapment syndrome, nerve root compression/spinal stenosis, and lower limb osteoarthritis. However, less than 25% of people with diabetes and PAD present with symptoms of claudication in part due to the predominantly crural vessel distribution of the

Table 14.1 Classification of peripheral arterial disease: Rutherford categories (Norgren et al. 2007)

Grade	Category	Clinical
0	0	Asymptomatic
I	1	Mild claudication
I	2	Moderate claudication
I	3	Severe claudication
II	4	Ischemic rest pain
III	5	Minor tissue loss
III	6	Major tissue loss

disease (http://www.iwgdf.org/, Diehm et al. 2008). Furthermore, some patients with diabetes and PAD will have atypical symptoms, which in part may be due to the presence of peripheral neuropathy with its associated impaired sensory feedback. Patients may, however, present with more subtle symptoms, which may include leg fatigue or a slower walking speed. A study by Dolan et al. found that patients with PAD and diabetes had poorer lower extremity function than those with PAD alone, which was in part due to neuropathy but also due to a greater cardiovascular disease burden limiting their overall physical ability (Dolan et al. 2002).

A number of screening tools are in use for determining the presence of claudication. One of the most commonly used questionnaires is the Edinburgh claudication questionnaire (ECQ), which has been extensively used within epidemiological studies (Leng & Fowkes 1992). However, the nature of the more atypical symptoms seen within the population with diabetes may limit its use. This is born out in a study by Rabia and Khoo that assessed the accuracy of the ECQ in a population with diabetes, with the questionnaire showing a high specificity (99.4%) but an extremely low sensitivity (25%) when compared with ABPI (Rabia & Khoo).

Critical limb ischemia

Critical limb ischemia (CLI) represents the most severe end of the spectrum with regard to PAD. The definition of CLI has evolved over time, but essentially CLI is defined not only by the clinical presentation but also by an objective measurement of impaired blood flow (Becker et al. 2011). The TASC II document defines CLI as the presence of symptoms (chronic ischemic rest pain, ulcers or gangrene) attributable to objectively proven arterial disease that has been present for at least 2 weeks (Norgren et al. 2007). The diagnosis should be confirmed by the ABPI or toe systolic pressure with an ankle pressure of Norgren et al. (2007). These hemodynamic parameters may be less reliable in patients with diabetes because arterial wall calcification can impair compression by a blood pressure cuff and produce systolic pressure measurements that are greater than the actual levels.

In CLI, essentially, the macrovascular disease is so great that the perfusion pressure is not sufficient enough to deliver nutritional blood flow to the most distal tissues of the foot. Pedal pain is the dominant symptom, most typically occurring initially at night (the limb no longer being in a dependent position with an associated reduced cardiac output during sleep) that is relieved by dependency before typically progressing to continuous pain as time progresses. The pain usually affects the most distal aspect of the foot initially slowly progressing more proximally.

The differential diagnosis of rest pain associated with CLI includes diabetes-related neuropathy, complex regional pain syndrome, nerve root compression, night cramps, Buerger's disease, and a number of other local inflammatory conditions of the foot.

Occasionally, a diagnostic dilemma can occur in a cohort of patients with diabetes who present with evidence of PAD but a history of pain that is not typical of CLI. Often the pain is due to the neuropathy itself, presenting with a burning or shooting pain within the leg/foot often worse at night. Often, however, there is a symmetrical distribution and making the leg dependent brings no relief. A trial of neuroleptic medication may help determine the diagnosis.

In patients with diabetes, however, the clinical presentation is somewhat blurred by the presence of such neuropathy. Neuropathy also typically affects the most distal aspect of the limb first and thus such patients may not experience the pain of CLI despite having a significant burden of lower limb arterial disease. The impairment of such sensory feedback allows continued progression of ischemia to occur. As such, the first presentation in patients with diabetes tends to be with a neuroischemic type ulcer or distal gangrene often with the precipitant being poorly fitting shoes or minor trauma.

Ulceration can occur primarily due to the combination or PAD and diabetes either causing purely ischemic ulceration or combined neuroischemic ulceration. However, ulceration can occur due to other common causes, including venous ulceration, with the suboptimal arterial flow not permitting ulcer healing to occur. The combination of three concurrent pathological processes adds further complexities to the management. Common causes of lower limb ulceration can be seen in **Table 14.2**. Indeed, healing requires tissue perfusion above and beyond that which is required to support and maintain intact skin. In venous ulceration, an ABPI >0.8 is deemed suitable to apply some form of compression bandaging (albeit 3-layer compression) (Vowden & Vowden). An ABPI >0.5 is out with a diagnosis of CLI but an arbitrary ABPI at which a diabetic foot ulcer will heal is not available. This is in part due to the burden of microcirculatory disease as well as the frequent coexistence of infection. A multidisciplinary approach to treating diabetic foot ulcers is required and 'in line' flow (i.e. at least one artery directly filling the foot without a critical stenosis or occlusion) has been traditionally thought necessary by vascular surgeons to get ulcers to heal (although lacks any real evidence base).

CLINICAL EXAMINATION

Examination of the patient with PAD should involve a comprehensive assessment of the cardiovascular system including measurement of

Table 14.2 Common causes of lower limb ulceration

Etiology	Location	Pain	Appearance
Arterial	Toe, foot, ankle	Severe	Various shapes, pale base dry
Neuropathic	Foot / plantar surface	None	Surrounding callous, often deep, infected.
Neuroischemic	Common sites with regard to arterial and neuropathic	Reduced	As arterial
Venous	Usually medial malleolus	Mild	Irregular, pink base, moist, surrounding stigmata of venous hypertension – hemosiderin deposition, lipodermatosclerosis
Mixed venous/ arterial	Usually medial malleolus	Mild	Usually similar to pure venous ulceration

Adapted from the TASC II guidelines (Norgren et al. 2007).

blood pressure in both arms, cardiac auscultation and palpation for an abdominal aortic aneurysm.

Specific examination of the lower limb vasculature requires examination of the femoral, popliteal, dorsalis pedis, and posterior tibial arteries. In a small proportion of people, the dorsalis pedis artery is not palpable due to its branching above the level of the ankle joint. Grading of the quality of the pulse is usually determined as 0 (absent), 1 (diminished), and 2 (normal). The finding of an absent pulses does, however, tend to overdiagnose PAD, and the presence of an absent pulse on a background of symptomatic PAD requires further objective investigation. An attempt to determine the value of pulse examination was undertaken by Khan et al (2006). Their meta-analysis concluded that clinical examination findings were not independently sufficient to include or exclude a diagnosis of PAD with certainty.

The presence of a bruit in the femoral artery is suggestive of flow turbulence and thus significant arterial disease. More subjective signs include changes in color and temperature of the skin of the feet, muscle atrophy from inability to exercise, decreased hair growth, and hypertrophied, slow-growing nails.

There is also a subgroup of patients who present with a good history of claudication and yet a full complement of palpable pulses at rest. These patients often have stenotic disease of either the common or external iliac system. Exercise and the precipitation of symptoms tend to result in loss of palpable pedal pulses due to the inability of the large vessels to provide sufficient flow to maintain distal pressure with muscle vasodilation during exercise.

All patients with diabetes and a foot ulcer or a history suggestive of severe lower limb ischemia should have an objective assessment of their vascular status at first presentation and with continued assessments on a regular basis thereafter.

Initial clinical inspection of the foot may find a relatively warm pink foot. This is often due to autonomic neuropathy with the associated increase in arteriovenous shunting of blood flow. In the 'acute foot,' there may be evidence of ulceration/gangrene with superimposed cellulitis. Sometimes, however, it is difficult to differentiate the infected foot from a foot with acute Charcot arthropathy. Associated edema is often present either in relation to the surrounding acute inflammation or as a result of persistent dependency of the leg, which is often seen in patients with severe CLI.

On the whole, diabetic foot ulceration is either ischemic, neuropathic, or neuroischemic in origin (**Table 14.2**). The distribution of diabetic foot ulceration is in part determined by the degree of neuropathy. The neuropathy does not only affect sensory nerves but also affects motor nerves causing changes with the function of the small muscles of the foot, which leads to alteration in the shape of the foot. As such, the majority of the ulcers affect the plantar aspect of the foot, specifically over pressure areas. Care also needs to be provided in those patients with diabetes who are bed bound as they are at high risk of developing pressure-related ulceration around the heel that is notoriously difficult to treat/heal.

ANKLE BRACHIAL PRESSURE INDEX

The American Diabetes Association consensus statement on PAD recommends screening of patients over the age of 50 years for PAD using the ABPI (Mayfield et al. 2004). This in itself may cause difficulties in the diagnosis of PAD, but the demonstration of PAD is important because not only does it highlight a possible/probable 'at risk' diabetic foot, but it is also a mark of global atherosclerotic disease and as such indicates the need for aggressive cardiovascular risk factor management.

The ABPI was initially introduced in the 1960s and since then has become a well-recognized measure of (reduced) blood flow to the lower limbs. As such, it is an effective test used to document the presence of PAD within both a clinical and scientific setting. It essentially determines the ratio of the systolic blood pressure within the lower legs when compared with that of the arms. In subjects without PAD, the ankle systolic pressure is expected to be 10–15% higher than that found in the arm. Classically, patients with PAD have been defined as having an ABPI (McDermott et al. 2005). Furthermore, subjects with an ABPI between 0.9 and 0.99 were found to have a higher incidence of claudication than those with an ABPI >1.0 (Wang et al. 2005). As such, the ABPI value needs to be combined with clinical findings and not used as a sole diagnosis of PAD specifically with values between 0.9 and 1.0.

Measurement of the ABPI

To measure the ABPI, the subject needs to be supine and to have rested for at least a 5-minute period. A sphygmomanometer cuff is placed around the ankle of the subject and a handheld Doppler probe (5–10 MHz) placed over the poster tibial artery and the dorsalis pedis artery in turn. The cuff is inflated until the audible Doppler signal is lost and the cuff then slowly deflated. The pressure at which the audible signal returns is the ankle systolic pressure. The brachial pressure can be determined in the same fashion. The ABPI is determined by dividing the higher ankle pressure (either the dorsalis pedis or posterior tibial) by the highest pressure from the arms. Reproducibility of ABPI measurement has been found to be good (Holland-Letz et al. 2007). **Table 14.3** shows how PAD severity is defined using the ABPI measurement. Therefore, not only is the ABPI a marker of disease severity, but it can also aid in the diagnosis of patients presenting with atypical symptoms of PAD. By nature of the test, it is in part user dependent. Skilled operators are required to produce consistent results. The reproducibility of the ABI varies in the literature, but it is significant enough that reporting standards require a change of 0.15 in an isolated measurement for it to be considered clinically relevant, or 0.10 if associated with a change in clinical status (Cao et al. 2011, Holland-Letz et al. 2007, Jeelani et al. 2000, Resnick et al. 2004). This potential lack of reliability is somewhat caused by a lack of standardized protocols. These requirements have put off a number of primary care physicians from performing what is a relatively speedy and accurate examination that confers a large amount of information about the limb specific and general status of the patient.

The one main caveat with regard to the use of ABPI as a marker for PAD in patients with diabetes is that of medial arterial calcification (MAC). This tends to lead to poorly compressible vessels and associated spuriously elevated ABPI levels. This is particularly frequent in patients

Table 14.3 Correlation of ABPI values with symptoms experienced

ABPI value	
0.91–1.30	Normal
0.70–0.9	Mild claudication
0.5–0.69	Moderate/severe claudication
<0.5	Critical limb ischemia
>1.3	Poorly compressible vessels

ABPI, ankle brachial pressure index.

with concomitant renal disease, neuropathy, and foot lesions and as such tends to correlate with patients with longer duration and increased severity of diabetes mellitus (Bosevski & Soedamah-Muthu 2012, Caruana et al. 2005, Everhart et al. 1988, Goss et al. 1989).

The ABPI does still have a role in the diagnosis of PAD in people with diabetes but the results need to be determined within the context of the individual patients. In patients with 'intermediate' vascular risk and no neuropathy, the ABPI has a sensitivity of between 63% and 100% and a specificity of between 88% and 97% with regard to the diagnosis of PAD. However, when the ABPI is compared with more formal imaging of the lower limb arterial tree in patients with more severe cardiovascular risk, neuropathy, or the presence of a foot ulcer, the sensitivities drop to 50–71% and the specificity to 30–97% (Potier et al. 2011). The effect of MAC also means that ABPI values between 0.9 and 1.3 should be considered with caution in this higher risk group of patients. Furthermore, patients with an ABPI >1.4 or incompressible vessels should be considered as having PAD unless proven otherwise.

Traditionally, the ABPI is measured using a traditional sphygmometer. More recent studies have investigated the role of automated devices. Such studies have shown that these automated devices correlate well with the gold standard ABPI measurement with good reproducibility (Rosenbaum et al. 2012).

Prognostic value of ABPI

In the general population as a whole, both low and high ABPI is associated with increased mortality rate (O'Hare et al. 2006, Weatherley et al. 2006). This is borne out by a subgroup analysis of the Strong Heart Study that demonstrated a U-shaped association between ABPI value and mortality. This trend is also seen in people with diabetes. The BARI two-dimensional trial analyzed 2368 patients with type II diabetes in whom ABPI was recorded at their baseline visit (mean follow-up of 4.3 years). An initial low ABPI (Abbott et al. 2012). Furthermore, the Fremantle diabetes study found similar findings with a low ABPI being shown to increase the overall risk of cardiac death by 67%, and another long-term prospective study from Sweden with 14 years follow-up showed similar results (Ogren et al. 2005). The ABPI also has the potential to provide additional risk stratification. This is specifically the case in those patients classified as having a Framingham risk score between 10% and 20% in 10 years. An abnormal ABPI in this intermediate-risk group moves the patient to the 'high risk' bracket and thus requirement for aggressive cardiovascular risk factor management.

Overall, the ABPI is a valuable test to perform. It confirms the presence of PAD, and provides key information on longer-term prognosis (with a lower ABPI conferring worse prognosis) providing a window of opportunity to deliver appropriate cardiovascular risk factor management.

The pole test

The pole test is an alternative method to assess lower limb blood flow in patients with difficult to compress crural vessels (Jachertz et al. 2000). It allows assessment of the hydrostatic blood pressure and is performed by elevating the leg and determining the height at which the Doppler signal disappears by means of a calibrated pole, which allows recalculation of cm H_2O for mmHg. This assessment method has been shown to be easy to perform as well as being an inexpensive yet able to provide meaningful, quantitative data determining the severity of lower limb arterial disease independent of the compressibility of the arteries.

Treadmill test

In certain situations, usually with iliac stenotic disease, the history may be characteristic of intermittent claudication but the resting parameters of lower limb ischemia (namely palpable pedal pulses and a normal resting ABPI) may be within normal limits. A treadmill test mimics the physiological experience of walking and allows measurement of the ABPI before and after the onset of claudication pain. This is especially important when there is doubt as to whether the symptoms are vasculogenic or neurogenic in nature. The treadmill test consists of a patients walking on a treadmill at a steady speed (2.5 km/h) on an incline (10°) for up to a maximum of 5 minutes duration. Patients with vascular claudication will experience a fall in their ABPI on walking (this does not occur in subjects without PAD). The magnitude of the fall reflects the severity of the arterial disease.

TOE PRESSURE MEASUREMENT

Toe pressure measurements and the subsequent calculation of the toe brachial index (TBI) are a frequently used test in patients with diabetes to assess the lower limb circulation. This is mainly due to the higher ankle systolic pressure readings often seen in this cohort of patients due to medial calcification. The digital arteries are often spared from such calcification and as such have the potential to offer a more accurate assessment of the arterial supply to the lower limb. Specifically, toe pressure measurements are a more accurate reflection of lower limb blood flow (when compared with ankle systolic pressure) in patients with diabetes who have either elevated ankle pressures or where there was evidence of peripheral neuropathy (Williams et al., 2005; Brooks et al., 2001). As such, it has been suggested that all patients with clinically suspected CLI and diabetes should undergo toe pressure measurement.

Toe pressure measurements are obtained by placing a small occlusive cuff around the proximal aspect of the toe and a sensor beyond the cuff to assess flow. Difficulties occur in patients with marked deformity of the toes, patients with significant tissue loss, and in those with previous digital amputations. The principle is the same as for measurement of the ankle systolic pressure, with the TBI being calculated again in the same manner as the ABPI.

Flow can be detected within the toes using either photo-plethysmography (PPG) or laser Doppler (LD) (Venermo et al. 2012). PPG detects changes in the blood filling of the digital arteries and arterioles. The PPG sensors emit an infrared light that penetrates the tissues under the probe and is reflected by blood cells. The LD perfusion signal is derived from the Doppler shift undergone by the emitted infrared laser light after reflection from moving particles (in this case the red blood cells). The PPG detectors need a pulsatile flow, whereas the LD sensors detect minor movements of red blood cells and thus allow lower values of toe pressure to be measured. As with ABPI measurement, there are issues with regard to reproducibility and environmental issues, such as room temperature, can affect the results.

A normal systolic toe pressure is usually found to be approximately 30 mmHg below that of the ankle systolic pressure. As such, a TBI >0.75 is usually defined as being normal. Certainly TBI values values <0.7 would be classified as being abnormal and either a TBI <0.25 or an absolute value of < 30 mmHg would equate to severe limb ischaemia.

Toe pressures are often used as part of the definition of CLI – defined as a pressure less than either 30 or 50 mmHg depending on the consensus document used and whether this is in the presence of tissue loss or not. Of note, TASC II requires toe pressures of <50 mmHg to confirm a diagnosis of CLI in diabetic patients (www.tasc-2-pad.org/).

In clinical practice, there is often debate as to whether the lower limb arterial circulation is sufficient to permit healing of a digital amputation site or to allow ulcer healing. Absolute toe pressures of [3] 55mmHg have been suggested to be predictive of ulcer healing, although a study by Apelqvist et al. showed that of 164 patients who healed their foot ulcers, 85% of them did so with a toe pressure >45 mmHg, whereas only 43 out of 117 patients (36%) did so with a toe pressure (Apelqvist et al. 1989).

TISSUE PERFUSION

Transcutaneous oxygen tension ($tcPO_2$) measurements within peripheral tissues have been extensively used in patients with both diabetes and PAD as an assessment of metabolic activity (Abou-Zamzam et al. 2007, Frykberg et al. 2000). Essentially, a probe is placed on the foot/leg and a point on the chest is used as a reference site. Each probe consists of a circular silver–silver chloride anode surrounding a central platinum cathode. Oxygen diffusion to the skin is reduced at the cathode to produce a current proportional to the partial pressure of oxygen. Common areas for investigation include the dorsum of the foot and the anteromedial aspect of the calf. A normal $tcPO_2$ level is approximately 60 mmHg (Andersen & Vasc 2010). A $tcPO_2$ level of <30 mmHg in patients with non-healing foot ulcers or diabetic foot (www.tasc-2-pad.org/). The addition of an 'oxygen challenge' may determine whether hyperbaric oxygen therapy may be a suitable treatment modality. $TcPO_2$ measurements have greatest clinical input in cases with severe limb ischemia and may play a role in determining optimal level of amputation healing in patients with diabetes. Furthermore, it has the advantage of the potential of measuring a number of differing points on the limb at the same time as well as being able to measure flow near to ulcers themselves.

The reliability of the test, however, is limited by numerous factors including skin temperature, sympathetic tone, the presence of cellulitis, hyperkeratosis, and edema. Furthermore, the test is of limited value given the frequent difficulty of patients with severe CLI to lie flat long enough to complete the test (Cao et al. 2011).

The measurement of skin perfusion pressure (SPP) is a further method to assess the microcirculation (Yamada et al. 2008). The SPP is the blood pressure required to restore microcirculatory/capillary flow after inducing controlled arterial occlusion. It is measured using a LD. SPP is not as accurate at predicting amputation healing as $tcpO_2$ measurement. A value of 50–70 mmHg is deemed normal with severe ischemia equating to a value <30 mmHg. SPP is not frequently available within the vascular lab setting.

AREAS OF CONTROVERSY AND/OR FUTURE RESEARCH

The following questions remain to be addressed:
- Which measures (singularly or in combination) with regard to lower limb/tissue perfusion will predict wound healing in patients with diabetes?
- Is there a perfusion level that is required for wounds to heal?
- Do anatomical measures of PAD in patients with diabetes accurately reflect tissue perfusion?
- What is the role of the angiosome in diabetic foot ulceration?
- Is duplex a suitable imaging modality to assess crural vessel patency in patients with diabetic-related PAD?

IMPORTANT FURTHER READING

Becker F, Robert-Ebadi H, Ricco JB, et al. Chapter I: Definitions, epidemiology, clinical presentation and prognosis. Eur J Vasc Endovasc Surg 2011; 42:S4–12.

Cao P, Eckstein HH, De Rango P, et al. Chapter II: Diagnostic methods. Eur J Vasc Endovasc Surg 2011; 42:S13–32.

Criqui MH, Fronek A, Barrett-Connor E, et al. The prevalence of peripheral arterial disease in a defined population. Circulation 1985; 71:510–551.

Holland-Letz T, Endres HG, Biedermann S, et al. Raised ankle/brachial pressure index in insulin-treated diabetic patients. Diabet Med 1989; 6:576–578.

Potier L, Abi Khalil C, Mohammedi K, Roussel R. Use and utility of ankle brachial index in patients with diabetes. Eur J Vasc Endovasc Surg 2011; 41:110–116.

von Bilderling P, Sternitzky R, Diehm C. Reproducibility and reliability of the ankle-brachial index as assessed by vascular experts, family physicians and nurses. Vasc Med 2007; 12:105–112.

REFERENCES

Abbott JD, Lombardero MS, Barsness GW, et al. Ankle-brachial index and cardiovascular outcomes in the Bypass Angioplasty Revascularization Investigation 2 Diabetes trial. Am Heart J 2012; 164:585–590.

Abou-Zamzam AM Jr, Gomez NR, Molkara A, et al. A prospective analysis of critical limb ischemia: factors leading to major primary amputation versus revascularization. Ann Vasc Surg 2007; 21:458–463.

Andersen CA. Noninvasive assessment of lower extremity hemodynamics in individuals with diabetes mellitus. J Vasc Surg 2010; 52:76S–80S.

Apelqvist J, Castenfors J, Larsson J, Stenström A, Agardh CD. Prognostic value of systolic ankle and toe blood pressure levels in outcome of diabetic foot ulcer. Diabetes Care 1989; 12:373–378.

Becker F, Robert-Ebadi H, Ricco JB, et al. Chapter I: Definitions, epidemiology, clinical presentation and prognosis. Eur J Vasc Endovasc Surg 2011; 42:S4–12.

Bosevski M, Soedamah-Muthu SS. Blood urea level and diabetes duration are independently associated with ankle-brachial index in type 2 diabetic patients. Diabetes Metab Syndr 2012; 6:32–35.

Bozkurt AK, Tasci I, Tabak O, Gumus M, Kaplan Y. Peripheral artery disease assessed by ankle-brachial index in patients with established cardiovascular disease or at least one risk factor for atherothrombosis--CAREFUL study: a national, multi-center, cross-sectional observational study. BMC Cardiovasc Disord 2011; 11:4.

Britton KA, Mukamal KJ, Ix JH, et al. 201 Insulin resistance and incident peripheral artery disease in the Cardiovascular Health Study. Vasc Med 2012; 17:85–93.

Brooks B, Dean R, Patel S, et al. TBI or not TBI: that is the question. Is it better to measure toe pressure than ankle pressure in diabetic patients? Diabet Med 2001; 18:528–532.

Cao P, Eckstein HH, De Rango P, et al. Chapter II: Diagnostic methods. Eur J Vasc Endovasc Surg 2011; 42:S13–32.

Caruana MF, Bradbury AW, Adam DJ. The validity, reliability, reproducibility and extended utility of ankle to brachial pressure index in current vascular surgical practice. Eur J Vasc Endovasc Surg 2005; 29:443–451.

Criqui MH, Fronek A, Barrett-Connor E, Klauber MR, Gabriel S, Goodman D. The prevalence of peripheral arterial disease in a defined population. Circulation 1985; 71:510–551.

Diehm N, Rohrer S, Baumgartner I, et al. Distribution pattern of infrageniculate arterial obstructions in patients with diabetes mellitus and renal insufficiency – implications for revascularization. Vasa 2008; 37:265–273.

Dolan NC, Liu K, Criqui MH, et al. Peripheral artery disease, diabetes, and reduced lower extremity functioning. Diabetes Care 2002; 25:113–120.

Eraso LH, Fukaya E, Mohler ER 3rd, et al. Peripheral arterial disease, prevalence and cumulative risk factor profile analysis. Eur J Prev Cardiol 2012; Jun 27 [Epub ahead of print].

Everhart JE, Pettitt DJ, Knowler WC, Rose FA, Bennett PH. Medial arterial calcification and its association with mortality and complications of diabetes. Diabetologia 1988; 31:16–23.

Frykberg RG, Armstrong DG, Giurini J, et al.; American College of Foot and Ankle Surgeons. Diabetic foot disorders: a clinical practice guideline. American College of Foot and Ankle Surgeons. J Foot Ankle Surg 2000; 39:S1–60. Review.

Goss DE, de Trafford J, Roberts VC, et al. Raised ankle/brachial pressure index in insulin-treated diabetic patients. Diabet Med 1989; 6:576–578.

Hiatt WR, Hoag S, Hamman RF. Effect of diagnostic criteria on the prevalence of peripheral arterial disease. The San Luis Valley Diabetes Study. Circulation 1995; 91:1472–1479.

Holland-Letz T, Endres HG, Biedermann S, et al. Reproducibility and reliability of the ankle-brachial index as assessed by vascular experts, family physicians and nurses. Vasc Med 2007; 12:105–112.

Holland-Letz T, Endres HG, Biedermann S, et al. Reproducibility and reliability of the ankle-brachial index as assessed by vascular experts, family physicians and nurses. Vasc Med 2007; 12:105–112.

http://www.diabetes.org/living-with-diabetes/complications/peripheral-arterial-disease.html

http://www.iwgdf.org/

Jachertz G, Stappler T, Do DD, Mahler F. The pole-pressure test: an easy alternative in patients with ischemic legs and incompressible arteries. Vasa 2000; 29:59–61.

Jeelani NU, Braithwaite BD, Tomlin C, MacSweeney ST. Variation of method for measurement of brachial artery pressure significantly affects ankle-brachial pressure index values. Eur J Vasc Endovasc Surg 2000; 20:25–28.

Khan NA, Rahim SA, Anand SS, Simel DL, Panju A. Does the clinical examination predict lower extremity peripheral arterial disease? JAMA 2006; 295:536–546.

Leng GC, Fowkes FG. The Edinburgh Claudication Questionnaire: an improved version of the WHO/Rose Questionnaire for use in epidemiological surveys. J Clin Epidemiol. 1992; 45:1101–1109.

Mayfield JA, Reiber GE, Sanders LJ, Janisse D, Pogach LM. Preventive foot care in diabetes. Diabetes Care 2004; 27:S63–S64.

McDermott MM, Liu K, Criqui MH, et al. Ankle-brachial index and subclinical cardiac and carotid disease: the multi-ethnic study of atherosclerosis. Am J Epidemiol 2005; 162:33–41.

Muntner P, Wildman RP, Reynolds K, et al. Relationship between HbA1c level and peripheral arterial disease. Diabetes Care 2005; 28:1981–1987.

Norgren L, Hiatt WR, Dormandy JA, et al.; TASC II Working Group. Inter-Society Consensus for the Management of Peripheral Arterial Disease (TASC II). J Vasc Surg 2007; 45:S5–67.

Ogren M, Hedblad B, Engström G, Janzon L. Prevalence and prognostic significance of asymptomatic peripheral arterial disease in 68-year-old men with diabetes. Results from the population study 'Men born in 1914' from Malmö, Sweden. Eur J Vasc Endovasc Surg 2005; 29:182–189.

O'Hare AM, Katz R, Shlipak MG, Cushman M, Newman AB. Mortality and cardiovascular risk across the ankle-arm index spectrum: results from the Cardiovascular Health Study. Circulation 2006; 113:388–393.

Potier L, Abi Khalil C, Mohammedi K, Roussel R. Use and utility of ankle brachial index in patients with diabetes. Eur J Vasc Endovasc Surg 2011; 41:110–116.

Rabia K, Khoo EM. Is the Edinburgh Claudication Questionnaire a good screening tool for detection of peripheral arterial disease in diabetic patients? Asia-PA J Fam Med 6, 2007.

Resnick HE, Lindsay RS, McDermott MM, et al. Relationship of high and low ankle brachial index to all-cause and cardiovascular disease mortality: the Strong Heart Study. Circulation 2004; 109:733–739.

Rosenbaum D, Rodriguez-Carranza S, Laroche P, et al. Accuracy of the ankle-brachial index using the SCVL(®), an arm and ankle automated device with synchronized cuffs, in a population with increased cardiovascular risk. Vasc Health Risk Manag 2012; 8:239–246.

Selvin E, Erlinger TP. Prevalence of and risk factors for peripheral arterial disease in the United States: results from the National Health and Nutrition Examination Survey, 1999–2000. Circulation 2004; 110:738–743.

Selvin E, Marinopoulos S, Berkenblit G, et al. Meta-analysis: glycosylated hemoglobin and cardiovascular disease in diabetes mellitus. Ann Intern Med 2004; 141:421–431.

Venermo M, Vikatmaa P, Terasaki H, Sugano N. Vascular laboratory for critical limb ischaemia. Scand J Surg 2012; 101:86–93.

Vowden P, Vowden K. Doppler assessment and ABPI: Interpretation in the management of leg ulceration, 2001. http://www.worldwidewounds.com/2001/march/Vowden/Doppler-assessment-and-ABPI.html

Wang JC, Criqui MH, Denenberg JO, et al. Exertional leg pain in patients with and without peripheral arterial disease. Circulation 2005; 112:3501–3508.

Weatherley BD, Chambless LE, Heiss G, Catellier DJ, Ellison CR. The reliability of the ankle-brachial index in the Atherosclerosis Risk in Communities (ARIC) study and the NHLBI Family Heart Study (FHS). BMC Cardiovasc Disord 2006; 6:7.

Williams DT, Harding KG, Price P. An evaluation of the efficacy of methods used in screening for lower-limb arterial disease in diabetes. Diabetes Care 2005; 28:2206–2210.

Yamada T, Ohta T, Ishibashi H, et al. Clinical reliability and utility of skin perfusion pressure measurement in ischemic limbs--comparison with other noninvasive diagnostic methods. J Vasc Surg 2008; 47:318–323.

Chapter 15

Imaging of peripheral arterial disease

Gerard S. Goh

SUMMARY

- Imaging of peripheral arterial disease (PAD) is an important adjunct to a thorough clinical history and examination
- Imaging may be noninvasive or invasive, and each modality has its own advantages and limitations
- The most commonly used noninvasive imaging modalities include ultrasound, computed tomography angiography, and magnetic resonance angiography (MRA)
- Digital subtraction angiography remains the gold standard for imaging PAD
- Newer technologies and imaging methods have their roles in certain applications

INTRODUCTION

The imaging of PAD is important, in association with a thorough clinical history and examination, in patient investigation and subsequent management. Imaging is increasingly used to assist with procedural planning and determining whether treatment should be undertaken with an endovascular, surgical, or hybrid approach. Knowledge of the different imaging techniques, advantages, and potential drawbacks is important in choosing the most appropriate method of imaging of a patient.

The methods of imaging PAD have evolved and been refined over time. Patients can be imaged by either noninvasive or invasive methods. Noninvasive methods include bedside tests, such as toe-brachial and ankle-brachial indices, segmental pressures, and pulse volumes measurements, as described in Chapter 14, as well as Doppler assessment of blood flow, ultrasonography assessment of blood vessels, computed tomography angiography (CTA), and magnetic resonance angiography (MRA). Invasive methods include catheter digital subtraction angiography (DSA), intravascular ultrasound (IVUS), and optical coherence tomography (OCT). Cost and availability, as well as keeping radiation exposure to a minimum, should be considered when choosing an imaging modality.

ULTRASONOGRAPHY

Modalities

B-mode ultrasound

Ultrasonography utilizes the principles of sound wave generation from a piezoelectric crystal and the reflection of these sound waves from tissues to form an image. The ultrasound transducer emits pulses of high-frequency sound waves (1–10 MHz) that enter the body and are reflected according to the different acoustic impedances of different tissues. Some sound waves are reflected while some travel deeper into the tissues. A computer analyzes the reflected sound energy intensity and the time taken to reach the transducer and creates a two-dimensional (2D) grayscale image based on these differences in acoustic impedance.

Doppler

The Doppler principle allows velocity measurements to be made, and in the case of PAD, blood velocity can be measured. Moving red blood cells constantly change the frequency of reflected ultrasound waves depending on their velocity and whether their motion is toward or away from the transducer. As blood flow in part of a of vessel is reduced due to a stenosis, the velocity increases. An occlusion or severe stenosis can demonstrate reduced velocities and monophasic Doppler wave patterns distal to this region.

Continuous-wave Doppler measures the reflected echoes by using a specialized separate transducer in the probe. Pulsed-wave Doppler (duplex) uses the same transducer to emit and receive sound waves. A transducer generates a short emission of sound waves in emission mode before converting to receiver mode and receiving the reflected waves, the process being continuously repeated. Pulse wave Doppler allows the user to measure the Doppler signal in a specific area of vessel and provides both systolic and diastolic velocities as well as information about the waveform pattern of the Doppler spectrum produced (**Figure 15.1**).

Spectral waveform patterns provide information about the direction, phasic quality of the blood flow, changes in velocities during systole and diastole, and the spectrum of velocities at the point of interest. Stenoses cause an increase in systolic velocity as well as spectral broadening. If the waveform is monophasic instead of triphasic, this indicates of a significant stenosis proximal to the region being imaged. Severe stenoses and occlusions can be difficult

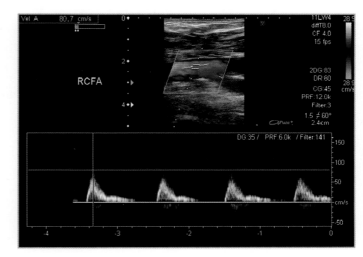

Figure 15.1 Duplex arterial ultrasound. The normal Doppler waveform pattern of a nondiseased right common femoral artery demonstrates an initial peak systolic wave followed immediately by a lower velocity diastolic wave.

to distinguish from each other. A marked reduction in the peak systolic velocity (PSV) may occur immediately proximal to a total occlusion unless there is a large collateral vessel.

Color Doppler

The Doppler shift, or change in velocity, can also be demonstrated as color, spectral waveforms, or audible sound. Color is usually displayed in red and blue, depending on the direction of flow, with different intensities of color representing different flow velocities. The color is superimposed over the grayscale image, with red conventionally used to represent flow towards the transducer and blue representing flow away from the transducer. This allows the operator to gain a quick overview of the vessel and to select areas of turbulent flow for further investigation with duplex.

Contrast-enhanced ultrasound

Ultrasound contrast agents are designed to reflect sound waves to allow differentiation of the contrast agent from other structures. These agents are gas-filled microbubbles that are administered intravenously (IV). The gas within the microbubbles reflects sound waves strongly and has a high degree of echogenicity. The contrast agents are composed of an exterior shell and gas-filled core. The exterior shell is generally hydrophobic to increase the time duration within the circulation before being taken up by the immune system and is commonly made up of albumin, galactose, lipid, or polymers (Lindner 2004). The gas-filled core is usually air, nitrogen, or perfluorocarbon. The size of the contrast particles is usually 1–4 μm. Contrast-enhanced

ultrasound allows the measurement of blood flow rate or end-organ perfusion. Contrast-enhanced ultrasound has been demonstrated to improve the agreement between arterial duplex scanning and contrast angiography of the tibial vessels (Coffi et al. 2004). Continued research into the development of ligand-specific binding agents holds promise for tissue- or inflammation-specific imaging. Contrast agents may be able to highlight areas of active plaque in atherosclerotic disease, thus enabling targeted treatment of these areas.

Advantages and limitations of ultrasound

Ultrasound requires an experienced vascular technologist or vascular interventionalist to achieve accurate results. Imaging of the proximal aortoiliac segment is performed with a low-frequency transducer (2–3.5 MHz), and the lower extremity is imaged with a high-frequency transducer (5–10 MHz). A full examination from the distal abdominal aorta to pedal arteries can be time intensive, requiring up to 2 hours per examination, although this may be shortened to 25–45 minutes in very experienced users (Hingorani et al. 2008) (**Figure 15.2**). Arterial duplex is commonly used for postintervention monitoring because of its reliability, repeatability, noninvasive nature, and low cost.

The predictive value of duplex ultrasound for the tibial vessels is not as good as for the aortoiliac or femoral–popliteal segments; however, patent tibial vessels are occasionally visualized by arterial duplex but not by DSA, especially in patients with critical limb ischemia (CLI) and multilevel disease (Favaretto et al. 2007, Hingorani et al. 2008). The pedal arteries may be visualized using arterial duplex; however, their superficial course renders them easily compressed by the transducer, which may

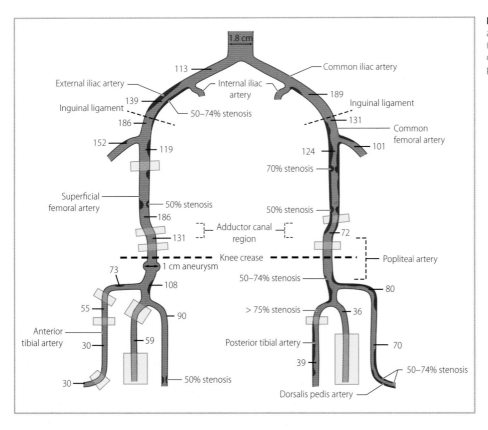

Figure 15.2 Ultrasound of lower limb arterial assessment. Numbers represent peak systolic velocity (cm/s) and the hatched areas show regions of heavy calcification where ultrasound analysis was not possible.

affect flow velocities. In addition, it is difficult to assess the entire pedal arch and the quality of the runoff within the foot (Langer et al. 2009).

Other limitations, such as obesity, bowel gas, leg edema, wound dressings, skin ulceration, vessel calcification, and severe ischemic pain, can inhibit obtaining an accurate arterial duplex examination. The image quality reduces the more tissue or dressings the ultrasound waves have to travel through. Bowel gas limiting visualization of the aortoiliac segment can be combated by having the patient present for the first morning examination having fasted since midnight. Leg edema can sometimes be treated by in-hospital leg elevation.

Ultrasonography can successfully be used as a screening tool to decrease the necessity for contrast angiography (Elgzyri et al. 2008) in CTA and DSA. It may also be used as the single preprocedural imaging modality prior to intervention in approximately 90% of patients (Hingorani et al. 2008, Schwarcz et al. 2009). The consistency of duplex ultrasound arterial mapping with DSA is 94.6% (Gabriel et al. 2012). The overall sensitivity and specificity for the detection and determination of stenosis in PAD ranges between 70% and 90% (Favaretto et al. 2007, Schwarcz et al. 2009); however, in identifying lesions requiring intervention, a sensitivity of 97% and specificity of 98% have been reported (Sultan et al. 2013).

Ultrasound can display various features of an artery and atherosclerosis. These include assessment of:

1. Vessel diameter: Ultrasound is able to give a measurement of the vessel diameter to aid decision-making in endovascular intervention or bypass. This can be measured by the use of the calipers on the machine.
2. Plaque morphology: The shape and size of a plaque can be determined. In DSA, this requires the imaging of a vessel in multiple planes, whereas ultrasound allows easy assessment of the plaque shape
3. The degree of stenosis: This can be measured but it may not always be possible if there is atherosclerotic calcification present that can obscure imaging. An alternative method to measure stenoses when encountering such limitations is to measure the velocities and velocity ratios proximal and distal to the region of interest, as well as to analyze the wave flow patterns to estimate the degree of vessel stenosis. Peak systolic velocities and velocity ratios aid in determining the degree of stenosis, and this information can be used in conjunction with the visual estimation of stenosis
4. Calcification: The presence of calcification (a common feature in patients with PAD and diabetes) strongly reflects sound waves, and the degree of calcification within an artery can be subjectively measured. The presence of heavy calcification within a region of an artery may help to indicate where endovascular intervention or bypass may not be so successful

As ultrasound is noninvasive, cost-effective, and quick to perform, it is often recommended as a first-line investigation for PAD. Ultrasound is also particularly useful in distal bypass. Vein mapping can be performed in the arms and legs to assess vein size and suitability for bypass grafting. Surveillance of distal bypass is another useful and commonly applied application of ultrasound. Other common applications include carotid duplex imaging and abdominal aortic aneurysm surveillance.

COMPUTED TOMOGRAPHY ANGIOGRAPHY

Basic technology and principles

Computed tomography angiography provides cross-sectional images of the peripheral arterial system as well as the adjacent nonvascular structures. Advances in both hardware and software have resulted in reduced acquisition times while improving image quality by enhancing resolution and decreasing motion artifact.

Iodinated contrast is injected intravenously by an injector pump, and once the contrast reaches the arterial circulation in sufficient concentration, CT data are acquired. An X-ray tube and detector array rotate through 360° around the patient as the CT gantry/table advances and acquires volumetric data. A computer then mathematically converts this information via a Fourier transformation into an image that can be viewed in multiple planes (e.g. axial, coronal, and sagittal).

Optimizing contrast exposure

Original single-detector CT systems were limited in their application by only being able to assess large vessels and small sections of vasculature due to long scanning times and low z-axis resolution. Often, contrast would travel through the peripheral arterial system more quickly than the CT scanner could acquire images. With the advent of multidetector systems, the application of CTA in imaging the peripheral arterial tree has advanced significantly. Multidetector CT (MDCT) allows coverage of a larger area of the patient per rotation of the tube/detector array and therefore allows rapid imaging of large anatomic areas. Sixteen-detector scanners had adequate diagnostic accuracy when compared with DSA but produced images that were significantly limited by calcification in the tibial arteries (Willmann et al. 2005, Hingorani et al. 2007). The newer generation MDCT scanners have 64, 128, and even 256 detector arrays that allow a reduction in scan time, radiation exposure, and contrast volume as well as an increase in resolution. Current protocols for 64-detector scanners involve a scan time of 15–20 seconds, a radiation dose of approximately 5 mSv, and a contrast volume of 80–130 mL of iodinated contrast (Cernic et al. 2009, Shareghi et al. 2010). Some centers include a normal saline bolus at the end of the contrast injection to maintain arterial forward flow and to promote the intravascular transit of contrast once administered. A delayed timed peripheral scan may be necessary to obtain optimal contrast opacification within the tibial vessels, especially in patients with long-segment upstream occlusions.

Radiation exposure

CTA produces a large amount of radiation exposure to the patient in a short period of time. It has been suggested that the radiation dose of CTA is of less clinical significance as patients with aortoiliac disease are typically older with shorter life expectancies. Despite this, major radiation protection agencies, including the International Commission on Radiation Protection, recommend using the ALARA principle (as low as reasonably achievable), meaning that radiation doses should be minimized wherever possible.

Radiation exposure can be measured in grays (Gy) or sieverts (Sv), where 1 Gy or 1 Sv = 1 J/kg. The sievert also takes into account biological tissue susceptibility by adding a multiplication factor, depending on the relative radiosensitivity of the tissue being scanned (e.g. gonads have a higher multiplier than skin). This allows a comparison of different tissue exposures between tissues with different radiation susceptibility. The levels of radiation exposure for a few common scenarios and diagnostic tests are listed in **Table 15.1**.

One of the initial studies into radiation exposure with CTA of the peripheral arteries found that the average dose was 9.3 mSv (Rubin et al. 2001). With the advent of further CT technology, low-dose protocols, and algorithms, radiation exposure levels have been dropping, with doses reaching 3–6 mSv while still retaining good concordance of findings between DSA and CT.

Table 15.1 Radiation dose

Source of exposure	Radiation dose (millisieverts)
Dental X-ray	0.005
135 g of Brazil nuts	0.005
Chest X-ray	0.02
4 hours on a transatlantic flight	0.02
CT scan of the head	1.4
UK average background radiation	2.7
US average background radiation	6.2
CT scan of the chest	6.6
CT scan of the chest, abdomen and pelvis	10
Annual exposure limit for medical radiation workers	20
Changes in blood cells can be readily observed	100
Acute radiation effects, e.g. nausea, reduction in white cell count	1000
Dose that would kill half of those receiving it within 1 month	5000

CT, computed tomography.

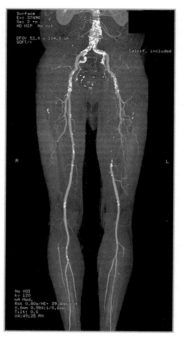

Figure 15.3 Coronal maximum image projection of computed tomography angiography (CTA). Representation of the entire length of the leg arteries can be displayed by CT post processing. Note the heavily calcified atherosclerotic disease throughout and occlusions of the left superficial femoral artery, proximal left anterior tibial artery, and mid to distal right anterior tibial artery.

Post-processing

Further developments have been made in CT software and raw data processing including various techniques for the manipulation and analysis of an image. Accurate assessment of the lower extremity vasculature requires analysis of the axial images, as well as the use of post-processing algorithms, which may include maximum-intensity projection (MIP), multiplanar reformat slices in coronal, sagittal, and oblique views, as well as three-dimensional (3D) volume rendering (Shareghi et al. 2010, **Figure 15.3**). MIP allows the representation of contrast to be highlighted against the surrounding soft tissues. Multiplanar reconstructions help to understand the anatomical relationships between the arterial vasculature and other structures with 3D volume rendering giving an overview of the anatomy. Curved multiplanar reformatting displays a vessel throughout its course in its middle section, factoring in curves. Other software applications include volume rendering, calcium scoring, and 3D reconstructions with soft tissue subtraction (**Figure 15.4**). Calcium scoring quantifies the degree of calcification within atherosclerotic plaques and areas of disease. Manually adjusting windowing levels aids in the differentiation between enhancing vessels, calcification, and surgical clips. Different protocols for bone subtraction exist and will continue to be refined in the future to allow better luminal resolution of calcified arteries (Brockmann et al. 2009).

Uses in PAD

Like arterial duplex, but unlike MRA and DSA, which are primarily luminal-based imaging modalities, CTA also gives an evaluation of the arterial wall and surrounding tissue. This includes the detection of peripheral aneurysms, as well as detailing plaque characteristics, calcification, ulceration, thrombus or soft plaque, intimal hyperplasia, in-stent restenosis, and stent fracture (Tang et al. 2010). The degree of stenosis and/or occlusion is illustrated, and an estimation of the degree of stenosis can be made in reference to the native vessel. Extraluminal

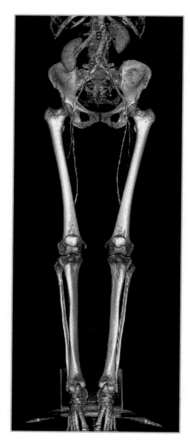

Figure 15.4 3D computed tomography (CT) bone and vessel reconstructions. A rotating 3D model can be created from the acquired CT data to aid surgeons in localizing lesions in relation to anatomical landmarks.

information can also be obtained, such as detailing any structures or pathology causing extrinsic compression of the arteries or the anatomy of anomalous vasculature in relation to the native vessels.

Advantages and limitations of CTA

The sensitivity and specificity to detect a > 50% stenosis or occlusion using CTA are in the range 95–99% (Cernic et al. 2009, Shareghi et al. 2010). In a meta-analysis by Met et al. in 2009, multidetector CTA for the evaluation of PAD was analyzed and the sensitivity of CTA for detecting >50% stenosis or occlusion was 95% and specificity was 96%. CTA correctly identified occlusions in 94%, the presence of >50% stenosis in 87%, and the absence of significant stenosis in 96% of segments. It should be noted that the majority of studies comparing CTA with DSA were in patients with claudication (68%) rather than in patients with CLI (32%) (Met et al. 2009). Patients with CLI often have greater disease burdens, and contrast transit time may subsequently be slower. There have yet to be any studies to determine this impact on the image quality of CTA.

The presence of heavy calcification, especially in the smaller crural vessels distally, can make differentiation between calcification and contrast difficult. Extensive calcification may mask any underlying contrast opacification or may even mimic the presence of contrast opacification where there is none, leading to misrepresentation of the disease state of the arteries.

MAGNETIC RESONANCE ANGIOGRAPHY

Basic technology and principles

Magnetic resonance imaging (MRI) physics is complicated. MRI uses the principle that all atoms spin along an axis and generate a very weak magnetic field. When these atoms are subject to an external magnetic field, they align along an axis in the magnetic field either pointing 'along with' or 'against' the direction of the magnetic field. There is a minute excess of atoms that point in one direction and a resultant net magnetic vector is created. This vector can be manipulated by the application of radio frequency energy pulses at different time and time length intervals. The atoms absorb this radio frequency energy, which alters their spin pattern. The absorbed energy is then released and emitted as a radio frequency signal when the atoms return to their normal resting spin pattern. This emitted radio frequency signal is detected by the MRI machine detectors. Differences in tissue compositions are able to be distinguished by the different number of atoms in a tissue type (e.g. fat, bone, and muscle all have different atomic compositions and quantities). As hydrogen is the most abundant atom in the human body, this atom is specifically targeted in MRI.

MRA sequences are generated by the detection of the flow of blood. The signal generated by relatively static tissue, such as muscle, bone, and fat, can be differentiated from flowing fluid using specialized techniques. MRA sequences are flow-sensitive acquisition methods that suffer from long acquisition times and overestimation of vessel stenosis in smaller peripheral vessels, making it an imperfect tool for evaluating PAD (Dellegrottaglie et al. 2007). Current advances in MRA, such as the development of novel MRA sequences, higher magnetic field strength, improved scanner hardware, software and coil technologies, have led to significantly improved image quality and acquisition times (Koelemay et al. 2001) (**Figure 15.5**). Contrast-enhanced sequences have also vastly improved vascular imaging capability in MRA.

Traditional 2D time-of-flight (TOF) MRA is performed without the use of contrast. The flow-related enhancement occurs when an

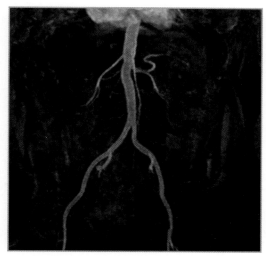

Figure 15.5 Magnetic resonance angiography (MRA) abdominal aorta and iliac arteries. An MRA of a normal abdominal aorta and iliac arteries.

influx of spinning atoms enters the imaging plane between two radio frequency pulses. MIPs and volume rendering can be performed on the data acquired, and images are generated to detect stenoses. 2D TOF imaging generally suffers from poorer resolution and longer imaging times, with a consequent increased risk of patient motion artifact. Contrast-enhanced MRA utilizes T1 shortening agents such as gadolinium-labeled diethylenetriamine penta-acetic acid (Gd-DTPA). This allows imaging of the arterial vessels as well as differentiation of the vessel from the surrounding structures when contrast-enhanced images are subtracted from precontrast images. This results in superior image acquisition compared with 2D TOF.

Studies in the 1990s comparing 2D TOF MRA with DSA demonstrated promising results with sensitivities ranging from 86% to 97% and specificities from 88% to99% for identifying <50% stenoses in patients with symptomatic PAD (Yucel et al. 1993, Glickerman et al. 1996, Sueyoshi et al. 1999). A meta-analysis of both 2D and 3D contrast-enhanced MRA in 2000 found that 3D techniques improved diagnostic performance (Nelemans et al. 2000). The sensitivity and specificity of arterial stenoses using contrast-enhanced MRA compared with DSA are in the range 80 to 90%, respectively (Bui et al. 2010), and the technique is comparable with DSA (Burbelko et al. 2013).

Newer generation machines feature higher magnetic strength such as 3 Tesla that can improve spatial resolution without requiring an increase in the length of time of an examination. The field of view is generally smaller than with 1.5 T units; in taller patients, four imaging stations may be required for the standard abdomen, pelvis, and lower extremity runoff views (Berg et al. 2008). Dedicated coil systems for peripheral arterial imaging are available and also increase spatial resolution (Kramer et al. 2007). Novel contrast agents are being developed that will also improve distal imaging (Gerretsen et al. 2010).

Uses in PAD

MRA provides similar information regarding the vascular patency compared with CTA and also provides some information about the surrounding structures.

Advantages and limitations of MRA

MRA has several advantages for imaging the peripheral arterial system over CTA and DSA. As calcium has a very different signal characteristic to time-of-flow sequences on MRA and more similar density to contrast on CTA, there is less confusion between calcification and contrast enhancement in MRA. There is no ionizing radiation exposure to the patient, and the gadolinium-based contrast agents used are less nephrotoxic than the iodinated contrast media used in CTA and DSA (Leiner et al. 2005). Gadolinium, however, has the potential to cause nephrogenic systemic fibrosis (NSF) in patients with renal failure, which is covered later in this chapter.

MRA has several limitations. It is generally more costly and less readily available than ultrasound, CTA, and DSA in most centers. MRA is very sensitive to motion artifact and even slight movements during image acquisition can significantly degrade image quality. Image acquisition time is long compared with the other modalities, with some examinations lasting up to 60 minutes. Furthermore, patients are required to stay very still for each sequence. Patients lie on the MRI gantry enclosed within a small tunnel-like setup that can provoke claustrophobia, especially in lengthy examinations. Contraindicated to MRI and MRA are patients with pacemakers, implanted cardiac defibrillators, cochlear implants, certain types of stent grafts, and aneurysm clips. Ferromagnetic blooming artifact from prior intra-arterial stents precludes evaluation of the stented area, which can easily be misinterpreted as an occlusion by physicians inexperienced in MRI and MRA interpretation (Leiner 2005). Venous contamination of the tibial-level images in MRA with contrast can be a problem especially in patients with CLI and diabetic foot ulcers (Dinter et al. 2009).

MRA is also limited in most centers to patients with glomerular filtration rates (GFRs) >30–35 mL/min secondary to reports of NSF developing in patients with either end-stage renal disease or declining renal function when exposed to gadolinium (Wertman et al. 2008, Weinreb et al. 2009). The risk is likely to be greater with certain formulations of gadolinium (Wertman et al. 2008), although the development of newer ferrous-based contrast agents may eventually prevent this problem. Metallic stents will appear as areas of vascular void on MRA, and this may confuse some inexperienced doctors interpreting MRA, leading them to believe that an area of occlusion is present.

GADOLINIUM

Gadolinium chelates are a type of MRI contrast that shortens the T1 relaxation time of nearby atoms. Gadolinium chelates have been used in the parenteral route since the late 1980s. Gadolinium chelates are extremely well tolerated by the vast majority of patients in whom they are administered. Acute adverse reactions are encountered with a lower frequency rate than with iodinated contrast media.

The frequency of all acute adverse events, after an injection of 0.1 or 0.2 mmol/kg of gadolinium chelate, ranges from 0.07% to 2.4%. The vast majority of these reactions are mild, including coldness at the injection site, nausea with or without vomiting, headache, warmth or pain at the injection site, paresthesias, dizziness, and itching. Severe, life-threatening anaphylactoid or non-allergic anaphylactic reactions are exceedingly rare, occurring in 0.001–0.01% of patients. Gadolinium chelates administered to patients with acute renal failure or severe chronic kidney disease (CKD) can result in a condition called NSF.

NSF is a fibrosing disease that predominantly involves the skin and subcutaneous tissues, but it is also known to involve other organs such as the heart, lungs, esophagus, and skeletal muscles. Initial symptoms include skin thickening and/or pruritis. The symptoms and signs of NSF may develop and progress rapidly, and some patients may develop contractures and joint immobility. In some patients,

the disease may be fatal. The time between injection of gadolinium-based contrast agent and the onset of NSF symptoms is within days to months in the vast majority of patients (Grobner 2006, Marckmann et al. 2006, Sadowski et al. 2007, Wertman et al. 2008). However, in rare cases, symptoms have appeared years after the last reported exposure (Shabana et al. 2008). It is estimated that patients with end-stage CKD (eGFR < 15 mL/min/1.73m^2) and severe CKD (eGFR 15–29 mL/min/1.73 m^2) have a 1–7% chance of developing NSF after one or more exposures to some gadolinium-based contrast agents (Marckmann et al. 2006, Sadowski et al. 2007, Collidge et al. 2007, Wertman et al. 2008).

DIGITAL SUBTRACTION ANGIOGRAPHY

Basic technology and principles

Arteriography was first performed by Dos Santos et al. in 1929. Along with the development of the Seldinger technique (Seldinger 1953), arteriography has advanced tremendously, both technically and technologically. Modern techniques are safe and have low complication rates.

The DSA remains the gold standard by which other imaging modalities are compared. DSA provides real-time X-ray imaging using fluoroscopy and allows the digital subtraction of soft tissue and bone before the acquisition of an arteriogram improving visualization of the arteries. Modern DSA systems employ image intensification to improve image quality and charge-coupled device (CCD) video displays to display the images obtained to the practitioner. Although DSA still has a lower resolution than that of a traditional X-ray, the ability of DSA to rapidly acquire images and instantly subtract and display an image on a screen, in addition to the ability to manipulate the image appearance, negates this disadvantage. Traditional X-ray filming is mechanical and slow compared with almost instantaneous DSA fluoroscopy imaging.

Contrast and contrast toxicity

Contrast agents are used to help differentiate different tissue structures within the body. There are different rates of uptake of iodinated contrast agents within each body organ and tissue. There are two major classes of iodinated IV contrast agents used in CT: nonionic and ionic. Ionic contrast agents contain a nonradiopaque cation that results in a low viscosity but high osmolality. Nonionic contrasts agents are not charged and do not contain a cation, which leads to a lower osmolality but increased viscosity of the agent. Higher osmolality is thought to be a major contributing factor to adverse reactions, and lower osmolality contrast agents also reduce the rate of nonallergy-related nonidiosyncratic physiological reactions. As a result, nonionic contrast agents are more frequently used.

A large nonrandomized, nonblinded study suggested a significantly greater safety of nonionic contrast agents over ionic contrast agents (Katayama et al. 1990). Other nonrandomized trials have shown similar results (Lasser et al. 1989); however, there still remain no definitive, unbiased, randomized clinical trials that demonstrate a significant reduction in severe reactions and fatality rates (Lasser et al. 1989).

The two major adverse reactions to iodinated contrast are anaphylaxis and contrast-induced renal failure. Anaphylaxis is a medical emergency, and all personnel involved with contrast administration should be trained in resuscitation and advanced life support, or be in the presence of staff with these skills. The incidence of life-threatening anaphylaxis is approximately 1 in 40,000–170,000. The most common cause of contrast-related mortality is airways obstruction due to angioedema. Fortunately, the majority of adverse reactions to iodinated contrast are minor, such as pain/discomfort or nausea (Stacul 2001, Tramer et al. 2006). Other minor adverse reactions include urticaria and mild angioedema, such as erythema, bronchospasm, tongue swelling, and transient hypotension with tachycardia. Nausea and vomiting are believed to be related to a central nervous system mechanism and are more frequent with venous injections. Complications may occur up to a week postadministration of iodinated contrast and are rare. These include rash, urticaria, and parotitis (Webb et al. 2006).

A history of allergy-like contrast reaction is associated with an up to fivefold increased likelihood of the patient experiencing a subsequent reaction (Katayama et al. 1990). A history of asthma may indicate an increased likelihood of a contrast reaction (Katayama et al. 1990). Specific allergies to shellfish or dairy products, previously thought to be helpful and predictive of contrast allergy, are unreliable in determining allergenic propensity (Coakley & Panicek 1997, Lieberman & Seigle 1999). Patients with significant cardiac disease may be at increased risk of contrast reactions, including symptomatic patients (e.g. patients with angina or congestive heart failure symptoms with minimal exertion) and also patients with severe aortic stenosis, primary pulmonary hypertension, or severe but well-compensated cardiomyopathy. In all such patients, attention should be paid to limit the volume and osmolality of the contrast media.

If a patient with prior contrast reaction requires IV contrast, patients should receive nonionic contrast and be considered for pharmacologic prophylaxis beginning at least 12 hours prior to the administration of contrast agent (Tramer et al. 2006). Unfortunately, studies have thus far indicated that the majority of contrast reactions that benefit from premedication are minor reactions that require no or minimal medical intervention (Lasser et al. 1994). No randomized controlled clinical trials have demonstrated premedication protection against severe life-threatening adverse reactions (Brockow et al. 2005, Morcos 2005, Tramer et al. 2006). One example protocol included administration of 50-mg oral prednisolone 13 hours prior, 50-mg prednisolone 7 hours prior, and 50-mg prednisolone 1 hour prior to the injection of contrast agent (e.g. for CTA) (Greenberger et al. 1986).

■ Contrast-induced nephrotoxicity

Contrast-induced nephrotoxicity (CIN) is a sudden deterioration in renal function after a recent intravascular administration of iodinated contrast in the absence of another nephrotoxic event. The pathophysiology of CIN is not entirely understood, and etiological factors that have been suggested include renal hemodynamic changes (vasoconstriction) and direct tubular toxicity. There may be some involvement of osmotic and chemotoxic mechanisms, and some investigations have suggested agent-specific chemotoxicity. The administration of IV contrast limits the use of CTA for patients with moderate or severe renal insufficiency who are not on dialysis.

There is consensus that the most important risk factor for CIN is pre-existing renal insufficiency. Multiple others risk factors have been proposed, including diabetes mellitus, dehydration, cardiovascular disease, diuretic use, advanced age, multiple myeloma, hypertension, hyperuricemia, and multiple iodinated contrast medium doses in a short time interval (<24 hours) (Lasser et al. 1994, Brockow et al. 2005, Tramer et al. 2006). Two studies have shown that CIN may occur after two closely spaced doses (Lasser et al. 1994, Tramer et al. 2006).

There is no universally agreed threshold of elevated serum creatinine/degree of renal dysfunction above which iodinated contrast agents should not be administered. Serum creatinine levels are commonly used as a measure of renal function, but this has limitations as an accurate measurement of GFR as it is influenced by the patient's gender, ethnicity, muscle mass, nutritional status, and age. A reduction in GFR of approximately 50% often maintains a normal serum creatinine level. The most commonly used estimation of GFR (eGFR) is the Modification of Diet in Renal Disease formula (Levey et al. 1999) (see **Box 15.1**).

> **Box 15.1 Modification of the diet in renal disease formula for determining eGFR**
>
> eGFR (mL/min/1.73 m^2) = 175 × (serum creatinine in mg/dL)$^{-1.154}$ × (age in years)$^{-0.0203}$ × (0.742 if female) × (1.212 if African American)

The risk of CIN in patients undergoing CT with IV contrast was found to be 0.6% in patients with an eGFR > 40 mL/min/1.73 m^2, 4.6% in patients with an eGFR of 30–40 mL/min/1.73 m^2, and 7.8% in patients with an eGFR < 30 mL/min/1.73 m^2. Kim et al. in 2010 examined 520 patients undergoing contrast-enhanced CT, 0/253 patients who had an eGFR between 45 and 59 mL/min/1.73 m^2 developed CIN, 6/209 (2.9%) patients with an eGFR between 30 and 44 mL/min/1.73 m^2 and 7/58 (12.1%) patients with an eGFR < 30 mL/min/1.73 m^2 developed CIN. Thomsen and Morcos in 2009 described 421 patients with an eGFR < 60 mL/min/1.73 m^2 who did not have end-stage kidney disease. Weisbord et al. in 2008 described that the rate of CIN following contrast-enhanced CT was 2.5% (8/316) in those patients who had an eGFR > 45 mL/min/1.73 m^2 and 9.8% (5/51) in patients with an eGFR between 30 and 45 mL/min/1.73 m^2.

Patients with mild renal impairment will frequently tolerate 80–100 mL contrast loads with appropriate prehydration. Solomon et al. in 2007 studied adult patients with CKD who underwent cardiac angiography. The reported incidence of CIN was decreased by prehydration (0.45% or 0.9% IV saline, 100 mL/h, 12 hours before to 12 hours after intravascular contrast administration).

The efficacy of *N*-acetylcysteine (NAC) to reduce the incidence of CIN is controversial. There is disagreement among multiple studies and meta-analyses as to whether this agent reduces the risk of CIN (Vaitkus & Brar 2007, Stenstrom et al. 2008). There is some evidence that NAC reduces the serum creatinine in normal volunteers without changing cystatin-C (cystatin-C is reported to be a better marker of GFR than serum creatinine). This raises the possibility that NAC might be lowering serum creatinine and not preventing renal injury. There is insufficient evidence of the efficacy of NAC to make a definitive recommendation.

Metformin is a biguanide oral antihyperglycemic agent used to treat patients with noninsulin-dependent diabetes mellitus. Metformin has the potential for the development of metformin-associated lactic acidosis in susceptible patients. The kidneys excrete metformin, probably by both glomerular filtration and tubular excretion. Any factors that decrease metformin excretion or increase blood lactate levels are important risk factors for lactic acidosis. Renal insufficiency with concurrent iodinated contrast administration is therefore a major consideration, and some guidelines for metformin and iodinated contrast are listed in **Table 15.2**.

■ Uses in PAD

DSA is considered as the reference standard for evaluating arterial stenosis or occlusion in patients with PAD (Norgren et al. 2007)

Table 15.2 Guidelines for metformin with iodinated contrast injection

Category	Renal function	Risk factors	Metformin guidelines
1	Normal	None	No change
2	Normal	Multiple	Discontinue for 48 hours
3	Abnormal	Multiple	Discontinue for 48 hours and repeat creatinine measurement

Risk factors: (1) Comorbidities for lactic acidosis with use of metformin: decreased metabolism of lactate, liver dysfunction, alcohol abuse. (2) Increase anaerobic metabolism: cardiac failure, myocardial or peripheral muscle ischemia, sepsis, or severe infection.

(**Figure 15.6**). In current practice however, DSA is not used as a diagnostic tool due to the invasive character and risk of complications (Singh et al. 2003). There have been meta-analyses that have demonstrated that CTA (Met et al. 2009) and contrast-enhanced MRA (Menke & Larsen 2010) are highly accurate noninvasive imaging modalities. Some studies have even suggested that contrast-enhanced MRA is superior to DSA in visualizing arteries of the lower leg and foot

(Dorweiler et al. 2002, Leiner et al. 2004). Despite this evidence, DSA remains the gold standard for imaging the peripheral arterial tree with the added option of intervention at the time should this be required.

Advantages and limitations of DSA

DSA is the most costly of the imaging strategies, involves iodinated contrast administration and radiation exposure, is invasive, and may result in iatrogenic arterial injury (Eslami et al. 2009). Patients must be able to lie flat for an extended period of time both during the procedure and during the postprocedural period, which may be up to 6 hours. In patients with conditions such as orthopnea, congestive cardiac failure, or chronic back pain, this may be challenging. The use of vascular closure devices may help to reduce the time before ambulation and has also been shown to reduce the rate of major vascular complications in percutaneous coronary interventions (Marso et al. 2010). Vascular closure devices should not be used in patients with significant plaque at the access site or in inappropriate access locations.

Smaller sheath sizes, ultrasound-guided access, and the use of preprocedure noninvasive imaging to select the access site will likely

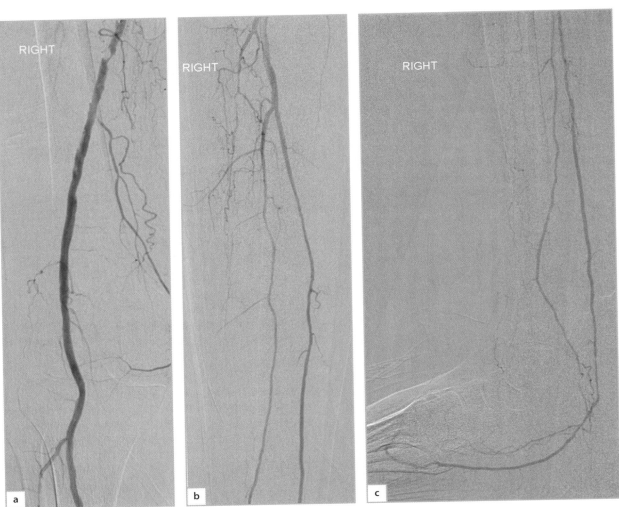

Figure 15.6 Digital subtraction angiography of the superficial femoral artery, crural arteries, and foot. (a) More than 90% stenosis in the distal superficial femoral artery above the adductor canal. (b) Crural vessels with an occluded anterior tibial artery but patent peroneal and posterior tibial arteries. (c) Lateral foot demonstrating an occluded anterior tibial artery and dorsal pedal arch but patent peroneal and posterior tibial arteries and patent plantar pedal arch.

decrease access site-related complications, such as hematoma, pseudoaneurysm, arteriovenous fistula, dissection, and embolization.

Subtraction of heavily calcified vessels gives DSA an advantage over ultrasound, CTA, and MRA, as these vessels are often difficult or impossible to image with these other modalities. It should be noted that DSA evaluates arterial lumina, and it may underestimate the presence of plaque in an artery that has undergone outward adaptive remodeling or partially thrombosed aneurysms. As the images acquired are displayed in a 2D plane, significant eccentric plaque may be undetected without special views (Kashyap et al. 2008). Angled views may be required to adequately image significantly stenotic plaque that lies on the anterior or posterior arterial walls and that may not be easily appreciated in an anteroposterior plane. Similar to the other imaging modalities, the presence of slow flow in distal arteries, such as the pedal arteries, makes imaging more challenging as a patient has to remain still for a longer period of time to reduce motion and subtraction artifacts while contrast reaches the pedal vessels. Subtraction artifacts are also caused by respiratory motion and bowel artifact in the aortoiliac segments (**Figure 15.7**). Patients with extensive PAD pose a further challenge to imaging of the distal peripheral arterial tree as arterial blood flow is slowed even further. This may be overcome by administering a saline bolus after the injection of contrast to increase the rate of flow.

Adequate patient preparation is required prior to DSA. A patient's platelet count, international normalized ratio (INR), activated partial thromboplastin time (APTT), and serum creatinine should be measured before angiography. A low platelet count is the single most important predictor of post- and preprocedural bleeding complications (Darcy et al. 1996). Consideration of a patient's pregnancy status should also be undertaken prior to exposure to ionizing radiation.

■ CO_2 ANGIOGRAPHY

In the 1970s, CO_2 was first used as an intra-arterial contrast agent. With the development of DSA in 1980, CO_2 angiography became a useful diagnostic technique. CO_2 angiography offers a safe, reliable alternative to contrast DSA (Hawkings & Caridi 1998). This is especially useful in patients with renal insufficiency to eliminate or reduce iodinated contrast load to avoid or reduce the incidence of contrast-induced nephropathy. CO_2 angiography offers an alternative imaging method in patients who are allergic to iodinated contrast media. Having a lower radiodensity than soft tissue and fluid, CO_2 displaces blood from the artery lumen and acts as a 'negative' contrast agent, allowing images to be obtained using traditional DSA techniques.

Faster X-ray acquisition frame rates (e.g. 6/s) and specialized equipment are needed that may not always be available at all institutions. A dedicated CO_2 injector system is required for aortoiliac imaging; however, it is not essential in the femoral arteries and below, where syringe injections of CO_2 can be used. CO_2 angiography is uncomfortable and patients often describe an intense burning sensation in the legs and feet that usually lasts for less than half a minute, and then subsides. CO_2 is compressible during injection; it expands in the vessel as it exits the catheter. This rapid expansion after injection is unlikely to cause vascular damage, but it may contribute to discomfort during the injection.

CO_2 is approximately 20 times more soluble than oxygen. When injected into a vessel, CO_2 bubbles completely dissolve within 2–3 minutes by combining with water to produce carbonic acid. In the bloodstream, it forms a hydrogen ion (H^+) and a bicarbonate ion (HCO_3^-) that reverts to CO_2 before being expelled out of capillaries into the lung. Carbonic anhydrase catalyzes the conversion of CO_2 to bicarbonate and protons, and CO_2 is eliminated by the lungs in a single pass. Two to three minutes should be left between injections of CO_2 to prevent the accumulation of gas bubbles, which may produce a significant gas embolism.

Care must be taken in using CO_2 angiography in patients with abdominal aortic aneurysms. If CO_2 gas becomes trapped in a large abdominal aneurysm, it may persist, allowing gas exchange between the CO_2 and nitrogen in the blood. As nitrogen is less readily absorbed in the blood, this may result in occlusion of the inferior mesenteric artery by a gas bubble, which, in turn, can lead to colonic ischemic and infarction.

The utility of CO_2 angiography has been well described for aortic imaging. In >90% of images obtained of the aortoiliac, common femoral, superficial femoral, and profunda arteries CO_2 angiography produced images of excellent or good quality (Seeger et al. 1993). Detailed tibial- and pedal level imaging, especially in the face of long segment proximal occlusions, generally require contrast (Madhusudhan et al. 2009).

■ ROTATIONAL ANGIOGRAPHY/ CONE BEAM CT

Rotational angiography/cone beam CT has been used successfully in neuroradiological interventions and is gaining widespread use in peripheral applications. The information is acquired by a complete rotation of the C-arm, while a continuous fluoroscopic acquisition is performed, which usually takes around 8 seconds. This information generates a 3D volume similar, but slightly more inferior, to a CT 3D volume that can be manipulated in the same way that CT images can. This allows 3D assessment of the target vessel and can aid in periprocedural treatment planning and assessment. This technique is particularly well suited for complex aortoiliac interventions as it allows appropriate sizing of stents, depicts tortuosity of the aortoiliac segment, and accurately demonstrates plaque morphology.

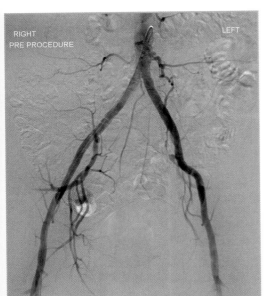

RIGHT
PRE PROCEDURE

LEFT

Figure 15.7
Digital subtraction angiography of the aortoiliac segment. Note small areas of movement artifact adjacent to the bowel loops within the abdomen.

Several companies provide this technology including Siemens (DynaCT) and Philips (XperCT). These systems are also available with a variety of software packages such as 'virtual' stent, where measurement and deployment of a stent are predicted on the basis of the virtual measurements. Pozzi-Mucelli et al. 2004 found a good level of agreement between the measurements of virtual stenting and the actual deployed stents.

Errors in measurements of rotational angiography/cone beam CT are <2%; if one considers that target vessels in peripheral interventions are no larger than 10 mm, the errors are small and <0.5 mm (Van den Berg & Moll 2003). To date, there is no evidence that demonstrates rotational angiography/cone beam CT leads to improved outcomes; however, there seems to be potential to more accurately represent complex anatomies and therefore to aid diagnosis and intervention.

INTRAVASCULAR ULTRASOUND

Basic technology and principles

Intravascular ultrasound (IVUS) was first introduced in the early 1990s and has since gained acceptance as a tool for diagnosing and treating an array of vascular diseases including coronary artery disease when used as an adjunct to angiography (Nissen & Yock 2001). IVUS utilizes a small ultrasound probe that is introduced into the lumen of an artery, usually mounted on a catheter, and a real-time 360° ultrasound image is obtained. Visualization of the lumen area and stenosis can be easily obtained, and the images can be recorded and played back.

Uses in PAD

IVUS is useful in the detailed evaluation of specific segments of arteries. IVUS is invasive compared with duplex ultrasound, is costly, requires a large sheath for access and takes longer to assess arteries compared with the other modalities. However, it gives superior assessment of plaque morphology and lesion length. This is particularly useful in assessing segments of artery that are indeterminate in evaluating in-stent restenosis.

Advantage and limitations of IVUS

Most evidence in IVUS comes from its use in coronary arteries. In a study comparing IVUS with DSA in PAD, stenosis was measured at an average of 10% greater by IVUS than by DSA (Arthurs et al. 2010). Studies examining IVUS in the coronary arteries have shown that DSA underestimated residual atheroma burden following atherectomy compared with IVUS (Koschyk et al. 2000). IVUS identified residual plaque burden and minimal lumen diameter as the most powerful predictors of clinical outcome (restenosis) in coronary arteries (Sgura & Di Mario 2001); however, it must be kept in mind that coronary artery disease is a different entity to PAD. These findings have not been studied in PAD.

OPTICAL COHERENCE TOMOGRAPHY

Optical coherence tomography utilizes a catheter with optical fibers that emit near-infrared light the back-reflections of which are then measured, similar in principle to B-mode ultrasound imaging. This information is used by a computer to generate images. The near-infrared light waves provide a much higher spatial resolution of 10 μm, which is 10–20x greater than that of ultrasound imaging. As a result, the resolution and imaging of plaque and intima is far superior to ultrasound; however, light is easily scattered and absorbed by biological tissue so tissue penetration is only very superficial (2–3 mm) compared with ultrasound waves that can penetrate deeply (Brezinski et al. 2001.). OCT is therefore used intraluminally via a catheter.

The majority of evidence is based on cerebral, carotid, and cerebral vessels. Meissner et al. 2006 studied the potential role of OCT in PAD and showed that findings were comparable with those reported for coronary arteries. There was high correlation of OCT findings between observers (K 0.84–0.87), and these findings were in agreement with histopathological findings in different atherosclerotic plaques (Meissner et al. 2006).

MOLECULAR IMAGING

Molecular imaging is a rapidly emerging field that allows visualization of structures on the molecular level rather than the macroscopic level. The rationale behind its application in imaging atherosclerosis is the recognition that molecular and cellular processes play a role in every stage of atherogenesis, including inflammation and rupture (Jaffer et al. 2006). Specific molecular markers can be attached to radiographic marker agents, such as radionuclides or magnetic nanoparticles. While current atherosclerosis imaging technologies focus mainly on the structural components of atherosclerotic plaque, molecular imaging of specific cellular processes in plaques raises the possibility of diagnosis of high-risk plaques before symptom onset, personalized medicine with molecularly based therapies, and new imaging endpoints for new therapeutic trials (Osborn & Jaffer 2008). Agents that can be used include magnetically charge nanoparticles or radioisotopes with cell-specific ligands. Images may then be acquired using single or combined systems of MRI, positron emission tomography (PET), single-photon emission computed tomography (SPECT), CT, ultrasound, and optical imaging.

The future possibilities for molecular imaging in atherosclerosis abound; however, most of the currently developing modalities will require multiple phases of trials and development with substantial cost before they can become applicable at the bedside (Jaffer et al. 2006).

AREAS OF CONTROVERSY AND/OR FUTURE RESEARCH

- Ultrasound with Doppler, when performed well, is a noninvasive, fast, and cost-effective way of imaging PAD and allows identification of patients requiring further imaging with CTA, MRA, or DSA
- CTA and MRA are both good noninvasive tests that have several advantages and limitations, and there is no overall clear advantage of using one method over the other
- DSA remains the gold standard for imaging PAD and allows endovascular treatment at the same time; however, using DSA as a first line imaging technique can be costly and resource intensive
- Iodinated contrast and gadolinium-based contrast agents are essential in some imaging modalities; however, knowledge of the side effects and complications of their use, particularly in patients with renal failure, is vital
- Other imaging methods such as rotational angiography/cone beam CT, IVUS, and OCT have their roles in specific applications

Chapter 17 Distal bypass techniques

Himanshu Verma, Robbie K. George, Ramesh K. Tripathi

SUMMARY

A successful distal bypass is dependent on good inflow, appropriate graft conduit and good outflow vessels. This chapter describes the following key points about distal bypass techniques for revascularization of the ischaemic diabetic foot.

- Dealing with iliac artery (inflow) stenosis before distal bypass
- Selecting the inflow site
- The anatomic exposure of inflow as well as outflow vessels
- Conduit options and handling techniques
- Techniques for tunneling bypass conduits
- Adjunctive procedures in distal bypasses
- Follow-up treatment and surveillance after distal bypass

INTRODUCTION

Around 50% of patients with diabetes and a foot ulcer have peripheral arterial disease (PAD). For some of these patients, the PAD is of mild severity with only a small perfusion deficit. For others, PAD is more severe and the diabetic foot ulcer has little chance of healing without the restoration of perfusion. For these patients, revascularization should be considered. The distribution of PAD in diabetes is often distal, comprising long occlusions, especially of the crural vessels. Although endovascular techniques have an increasing role to play, the gold standard revascularization technique remains distal bypass.

- Distal bypasses have been the gold standard for revascularization of ischemic limbs
- Different techniques have been described with varying degrees of success
- With an expanding population of patients with diabetes and growing sophistication of distal bypass procedures, the pool of patients with reconstructible arteries has expanded as the 'inoperable' or 'nonreconstructible' group has contracted
- There is universal agreement among vascular surgeons that all attempts to salvage a limb by vascular reconstruction are justified if the limb is threatened because of anatomically correctable occlusive vascular disease and can continue to be a useful functional organ after surgical intervention
- The merits or otherwise of the surgical options are reviewed in this chapter, but the indications and contraindica
  - Indications
    - Infrainguinal peripheral arterialocclusive disease with symptomatic lower extremity ischemia (disabling claudication, rest pain, pregangrene, tissue loss (gangrene, nonhealing ulcer)
    - Aneurysmal disease [superficial femoral artery (SFA) /popliteal aneurysm; >2-cm diameter]
    - Traumatic arterial injury
  - Contraindications
    - Debilitated patient with severe comorbidities
    - Lack of an appropriate distal target for revascularization

- Unaddressed inflow disease
- Severe joint contractures
- Nonambulatory patient

BYPASS TECHNIQUES

To achieve satisfactory results after any bypass procedure, it is essential to optimize three factors:
1. Inflow
2. Conduit
3. Outflow

Problems with any of these components may result in suboptimal outcomes and failure or early occlusion of the bypass graft.

Selecting inflow site

The common femoral artery (CFA) is the most common inflow origin for infrainguinal bypasses. However, an in-line patent distal SFA or popliteal artery can also be utilized as the inflow vessel. The following should be taken into consideration while selecting the inflow artery for any lower limb bypass procedure.

Concomitant iliac stenosis

Diabetes typically involves infragenicular vessels; however, involvement of proximal vessels (e.g. femoral and iliac arteries) is not uncommon. In the presence of significant iliac artery stenosis, the inflow into the graft is poor and the likelihood of failure is high. This should be addressed by an endovascular procedure like an iliac artery angioplasty with or without stenting or a surgical procedure before the bypass is constructed. This may be done as a single-step hybrid procedure (Liu et al. 2001, Schneider 2003, Mousa et al. 2010).

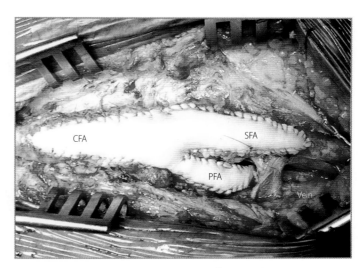

Figure 17.1 Femoral endarterectomy with profunda patch plasty using bovine pericardial patch.

Femoral and profunda femoris artery disease and exposure

Coexistent PAD in the CFA and especially profunda femoris artery (PFA) origin must be surgically addressed. The CFA responds poorly to endovascular interventions and will need an endarterectomy with patch closure (Kang et al. 2008, Ballotta et al. 2010, Bosier & Deloose 2009). If the disease involves PFA origin, patch profundaplasty must also be carried out (**Figure 17.1**). Preservation of PFA flow is essential as it serves as an excellent source of collateral supply in case a graft bypassing an occluded SFA was to occlude.

Most surgeons employ a vertical incision directly over the femoral pulse to secure control of the femoral arterial system. Others advocate laterally-based vertical incisions. Whichever incision is employed, great consideration must be given to avoiding division of lymph nodes, ligation of lymphatic rich tissue, and extensive use of diathermy.

Oblique incisions are popular for femoral exposure in endo-vascular procedures as they have fewer wound complications in the groin (Swinnen et al. 2010); however, their use in reconstructive procedures is limited due to limited exposure and an inability to extend them cranially or caudally if needed. However, there have been reports in support of oblique incision causing a lower incidence of wound infection and lymphorrhea. Low oblique incision could be considered in obese patients if an adequate SFA exists for inflow.

Access to a remote PFA is a useful alternative, especially when dealing with a heavily scarred or infected groin. It is surgically accessible for a considerable length and can serve as an adequate source of inflow to a distal bypass in selected cases. By carefully dividing profunda vein branches anterior to the PFA origin and retracting motor nerves to the sartorius and rectus femoris muscles, a considerable length of PFA can be obtained to serve as an inflow vessel.

In a surgically challenging groin (especially when there has previous groin/arterial surgery), the mid- and distal-PFA can be approached laterally, which requires incision over the lateral border of the sartorius muscle, medial retraction of the latter and dissection along the lateral border of the rectus femoris muscle. Division of the lateral circumflex vein enables mobilization of the PFA.

Distal SFA and popliteal artery as inflow source

When available, using the distal SFA or popliteal artery as inflow vessels decreases the length of bypass conduit required and is associated with excellent outcomes, with similar long-term patency when compared with the CFA as the source of inflow. However, radiological evaluation of the upstream CFA, SFA, and popliteal artery is essential to rule out significant inflow disease.

SFA inflow can be obtained in the groin or from the distal SFA in the thigh, depending on the level of arterial occlusion. In the presence of proximal disease, prior or simultaneous SFA angioplasty/stenting followed by distal SFA or popliteal artery origin distal bypass provide long-term primary and secondary patency rates equal to femorodistal bypass (Veith et al. 1981, Balotta et al. 2004a, Reed 2009).

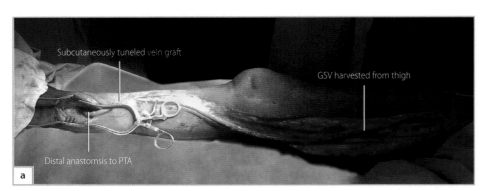

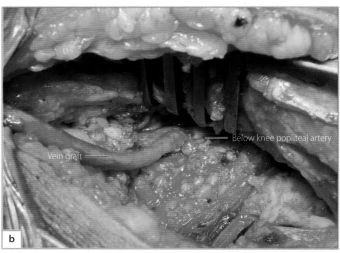

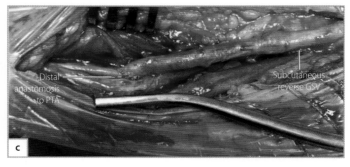

Figure 17.2 Below-knee popliteal–posterior tibial artery bypass (at ankle) with reversed great saphenous vein.

Henke PK, Blackburn S, Proctor MC, et al. Patients undergoing infrainguinal bypass to treat atherosclerotic vascular disease are underprescribed cardioprotective medications: effect on graft patency, limb salvage, and mortality. J Vasc Surg 2004; 39:357–365.

Hingorani AP, Ascher E, Marks NA, et al. A 10-year experience with complementary distal arteriovenous fistula and deep vein interposition for infrapopliteal prosthetic bypasses. Vasc Endovascular Surg 2005; 39:401–409.

Hocking KM, Brophy C, Rizvi SZ, et al. Detrimental effects of mechanical stretch on smooth muscle function in saphenous veins. J Vasc Surg 2011; 53:454–460.

Hofmann WJ, Magometschnigg H. Pedal artery bypass. Acta Chir Belg 2004; 104:654–658.

Julliard W, Katzen J, Nabozny M, et al Long-term results of endoscopic versus open saphenous vein harvest for lower extremity bypass. Ann Vasc Surg 2011;101–107. doi: 10.1016/j.avsg.2010.10.013.

Kapadia MR, Popowich DA, Kibbe MR. Modified prosthetic vascular conduits. Circulation 2008; 117:1873–1882.

Khaleel MS, Dorheim TA, Duryee MJ, et al. High-pressure distention of the saphenous vein during preparation results in increased markers of inflammation: a potential mechanism for graft failure. Ann Thorac Surg 2012; 93:552–558.

Klinkert P, Post PN, Breslau PJ, van Bockel JH. Saphenous vein versus PTFE for above-knee femoropopliteal bypass. A review of the literature. Eur J Vasc Endovasc Surg 2004; 27:357–362.

Kunlin J. Le Traitement de l'arterite obtitrante par la greffe veineuse. Arch Mal Coeur 1949; 42:371. [in French].

Lancaster RT, Conrad MF, Patel VI, Cambria RP, LaMuraglia GM. Predictors of early graft failure after infrainguinal bypass surgery: a risk-adjusted analysis from the NSQIP. Eur J Vasc Endovasc Surg 2012; 43:549–555.

Laurila K, Lepäntalo M, Teittinen K, et al. Does an adjuvant AV-fistula improve the patency of a femorocrural PTFE bypass with distal vein cuff in critical leg ischaemia?--a prospective randomised multicentre trial. Eur J Vasc Endovasc Surg 2004; 27:180–185.

Laurila K, Luther M, Roth WD, et al. Adjuvant arteriovenous fistula as means of rescue for infrapopliteal venous bypass with poor runoff. J Vasc Surg 2006; 44:985–991.

Liu C, Guan H, Li Y, Zheng Y, Liu W. Combined intraoperative iliac artery stents and femoro-popliteal bypass for multilevel atherosclerotic occlusive disease. Chin Med Sci J. 2001; 16:165–168.

Luckraz H, Lowe J, Pugh N, Azzu AA. Pre-operative long saphenous vein mapping predicts vein anatomy and quality leading to improved post-operative leg morbidity. Interact Cardiovasc Thorac Surg 2008; 7:188–191.

Lundgren F SCAMICOS (Scandinavian Miller Collar Study). Does patency after a vein collar and PTFE-bypass depend on sex and age? Re-analysis of a randomised trial. Int Angiol 2012; 31:156–162.

Malmstedt J, Takolander R, Wahlberg E. A randomized prospective study of valvulotome efficacy in in situ reconstructions. Eur J Vasc Endovasc Surg 2005; 30:52–56.

Mani K, Campbell A, Fitzpatrick J, et al. A novel reverse thermosensitive polymer to achieve temporary atraumatic vessel occlusion in infra-popliteal bypasses. Eur J Vasc Endovasc Surg 2013; 45:51–56.

Maruf MF, Sabur S, Akter T, Hakim E, Ahsan N. Improved preservation of saphenous venous conduits by the use of papaverine mixed heparinized blood solution during harvesting. Cardiovasc J 2011; 4:3–7.

Mousa A, Abdel-Hamid M, Ewida A, Saad M, Sahrabi A. Combined percutaneous endovascular iliac angioplasty and infrainguinal surgical revascularization for chronic lower extremity ischemia: preliminary result. Vascular 2010; 18:71–76.

Nakajima H, Kobayashi J, Tagusari O, et al. Competitive flow in arterial composite grafts and effect of graft arrangement in Off-Pump coronary revascularization. Ann Thorac Surg 2004; 78:481–486.

Nehler MR, Brass EP, Anthony R, et al; Circulase investigators. Adjunctive parenteral therapy with lipo-ecraprost, a prostaglandin E1 analog, in patients with critical limb ischemia undergoing distal revascularization does not improve 6-month outcomes. J Vasc Surg 2007; 45:953–960; discussion 960–961. Epub 2007 Mar 9.

Panetta TF, Marin ML, Veith FJ, et al. Unsuspected preexisting saphenous vein disease: an unrecognized cause of vein bypass failure. J Vasc Surg 1992; 15:102–110.

Randon C, Jacobs B, De Ryck F, Beele H, Vermassen F. Fifteen years of infrapopliteal arterial reconstructions with cryopreserved venous allografts for limb salvage. J Vasc Surg 2010; 51:869–877.

Reed AB. Endovascular as an open adjunct: use of hybrid endovascular treatment in the SFA. Semin Vasc Surg 2008; 21:200–203.

Reed AB. Hybrid procedures and distal origin grafts. Semin Vasc Surg 2009; 22:240–244.

Robin C, Lermusiaux P, Bleuet F, Martinez R. Distal bypass for limb salvage: should the contralateral great saphenous vein be harvested? Ann Vasc Surg 2006; 20:761–766.

Ruffolo AJ, Romano M, Ciapponi A. Prostanoids for critical limb ischaemia. Cochrane Database Syst Rev. 2010 Jan 20;CD006544

Rush DS, Frame SB, Bell RM, et al. Does open fasciotomy contribute to morbidity and mortality after acute lower extremity ischemia and revascularization? J Vasc Surg 1989; 10:343–350.

Schanzer A, Hevelone N, Owens CD, et al. Technical factors affecting autogenous vein graft failure: observations from a large multicenter trial. J Vasc Surg 2007; 46:1180–1190.

Schneider PA. Iliac angioplasty and stenting in association with infrainguinal bypasses: timing and techniques. Semin Vasc Surg 2003; 16:291–299.

Shah DM, Darling RC 3rd, Chang BB, et al. Long-term results of in situ saphenous vein bypass. Analysis of 2058 cases. Ann Surg 1995; 222:438–446; discussion 446–448.

Soong CV, Barros B'Sa AA. Lower limb oedema following distal arterial bypass grafting. Eur J Vasc Endovasc Surg. 1998; 16:465–471.

Sonnenfeld T, Cronestrand R. Pharmacological vasodilation during reconstructive vascular surgery. Acta Chir Scand 1980; 146:9–14.

Swinnen J, Chao A, Tiwari A, et al. Vertical or transverse incisions for access to the femoral artery: a randomized control study. Ann Vasc Surg 2010; 24:336–341.

te Slaa A, Dolmans DE, Ho GH, Mulder PG, van der Waal JC, et al. Prospective randomized controlled trial to analyze the effects of intermittent pneumatic compression on edema following autologous femoropopliteal bypass surgery. World J Surg 2011; 35:446–454.

Tarry WC, Walsh DB, Birkmeyer NJ, Fillinger MF, Zwolak RM, Cronenwett JL.Fate of the contralateral leg after infrainguinal bypass J Vasc Surg 1998:1039–1047; discussion 1047– 1048.

Tiwari A, Cheng KS, Salacinski H, Hamilton G, Seifalian AM. Improving the patency of vascular bypass grafts: the role of suture materials and surgical techniques on reducing anastomotic compliance mismatch. Eur J Vasc Endovasc Surg 2003; 25:287–295.

Twine CP, McLain AD. Graft type for femoro-popliteal bypass surgery. Cochrane Database Syst Rev. 2010:CD001487

Veith FJ, Gupta SK, Samson RH, et al. Superficial femoral and popliteal arteries as inflow sites for distal bypasses. Surgery 1981; 90:980–990.

Veith FJ, Gupta SK, Ascer E, White-Flores S, Samson RH. Six-year prospective multicenter randomized comparison of autologous saphenous vein and expanded polytetrafluoroethylene grafts in infrainguinal arterial reconstructions. J Vasc Surg 1986; 3:104–114.

Wengerter KR, Veith FJ, Gupta SK, Goldsmith J, Farrell E, Prospective randomized multicenter comparison of in situ and reversed vein infrapopliteal bypasses. J Vasc Surg 1991; 13:189–197.

Westerband A, Mills JL, Kistler S, et al. Prospective validation of threshold criteria for intervention in infrainguinal vein grafts undergoing duplex surveillance. Ann Vasc Surg 1997; 11:44–48.

Ziegler KR, Muto A, Eghbalieh SD, Dardik A. Basic data related to surgical infrainguinal revascularization procedures: a twenty year update. Ann Vasc Surg 2011; 25:413–422.

Chapter 18   Angioplasty techniques

Ezio Faglia, Giacomo Clerici, Flavio Airoldi

SUMMARY

- Percutaneous transluminal angioplasty (PTA) is a minimally invasive therapy for managing patients with chronic limb ischemia (CLI) to relieve rest pain and prevent limb loss
- Subintimal angioplasty (SIA) may be intentionally selected to attempt recanalization of long, noncalcified superficial femoral artery (SFA) occlusions, with a large and disease-free target re-entry site in the distal SFA/popliteal artery
- Advantages of PTA include:
  - Minimizing surgical stress
  - No need for general anesthesia
  - Very short hospital stay
  - Absence of surgical wounds
- Revascularization and restoration of ideally direct pulsatile flow to at least one of the foot arteries is generally thought to be an important step in the management of healing of foot ulcers
- Restenosis is a limitation for endovascular therapy; however, repeat interventions can be easily performed if necessary
- Ipsilateral antegrade femoral access enables access to very distal vessels (e.g. plantar or pedal arteries), which are almost always in peripheral arterial disease (PAD) in patients with diabetes
- Retrograde popliteal, tibial, or pedal access has been used effectively and safely in some patients with diabetes to heal ulcers and prevent amputation
- Stent implantation should be limited to cases of residual stenosis of flow-limiting dissections after balloon angioplasty. Elective stenting of all of the treated segments is not applicable in the presence of diffuse disease or the involvement of multiple vessels both above and below the knee

INTRODUCTION

Percutaneous transluminal angioplasty is a minimally invasive therapy for the treatment of patients with PAD. The appropriateness of this therapy in managing patients with CLI to prevent limb loss and accompanying disabilities is unquestioned; however, PTA is also often selected for the treatment of patients with claudication.

This technique was first described by Dotter and Judkins in a paper published in the journal Circulation in 1964. Gruentzig (Gruntzig 1978) subsequently demonstrated its feasibility to address lesions in coronary arteries (percutaneous transluminal coronary angioplasty: PTCA). Although PTA was the pioneering procedure, PTCA rapidly became a widely performed technique in the 1980s (Nicod & Scherrer 1993). It was during the 1990s that PTA proved its worth as a successful revascularization technique (Isner & Rosenfield 1993) and, in the 2000s it became the most commonly used approach to lower limb revascularization (Goodney 2009). At present, PTA is regarded by some specialists as the first choice procedure for lower limb revascularization (Kudo et al. 2005, DeRubertis et al. 2007, Conrad et al. 2009).

INDICATIONS FOR PTA

Revascularization is an appropriate therapy for patients with CLI directed at relieve ischemic pain and heal (neuro)ischemic ulcers: both the TransAtlantic Inter-Society Consensus (TASC) 2000 (Dormandy & Rutherford 2000) and TASC 2007 (Norgren et al. 2007) report this statement. PTA is undoubtedly a revascularization procedure that is effective in preventing both rest pain and limb loss. Revascularization is also used for the treatment of patients with claudication: this in contrast with the TASC indications, which recommend for these patients a treatment based on intensive management of risk factors and supervised exercise. In patients with diabetes the most frequent manifestation of PAD is in association with ulceration or wounds on the foot and not as claudication.

In 2000, the TASC outlined detailed criteria to select the appropriate revascularization procedure (angioplasty or bypass) for patients with CLI. Such guidelines had provided very analytical criteria, which were based on a morphological stratification of the lesions (length, stenosis, or occlusion), both for the femoral popliteal and infrapopliteal segments. In 2007, a second edition – TASC II – was published. In these guidelines, the morphological stratification for the femoral and popliteal area was confirmed; however, criteria on the length of occlusions had changed, and criteria for selecting PTA as a first choice revascularization procedure became less restrictive. For type B lesions, the previous statement 'more evidence' was replaced by the 'first choice' indication. For type C lesions, the length of the occlusions requiring surgery as a first option was increased and accompanied by the introduction of the concept of 'good-risk patients'. For type D lesions, the length of the occlusion in the SFA that excluded PTA as a first option was raised from >5 to >20 cm, but the indications for the surgical approach to total occlusion of the popliteal artery and proximal trifurcation were maintained. **Table 18.1** summarizes a comparison between the recommendations for selecting PTA or bypass graft (BPG) as the first choice revascularization procedure according to the two editions of the TASC guidelines.

Indications for revascularization of the infrapopliteal artery lesions completely changed. The stratification of type A, B, C, and D lesions according to the TASC 2000 was abandoned, and, consequently, indications on the length of obstructions disappeared: in particular, the TASC 2000 indication for surgery as a first option in type D occlusions >2 cm was missing in TASC 2007.

These indications are of particular importance for patients with diabetes, as their peripheral arteries have a very peculiar morphology. One of the most important indications for revascularization is the presence of multiple lesions spreading both in femoropopliteal and infrapopliteal segments. A large percentage of patients with diabetes have more occlusions than stenoses, and the occlusions are often long, both in the femoral segment and, above all, in the infrapopliteal segment. The high prevalence of long occlusions in the tibial arteries is the most relevant issue for the feasibility of revascularization. In all our case studies of patients with diabetes and CLI treated during the year 2000: occlusions in the femoropopliteal segment were less than a half of the number of stenoses in that segment; however, occlusions

Table 18.1 Classification of femoropopliteal lesions and recommended treatment options according to TASC 2000 and TASC 2007 guidelines

TASC 2000: classification of femoropopliteal lesions		TASC 2007: classification of femoropopliteal lesions	
Type A single stenosis, up to 3 cm in length, which is not at the superficial femoral origin or distal portion of the popliteal artery	PTA first choice	Type A single stenosis >10 cm in length, single occlusion > 5 cm in length	PTA first choice
Type B single stenosis 3–10 cm in length, not involving the distal popliteal artery: heavily calcified stenosis, up to 3 cm in length. Multiple lesions in the absence of continuous tibial runoff to improve inflow for distal surgical bypass	More evidence	Type B multiple lesions (stenoses or occlusions), each >5 cm; single stenosis or occlusion >5 cm not involving the infrageniculate popliteal artery; single or multiple lesions in the absence of continuous tibial vessels to improve inflow for a distal bypass; heavily calcified occlusion >5 cm in length; single popliteal stenosis	PTA first choice
Type C single stenosis or occlusion >5 cm. Multiple stenosis or occlusions, each 3–5 cm, with or without heavy calcification	Stenosis 5–10 cm, or occlusions 3–5 cm: surgery preferred	Type C multiple stenoses or occlusions totaling >15 cm with or without heavy calcification or recurrent stenoses or occlusions that need treatment after two endovascular interventions	Stenosis or occlusion >15 cm: surgery preferred (good-risk patients)
Type D complete common femoral artery or superficial femoral artery occlusions or complete popliteal and proximal trifurcation occlusions	Occlusion > 5 cm: surgery first choice	Type D chronic total occlusion of the superficial femoral artery (>20 cm, involving the popliteal artery). Chronic total occlusion of popliteal artery and proximal trifurcation vessels	Occlusion >20 cm: surgery first choice

PTA, percutaneous transluminal angioplasty; TASC, TransAtlantic Inter-Society Consensus.

of the tibial arteries were the most common types of lesions found in the infrapopliteal segment (Faglia 2012b). **Figure 18.1** shows the type and length of obstructions observed in 360 limbs of 344 patients with diabetes hospitalized because of CLI in 2009.

These morphological peculiarities of PAD in patients with diabetes prompt discussion on what we believe are the most important criteria for selecting PTA as the first-choice revascularization procedure: the revascularization feasibility.

■ REVASCULARIZATION FEASIBILITY

Increased rates of revascularization have been shown to decrease above-the-ankle amputations (LoGerfo et al. 1992). If revascularization reduces the rate of amputations, it is obvious that the feasibility of this procedure plays an important role in minimizing amputation risk.

Many trials have reported the outcomes of revascularized patients (Aulivola & Pomposelli 2004, Awad et al. 2006), whereas only a few studies have assessed the revascularization feasibility and the outcomes of revascularized and nonrevascularized patients with diabetes and CLI (Faglia 2012a).

As previously mentioned, patients with diabetes and CLI have PAD with peculiar morphological characteristics: in skilled hands, PTA is feasible even in patients presenting with long calcified occlusions of both the femoral and infrapopliteal arteries. Moreover, there are no particular contraindications to this procedure in patients deemed to be high surgical risk candidates. The main obstacle to limb revascularization by PTA is the presence of a calcified vessel that is completely occluded, which therefore prevents balloon catheter access. In our experience, PTA down to the foot is feasible in about 80% of cases.

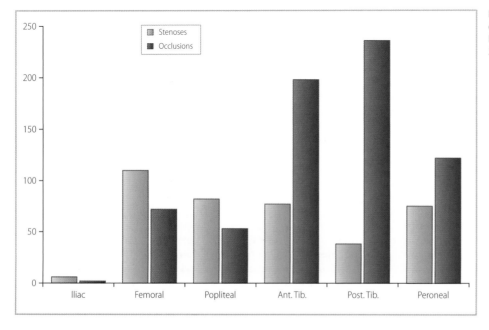

Figure 18.1 Type and length of obstructions observed in 360 limbs of 344 patients with diabetes hospitalized because of chronic limb ischemia in 2009.

segment is then dilated with a balloon. The guidewire should be advanced into the vessel wall with the added support of the catheter (usually a 4–6 F diagnostic catheter), carefully avoiding any large collateral branches arising from the main vessel. The advancement of the wire, whose loop at the tip should be 3–5 cm in length, is usually performed with little resistance. The resistance, however, can increase greatly in the presence of significant calcification. In these cases, operators may use a stiff hydrophilic guidewire to increase the 'pushability' of the system and, whenever the advancement of the catheter is also prevented by heavy calcification, a hydrophilic catheter or a 0.035-inch compatible lubricant-coated micro-catheter and sharp, tapered tip can be used. Re-entering into the true lumen is sometimes accomplished by simply pushing and advancing the guidewire, since it may pass into the lumen following the path of least resistance. However, in as many as 30% of the lesions, re-entry into the true lumen can be difficult. Successful re-entry may be achieved by rotating and repositioning the guidewire wire and catheter to create a different dissection plane in the subintimal space, or by using a preshaped angulated catheter (BER I, BER II, RCA, C2) to direct the tip or loop of the guidewire toward the true lumen. These maneuvers should be performed taking at least two orthogonal views of the re-entry site to properly discriminate between the subintimal space and the true lumen to accurately direct the device toward the true lumen. A roadmap or, alternatively, a radiopaque ruler should also be used to precisely assess the vessel lumen patency and therefore avoid re-entry of the guidewire at a distance well beyond the end of the occlusion (**Figure 18.4**). Propagation of a dissection over the proper entry site may affect collateral branches or vascular segments in areas that are not involved in the occlusion and may be potential targets for vascular surgery. SIA was first described in 1989 by Bolia as a valuable technique in the management of femoropopliteal occlusive disease in patients with intermittent claudication. Since then, indications for this technique have been extended to include occlusions in other areas,

such as the BTK arteries. SIA has been found to play an important role in the management of critically ischemic limbs and, over the last few years, has had an increasingly important role in these clinical settings. The greatest merit of this technique is that it attempts to overcome the problems of a standard intraluminal angioplasty, thus enabling treatment of complex disease patterns that are frequently encountered in CLI patients. This technique is best suited to the treatment of heavily calcified occlusions, long-term atherosclerotic occlusions, and SFA occlusions after prior failure of PTA or BPG. Although preferable, intraluminal crossing in these settings may not be feasible, because wires follow the path of least resistance between the intimal plaque and the adventitia (Alexandrescu et al. 2009). SIA also has the advantages of being an easily performed and low-cost technique, which provides good outcomes in both the short and long term. There have been no randomized controlled trials in which SIA was compared with any other treatment (Chang & Liu 2013).

■ Retrograde popliteal access

Retrograde popliteal access has been proposed as a safe and effective procedure to increase the success rate of PTA performed for SFA occlusions after failed antegrade attempts via ipsilateral or contralateral femoral access (**Figure 18.5**). The rationale for the increased success rate is that the distal occlusion stump is usually tapered, thus increasing the chance of a successful intraluminal passage of guidewires. This approach, first described by Tønnesen et al. in 1988, raised some concerns about the possible increase in arterial puncture site complications, such as large hematoma, pseudohematoma, vessel rupture, dissection, and arteriovenous fistula. However, it should be noted that large sheaths were used in many of these studies, but this technique is performed today using 3- or 4-F sheaths, or even adopting a sheathless approach using a 0.018-inch guidewire (Fanelli et al. 2011, Nishino et al. 2012) and compatible

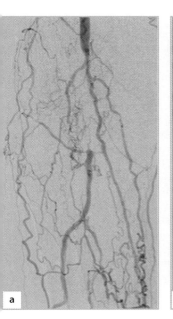
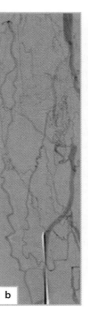
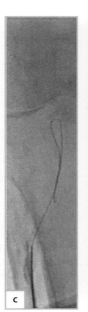
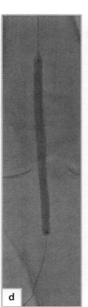
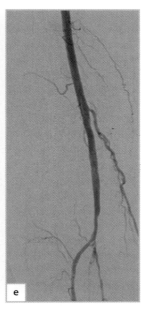

Figure 18.5 Retrograde recanalization of an occluded popliteal artery. (a) The angiogram shows an occlusion of the popliteal artery. The absence of a stump and a large collateral branch arising at the level of the occlusion prevent a successful antegrade recanalization. (b) Percutaneous puncture of the proximal portion of the anterior tibial artery performed with a 21-G needle under fluoroscopic guidance. (c) Sheathless retrograde approach with a 0.018-inch wire (Connect flex; Abbott Vascular, Redwood City, CA) and a coaxial microcatheter with successful chronic total occlusion recanalization. (d, e) Final angiographic result after prolonged (2 minutes) inflation of a 5.0 × 100-mm balloon.

microcatheters. To minimize vessel trauma, the desired puncture site can be accurately identified by duplex scanning under fluoroscopic guidance coupled to a roadmap image generated by the injection of contrast into the proximal femoral artery. According to quoted studies, retrograde access may result in higher success rates (up to 90–96%) compared with those obtained when only an antegrade approach is used (75–80%). Despite the recognized worth of this approach and the increased procedural safety, its use is usually limited by the need to frequently change the patient's position during the procedure: in fact, the patient has to change their position from supine to prone or lateral decubitus during the popliteal artery puncture, and back again to supine to complete the intervention. Such repositioning is not suited to subjects with respiratory problems, obesity, and/or mental impairment. This approach time-consuming, even when performed perfectly with no complications, and patients may well experience some discomfort as a result. Recently, a modification of this technique has been proposed to obtain femoral access with no need to change the patient's position. Patients may be maintained in the supine position, with the knee gently flexed and medially rotated: with this modality, the authors have achieved successful vascular access in all patients. Other alternative techniques for retrograde recanalization of chronic total SFA occlusions have been proposed to facilitate vascular access into a patent vessel segment distal to the occlusion with the patient maintaining the supine position. Schmidt et al. (2012) described a direct puncture of the distal SFA through an anteromedial access into the distal thigh without knee flexion. The main advantages of this approach over the traditional retrograde approach include the possibility to keep patients in the supine position, easy access to the vessel, and the possibility of performing manipulations of guidewires and balloon catheters inserted simultaneously from antegrade and retrograde directions into the occlusion. This technique is indicated only in patients with occlusions that do not extend distally to the level of adductor canal, and in obese patients with femoral arteries buried deep underneath the fatty tissue. The authors also described a retrograde approach in which the puncture was attempted at the proximal portion of the tibial artery (Montero-Baker et al. 2008). This innovative approach broadens the indications for a retrograde approach to a larger patient population, being the only procedure that is also suitable for patients with occluded or diseased popliteal arteries. In this procedure, guidewires may be advanced and microcatheters or over-the-wire balloon catheters may be threaded over the guidewire without using a sheath: prolonged balloon inflation from above may be sufficient to provide hemostasis.

■ Dedicated devices for revascularization of femoropopliteal occlusions

The above-described techniques allow successful recanalization of many long femoropopliteal occlusions using traditional devices (such as catheters, balloons, guidewires) and technologies. Nevertheless, considerable advances have been made over the last decade in the development of new endovascular device. These devices belong to two main categories:

1. Devices designed to remain in the true lumen
2. Devices designed to improve re-entry into the distal true lumen after subintimal recanalization

The indications for their use are still controversial. At present, several studies report clinical and technical outcomes obtained in relatively small case series of lesions treated using different devices.

These are prospective series of consecutive lesions; however, most frequently, they are retrospective evaluations of lesions that were selected according to operators' preference, rather than prespecified criteria. Moreover, these studies include both claudicating and CLI patients, with or without diabetes. It is therefore difficult to judge the performance of these devices for the endovascular management of CLI patients per se.

Devices designed to remain in the true lumen

The Crosser CTO recanalization system (Bard Peripheral Vascular, Inc, Tempe, AZ) consists of a transducer with piezoelectric crystals that convert the amplified alternating current supplied by the generator into high-frequency vibrations, which are then propagated at 21,000 cycles/s to the catheter's metal tip (**Figure 18.6a**). The very rapid reciprocal (back and forth) stroke (20-μm depth) disrupts and channels through the fibrocalcific plaque without harming the vessel wall, thus facilitating the penetration of hard or calcified lesions and assisting in the recanalization of an occluded artery. An irrigation line is required during device activation to cool the system and provide a medium for cavitation at the catheter tip. Three different versions of this monorail hydrophilic catheter are available. The TruePath device (Boston Scientific Corporation, Natick, MA) is designed to penetrate hard or calcified occlusions and create microdissection in CTOs to facilitate access to the distal true lumen (**Figure 18.6b**). It is a 0.018-inch wire with a diamond-coated tip that rotates at 13,000 rpm. The wire has a working length of 165 cm that tapers over the distal 9 cm to optimize flexibility. The tip of the device has a 3° angle, which can be shaped to a 15° angle. A support catheter is generally used to advance the TruePath to the lesion.

The Wildcat device (Avinger, Inc, Redwood City, CA) is a 0.035-inch catheter that has a hydrophilic coating that facilitates tracking through complex lesions in the SFA (**Figure 18.6c**). The rotatable tip assumes both passive (wedges in) and active (wedges out) configurations. The tip may be rotated manually or with a handheld motorized unit. A 0.014-inch version of the device (Kittycat) is also available and provides smaller crossing profiles and longer working lengths for BTK vessels. The latest evolution of the device is the Ocelot, which is derived from the Wildcat and incorporates real-time optical coherence tomography built into the catheter to guide intraluminal crossing.

The Viance Crossing Catheter Enteer Re-entry System (Covidien, Plymouth, MN) is composed of a crossing catheter that facilitates both intraluminal and subintimal recanalization of the lesion and a re-entry device to facilitate access to the distal true lumen. The crossing catheter has a working length of 150 cm. It has a coiled shaft and an atraumatic distal tip to prevent vessel exit. Using a torque device, the catheter is rapidly spun in either direction to facilitate advancement through the lesion.

The ENABLER-P (Endocross, Yokneam Illit, Israel) balloon catheter system consists of two main components: a dual lumen balloon and a control unit. The balloon is manually inflated to anchor it against the vessel wall a few millimeters proximal to the lesion. The control unit sets an automated cyclical modulation of the balloon pressure (2.5 times per second). As the pressure increases (max 6 atm), the balloon grabs the guidewire and cyclically elongates to facilitate the wire advancement into the vessel occlusion. With each inflation the guidewire advances up to 3 mm. During the whole procedure, the operator maintains control over the guidewire and is able to retract, advance, or torque the wire.

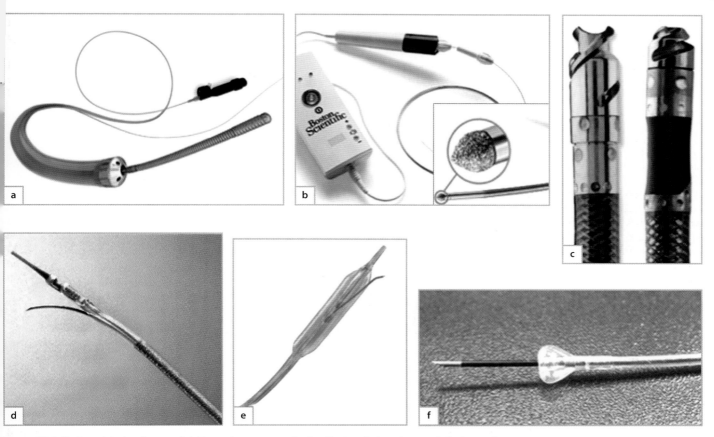

Figure 18.6 Dedicated devices for superficial femoral artery recanalization. Devices designed to remain in the true lumen.

Devices designed to facilitate re-entry into the distal true lumen

Pioneer (Medtronic Inc, Minneapolis, MN) is a 6-F catheter with two-wire ports, each 0.014-inch compatible. One port houses a hollow-core nitinol needle that is guided by an integrated 64-element, phased-array intravascular ultrasound device and is connected to a Volcano s5i Imaging System console (Volcano Corporation, Rancho Cordova, CA), which enables vessel imaging. The re-entry device is delivered through the subintimal plane and is placed with the distal tip at the level of the SFA re-entry site. By slowly rotating the catheter, the operator maneuvers the nitinol needle until its tip is oriented toward the true lumen and is lined up at the 12-o'clock position on the ultrasonographic image. Finally, the needle is plunged into the true lumen at a controlled depth (**Figure 18.6d**).

The Enteer Re-entry Catheter system (Covidien, Plymouth, MN) is a re-entry system composed of two components: an orienting balloon catheter and a re-entry guidewire. The balloon has a flat shape, which is designed to self-orient one of two 180° offset exit ports toward the vessel true lumen upon low-pressure inflation. The balloon is available in two sizes (3.75 × 20 mm and 2.75 × 20 mm). This is the only re-entry device designed for BTK use (**Figure 18.6e**).

The OffRoad (Boston Sc., Natick, MA) system consists of two separate components: a dedicated balloon catheter and a lancet-tip microcatheter. The semicompliant balloon reaches a maximum diameter of 5.7 mm, is ultrashort, and has a unique design characterized by a tip-less triangular shape. It is mounted on a 5-F over-the-wire (OTW) 60-mm-long shaft and is compatible with a 6-F

sheath. The microcatheter, which is coaxially advanced in the balloon lumen after wire removal, has a 0.031-inch outer lumen and is able to accommodate a 0.014-inch guidewire. The balloon is inflated at 2–3 atm and gently pushed until its tip is addressed to the distal patent vessel. The correct positioning is controlled under fluoroscopic guidance (**Figure 18.6f**).

■ POPLITEAL ARTERY

The results of endovascular treatment of the popliteal artery lesions have been commonly associated with those obtained in the treatment of SFA lesions. However, because of its distinct anatomy, this artery is exposed to high mechanical forces during normal activity, which are completely different from those applied to other arterial segments. For this reason, we believe that the outcomes of endovascular treatment of popliteal artery lesions should be analyzed separately from those obtained after revascularization of other lower limb artery occlusions. Endovascular stenting for popliteal artery stenoses using standard nitinol stents has been associated with higher rates of stent fracture (Chang et al. 2011, León et al. 2013). Moreover, early restenosis and vessel thrombosis more frequently occur in the popliteal than in femoral segments. For this reason, when treating popliteal artery occlusions, many operators may prefer a more conservative strategy, performing a simple, plain angioplasty. Therefore, endovascular stenting for popliteal artery stenoses is limited to the treatment of occlusions carrying a significant risk of vessel dissection or immediate elastic recoil with critical stenosis. Thus, in selecting the type of approach, endovascular specialists have to carefully weigh

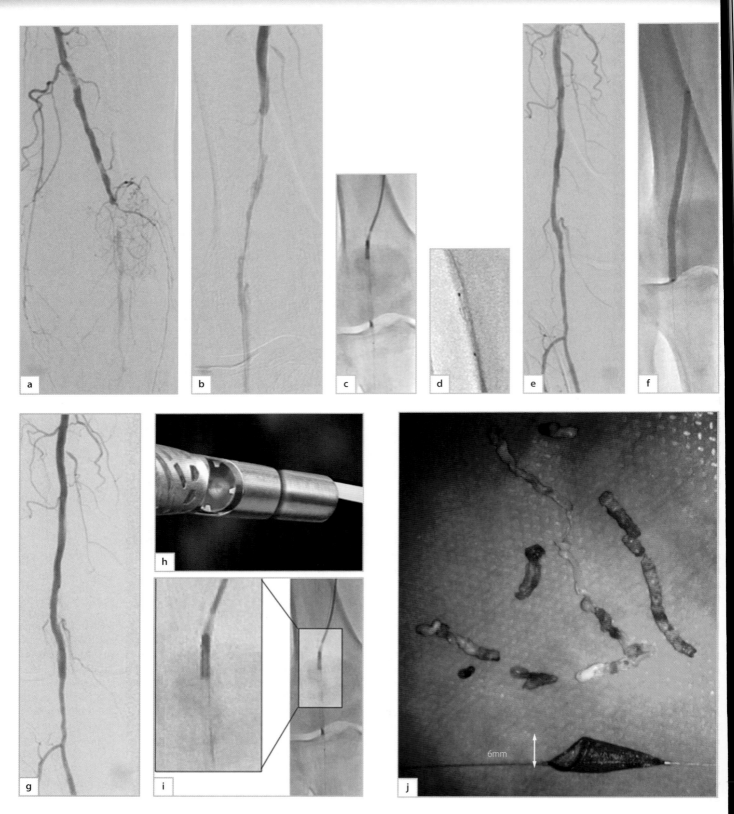

Figure 18.7 Atherectomy of an occluded popliteal artery. (a) Angiogram showing an occlusion of the popliteal artery. The lesion is crossed and predilated with a 2.5-m balloon (b) to make possible the transit of the atherectomy device (TurboHawk; Covidien, Plymouth, MN) (c) The procedure is performed with an antiembolic distal protection filter (Spider FX, 6 mm; Covidien) (d). (e) Angiogram showing the result after six passages of the atherectomy device. (f) A prolonged balloon inflation at low pressure (5.0 × 100 mm inflated for 2 minutes at 6 atm) is performed. (g) Final angiogram of the popliteal artery after directional atherectomy and balloon inflation. Detail of the rotating blade of the atherectomy device (h) and its fluoroscopic appearance (i). (j) The debulked plaque extracted from the TurboHawk after six passages; a small amount of plaque material has also been collected into the distal protection device placed to prevent embolization.

he relatively poor outcomes after plain balloon angioplasty against he use of a standard nitinol stent, which has not been specifically lesigned for this arterial segment. More recently, two different alternatives have been proposed:

1. Use of a stent with high resistance to mechanical stress (Supera; IDEV, Karlsruhe, Germany)
2. Use of a plaque excision system catheter for peripheral atherectomy (TurboHawk; Covidien, Plymouth, MN)

The Supera stent is a nitinol device with an original helical design hat reduces the risk of kinking and strut fractures, and increases the adial force. The advantage of this device is the high resistance to stress forces created by repetitive flexion and extension of the knee. A limitation with this stent may be the difficulty encountered in lelivering it since its particular design may lead to uneven stent struts listribution and stretching. A learning curve is mandatory, and the use of long devices (180 mm) may increase the risk of incorrect stent implantation (Goltz et al.2012).

At present, three devices are available for endovascular atherectomy TurboHawk or Silverhawk; Covidien, Plymouth, MN, Rotarex; Straub Medical, Wang, Switzerland, Jetstream; Medrad, Warrendale, PA). In all of these, the atherectomy catheter is used to debulk the complex esion in the popliteal artery, thus facilitating successful angioplasty and minimizing the need for stenting. With this technique, the plaque is excised without placing a metal foreign body. On 10 October 2012 at the Vascular InterVentional Advances meeting in Las Vegas, the final 12-month results from the DEFINITIVE LE (Determination of Effectiveness of SilverHawk/TurboHawk Peripheral Plaque Excision Systems for the Treatment of Infrainguinal Vessels/Lower Extremities) rial was presented. This was a large study conducted on 800 patients with femoropopliteal lesions treated with atherectomy: stents were used only in 3.1% of patients. An angiographically satisfactory result <30% residual stenosis) was obtained in all of the remaining lesions reated without the need for stents (**Figure 18.7**).

BTK ARTERIES

At least one occlusion of a BTK vessel is evident in at least 90% of the angiograms performed in patients with diabetes and CLI. Different echniques and instruments have been developed to specifically address BTK lesions, according to the length of the lesions and the frequent presence of long calcified occlusions.

Standard approach

Lesions are usually crossed with polymeric coated wires. Vascular surgeons may select between two different wire calibers: 0.014-inch Hi-Torque Pilot; Abbott Vascular, Redwood City, CA, ChoICE PT; Boston Scientific, Natick, MA) or 0.018-inch (Hi-Torque Connect; Abbott Vascular, Redwood City, CA, V-18 Control Wire; Boston Scientific, Natick, MA). Due to its limited 'pushability', the wire should never be advanced alone from the sheath to the target BTK lesion. To enhance both pushability and trackability, the wire is usually ntroduced and advanced with the help of a 4-F support catheter with a very short angled curve (usually BER I or BER II) along with a dedicated microcatheter (CXI; Cook Medical, Bloomington, IN or TrailBlazer; Covidien, Plymouth, MN) or an OTW balloon. Balloon nflations are performed at different pressures according to the type of esion. Several guidewires are available that are specifically designed to cross CTOs. Some of these devices originate from the coronary experience (Miracle, Confianza and Confianza Pro; Asahi Intecc, Nagoya, Japan, High-Torque Cross-it; Abbott Vascular, Redwood City, CA, Persuader 9; Medtronic Inc, Minneapolis, MN), whereas

others have been specifically developed for peripheral interventions (Approach CTO; Cook Medical, Bloomington, IN, Connect 250T, Abbott Vascular, Redwood City, CA; Astato 20, Astato 30, and Treasure 12; Asahi Intecc, Nagoya, Japan). The common denominator of most of these guidewires is an uncoated tapered stiff tip that is specifically designed to drill or break through fibrous caps and calcium deposits.

Crossing CTOs requires the use of an OTW catheter or balloon to support and remove the guidewire, to change it or modify its tip curve. Once the lesion is crossed, balloon inflation to nominal pressures (8–14 atm) is often sufficient to achieve good balloon expansion; however, a pressure > 20 atm may sometimes be required. The 2.0-mm-diameter balloon is optimal for dilating foot arteries, and a 3.0-mm-diameter balloon is optimal for dilating tibial vessels. The length varies greatly from 20 to 300 mm and should be tailored to the lesion extension to minimize the number of inflations and avoid barotrauma in healthy or nonstenosed segments. The optimal duration of balloon inflations is still matter of debate. Although it is usually stated that prolonged balloon inflation (>2 minutes) may improve immediate and long-term outcomes, there is no solid evidence to substantiate these claims. Therefore, we suggest performing prolonged balloon inflation only in cases where suboptimal results were obtained after standard primary dilation. When addressing BTK lesions using an antegrade approach, a guidewire length ranging from 180 to 200 cm is usually required. In the case of a crossover or brachial approach, longer guidewire lengths (260–300 cm) should be preferred to safely maintain the wire in position during catheter and balloon removal. During antegrade access, catheters and balloons should have a shaft length of at least 120 cm to reach foot vessels from the groin or at least 150 cm when a crossover maneuver is to be performed. BTK angioplasty can also be performed by abrachial approach using 0.018-inch compatible balloons with a 180-cm-long shaft (Amphirion deep; Medtronic Inc, Minneapolis, MN). This latter approach can only be successful if it is used to address simple lesions or noncalcified occlusions due to loss of pushability and maneuverability of wires and balloons over such a long route.

Subintimal recanalization

The subintimal approach is frequently used to perform recanalization of BTK lesions. The technique is similar to that described to address femoropopliteal lesions, with the only difference being the size of the material used. In our practice, BTK lesions are treated with a 0.018-inch guidewire with a polymeric, hydrophilic coating (Connect; Abbott Vascular, Redwood City, CA, V-18 Control Wire; Boston Scientific, Natick, MA) used in combination with a 100-mm OTW balloon. A longer balloon may create higher friction, especially if it has been already inflated. Some interventionists prefer a 0.35-inch hydrophilic wire (Terumo Medical, Japan). However, we believe that the use of large devices in these small arteries may increase the risk of vessel rupture. The success rate of subintimal recanalizations dramatically falls in the presence of complex re-entry situations, due particularly to local calcification, as the presence of calcium may be an obstacle to the creation of a communication channel between the false and true lumen. Dedicated re-entry devices are not available; however, re-entry into the true lumen may be attempted by exchanging the polymeric wire adopted for subintimal tracking for a stiff, tapered wire, with a short 45° C-shaped curve.

Retrograde approach

Although revascularization of BTK lesions may be performed using all of the above-described techniques, and a large variety of dedicated interventional devices are available for this purpose, the failure rate in the treatment of long chronic infrapopliteal disease ranges from 10% to 40%. The age and the length of the occlusion, the presence of heavy calcifications and/or large collaterals arising at the level of the occlusion are significant independent predictors of failure of endovascular revascularization for critical limb ischemia. Percutaneous intervention with a retrograde approach after antegrade failure has been demonstrated to increase the success rate in recanalization of BTK lesions. However, this technique is not considered as a first-line approach, and is generally used after prior failed attempts. The rationale for this alternative approach originates from the histological finding that the distal portion of the occlusive plaque is often softer than the proximal one, and therefore, it can be penetrated more easily by guidewires. Retrograde access (Gandini et al. 2012) to the occlusion can be achieved through two main strategies:

1. By entering into relatively distal, healthy segment of target artery
2. By using the pedal–plantar loop technique

Retrograde tibial access

For the retrograde approach to recanalization of tibial lesions, puncture may be attempted in the distal portion of the anterior or posterior tibial artery, or in the proximal portion of the pedal artery. There have been anecdotal reports of direct retrograde puncture of the peroneal artery. An important technical aspect that should be considered first is the modality used for imaging peripheral vascular problems. Different options are available, and the interventionists' selection should be made according to clinical experience, local facilities, and personal preferences. The puncture site can be identified with duplex scan imaging. This approach has the advantage of limiting X-ray exposure; however, it requires high technical skills for diagnostic scanning and the availability of ultrasound pulse-echo apparatus in the catheterization laboratory. Alternatively, fluoroscopy (by injecting contrast material into the groin) can be used to visualize the target vessel correctly. In this case, keeping radiation doses as low as reasonably possible and using appropriate protective shields can minimize direct exposure of interventionist's hands to X-rays. Puncture needles should be smaller than those used for standard femoral punctures. As a result of experience gleaned from thousands of radial catheterizations, a 21-G needle is normally considered to be suitable to confirm good backflow on aspiration and minimize vessel trauma. Micropuncture introducer sets, which include an outer 4-Fr catheter, have been specifically designed for this type of catheterization; however, using the 'sheathless approach' may further reduce the size of the puncture hole. This approach is best suited to all kinds of retrograde access techniques. The sheathless approach consists of inserting a long guidewire (0.018-inch or even 0.014-inch) through the puncture needle, followed by one of the above-mentioned microcatheters. The maximum diameter of these devices varies slightly from 2.1 to 2.6 Fr according to the guidewire diameter. Once the wire has crossed the BTK occlusion, it can be snared using a gooseneck device or advanced into an angled 4-Fr catheter inserted from the groin. The steps are as follows: (a) progression with the microcatheter out of the femoral sheath, (b) removal of the retrograde wire, (c) reinsertion of the wire antegradely through the same microcatheter, (d) removal of the microcatheter from the entry site. The rest of the intervention can be performed as it would be in the standard procedure. Hemostasis is achieved with prolonged balloon inflation from above, and a final angiogram should be performed to confirm the absence of active bleeding (**Figure 18.8**).

Hybrid tibial access

In some cases, distal tibial arterial access to perform angioplasty can be difficult even it is performed under duplex-scan guidance and may result in vessel damage. This is an even more critical issue when the target vessel is the single infragenicular artery remaining in the leg and the puncture site presents a large plaque burden. In these cases, a hybrid approach that combines endovascular and surgical expertise may be preferred (Airoldi et al. 2010) (**Figure 18.9**).

After surgical exposure of the distal tibial artery, trauma to the vessel wall is limited to a single needle puncture, and hemostasis achieved with prolonged balloon inflation thus reducing the risks of local hematoma. The hybrid approach for retrograde tibial access can be a time-consuming procedure and may increase the risk of wound infection; however, skilled vascular surgeons perform the procedure within a few minutes, and surgical trauma is minimized, since the small skin incision is performed under local anesthesia and does not require prolonged hospitalization.

Pedal–plantar loop-technique

With this technique, the lesion in the tibial artery is approached via retrograde puncture of the other patent tibial artery (Manzi et al. 2009).

The technique takes advantage of the normal anatomic relationships between the two tibial arteries. By definition, this approach allows the recanalization of one tibial artery occlusion if the other tibial artery provides an adequate blood supply to the foot. For this reason, this technique should only be attempted to recanalize lesions in arteries directly feeding an ischemic region according to the angiosome model. Moreover, the arterial network supplying the foot may differ between patients. In some cases it can be diffusely diseased and therefore not be amenable to endovascular intervention.

The procedure is performed as follows: the wire–balloon assembly is advanced through the pedal–plantar arch toward the tibial arteries. Short low-profile balloons or microcatheters may be used to reduce difficulties in advancing the system. Multiple balloon inflations can be performed to dilate collateral vessels and allow balloon or catheter advancement. In this situation, friction of materials inside the vessel can be extraordinarily high. Strong push or traction forces must be avoided as they may damage foot vessels. Once the wire has retrogradely crossed the occlusion, it can be snared using the femoral access or by advancing into an angled catheter antegradely inserted into the femoropopliteal artery. The wire is then removed and inverted, the OTW balloon or microcatheter is removed, and the intervention is performed antegradely as previously described. The loop wire should not be removed without an OTW balloon or catheter protecting the vessel (**Figure 18.10**).

NITINOL STENTS

Self-expandable nitinol stents are available: their length varies from 20 to 200 mm and their diameters range from 3 to 12 mm. Most require the use of a 6-Fr sheath; however, smaller devices have been developed that allow the use of a 4-Fr sheath. Reducing wire lumen (0.014–0.018 inch) and struts thickness has allowed the development of low-profile devices. Reduction in struts thickness may result in lower radial force. Calcified lesions may require the use of a 6-Fr compatible stent with high radial force to maximize the acute gain in luminal dimensions and reduce the risk of stent fractures. Nitinol stents have been designed to maximize flexibility and provide 'scaffolding' at the site of implantation. Great enthusiasm was shown

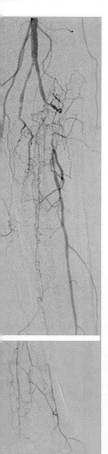
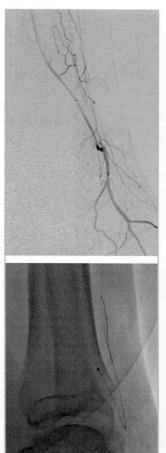
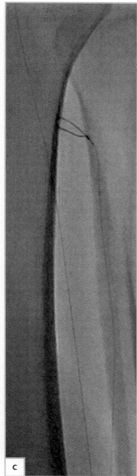
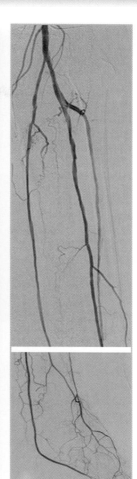

a b c d

Figure 18.8 Retrograde anterior tibial artery recanalization performed through collateral branches. (a) Angiogram demonstrating a short occlusion of the peroneal artery and long occlusions of both anterior tibial (AT) artery and posterior tibial (PT) artery. (b) Recanalization of the peroneal artery is performed and an unsuccessful antegrade recanalization of the anterior tibial artery is attempted. (c) The 0.014-inch wire (Pilot 50; Abbott Vascular, Redwood City, CA) is retrogradely advanced into the AT artery through the pre-existing collaterals connecting the anterior perforating branch of the peroneal artery to the AT artery. The PT artery is successful recanalized with subintimal tracking using a 0.018-inch wire (Control V 18; Boston Scientific, Natick, MA). (d) The final angiogram shows patency of all the three below-the-knee vessels and of the foot arteries. (e) The final angiogram shows patency of all three below-the-knee vessels and of the foot arteries.

by many interventionists when these products were first introduced to the market; however, their use has revealed several flaws. The capability to fix dissection and expand residual stenosis allows a wide and predictable lumen enlargement at the time of implantation, but long-term outcomes are subject to significant restenosis rates (20–80%). The reason for such a high variability lies in the fact that results largely differ according to the clinical and morphological characteristics of the lesions. Diabetes, extension of the lesion, and the presence of calcification and occlusion are all common in CLI, and are the most significant predictors of restenosis. Therefore, nitinol stents should only really be considered as a 'bailout' option when there has been a complication or a suboptimal result using angioplasty (Rastan et al. 2012, Scheinert et al. 2012).

DRUG ELUTING STENTS (DES) FOR BELOW-THE-KNEE ARTERIES

Drug eluting stents have undeniably revolutionized coronary artery intervention over the past decade. The drug eluting technology is intended to reduce intimal hyperplasia, which commonly results in restenosis (Boisiers et al 2012). Data on BTK vessels suggest they are associated with a significant reduction in target lesion revascularization and binary restenosis compared with either balloon

angioplasty or bare-metal stents. The trials have not been of sufficient power to detect a difference in major amputation. The most recent randomized trials include the ACHILLES, DESTINY, and YUKON-BTK trials, all of which demonstrated favorable radiological outcomes (binary restenosis and patency) with DESs.

Despite these extremely positive results, DESs are only used in a minority of lesions and patients. This is because lesions in patients with CLI are often long, whereas these stents (and trials) were performed in patients with short lesions (<4.0 cm in length) In our practice, DESs are used in relatively short lesions localized at the proximal portion of BTK vessels or in the tibioperoneal trunk. Bifurcation lesions may be treated with standard techniques proposed for the management of patients with coronary artery disease. The simplest option consists of the use of a stent in one branch and balloon dilatation in the other branch through the stent struts. More rarely, when both branches need to be covered by stents a 'V,' 'T' or a 'culotte' stenting technique may be adopted as described elsewhere (**Figure 18.11**). All of these techniques require simultaneous balloon inflations in the two branches of the bifurcation, and a 5-Fr sheath or 6-Fr guiding catheter should be used.

Drug eluting balloons that are much longer may improve longer-term outcomes by reducing intimal hyperplasia and are coming into widespread use. Data are encouraging, but longer-term data including those on limb salvage and major amputations are still awaited.

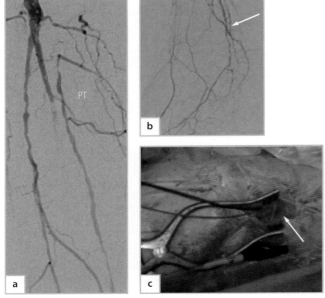
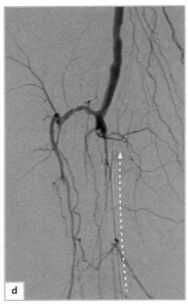
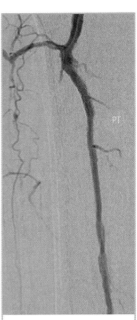
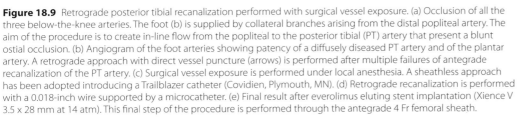
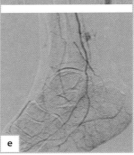

Figure 18.9 Retrograde posterior tibial recanalization performed with surgical vessel exposure. (a) Occlusion of all the three below-the-knee arteries. The foot (b) is supplied by collateral branches arising from the distal popliteal artery. The aim of the procedure is to create in-line flow from the popliteal to the posterior tibial (PT) artery that present a blunt ostial occlusion. (b) Angiogram of the foot arteries showing patency of a diffusely diseased PT artery and of the plantar artery. A retrograde approach with direct vessel puncture (arrows) is performed after multiple failures of antegrade recanalization of the PT artery. (c) Surgical vessel exposure is performed under local anesthesia. A sheathless approach has been adopted introducing a Trailblazer catheter (Covidien, Plymouth, MN). (d) Retrograde recanalization is performed with a 0.018-inch wire supported by a microcatheter. (e) Final result after everolimus eluting stent implantation (Xience V 3.5 x 28 mm at 14 atm). This final step of the procedure is performed through the antegrade 4 Fr femoral sheath.

■ AREAS OF CONTROVERSY AND/OR FUTURE RESEARCH

- The following areas need further investigation:
- The recognition of the morphological and clinical features of PAD in those with and without diabetes
- The optimal way to revascularize patients with PAD and diabetes
- The criteria used to choose the type of revascularization for total occlusions in femoral, popliteal and the crural vessels
- The relative merits of subintimal versus endoluminal angioplasty
- The role of elective stenting in femoral, popliteal, and above-knee lesions
- The role of atherectomy alone or in combination with drug eluting technologies
- The relevance of symptomatic restenosis (clinically evident) and of asymptomatic restenosis (only morphological) in the treatment and prognosis of patients with diabetes
- The type and optimal duration of antithrombotic regimens after percutaneous interventions

■ IMPORTANT FURTHER READING

Airoldi F, Faglia E, Losa S, et al. Antegrade approach for percutaneous interventions of ostial superficial femoral artery: outcomes from a prospective series of diabetic patients presenting with critical limb ischemia. Cardiovasc Revasc Med 2012; 13:20–24.

Airoldi F, Vitiello R, Losa S, et al. Retrograde recanalization of the anterior tibial artery following surgical vessel exposure: a combined approach for single remaining infragenicular vessel. J Vasc Interv Radiol 2010; 21:949–950.

Chang ZH, Liu ZY. Subintimal angioplasty for chronic lower limb arterial occlusion. Cochrane Database Syst Rev 2013; 3:CD009418.

Dick F, Diehm N, Galimanis A, et al. Surgical or endovascular revascularization in patients with critical limb ischemia: influence of diabetes mellitus on clinical outcome. J Vasc Surg 2007; 45:751–761.

Faglia E, Clerici G, Clerissi J, et al. When is a technically successful peripheral angioplasty effective in preventing above-the-ankle amputation in diabetic patients with critical limb ischaemia? Diabet Med 2007; 24:823–829.

Faglia E, Clerici G, Losa S, et al. Limb revascularization feasibility in diabetic patients with critical limb ischemia: results from a cohort of 344 consecutive unselected diabetic patients evaluated in 2009. Diabetes Res Clin Pract 2012a; 95:3643–3671.

Vogel TR, Dombrovskiy VY, Haser PB, Graham AM. Evaluating preventable adverse safety events after elective lower extremity procedures. J Vasc Surg 2011; 54:706–713.

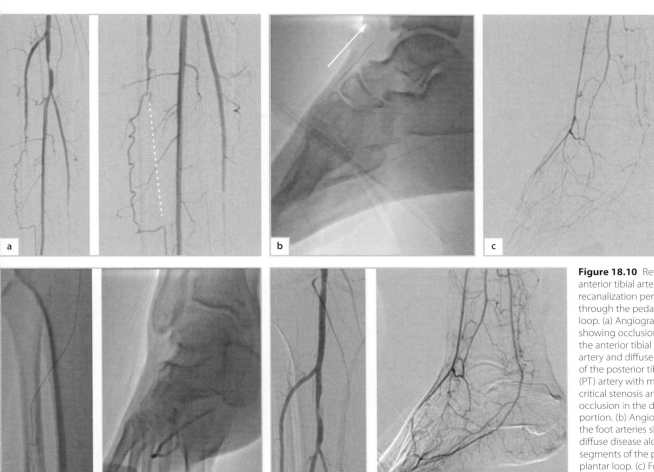

Figure 18.10 Retrograde anterior tibial artery recanalization performed through the pedal–plantar loop. (a) Angiogram showing occlusion of the anterior tibial (AT) artery and diffuse disease of the posterior tibial (PT) artery with multiple critical stenosis and a short occlusion in the distal portion. (b) Angiogram of the foot arteries showing diffuse disease along all the segments of the pedal–plantar loop. (c) Following unsuccessful attempt of antegrade recanalization of the AT artery, a wire (Contact, Abbott Vascular, Redwood city, CA) is advanced from the PT artery into the pedal–plantar loop supported by an over-the-wire balloon. The AT artery occlusion is successfully retrogradely crossed and multiple balloon inflations are performed. (d) Final angiogram showing the patency of all the three below-the-knee vessels and of the foot arteries.

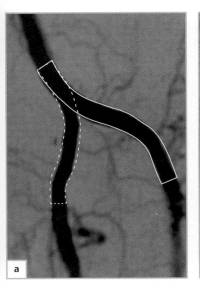
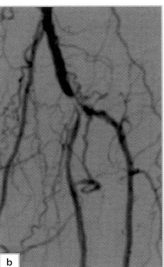
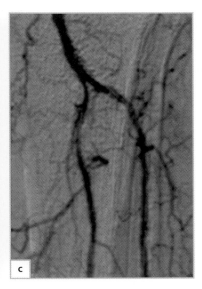

Figure 18.11 Drug eluting stent implantation in a crural bifurcational lesion. (a) Baseline angiogram showing the popliteal artery and its bifurcation into the anterior tibial (AT) artery and tibioperoneal (TP) trunk. (b) Angiographic result after balloon angioplasty (3.0 x 20-mm long balloons at 12 atm) on both branches. (c) Schematic representation of stent strut distribution after culotte stenting with two drug eluting stents (Taxus 3.5 x 32 mm; Boston Scientific, Natick, MA). The first stent is implanted in the anterior tibial artery (continuous line), and second stent in the TP trunk (dotted line). The first struts of the two stents are overlapped in the distal portion of the popliteal artery. This technique provides a complete vessel scaffolding of both branches. (d) Final kissing balloon inflation (3.5 x 20 mm at 24 atm). (e) Final results after kissing balloon inflation. (f) One-year angiographic follow-up showing patency of both stented vessels with moderate stenosis limited to the ostium of the TP trunk.

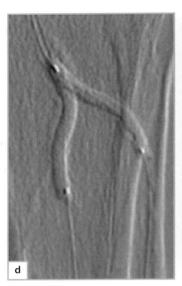
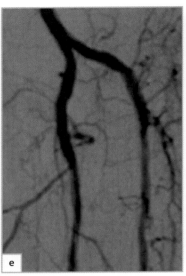
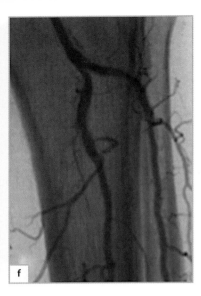

Figure 18.11 *Continued*

■ REFERENCES

Airoldi F, Faglia E, Losa S, et al. Antegrade approach for percutaneous interventions of ostial superficial femoral artery: outcomes from a prospective series of diabetic patients presenting with critical limb ischemia. Cardiovasc Revasc Med 2012; 13:20–24.

Airoldi F, Vitiello R, Losa S, et al. Retrograde recanalization of the anterior tibial artery following surgical vessel exposure: a combined approach for single remaining infragenicular vessel. J Vasc Interv Radiol 2010; 21:949–950.

Alexandrescu V, Hubermont G, Philips Y, et al. Combined primary subintimal and endoluminal angioplasty for ischaemic inferior-limb ulcers in diabetic patients: 5-year practice in a multidisciplinary 'diabetic-foot' service. Eur J Vasc Endovasc Surg 2009; 37:448–456.

Al-Nouri O, Krezalek M, Hershberger R, et al. Failed superficial femoral artery intervention for advanced infrainguinal occlusive disease has a significant negative impact on limb salvage. J Vasc Surg 2012; 56:106–110.

Angiolillo DJ, Bhatt DL, Gurbel PA, Jennings LK. Advances in antiplatelet therapy: agents in clinical development. Prasugrel, ticagrelor, and cangrelor seem to offer some benefits from pharmacological and pharmacokinetic properties compared to clopidogrel. Am J Cardiol 2009; 103:40A–51A.

Aulivola B, Pomposelli FB. Dorsalis pedis, tarsal and plantar artery bypass. J Cardiovasc Surg (Torino) 2004; 45:203–212.

Awad S, Karkos CD, Serrachino-Inglott F, et al. The impact of diabetes on current revascularisation practice and clinical outcome in patients with critical lower limb ischaemia. Eur J Vasc Endovasc Surg 2006; 32:51–59.

Biondi-Zoccai GG, Agostoni P, Sangiorgi G, et al. Mastering the antegrade femoral artery access in patients with symptomatic lower limb ischemia: learning curve, complications, and technical tips and tricks. Catheter Cardiovasc Interv 2006; 68:835–842.

Bolia A, Brennan J, Bell PR. Recanalisation of femoro-popliteal occlusions: improving success rate by subintimal recanalisation. Clin Radiol 1989; 40:325.

Bosiers M, Scheinert D, Peeters P, et al. Randomized comparison of everolimus-eluting versus bare-metal stents in patients with critical limb ischemia and infrapopliteal arterial occlusive disease. J Vasc Surg 2012; 55:390–398.

Chang IS, Chee HK, Park SW, et al. The primary patency and fracture rates of self-expandable nitinol stents placed in the popliteal arteries, especially in the P2 and P3 segments, in Korean patients. Korean J Radiol 2011; 12:203–209.

Chang ZH, Liu ZY. Subintimal angioplasty for chronic lower limb arterial occlusion. Cochrane Database Syst Rev 2013; 3:CD009418.

Conrad MF, Kang J, Cambria RP, et al. Infrapopliteal balloon angioplasty for the treatment of chronic occlusive disease. J Vasc Surg 2009; 50:799–805.

DeRubertis BG, Pierce M, Chaer RA, et al. Lesion severity and treatment complexity are associated with outcome after percutaneous infra-inguinal intervention. J Vasc Surg 2007; 46:709–716.

Dick F, Diehm N, Galimanis A, et al. Surgical or endovascular revascularization in patients with critical limb ischemia: influence of diabetes mellitus on clinical outcome. J Vasc Surg 2007; 45:751–761.

Dormandy JA, Rutherford RB. Management of peripheral arterial disease (PAD). TASC Working Group. TransAtlantic Inter-Society Consensus (TASC). J Vasc Surg 2000; 31:S1–S296.

Dörffler-Melly J, Koopman MM, Prins MH, Büller HR. Antiplatelet and anticoagulant drugs for prevention of restenosis/reocclusion following peripheral endovascular treatment. Cochrane Database Syst Rev 2005; CD002071.

Dotter CT, Judkins MP. Transluminal treatment of arteriosclerotic obstruction. description of a new technic and a preliminary report of its application. Circulation 1964; 30:654–670.

Faglia E, Clerici G, Clerissi J, et al. When is a technically successful peripheral angioplasty effective in preventing above-the-ankle amputation in diabetic patients with critical limb ischaemia? Diabet Med 2007; 24:823–829.

Faglia E, Clerici G, Losa S, et al. Limb revascularization feasibility in diabetic patients with critical limb ischemia: results from a cohort of 344 consecutive unselected diabetic patients evaluated in 2009. Diabetes Res Clin Pract 2012a; 95:3643–3671.

Faglia E, Clerici G, Airoldi F, et al. Revascularization by angioplasty of type D femoropopliteal and long infrapopliteal lesion in diabetic patients with critical limb ischaemia: are TASC II recommendations suitable? a population-based cohort study. Int J Low Extrem Wounds 2012b; 11:277–285.

Fanelli F, Lucatelli P, Allegritti M, et al. Retrograde popliteal access in the supine patient for recanalization of the superficial femoral artery: initial results. J Endovasc Ther 2011; 18:503–509.

Gandini R, Uccioli L, Spinelli A, et al. Alternative techniques for treatment of complex below-the knee arterial occlusions in diabetic patients with critical limb ischemia. Cardiovasc Intervent Radiol 2013; 36:75–83.

Goodney PP, Beck AW, Nagle J, et al. National trends in lower extremity bypass surgery, endovascular interventions, and major amputations. J Vasc Surg 2009; 50:54–60.

Goltz JP, Ritter CO, Kellersmann R, et al. Endovascular treatment of popliteal artery segments P1 and P2 in patients with critical limb ischemia: initial experience using a helical nitinol stent with increased radial force. J Endovasc Ther 2012; 19:450–456.

Gruntzig A. Transluminal dilatation of coronary-artery stenosis. Lancet 1978; 1:263.

Ihnat DM, Duong ST, Taylor ZC, et al. Contemporary outcomes after superficial femoral artery angioplasty and stenting: the influence of TASC classification and runoff score. J Vasc Surg 2008; 47:967–974.

Isner JM, Rosenfield K. Redefining the treatment of peripheral artery disease. Role of percutaneous revascularization. Circulation 1993; 88:1534–1557.

Kudo T, Chandra FA, Ahn SS. The effectiveness of percutaneous transluminal angioplasty for the treatment of critical limb ischemia: a 10-year experience. J Vasc Surg 2005; 41:423–435.

León LR, Jr, Dieter RS, Gadd CL, et al. Preliminary results of the initial United States experience with the Supera woven nitinol stent in the popliteal artery. J Vasc Surg 2013; 57:1014–1022.

LoGerfo FW, Gibbons GW, Pomposelli FB J, et al. Trends in the care of the diabetic foot. Expanded role of arterial reconstruction. Arch Surg 1992; 127:617–620.

Manzi M, Fusaro M, Ceccacci T, et al. Clinical results of below-the knee intervention using pedal-plantar loop technique for the revascularization of foot arteries. J Cardiovasc Surg (Torino) 2009; 50:331–337.

Montero-Baker M, Schmidt A, Bräunlich S, et al. Retrograde approach for complex popliteal and tibioperoneal occlusions. J Endovasc Ther 2008; 15:594–604.

Nicod P, Scherrer U. Explosive growth of coronary angioplasty. Success story of a less than perfect procedure. Circulation 1993; 8:1749–1751.

Nishino M, Taniike M, Makino N, et al. Bidirectional endovascular treatment for chronic total occlusive lesions of the femoropopliteal arterial segment using a hand-carried ultrasound device and a retrograde microcatheter. J Vasc Surg 2012; 56:113–117.

Norgren L, Hiatt WR, Dormandy JA, et al. Inter-Society Consensus for the Management of Peripheral Arterial Disease (TASC II). Eur J Vasc Endovasc Surg 2007; 33:S1–S70.

Rastan A, Brechtel K, Krankenberg H, et al. Sirolimus-eluting stents for treatment of infrapopliteal arteries reduce clinical event rate compared to bare-metal stents: long-term results from a randomized trial. J Am Coll Cardiol 2012; 60:587–591.

Rooke TW, Hirsch AT, Misra S, et al. 2011 ACCF/AHA Focused Update of the Guideline for the Management of Patients With Peripheral Artery Disease (updating the 2005 guideline): a report of the American College of Cardiology Foundation/American Heart Association Task Force on Practice Guidelines. J Am Coll Cardiol 2011; 58:2020–2045.

Sandford RM, Bown MJ, Sayers RD, et al. Is infrainguinal bypass grafting successful following failed angioplasty? Eur J Vasc Endovasc Surg 2007; 34:29–34.

Scheinert D, Katsanos K, Zeller T, et al. A prospective randomized multicenter comparison of balloon angioplasty and infrapopliteal stenting with the sirolimus-eluting stent in patients with ischemic peripheral arterial disease: 1-year results from the Achilles trial. J Am Coll Cardiol 2012; 60:2290–2295.

Schillinger M, Minar E. Percutaneous treatment of peripheral artery disease: novel techniques. Circulation 2012; 126:2433–2440.

Schmidt A, Bausback Y, Piorkowski M, et al. Retrograde recanalization technique for use after failed antegrade angioplasty in chronic femoral artery occlusions. J Endovasc Ther 2012; 19:23–29.

Spectre G, Arnetz L, Östenson CG, et al. Twice daily dosing of aspirin improves platelet inhibition in whole blood in patients with type 2 diabetes mellitus and micro- or macrovascular complications. Thromb Haemost 2011; 106:491–499.

Tønnesen KH, Sager P, Karle A, et al. Percutaneous transluminal angioplasty of the superficial femoral artery by retrograde catheterization via the popliteal artery. Cardiovasc Intervent Radiol 1988; 11:127–131.

Vogel TR, Dombrovskiy VY, Haser PB, Graham AM. Evaluating preventable adverse safety events after elective lower extremity procedures. J Vasc Surg 2011; 54:706–713.

Wheatley BJ, Mansour MA, Grossman PM, et al. Complication rates for percutaneous lower extremity arterial antegrade access. Arch Surg 2011; 146:432–435.

Zayed HA, Fassiadis N, Jones KG, et al. Day-case angioplasty in diabetic patients with critical ischaemia. Int Angiol 2008; 27:232–238.

However, the question of long-term patency remains an issue in endovascular treatment, particularly in below-the-knee disease – primary patency at 1 year is around 58% after crural vessel angioplasty (Romiti et al. 2008).

In addition to straightforward plain balloon angioplasty, novel endovascular adjuncts have been developed on the basis of the principles and practice of coronary artery revascularization, to reduce the rate of restenosis and loss of patency after peripheral artery revascularization. These have been accepted to varying degrees within the vascular community and include bare metal stents, ePTFE stents, drug-eluting devices (DES), and drug-impregnated balloons.

Bare metal stents are widely used in aortoiliac and suprapopliteal disease, but their use in crural vessels is not well established. ePTFE-coated iliac stents (stent grafts) have been shown to offer higher rates of patency than angioplasty alone at 2 years. In theory, stents provide a barrier to early restenosis and can be a useful adjunct where there is recoil of angioplasty at the initial intervention. However, problems with in-stent stenosis due to thrombus and neointimal hyperplasia have led to the development of DES and drug-impregnated balloons. Initially used in the coronary circulation, DES provide slow-release local delivery of antiproliferative drugs (e.g. sirolimus and paclitaxel) to the vessel lumen, hence reducing the tendency for neointimal proliferation of vascular smooth muscle cells.

Various randomized trials have explored the use of stents, DES, and impregnated balloons, predominantly in femoropopliteal disease, and developments of second-generation devices are ongoing. Early evidence of their effectiveness in the context of occlusive PAD in femoropopliteal disease is emerging but drawbacks include stent fracture, late in-stent stenosis, and need for prolonged dual antiplatelet therapy. There is also concern about incomplete coverage of DES with antirestenotic drugs, meaning that unequal delivery of antiproliferative drugs to the vessel wall may lead to partial endothelialization. The STRIDES (SFA Treatment with Drug-Eluting Stents) trial evaluated self-expanding everolimus-eluting stents in occlusive femoropopliteal disease but demonstrated that the initial promising rate of primary patency at 6 months (94 +/- 2.3%) was unsustained at 12 months (68 +/- 4.6%) (Lammer et al. 2011).

To that end, the use of drug-impregnated angioplasty balloons may be more effective and this remains the most promising new technique. An antiproliferative drug coats the balloon, and a larger dose is delivered at the point of initial luminal contact with the balloon, with some lasting effect. This allows more widespread and equal coverage than drug-eluting stents and also negates the need for foreign body deployment. Short-term follow-up data suggest that drug-impregnated balloons are associated with a reduction in restenosis when compared with uncoated angioplasty, with no difference in safety profile (Cassese et al. 2012); however, there is no data on their effect on long-term clinical outcomes.

Endovascular brachytherapy using γ-emitting sources is another novel technique, which has been developed in the attempt to improve endovascular outcomes and has been shown to improve patency in femoropopliteal intervention (Norgren et al. 2007); however, large trials are lacking.

With regard to patients with diabetes and infragenicular arterial disease, there is no current data to support the use of these devices and techniques; however, trials are ongoing and the concepts remain promising. Current guidelines specify that such novel treatments should not be used outside the remit of established clinical trials, as there is no convincing overall data suggesting their superiority over traditional balloon angioplasty.

ALTERNATIVE THERAPIES IN NONREVASCULARIZABLE DISEASE: CELL-BASED THERAPY

Although bypass or angioplasty remains the mainstay of treatment for severe and limb-threatening PAD, we know that an alarming proportion of patients progress to amputation despite successful revascularization. Morbidity and mortality associated with major amputation is huge, with a perioperative mortality rate of around 17% in the case of major lower limb amputation and a 30–50% 5-year mortality rate, which is worse than many common cancers. As such, there is growing interest in the development of alternative or adjunctive treatments for nonrevascularizable severe and CLI, based on targeting the known cellular mechanisms of atherosclerosis and the replication of angiogenesis to provide collateral circulation.

Peripheral arterial disease is a result of progressive arteriosclerosis, culminating in stenotic and occlusive disease and resulting in inadequate tissue perfusion. However, some patients with even long femoropopliteal occlusions remain asymptomatic, and this can be explained by endogenous compensatory mechanisms, collectively known as 'angiogenesis.' The premise of cell therapy as a treatment for severe PAD is to replicate and enhance the already existing physiological compensatory mechanisms, using bone marrow-derived cells to induce arteriogenesis. This may be particularly relevant in patients with diabetes, whose regenerative capacity and rate of collateralization is poorer than those without diabetes.

Animal models and early human preclinical studies have demonstrated that the transplantation of bone marrow-derived mononuclear cells into the gastrocnemius muscle of an ischemic limb may improve ABPI or TcPO2, symptoms, and walking distance in the short term (Tateisha-Yuyama et al. 2002). Although the concept has gathered interest around the world, these novel cell techniques are clearly not without limitation. Small study size, heterogeneity of patient characteristics and perfusion deficits, and lack of standardized outcomes preclude confident conclusions to be drawn, whereas the potential side effects and ethical issues surrounding allogeneous bone marrow harvest and transplant add further to this dilemma. If cell therapy is found to be an effective alternative treatment for refractory PAD, its wider use is likely to be restricted due to the complexity of the technique, likely poor reproducibility in nonteaching hospitals and its expense.

OTHER APPROACHES: PRE-EMPTIVE REVASCULARIZATION

There is currently no evidence to support 'pre-emptive' revascularization, i.e. intervention before the patients develops an ulcer, and the role of early revascularization in DFU with mild or moderate PAD is yet to be established. However, ulceration and infection in the foot will increase the demand for oxygen, and thus, it follows that even a mild perfusion deficit may significantly compromise the healing of DFU. In addition, adverse biological factors that are commonly associated with diabetes – impaired humoral immunity, abnormal inflammatory responses, microvascular dysregulation – will further inhibit the healing process. Neuropathy and autonomic dysfunction can contribute to a painless but critically ischemic foot, meaning that patients with diabetes and severe disease may present much later with more advanced sequelae than patients without diabetes with the same perfusion deficit. Thus, revascularization in DFU often occurs later than it otherwise might.

In terms of angiographic findings, there is suggestion that arterial occlusions in patients with diabetes may result in more severe perfusion deficits than those without diabetes due to poor collateral circulation, arterial wall calcification, and arteriovenous shunting. Patients with diabetes seem to have less physiological compensatory mechanisms to cope with tissue ischemia. Arguably, then, it may be worthwhile to consider revascularization in patients with DFU and mild or moderate PAD, or indeed PAD in patients with diabetes but no ulceration.

VOLUME–OUTCOME RELATIONSHIP IN PERIPHERAL ARTERIAL SURGERY

In the present era, there is a drive toward improved transparency among the surgical community, with the advent of individual surgeon outcome reporting in the United Kingdom. Surgical outcomes vary between centers, but there is heterogeneity in outcome reporting, classification of disease, and standardization of outcomes. Therefore, any comparative results must be interpreted with caution.

However, there is evidence to show that higher volume hospitals are associated with better surgical outcomes, particularly as the complexity of the procedure increases. This has been demonstrated in surgery for PAD – a recent systematic review and meta-analysis found that amputation and mortality rates after lower limb arterial surgery are reduced in higher volume centers (Awopetu et al. 2010). Birkmeyer et al. (2003) showed a relationship between surgeon volume and outcomes in vascular procedures in the USA; therefore, choosing the right surgeon, in the right place at the right time, is an important premise for lower limb arterial surgery.

AREAS OF CONTROVERSY AND/OR FUTURE RESEARCH

- There is no evidence to support pre-emptive revascularization in those patients with diabetes and a high-risk foot (e.g. those with deformity or neuropathy) to prevent ulceration/amputation
- The benefit of revascularization in patients with DFU and mild PAD (perfusion deficit) is unclear; many of these patients will eventually heal with good wound and diabetes care
- There is no robust evidence comparing angioplasty versus bypass in patients with diabetes and severe limb ischemia. In clinical practice, comorbidity, the distribution of PAD and local expertise are important considerations in the decision to perform either technique
- Primary infrapopliteal angioplasty is becoming more popular in high-risk patients with distal disease and severe limb ischemia; however, there is no evidence to support an angioplasty-first approach, and technical success with long occlusions is limited in the crural segment
- Limb salvage at 1 year after revascularization for patients with a DFU is 85% for open surgical procedures and 78% for endovascular treatment, and there appears to be little overall difference in complete wound healing between the two techniques
- Autologous vein (preferably the GSV) should be used in all surgical bypass procedures when available, because the results of prosthetic grafts are poor
- Drug eluting balloons and stents may be the most useful adjunct to angioplasty, with evidence to suggest a reduction in restenosis rates when compared with plain balloon angioplasty. However, more robust clinically meaningful outcome data are lacking

IMPORTANT FURTHER READING

Albers M, Romiti M, Brochado-Neto FC, De Luccia N, Pereira CAB. Meta-analysis of popliteal-to-distal vein bypass grafts for critical ischaemia. J Vasc Surg 2006; 43:498–503.

Awad S, Karkos CD, Serrachino-Inglott F, et al. The impact of diabetes on current revascularization practice and clinical outcome in patients with critical lower limb ischaemia. Eur J Vasc Endovasc Surg 2006; 31:51–59.

Cassese S, Byrne RA, Ott I, et al. Paclitaxel-coated versus uncoated balloon angioplasty reduces target lesion revascularization in patients with femoropopliteal arterial disease: a meta-analysis of randomized trials. Circ Cardiovasc Interv 2012; 5:582–589.

Dick F, Diehm N, Galimanis A, et al. Surgical or endovascular revascularization in patients with critical limb ischaemia: influence of diabetes on clinical outcome. J Vasc Surg 2007; 45:751–761.

Hinchliffe RJ, Andros G, Apelqvist J, et al. A systematic review of the effectiveness of revascularization of the ulcerated foot in patients with diabetes and peripheral arterial disease. Diabetes Metab Res Rev 2012; 28:179–217.

Romiti M, Albers M, Brochado-Neto FC, et al. Meta-analysis of infrapopliteal angioplasty for chronic critical limb ischaemia. J Vasc Surg 2008; 47:975–981.

REFERENCES

AbuRahma AF, Robinson PA, Holt SM. Prospective controlled study of polytetrafluoroethylene versus saphenous vein in claudicant patients with bilateral above knee femoropopliteal bypasses. Surgery 1999; 126:594–602.

Adam DJ, Beard JD, Cleveland T, et al. Bypass versus angioplasty in severe ischaemia of the leg (BASIL): multicentre, randomized controlled trial. Lancet 2005; 366:1925–1934.

Albers M, Romiti M, Brochado-Neto FC, De Luccia N, Pereira CAB. Meta-analysis of popliteal-to-distal vein bypass grafts for critical ischaemia. J Vasc Surg 2006; 43:498–503.

Anandbabu S, Neville RF. Distal vein patch improves results in PTFE bypasses to tibial arteries. Acta Chir Belg 2006; 106:372–377.

Awad S, Karkos CD, Serrachino-Inglott F, et al. The impact of diabetes on current revascularization practice and clinical outcome in patients with critical lower limb ischaemia. Eur J Vasc Endovasc Surg 2006; 31:51–59.

Awopetu AI, Moxey P, Hinchliffe RJ, et al. Systematic review and meta-analysis of the relationship between hospital volume and outcome for lower limb arterial surgery. Br J Surg 2010;97:797–803.

Belch JJF, Dormandy J, CASPAR Writing Committee. Results of the randomized, placebo-controlled clopidogrel and acetylsalicylic acid in bypass surgery for peripheral artery disease (CASPAR) trial. J Vasc Surg 2010; 52:825–833.

Berceli SA, Chan AK, Pomposelli FB, et al. Efficacy of dorsal pedal artery bypass in limb salvage for ischemic heel ulcers. J Vasc Surg 1999; 30:499–508.

Bergan JJ, Veith FJ, Bernhard VM, et al. Randomization of autogenous vein and polytetrafluoroethylene grafts in femorodistal reconstruction. Surgery 1982; 92:921–930.

Birkmeyer JD, Stukel TA, Siewers AE, et al. Surgeon volume and operative mortality in the United States. N Engl J Med 2003;349: 2117–2127.

Bolia A. Subintimal angioplasty, the way forward. Acta Chir Belg 2004; 104:547–554.

Byrne J, Darling C, Chang B, et al. Infrainguinal arterial reconstruction for claudication: Is it worth the risk? An analysis of 409 procedures. J Vasc Surg 1999; 29:259–269.

Cassese S, Byrne RA, Ott I, et al. Paclitaxel-coated versus uncoated balloon angioplasty reduces target lesion revascularization in patients with femoropopliteal arterial disease: a meta-analysis of randomized trials. Circ Cardiovasc Interv 2012; 5:582–589.

Davies AH, Hawdon AJ, Sydes MR, Thompson SG. Is duplex surveillance of value after leg vein bypass grafting? Principal results of the vein graft surveillance randomized trial (VGST). Circulation 2005; 112:1985–1991.

Davies AH, Magee TR, Tennant SGW, Baird RN, Horrocks M. Criteria for indentification of the "at risk" infrainguinal bypass graft. Eur J Vasc Surg 1994; 8:315–319.

Dick F, Diehm N, Galimanis A, et al. Surgical or endovascular revascularization in patients with critical limb ischaemia: influence of diabetes on clinical outcome. J Vasc Surg 2007; 45:751–761.

Dolan NG, Lui K, Criqui MH, et al. Peripheral arterial disease, diabetes, and reduced lower extremity functioning. Diabetes Care 2002; 25:113–120.

Dutch Bypass Oral Anticoagulants or Asprin (BOA) Study Group. Efficacy of oral anticoagulants compared with aspirin after infrainguinal bypass surgery (The Dutch Bypass Oral Anticoagulant or Aspirin Study): a randomized trial. Lancet 2000; 355:346–351.

Faglia E, Dalla Paola L, Clerici G, et al. Peripheral angioplasty as the first-choice revascularization procedure in diabetic patients with critical limb ischaemia: prospective study of 993 consecutive patients hospitalized and followed between 1999 and 2003. Eur J Vasc Endovasc Surg 2005; 29:620–627.

Garcia S, Moritz TE, Ward HB, et al. The usefulness of revascularization of patients with multivessel coronary artery disease before elective vascular surgery for abdominal aortic and peripheral occlusive disease. Am J Cardiol 2008; 102:809–813.

Graziani L, BSC clinical edition, Issue 17, April 2006, Gosling, UK.

Green RM, Abbott WM, Matsumoto T, et al. Synthetic above-knee femoropopliteal bypass grafting: five year results of a randomized trial. J Vasc Surg 2000; 31:417–425.

Hinchliffe RJ, Andros G, Apelqvist J, et al. A systematic review of the effectiveness of revascularization of the ulcerated foot in patients with diabetes and peripheral arterial disease. Diabetes Metab Res Rev 2012; 28:x–xx.

Jeffcoate WJ. Wound healing – a practical algorithm. Diabetes Metab Res Rev 2012; 28:85–88.

Kapfer X, Meichelboek W, Groegler FM. Comparison of carbon-impregnated and standard ePTFE prostheses in extra-anatomical anterior tibial artery bypass: a prospective randomized multicentre study. Eur J Vasc Endovasc Surg 2006; 32:155–168.

Karthikesalingam A, Holt PJE, Moxey P, et al. A systematic review of scoring systems for diabetic foot ulcers. Diabet Med 2010; 27:544–549.

Kechagias A, Perala J, Ylonen K, Mahar MAA, Biancari F. Validation of the Finnvasc Score in infrainguinal percutaneous transluminal angioplasty for critical lower limb ischaemia. Ann Vasc Surg 2008; 22:547–551.

Klinkert P, Post PN, Breslau PJ, van Bockel JH. Saphenous vein versus PTFE for above-knee femoropopliteal bypass. A review of the literature. Eur J Vasc Endovasc Surg 2004; 27:357–362.

Lammer J, Bosiers M, Zeller T, et al. First clinical trial of self-expanding everolimus-eluting stent implantation for peripheral arterial occlusive disease. J Vasc Surg 2011; 54:394–401.

Lees T, Troeng T, Thomson IA, et al. International variations in infrainguinal bypass surgery – a VASCUNET report. Eur J Vasc Endovasc Surg 2012; 44:185–192.

Lepantalo M, Matzke S. Outcome of unreconstructed chronic critical leg ischaemia. Eur J Vasc Endovasc Surg 1996; 11:53–157.

Lindholt JS, Gottschalksen B, Johannesen N, et al. The Scandinavian Propaten(®) trial - 1-year patency of PTFE vascular prostheses with heparin-bonded luminal surfaces compared to ordinary pure PTFE vascular prostheses – a randomised clinical controlled multi-centre trial. Eur J Vasc Endovasc Surg 2011; 41:668–673.

Marston WA, Davies SW, Armstrong B, et al. Natural history of limbs with arterial insufficiency and chronic ulceration treated without revascularization. J Vasc Surg 2006; 44:108–114.

McQuade K, Gable D, Pearl G, Theune B, Black S. Four-year randomized prospective comparison of percutaneous ePTFE/nitinol self-expanding stent graft versus prosthetic femoro-popliteal bypass in the treatment of superficial femoral artery occlusive disease. J Vasc Surg 2010; 52:584–590.

Moxey PW, Hofman D, Hinchliffe RJ, et al. Trends and outcomes after surgical lower limb revascularization in England. Br J Surg 2011; 98:1373–1382.

Neville R, Singh N, Jamil T, et al. Revascularization for wound healing: are endovascular techniques as good as open bypass. Presented at the Society for Clinical Vascular Surgery 35th Annual Symposium, Naples, Florida, 2007.

Norgren L, Hiatt WR, Dormandy JA, et al. Inter-Society Consensus for the Management of Peripheral Arterial Disease (TASC II). J Vasc Surg. 2007; 45: S5–S6.

Prompers L, Huijberts M, Apelqvist J, et al. Delivery of care to diabetic patients with foot ulcers in daily practice: results of the Eurodiale Study, a prospective cohort study. Diabet Med 2008; 25:700–707.

Romiti M, Albers M, Brochado-Neto FC, et al. Meta-analysis of infrapopliteal angioplasty for chronic critical limb ischaemia. J Vasc Surg 2008; 47:975–981.

Saqib NU, Domenick N, Cho JS, et al. Predictors and outcomes of restenosis following tibial artery endovascular interventions for critical limb ischaemia. J Vasc Surg 2013; 57:692–699.

Schaper NC. Diabetic foot ulcer classification system for research purposes: a progress report on criteria for including patients in research studies. Diabetes Metab Res Rev 2004; 20:S90–S95.

Schaper NC, Andros G, Apelqvist J, et al. Diagnosis and treatment of peripheral arterial disease in diabetic patients with a foot ulcer. A progress report from the International Working Group on the Diabetic Foot. Diabetes Metab Res Rev 2012a; 28:218–224.

Schaper NC, Andros G, Apelqvist J, et al. Specific guidelines for the diagnosis and treatment of peripheral arterial disease in a patient with diabetes and ulceration of the foot 2011. Diabetes Metab Res Rev 2012b; 28:236–237.

Sumpio BE, Forsythe RO, Ziegler KR, et al. Clinical implications of the angiosome model in peripheral vascular disease. J Vasc Surg 2013; 58:814–826.

Tateisha-Yuyama E, Matsubara H, Murohara T, et al. Therapeutic angiogenesis for patients with limb ischaemia by autologous transplantation of bone-marrow cells: a pilot study and a randomized controlled trial. Lancet 2002; 360:427–435.

Taylor SM, Kalbaugh, Blackhurst DW, et al. Preoperative clinical factors predict postoperative functional outcomes after major lower limb amputation: an analysis of 553 consecutive patients. J Vasc Surg 2005; 42:227–235.

Twine CP, McLain AD. Graft type for femoro-popliteal bypass grafting. Cochrane Database Sys Rev 2010; 12:CD001487.

Vauclair F, Haller C, Marques-Vidal P, et al. Infrainguinal bypass for peripheral arterial occlusive disease: when arms save legs. Eur J Vasc Endovasc Surg 2012; 43:48–53.

Walker C. Durability of PTAs using pedal artery approaches. Presented at the 37th Annual VEITH Symposium, 18th November 2010, New York City, NY.

Wartman SM, Woo K, Herscu G, et al. Endoscopic vein harvest for infrainguinal arterial bypass. J Vasc Surg 2013; pii:S0741–5214(13)00012-8. doi: 10.1016/j.jvs.2012.12.029. [Epub ahead of print]

Xiao L, Huang D, Tong J, Shen J. Efficacy of endoluminal interventional therapy in diabetic peripheral arterial occlusive disease: a retrospective trial. Cardiovasc Diabetol 2012; 11:17.

Section 4

NEUROPATHY

Chapter 20 | Pathobiology of neuropathy

Ketan Dhatariya

SUMMARY

- A wide variation in the reported prevalence and incidence of diabetic neuropathy results from the many differences in defining the condition, the tests used to assess it, and the patient population under consideration

- In addition, there are considerable differences in the interpretation of the various tests used to determine the presence or absence of neuropathy

- Diabetes-related neuropathy can have serious adverse effects on a wide variety of normal body function

- Motor nerve dysfunction results in disturbances in posture and balance that can, in turn, lead to increased pressures within the foot

- Loss of sensory perception results in an inability to feel trauma that would have otherwise resulted in pain, thus inhibiting any early preventative action from being taken

- Loss of autonomic function in the lower limbs leads to a loss of sweating and hence very dry skin. This, in turn, leads to an increased risk of the skin cracking, allowing the entry of pathogens into the wound

- Autonomic dysregulation also disrupts the ability to control vascular blood flow

- It is extremely difficult to get accurate estimates of the incidence and prevalence of neuropathy

- The most important factors that determine the development of the condition are poor glycemic control and increasing duration of diabetes

- There remains debate over the exact pathological mechanisms that are responsible for the development of diabetic neuropathy

INTRODUCTION

In 1864, Marchal de Calvi first recognized that diabetes affect the nervous system (de Calvi 1864), but it was not until 1885 that diabetic polyneuropathy was first described (Pavy 1885). Pavy described many of the classic symptoms of hyperesthesia or anesthesia, as well as the loss of tendon reflexes. However, due to the lack of technological capability in the late 19th and early 20th centuries, it was not until 1945 that the first comprehensive description of autonomic neuropathy appeared (Rundles 1945). It was this same lack of technology, and the lack of formal definitions of neuropathy that have led to the delay in getting robust data on the incidence and prevalence of neuropathy in the diabetes population. The different rates of nerve fiber population involvement mean that it is often difficult to differentiate types of neuropathy. Furthermore, the long follow-up needed for a large number of patients whose glycemic control varies over time mean that, until recently, there are very few reliable data on neuropathy in people with diabetes; moreover, only in recent years it has become clear that nerve conduction slows with age even in those without diabetes.

Given the recognition that diabetes has been associated with peripheral neuropathy, regular foot examination, checking for loss of protective sensation, has long been part of the standard of care for people with diabetes. Examinations starting from the time of diagnosis for people with type 2 diabetes and after 5 years of diagnosis for those with type 1 diabetes have been advocated (American Diabetes Association 2013). An understanding of the pathobiology of neuropathy is important because of its strong association with premature cardiovascular death (Coppini et al. 2000, Forsblom et al. 1998). The association with several modifiable risk factors for cardiovascular disease means that the presence of neuropathy should prompt early and aggressive treatment to optimize these risk factors. However, there is debate about how neuropathy should be diagnosed.

There are numerous classifications of diabetic neuropathy based on clinical features, etiology, anatomical patterns, or pathogenesis. The classification originally proposed by Thomas (1997) has been advocated by the American Diabetes Association and other expert groups (Boulton et al. 2005, Tesfaye 2010). The condition that is termed 'neuropathy' is a heterogeneous group that varies by symptoms, underlying mechanisms, and patterns of neurological involvement (Dyck et al. 1993). In essence, neuropathy can be classified as motor or sensory, or large fiber or small fiber. Small fiber neuropathy often precedes large fiber disease and is manifest by the classic symptoms of pain, numbness, and loss of pinprick and light touch perception. The large fiber neuropathy results in the loss of vibration sense and muscle weakness, with loss of tendon reflexes. It is, however, rare to get isolated small or large fiber symptoms or signs, with most patients exhibiting a mixed picture.

THE ANATOMY OF THE PERIPHERAL NERVOUS SYSTEM

Briefly, the nervous system is divided into three main components – motor, sensory (together known as somatic nerves), and the autonomic nervous system. Each of these systems has a vital role to play in the development of diabetes-related foot disease. **Figure 20.1** shows a cross section of the thoracic spinal cord highlighting the major ascending and descending pathways.

Motor nerves

The motor nerves descend from the brain in a variety of specialized anatomical pathways, including the lateral corticospinal and rubrospinal tracts that carry the nerves responsible for voluntary movement. The ventromedial pathways includes the reticulospinal tract, which is primarily responsible for locomotion and posture, and the tectospinal and vestibulospinal tracts, which are responsible for control of movement within the head and neck.

Once the nerves have made connections with the peripheral motor nerves in the ventral horn of the spinal cord, the motor neurons then progress to skeletal muscle. The myelinated α-motoneurones form the major bulk of these peripheral nerves and end on skeletal muscle fibers in a motor end plate. The number of motoneurons per muscle fiber determines how fine the resultant movement should be. The more precise a movement, the fewer motor neurons it has. The constant low-grade ('background') activity of these motor nerves also maintains the

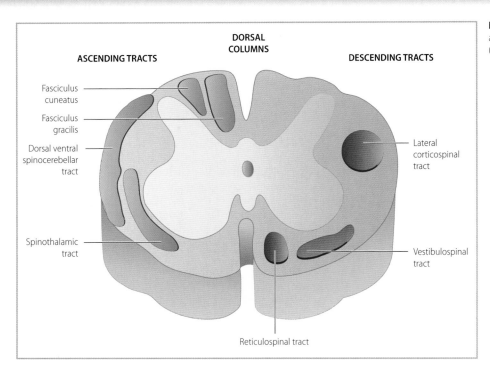

Figure 20.1 A cross section through the spinal cord at the thoracic level showing the major ascending (blue) and descending (red) tracts.

Labels in figure:
DORSAL COLUMNS
ASCENDING TRACTS
DESCENDING TRACTS
Fasciculus cuneatus
Fasciculus gracilis
Dorsal ventral spinocerebellar tract
Spinothalamic tract
Lateral corticospinal tract
Vestibulospinal tract
Reticulospinal tract

integrity of the muscles. This means that the muscles are constantly being stimulated and their strength maintained.

Sensory nerves

These nerves, often called the somatosensory nerves, bring nerves impulses from the periphery to the spinal cord and from there to the sensory areas within the cerebral cortex. The two main pathways within the spinal cord are the dorsal columns, which carry information about touch and proprioception, and the spinothalamic tracts, which convey information on pain and temperature.

There are three different forms of sensory receptors that relay information from the outside world into electrical impulses. These are the mechanoreceptors, which respond when they are moved (e.g. when a muscle changes position) or deformed under pressure. Thermoreceptors detect changes in temperature and nociceptors that detect stimuli, which would, under normal circumstances, be associated with tissue damage and is thus painful.

Together, these motor and sensory nerves make up the peripheral nerve fibers. Within these fibers are nerves of varying diameter – with all but the finest nerves being myelinated. The larger the diameter of the nerve, and the more associated myelin, the faster the nerve conduction velocity. The Aα fibers are the largest, ranging from 8 to 20 μm in diameter with a conduction velocity of between 44 and 120 m/s. The Aγ fibers that make up the motoneurons to individual muscle spindles have less myelin and are smaller in diameter than the Aα fibers, with a diameter of 3–8 μm and a slower conduction velocity of 18–48 m/s. The finest nerves are those without any myelin cover and thus have the slowest conduction speed. These are the C fibers associated with warmth and pain sensation with a diameter of <1.5 μm and a conduction velocity of 0.5–2 m/s. It is these thinnest fibers, which are often found furthest away from the central nervous system that is usually (but not always) affected first by diabetes.

Autonomic nerves

The autonomic nerves are integral to maintaining normal functioning in almost every organ in the body. They are vital to maintaining homeostasis. It is divided into the sympathetic and parasympathetic systems. The sympathetic nerves leave the spinal cord at all thoracic levels innervating many organs from the eye, the salivary glands to the heart, major abdominal organs, adrenal glands, and blood supply. It also innervates the bladder and reproductive organs. The parasympathetic nervous system leaves the central nervous system along several cranial nerves (III, VII, IX, and X) and through these innervates the eye, the salivary glands, the lungs and heart, and several major abdominal organs. The parasympathetic nerves also leave the sacral spinal cord to innervate the large bowel, the bladder, and reproductive organs. The long intra-abdominal path of the vagus nerve means that when this is affected, then gastrointestinal symptoms, such as early satiety, nausea and vomiting, constipation, and bloating, are more common.

The autonomic nervous system has several functions within the cardiovascular system. It regulates heart rate and allows the maintenance of blood pressure by maintaining vasoactive tone as well as sensing circulating blood volume in the baroreceptors. It controls the rate of transit of food from be oropharynx to the rectum. The parasympathetic nervous system in men is responsible for penile vasoconstriction, allowing an erection to be sustained, whereas the sympathetic system controls ejaculation. The skin is heavily innervated to allow for adequate thermoregulation, with the autonomic nervous system controlling peripheral vasodilatation and vasoconstriction, and sweating. Autonomic neuropathy leads to a loss of sympathetic constrictor tone. In the feet, this is typically associated with peripheral vasodilation and increased thermoregulatory blood flow, resulting in a relative warm foot with distended veins. However, if an injury occurs, there is an inability to allow for further vasodilation, leading to a 'relative reduction' in the necessary perfusion to allow for adequate wound healing. This is discussed later in this chapter. The presence of autonomic neuropathy is associated with a poor prognosis, with previous estimates of 2.5-year mortality being 44% (Ewing & Clarke 1982).

TESTING FOR NEUROPATHY

Although this is dealt with in more detail in the next chapter, one of the reasons for the wide variation in reported prevalence and incidence of diabetic neuropathy have been the many differences in defining the condition, the tests used to assess it, and the patient population under consideration. In addition, there are considerable differences in the interpretation of the various tests used to determine the presence or absence of neuropathy (Dyck et al. 2010). As a result of these findings, it is important for the clinician to choose a small set of tests designed to assess different modalities of sensation and stick to them. For example, tests to assess vibration perception could include a 128-Hz tuning fork or a neurothesiometer. It has been shown that in individuals who have a vibration perception threshold of ≥ 25 Hz have a greater than eightfold increase of developing ulceration (Young et al. 1994). Combinations of tests have been shown to have >87% sensitivity for detecting peripheral neuropathy (American Diabetes Association 2013). While outside the remit of this chapter, testing for evidence of peripheral vascular disease is also an integral part of the foot examination.

THE CONSEQUENCES OF NERVE DAMAGE IN THE LOWER LIMBS AND FEET

With these many functions in mind it can be seen that diabetes-related neuropathy can have serious adverse effects on a wide variety of normal body function. However, because this insidious condition tends to affect the longest axons, it is the feet that are affected first before proximal progression affects the hands. It is also usually the case that sensorimotor neuropathy becomes symptomatic before autonomic neuropathy. With respect to the feet, several different interactions come together to create potential problems.

Consequences of motor nerve dysfunction

As mentioned, the motor nerves are responsible for maintaining normal posture and balance. With the loss of neuronal activity, posture and balance diminish, leading to increased pressures within the foot in an attempt to maintain posture and balance.

In addition, the small muscles of the feet lose their strength due to the loss of the background neuronal activity. Due to the differential loss of strength between the extensor muscles and the flexor muscles, the extensors remain stronger than the flexors, and toes often become clawed. As illustrated in **Figure 20.2**, over time, this is thought to lead to the toes often dislocating, exposing the heads of the metatarsals. The head of the metatarsals are then pressing directly on the deeper skin structures. As a result, the shear stresses on the skin under the metatarsal heads increase, as the direct pressures are likely to increase the load over a smaller area. However, given that the toes also claw, the pressure distribution also becomes concentrated on the tips of the toes, resulting in higher pressures during the gait cycle. Thus, pressure ulcers can develop in a variety of sites across the foot.

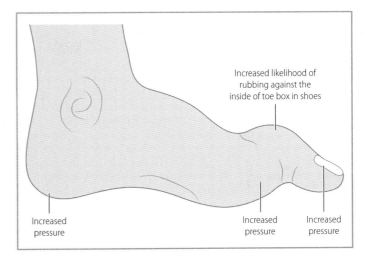

Figure 20.2 The shape of the foot with motor nerve dysfunction. The characteristic 'clawing' is due to the differential loss of strength between the extensor muscles and the flexor muscles leading to areas of high plantar pressures and an increased risk of the dorsal aspects of the toes rubbing against the inside of the toe box of a shoe.

It is at this stage that patient education is paramount, so that they are aware of their risk and take appropriate preventative action. This includes using correct foot wear to correctly redistribute the abnormal plantar pressures with the use of appropriate insoles and other pressure relieving devices. Without these, the increased pressures often lead to callus formation and ultimately lead to an increased risk of ulceration.

Consequences of sensory nerve dysfunction

The most obvious result of the loss of sensory perception is the inability to feel trauma that would have otherwise resulted in pain. This loss of sensation then results in preventative action not being taken (e.g. stepping on a pin and not feeling it). This often results in the protective barrier offered by the skin being breached and entry of pathogens into the subcutaneous tissues and infection ensuing.

The loss of protective sensation also means that in instances where the foot is in some way damaged (e.g. twisting an ankle) then that pain is not felt, and gait is not altered to allow healing of that area. In people with intact sensation, a person may limp, or keep their weight of the injured area; however, in neuropathy this does not occur, resulting in ongoing trauma to the injured area – making it worse.

The loss of proprioception means that the individual does not know where their foot is at any given time. This will eventually result in the classic 'high stepping' gait associated with a distal peripheral neuropathy. This results in abnormal pressure distributions on the plantar surface of the foot when it is put on the floor. Due to the sensory loss in combination with the motor dysfunction and loss of muscle strength, patients with diabetic neuropathy can have an abnormal and unstable walking pattern, with an increased tendency to fall. The postural instability and these spatiotemporal changes in gait are important, but frequently unrecognized, factors in the loss of quality of life in these patients.

Figures 20.3 and **20.4** show the consequences of distal symmetrical large fiber and small fiber polyneuropathy.

Consequences of autonomic nerve dysfunction

Loss of autonomic function in the lower limbs has two main consequences. First, sweating is important to maintain moisture within the skin. The loss of autonomic function leads to a loss of sweating and hence very dry skin. This leads to an increased risk of the skin cracking and allows the entry of skin organisms into the wound.

The other main effect of autonomic dysregulation is the loss of the ability to control vascular blood flow. If an injury occurs and the underlying tissues are exposed, then a variety of mechanisms lead to vasodilatation to encourage an increased blood supply to the site of injury. The immediate response to an injury is to vasoconstrict the surrounding blood vessels to stem the flow of blood loss, but very soon afterward, the blood flow increases to allow the materials in the blood that would heal the wound to be delivered more swiftly. Apart from local mediators, the autonomic nervous system allows for further vasoconstriction and then vasodilatation to occur. However, in autonomic neuropathy, these changes in blood flow do not occur. There is a loss of vasoconstriction and a loss of vasodilatation. These changes are thought to contribute to an impairment of wound healing.

EPIDEMIOLOGY

It is extremely difficult to get accurate estimates of the incidence and prevalence of neuropathy. Older data suggested that the annual incidence of neuropathy was between 2% and 3% (Partanen et al. 1995, Pirart 1978, UK Prospective Diabetes Study [UKPDS] Group 1998) and was the same for people with type 1 and type 2 diabetes (Young et al. 1994). A 1993 study suggested that the overall prevalence of neuropathy in 119 diabetes centers from around the United Kingdom was 28.5% (Young et al. 1993). The incidence increased with duration of diabetes, with 36.8% of the population having a diagnosis of neuropathy if diabetes had been present for ≥10 years. In addition, age was an important factor, with 44.2% of patients aged between 70 and 79 years being affected. These data are consistent with the 30–40% prevalence reported from other populations (Fedele et al. 1997, Tesfaye et al. 1996). Despite these data, the actual incidence may have been different, given that the vast majority of diabetes care was provided in the community most of whom are less likely to have complex diabetes-related end-organ damage than a secondary care population (Walters et al. 1992a). Further difficulties arise when one considers the large numbers of people with diabetes who remain undiagnosed (Walters et al. 1992b). In addition, given the difficulties on defining diabetes-related sensorimotor neuropathy, it is hard to get good estimates of prevalence (Dyck et al. 2010). However, some newer data have suggested that the prevalence of painful diabetic polyneuropathy in the community is approximately 16–26%. Quality of life is reduced in patients with painful neuropathy, with restrictions in the activities of daily living and social activities. In addition, painful neuropathy is associated with sleep disturbances, anxiety, and depression (Jude & Schaper 2007). These difficulties in diagnosing

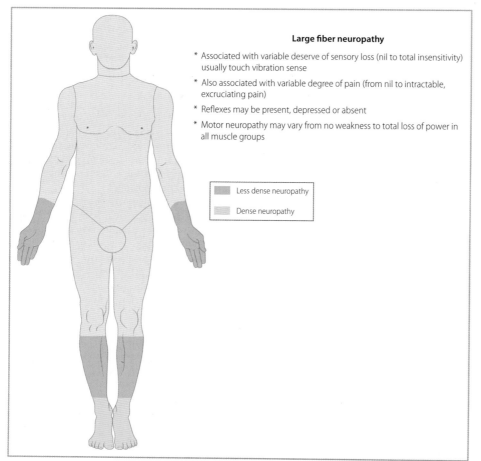

Large fiber neuropathy

* Associated with variable deserve of sensory loss (nil to total insensitivity) usually touch vibration sense

* Also associated with variable degree of pain (from nil to intractable, excruciating pain)

* Reflexes may be present, depressed or absent

* Motor neuropathy may vary from no weakness to total loss of power in all muscle groups

Less dense neuropathy

Dense neuropathy

Figure 20.3 The 'stocking and glove' distribution of the sensory defect seen with large fiber neuropathy.

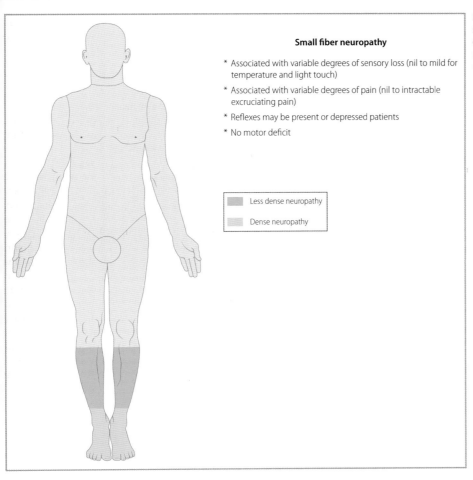

Small fiber neuropathy

* Associated with variable degrees of sensory loss (nil to mild for temperature and light touch)

* Associated with variable degrees of pain (nil to intractable excruciating pain)

* Reflexes may be present or depressed patients

* No motor deficit

Less dense neuropathy
Dense neuropathy

Figure 20.4 The distribution of the sensory defect seen with small fiber neuropathy. There is an overlap with the abnormalities seen with large fiber neuropathy, but clinical examination shows different neurological modalities being affected.

or defining neuropathy are further highlighted when considering the Diabetes Control and Complications Trial (DCCT) cohort. According to the theories about long-term chronic hyperglycemia, people with type 1 diabetes within 5 years of diagnosis should not develop a chronic complication; however, between 0.3% and 21.8% of that population had a degree of neuropathy, depending on the definitions used (The DCCT Research Group 1995).

In summary, the available data suggest that despite the improvements in controlling hyperglycemia, the prevalence of peripheral neuropathy remains high, with many people either not diagnosed correctly or not treated appropriately. It may well be that in the intervening years with the publication of the DCCT and the UKPDS, that as overall glycemic control of people with diabetes has improved, so the incidence and prevalence of diabetic neuropathy has declined (The DCCT Research Group 1993, UKPDS Group 1998).

DIFFERENTIAL DIAGNOSIS OF A DISTAL SYMMETRIC POLYNEUROPATHY

The differential diagnosis of distal symmetric polyneuropathy is large and is listed in **Table 20.1**. As with most conditions, a 'pathological sieve' should be used to exclude other causes.

■ PATHOLOGICAL MECHANISMS

Over the last few years, several metabolic, immune, microvascular, and neuroendocrine factors have emerged as contributing to the development of peripheral diabetic neuropathy. However, it has been recognized for several decades that the most important factors that determine the development of the condition are poor glycemic control and increasing duration of diabetes (Dyck et al. 1999, 2006, Pirart 1978).

There remains debate over the exact pathological mechanisms that are responsible for the development of diabetic neuropathy. Part of this comes from the DCCT data that showed that despite intensive glycemic control leading to a 60% reduction in neuropathy, the cumulative incidence or neuropathy remained high (15–21%), as did the cumulative incidence of abnormal nerve conduction (40–52%) (The DCCT Research Group 1995). These data suggest other factors may be responsible for the development of neuropathy in the face of tight glycemic control.

The DCCT data demonstrated that in those without neuropathy at baseline, but went on to develop it, there were statistically significant correlations with 'traditional' risk factors, such as HbA1c, age, duration of diabetes, body mass index, the presence of hypertension, microalbuminuria, retinopathy, and a history of cardiovascular disease (The DCCT Research Group 1995). Observational data of >1100 patients have shown that a change in glycemic control

Table 20.1 Some of the more common causes of distal symmetric polyneuropathy. As always, a good history and physical examination will help narrow down the differential diagnosis

Metabolic or endocrine	Diabetes mellitus
	Uremia
	Vitamin B12 deficiency
	Hypothyroidism
	Porphyria
Malignancy	Paraneoplastic syndromes
	Amyloid
	Myeloma
Vascular	Vasculitis
Congenital/familial	Charcot–Marie–Tooth disease
Trauma	Entrapment neuropathies
Inflammatory or infection	Sarcoid
	HIV
	Leprosy
	Syphilis
	Borrelia infection (Lyme disease)
Autoimmune	Type 1 diabetes mellitus
	Antiphospholipid/anticardiolipin syndrome
	Guillain–Barré syndrome
	Chronic inflammatory demyelinating neuropathy
Toxicity	Alcohol
	Chemotherapy
	Heavy metals

was associated with a change in risk of subsequently developing neuropathy over 7 years of follow-up. These authors found that with a rise in HbA1c of 16.3 mmol/mol (1.9%), the odds ratio of developing neuropathy increased by 2.48 (95% confidence interval 1.5–4.11) (Tesfaye et al. 2005). Although one study has shown a relationship between height and the risk of developing neuropathy (Gadia et al. 1987), other studies have found that there were significant associations with less established, potentially modifiable risk factors that remained significant after adjustment for the improvement in HbA1c over the duration of the trial. These included smoking, high levels of total cholesterol, low-density cholesterol and triglycerides, and low levels of high-density cholesterol (Maser et al. 1989, Mitchell et al.1990, Tesfaye et al. 2005, The DCCT Research Group 1995). What is less contentious is that it is thought that the chronic hyperglycemia leads to intracellular damage, much of which is probably reversible in the early stages of the condition, but that over time, becomes irreversible. Animal studies suggest that hyperglycemia affects several metabolic pathways, each with their own downstream pathways being affected. Thus, research has been focused on learning many of these pathways to see if anything – other than improving glycemic control – can be done to detect pathological changes early and if these changes can be prevented or reversed. Given that these irreversible changes occur before neuropathy is clinically detectable, this makes intervention and treatment very difficult indeed. However, it also gives further reasons (if any were needed) to ensure that glycemic control is held as close to the levels seen in people without diabetes as possible from the time of diagnosis for as long as possible.

■ Aldose reductase and the polyol pathway (Figure 20.5)

The oldest and perhaps best-known etiological hypothesis is the aldose reductase hypothesis (Brownlee 2001, Tomlinson & Gardiner 2008). Glucose entry into nervous tissue is independent of insulin and with increasing glucose concentrations aldose reductase is activated. Aldose reductase is the rate-limiting enzyme of the polyol pathway and is generally inactive when glucose levels are in the range of 3 to 6 mmol/L, because it has a low affinity for glucose. Glucose is preferentially metabolized by hexokinase, an enzyme with a much higher affinity for glucose, and rapidly transforms glucose into glucose-6-phosphate. When glucose levels rise in diabetes, the hexokinase pathway is saturated forcing more glucose down the sorbitol pathway where the enzyme aldose reductase converts the glucose to fructose via sorbitol using the enzyme sorbitol dehydrogenase. However, the conversion of sorbitol to fructose is very slow, leading to build up of sorbitol. This reaction uses nicotinamide adenine dinucleotide phosphate (NADPH) as a proton donor. However, NADPH is also used by glutathione reductase to convert reduced glutathione (GSH) to glutathione disulphide (GSSG). GSH is important because it removes hydrogen peroxide. The excessive use of NADPH by the sorbitol pathway results in lower levels of GSH and thus higher levels of hydrogen peroxide. The hydrogen peroxide is produced by normal mitochondrial respiration that produces free oxygen radicals that are themselves converted to hydrogen peroxide by superoxide dismutase. When levels of hydrogen peroxide build up, the Fenton reaction liberates the free radical superhydroxide that is damaging to the surrounding tissues (so called 'oxidative stress'). Thus, high glucose levels ultimately lead to a reduction in superoxide removal. It is these superoxide molecules that have been implicated in damaging strands of DNA. This, in turn, leads to reductions in intracellular NAD, thus slowing the rate of conversion of sorbitol to fructose, leading to a greater buildup of sorbitol. Sorbitol diffuses very slowly out through cell membranes, thus intracellular accumulation ultimately leads to irreversible cell damage and cell death.

Further damaging processes also occur as a result of high intracellular glucose. As mentioned above and shown in **Figure 20.5**, once the glucose is converted to glucose-6-phosphate, most of it is metabolized to fructose-6-phosphate. This molecule is metabolized in two main ways. First, fructose-6-phosphate is converted into glyceraldehyde-3-phosphate. This is metabolized into the highly damaging methylglyoxal. This molecule, as well as other reactive glucose metabolites, nonenzymatically attaches to other proteins, resulting in the accelerated formation of advanced glycation end products (AGEs) and so, cellular dysfunction. In addition, these proteins may extravasate, leading to progressive microvascular occlusion. Over time, as renal function deteriorates, AGE clearance is impaired, thus perpetuating the problem. AGEs can affect nerve function in two main ways. First, protein glycation affects structure and normal biological function. Second, the binding of AGE to cell surface receptors (RAGE) leads to activation of an inflammatory intracellular signaling cascade, increasing the oxidative stress.

The second pathway for fructose-6-phosphate is as a metabolite for the hexosamine pathway. This converts fructose-6-phosphate into uridine diphosphate-N-acetylhexosamine (UDP-GlcNAc). This molecule has an affinity for serine and threonine residues on proteins such as Sp1. This binding of UDP-GlcNAc to these proteins, in turn,

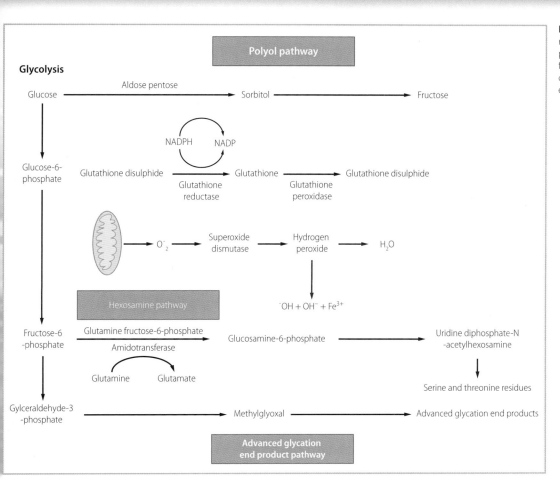

Figure 20.5 The aldose reductase and the polyol pathway showing the potential fate of glucose entering the cells. Please see text for a full explanation of the pathway.

adversely affects their structure and function and has been suggested as a contributory factor to the inflammation and endothelial injury seen in hyperglycemia.

The intracellular hyperglycemia and activation of the aldose reductase pathway described above is also associated with activation of intracellular signaling pathways mediated by the mitogen-activated protein kinases. These kinases are also activated by high levels of oxidized low-density lipoprotein (LDL) and RAGE. These molecules perform key roles in the intracellular signaling pathways, with at least two (p38 and JNK) being activated in the face of intracellular hyperglycemia. Activation is associated with phosphorylation of a variety of proteins, including ion channels, disrupting their function, and eventually causing measurable changes in cell damage and in nerve function.

With these multiple pathological mechanisms in mind, several agents have been tried to try and prevent the damage done by these processes. Aldose reductase inhibitors have been used, as have AGE inhibitors such as aminoguanidine and benfotiamine – all with limited success in neuropathy (Balakumar et al. 2010, Schemmel et al. 2010). However, the development of RAGE inhibitors remains an attractive therapeutic target.

Hypoxia

Given the microvascular damage associated with poorly controlled diabetes, it is unsurprising that this is a potential mechanism of neuropathic damage. Occlusion of the vasa nervorum (by the gradual accumulated extravasated AGEs described above) is associated with hypoxic damage to the endoneurium, leading to the neuropathy. This is along the same mechanism associated with the microvascular damage associated with diabetic retinopathy (Stevens et al. 1995).

Hyperlipidemia

The classic dyslipidemia of poorly controlled diabetes is the high levels of total cholesterol, high levels of LDL, low levels of high-density lipoprotein, and high levels of triglycerides. In addition to the high cardiovascular risk that these biochemical abnormalities confer, they are also significantly associated with the development of diabetic neuropathy (Vincent et al. 2011).

High free fatty acid levels are also associated with the development of neuropathy. High levels of free fatty acids are associated with a proinflammatory state, with increased levels of inflammatory cytokines, raising oxidative stress. Furthermore, the insulin-resistance and resultant hyperglycemia that characterizes type 2 diabetes is associated with intramuscular accumulations of free fatty acids – thus perpetuating the problems.

Although there are in vitro and animal data suggesting that dyslipidemia leads to accumulation of sorbitol and other intermediary metabolites, the exact mechanisms by which high lipid levels interfere with neuronal function remains to be elucidated.

■ AREAS OF CONTROVERSY AND/OR FUTURE RESEARCH

- Work continues to accurately identify the molecular causes of neuropathy – in particular painful neuropathy – and several drugs are in development that block the above described metabolic pathways and the accumulation of harmful molecules
- Understanding these metabolic pathways should allow the development of new agents to target appropriate receptors in an attempt to bring symptom relief to the millions of people around the world who continue to suffer as a result of this debilitating complication of diabetes
- An expanding research base is bringing together abnormalities in structure and function to determine the pathophysiology of diabetic neuropathy
- As the incidence and prevalence of diabetes continues unabated, especially in parts of the world where access to health care is limited, it is likely that there will be an increase in the number of people developing micro- and macrovascular complications, despite the awareness that good glycemic control and multiple risk factor management helps reduce the likelihood of them occurring
- The challenge for researchers and pharmaceutical companies is to make any new treatments developed accessible and affordable to those who are most at risk of developing these complications
- Until recently, due to the requirements of the regulatory authorities to develop new treatments compared with placebo, it has been difficult to determine which of the treatments is likely to be most beneficial
- Those treating patients with peripheral neuropathy are heartened to see some companies take the initiative and undertake comparative 'head-to-head' trials to help determine a realistic treatment algorithm
- With the advent of genomic medicine there is a hope that individualized treatments will become possible, to ensure that the most appropriate agents will be prescribed according to an individuals' genetic susceptibility

■ IMPORTANT FURTHER READING

American Diabetes Association. Standards of medical care in diabetes - 2013. Diabetes Care 2013; 36:S11–S66.

Brownlee M. Biochemistry and molecular cell biology of diabetic complications. Nature 2001; 414:813–820.

Dyck PJ, Davies JL, Wilson DM, et al. Risk factors for severity of diabetic polyneuropathy: intensive longitudinal assessment of the Rochester Diabetic Neuropathy Study cohort. Diabetes Care 1999; 22:1479–1486.

Ewing DJ, Clarke BF. Diagnosis and management of diabetic autonomic neuropathy. BMJ 1982; 285:916–918.

Partanen J, Niskanen L, Lehtinen J, et al. Natural history of peripheral neuropathy in patients with non-insulin-dependent diabetes mellitus. N Engl J Med 1995; 333:89–94.

Tesfaye S, Boulton AJ, Dyck PJ, et al. Diabetic neuropathies: update on definitions, diagnostic criteria, estimation of severity, and treatments. Diabetes Care 2010; 33:2285–2293.

■ REFERENCES

American Diabetes Association. Standards of medical care in diabetes - 2013. Diabetes Care 2013; 36:S11–S66.

Balakumar P, Rohilla A, Krishnan P, et al. The multifaceted therapeutic potential of benfotiamine. Pharmacol Res 2010; 61:482–488.

Boulton AJ, Vinik AI, Arezzo JC, et al. Diabetic neuropathies: a statement by the American Diabetes Association. Diabetes Care 2005; 28:956–962.

Brownlee M. Biochemistry and molecular cell biology of diabetic complications. Nature 2001; 414:813–820.

Coppini DV, Bowtell PA, Weng C, et al. Showing neuropathy is related to increased mortality in diabetic patients – a survival analysis using an accelerated failure time model. J Clin Epidemiol 2000; 53:519–523.

de Calvi CJM. Recherches sur les accidents diabétiques et essai d'une théorie générale du diabète. Publisher: P. Asselin. Paris 1864.

Dyck PJ, Davies JL, Clark VM, et al. Modeling chronic glycemic exposure variables as correlates and predictors of microvascular complications of diabetes. Diabetes Care 2006; 29:2282–2288.

Dyck PJ, Davies JL, Wilson DM, et al. Risk factors for severity of diabetic polyneuropathy: intensive longitudinal assessment of the Rochester Diabetic Neuropathy Study cohort. Diabetes Care 1999; 22:1479–1486.

Dyck P, Kratz KM, Karnes JL, et al. The prevalence by staged severity of various types of diabetic neuropathy, retinopathy, and nephropathy in a population-based cohort: the Rochester Diabetic Neuropathy Study. Neurology 1993; 43:817–825.

Dyck PJ, Overland CJ, Low PA, et al. Signs and symptoms versus nerve conduction studies to diagnose diabetic sensorimotor polyneuropathy: CI vs. NPhys trial. Muscle Nerve 2010; 42:157–164.

Ewing DJ, Clarke BF. Diagnosis and management of diabetic autonomic neuropathy. BMJ 1982; 285:916–918.

Fedele D, Comi G, Coscelli C, et al. A multicenter study on the prevalence of diabetic neuropathy in Italy. Diabetes Care 1997; 20:836–843.

Forsblom CM, Sane T, Groop PH, et al. Risk factors for mortality in Type II (non-insulin-dependent) diabetes: evidence of a role for neuropathy and a protective effect of HLA-DR4. Diabetologia 1998; 41:1253–1262.

Gadia MT, Natori N, Ramos LB, et al. Influence of height on quantitative sensory, nerve-conduction, and clinical indices of diabetic peripheral neuropathy. Diabetes Care 1987; 10:613–616.

Jude EB, Schaper N. Treating painful diabetic polyneuropathy. BMJ 2007; 335:57–58.

Maser RE, Steenkiste AR, Dorman JS, et al. Epidemiological correlates of diabetic neuropathy: report from Pittsburgh Epidemiology of Diabetes Complications Study. Diabetes 1989; 38:1456–1461.

Mitchell BD, Hawthorne VM, Vinik AI. Cigarette smoking and neuropathy in diabetic patients. Diabetes Care 1990; 13:434–437.

Partanen J, Niskanen L, Lehtinen J, et al. Natural history of peripheral neuropathy in patients with non-insulin-dependent diabetes mellitus. N Engl J Med 1995; 333:89–94.

Pavy FW. Introductory address to the discussion on the clinical aspect of glycosuria. Lancet 1885; 126:1085–1087.

Pirart J. Diabetes mellitus and its degenerative complications: a prospective study of 4,400 patients observed between 1947 and 1973. Diabetes Care 1978; 1:168–188.

Rundles RW. Diabetic neuropathy: general review with report of 125 cases. Medicine 1945; 24:111–160.

Schemmel KE, Padiyara RS, D'Souza JJ. Aldose reductase inhibitors in the treatment of diabetic peripheral neuropathy: a review. J Diabetes Complications 2010; 24:354–360.

Stevens MJ, Feldman EL, Greene DA. The aetiology of diabetic neuropathy: the combined roles of metabolic and vascular defects. Diabet Med 1995; 12:566–579.

Tesfaye S, Boulton AJ, Dyck PJ, et al. Diabetic neuropathies: update on definitions, diagnostic criteria, estimation of severity, and treatments. Diabetes Care 2010; 33:2285–2293.

Tesfaye S, Chaturvedi N, Eaton SE, et al. Vascular risk factors and diabetic neuropathy. N Engl J Med 2005; 352:341–350.

Tesfaye S, Stevens LK, Stephenson JM, et al. Prevalence of diabetic peripheral neuropathy and its relation to glycaemic control and potential risk factors: the EURODIAB IDDM Complications Study. Diabetologia 1996; 39:1377–1384.

The Diabetes Control and Complications Trial Research Group. The effect of intensive treatment of diabetes on the development and progression of long-term complications in insulin-dependent diabetes mellitus. New Engl J Med 1993; 329:977–986.

The Diabetes Control and Complications Trial Research Group. The effect of intensive diabetes therapy on the development and progression of neuropathy. Ann Intern Med 1995; 122:561–568.

Thomas PK. Classification, differential diagnosis, and staging of diabetic peripheral neuropathy. Diabetes 1997; 46:S54–S57.

Tomlinson DR Gardiner NJ. Diabetic neuropathies: components of etiology. J Peripher Nerv Syst 2008; 13:112–121.

UK Prospective Diabetes Study Group. Intensive blood-glucose control with sulphonylureas or insulin compared with conventional treatment and risk of complications in patients with type 2 diabetes (UKPDS 33). Lancet 1998; 352:837–853.

Vincent AM, Callaghan BC, Smith AL, Feldman EL. Diabetic neuropathy: cellular mechanisms as therapeutic targets. Nature Rev Neurol 2011; 7:573–583.

Walters DP, Gatling W, Mullee MA, Hill RD. The distribution and severity of diabetic foot disease: a community study with comparison to a non-diabetic group. Diabet Med 1992a; 9:354–358.

Walters DP, Gatling W, Mullee MA, Hill RD. The prevalence of diabetic distal sensory neuropathy in an English community. Diabet Med 1992b; 9:349–353.

Young MJ, Boulton AJ, Macleod AF, et al. A multicentre study of the prevalence of diabetic peripheral neuropathy in the United Kingdom hospital clinic population. Diabetologia 1993; 36:150–154.

Young MJ, Breddy JL, Veves A, Boulton AJ. The prediction of diabetic neuropathic foot ulceration using vibration perception thresholds: a prospective study. Diabetes Care 1994; 17:557–560.

Callaghan BC, Little AA, Feldman EL, Hughes RA. Enhanced glucose control for preventing and treating diabetic neuropathy. Cochrane Database Syst Rev 2012; 6:CD007543.

Caselli A, Pham H, Giurini JM, Armstrong DG, Veves A. The forefoot-to-rear foot plantar pressure ratio is increased in severe diabetic neuropathy and can predict foot ulceration. Diabetes Care 2002; 25:1066–1071.

Chalk C, Benstead TJ, Moore F. Aldose reductase inhibitors for the treatment of diabetic polyneuropathy. Cochrane Database Syst Rev 2007; 4:CD004572.

Cruccu G, Sommer C, Anand P, et al. EFNS guidelines on neuropathic pain assessment: revised 2009. Eur J Neurol 2010; 17:1010–1018.

Daousi C, MacFarlane IA, Woodward A, et al. Chronic painful peripheral neuropathy in an urban community: a controlled comparison of people with and without diabetes. Diabet Med 2004; 21:976–982.

Daousi C, McFarlane IA, Woodward A, et al. Chronic painful peripheral neuropathy in an urban community: a control comparison of people with and without diabetes. Diabet Med 2004; 21:976–982.

Davies M, Brophy S, Williams R, Taylor A. The prevalence, severity, and impact of painful diabetic peripheral neuropathy in type 2 diabetes. Diabetes Care 2006; 29:1518–1522.

Davies M, Brophy S, Williams R, Taylor A. The prevalence, severity, and impact of painful diabetic peripheral neuropathy in type 2 diabetes. Diabetes Care 2006; 29:1518–1522.

Diabetes UK. Putting feet first. www.diabetes.org.uk/putting-feet-first (accessed 06 March, 2014)

Dolan NC, Liu K, Criqui MH, et al. Peripheral artery disease, diabetes, and reduced lower extremity functioning. Diabetes Care 2002; 25:113–120.

Dros J, Wewerinke A, Bindels PJ, van Weert HC. Accuracy of monofilament testing to diagnose peripheral neuropathy: a systematic review. Ann Fam Med 2009; 7:555–558.

Dyck PJ, Kratz KM, Karnes JL, et al. The prevalence by staged severity of various types of diabetic neuropathy, retinopathy, and nephropathy in a population-based cohort: the Rochester Diabetic Neuropathy Study. Neurology 1993; 43:817–824.

Dyck PJ, Overland CJ, Low PA, et al. Signs and symptoms versus nerve conduction studies to diagnose diabetic sensorimotor polyneuropathy: CI vs. NPhys trial. Muscle Nerve 2010; 42:157–164.

Dyck PJ. Detection, characterization, and staging of polyneuropathy: assessed in diabetics. Muscle Nerve 1988; 11:21–32.

Edmonds ME, Morrison N, Laws JW, Watkins PJ. Medial arterial calcification and diabetic neuropathy. Br Med J 1982; 284:928–930.

England JD, Gronseth GS, Franklin G, et al. Distal symmetric polyneuropathy: a definition for clinical research: report of the American Academy of Neurology, the American Association of Electrodiagnostic Medicine, and the American Academy of Physical Medicine and Rehabilitation. Neurology 2005; 64:199–207.

Feng Y, Schlösser FJ, Sumpio BE. The Semmes Weinstein monofilament examination as a screening tool for diabetic peripheral neuropathy. J Vasc Surg 2009; 50:675–682.

Freeman R, Durso-Decruz E, Emir B. Efficacy, safety, and tolerability of pregabalin treatment for painful diabetic peripheral neuropathy: findings from seven randomized, controlled trials across a range of doses. Diabetes Care 2008; 31:1448–1454.

Freynhagen R, Baron R, Gockel U, Tölle TR. painDETECT: a new screening questionnaire to identify neuropathic components in patients with back pain. Curr Med Res Opin 2006; 22:1911–1920.

Frykberg RG, Lavery LA, Pham H, et al. Role of neuropathy and high foot pressures in diabetic foot ulceration. Diabetes Care 1998; 21:1714–1719.

Geerts M, Landewé-Cleuren SA, Kars M, Vrijhoef HJ, Schaper NC. Effective pharmacological treatment of painful diabetic neuropathy by nurse practitioners: results of an algorithm-based experience. Pain Med 2012; 13:1324–1333.

Gore M, Brandenburg NA, Dukes E, et al. Pain severity in diabetic peripheral neuropathy is associated with patient functioning, symptom levels of anxiety and depression, and sleep. J Pain Symptom Manage 2005; 30:374–385.

Gore M, Brandenburg NA, Hoffman DL, Tai KS, Stacey B. Burden of illness in painful diabetic peripheral neuropathy: the patients' perspectives. J Pain 2006; 7:892–900.

Greenman RL, Panasyuk S, Wang X, et al. Early changes in the skin microcirculation and muscle metabolism of the diabetic foot. Lancet 2005; 366:1711–1717.

Guldemond NA, Leffers P, Sanders AP, et al. Daily-life activities and in-shoe forefoot plantar pressure in patients with diabetes. Diabetes Res Clin Pract 2007; 77:203–209.

Ijzerman TH, Schaper NC, Melai T, et al. Lower extremity muscle strength is reduced in people with type 2 diabetes, with and without polyneuropathy, and is associated with impaired mobility and reduced quality of life. Diabetes Res Clin Pract 2012; 95:345–351.

Jensen TS, Backonja MM, Hernández Jiménez S, et al. New perspectives on the management diabetic peripheral neuropathic pain. Diab Vasc Dis Res 2006; 3:108–119.

Kanade RV, Van Deursen RW, Harding KG, Price PE. Investigation of standing balance in patients with diabetic neuropathy at different stages of foot complications. Clin Biomech 2008; 23:1183–1191.

Katoulis EC, Ebdon-Parry M, Hollis S, et al. Postural instability in diabetic neuropathic patients at risk of foot ulceration. Diabetic Med 1997; 14:296–300.

Kumar S, Ashe HA, Parnell LN, et al. The prevalence of foot ulceration and its correlates in type 2 diabetic patients: a population-based study. Diabet Med 1994; 5:480–484.

Lavery LA, Armstrong DG, Wunderlich RP, Tredwell J, Boulton AJ. Predictive value of foot pressure assessment as part of a population-based diabetes disease management program. Diabetes Care 2003; 26:1069–1073.

Lefrandt JD, Bosma E, Oomen PH, et al. Sympathetic mediated vasomotion and skin capillary permeability in diabetic patients with peripheral neuropathy. Diabetologia 2003; 46:40–47.

LeMaster JW, Mueller MJ, Reiber GE, et al. Effect of weight-bearing activity on foot ulcer incidence in people with diabetic peripheral neuropathy: feet first randomized controlled trial. Phys Ther 2008; 88:1385–1398.

Maser RE, Mitchell BD, Vinik AI, Freeman R. The association between cardiovascular autonomic neuropathy and mortality in individuals with diabetes: a meta-analysis. Diabetes Care 2003; 26:1895–1901.

Melai T, Schaper NC, Ijzerman TH, et al. Lower leg muscle strengthening does not redistribute plantar load in diabetic polyneuropathy: a randomised controlled trial. J Foot Ankle Res 2013; 6:41.

Meyer C, Milat F, McGrath BP, et al. Vascular dysfunction and autonomic neuropathy in Type 2 diabetes. Diabet Med 2004; 21:746–751.

Monteiro-Soares M, Boyko EJ, Ribeiro J, Ribeiro I, Dinis-Ribeiro M. Predictive factors for diabetic foot ulceration: a systematic review. Diabetes Metab Res Rev 2012; 28:574–600.

Morrison S, Colberg SR, Mariano M, Parson HK, Vinik AI. Balance training reduces falls risk in older individuals with type 2 diabetes. Diabetes Care 2010; 33:748–750.

Mueller MJ, Tuttle LJ, Lemaster JW, et al. Weight-bearing versus nonweight-bearing exercise for persons with diabetes and peripheral neuropathy: a randomized controlled trial. Arch Phys Med Rehabil 2013; 94:829–838.

Nabuurs-Franssen MH, Huijberts MS, Nieuwenhuijzen Kruseman AC, Willems J, Schaper NC. Health-related-quality-of-life of diabetic foot ulcer patients and their caregivers. Diabetologia 2005; 48:1906–1910.

Nabuurs-Franssen MH, Houben AJ, Tooke JE, Schaper NC. The effect of polyneuropathy on foot microcirculation in Type II diabetes. Diabetologia 2002; 45:1164–1171.

Nabuurs-Franssen MH, Sleegers R, Huijberts MS, et al. Total contact casting of the diabetic foot in daily practice: a prospective follow-up study. Diabetes Care 2005; 28:243–247.

Pambianco G, Costacou T, Strotmeyer E, Orchard TJ. The assessment of clinical distal symmetric polyneuropathy in type 1 diabetes: a comparison of methodologies from the Pittsburgh Epidemiology of Diabetes Complications Cohort. Diabetes Res Clin Pract 2011; 92:280–287. 15

Pataky Z, Assal JP, Conne P, Vuagnat H, Golay A. Plantar pressure distribution in Type 2 diabetic patients without peripheral neuropathy and peripheral vascular disease. Diabet Med 2005; 22:762–767.

Prompers L, Huijberts M, Apelqvist J, et al. High prevalence of ischaemia, infection and serious comorbidity in patients with diabetic foot disease in Europe. Baseline results from the Eurodiale study. Diabetologia 2007; 50:18–25.

Purewal TS, Goss DE, Watkins PJ, Edmonds ME. Lower limb venous pressure in diabetic neuropathy. Diabetes Care 1995; 18:377–381.

Richardson JK, Thies SB, Demott TK, Ashton-Miller JA. Gait analysis in a challenging environment differentiates between fallers and nonfallers among older patients with peripheral neuropathy. Arch Phys Med Rehabil 2005; 86:1539–1544.

Richardson JK. Factors associated with falls in older patients with diffuse polyneuropathy. J Am Geriatr Soc 2002; 50:1767–1773.

Rowbotham MC, Goli V, Kunz NR, Lei D. Venlafaxine extended release in the treatment of painful diabetic neuropathy: a double-blind, placebo-controlled study. Pain 2004; 110:697–706.

Savelberg HH, Schaper NC, Willems PJ, de Lange TL, Meijer K. Redistribution of joint moments is associated with changed plantar pressure in diabetic polyneuropathy. BMC Musculoskelet Disord 2009; 10:16.

Schaper NC, Havekes B. Diabetes: impaired damage control. Diabetologia 2012; 55:18–20.

Schaper NC, Huijberts M, Pickwell K. Neurovascular control and neurogenic inflammation in diabetes. Diabetes Metab Res Rev 2008; 24:S40—S44.

Selvarajah D, Wilkinson ID, Emery CJ, et al. Thalamic neuronal dysfunction and chronic sensorimotor distal symmetrical polyneuropathy in patients with type 1 diabetes mellitus. Diabetologia 2008; 51:2088–2092.

Selvarajah D, Wilkinson ID, Gandhi R, Griffiths PD, Tesfaye S. Microvascular perfusion abnormalities of the Thalamus in painful but not painless diabetic polyneuropathy: a clue to the pathogenesis of pain in type 1 diabetes. Diabetes Care 2011; 34:718–720.

Shepherd AJ, Downing JE, Miyan JA. Without nerves, immunology remains incomplete -in vivo veritas. Immunology 2005; 116:145–163.

Siersma V, Thorsen H, Holstein PE, et al. Importance of factors determining the low health-related quality of life in people presenting with a diabetic foot ulcer: the Eurodiale study. Diabet Med 2013; 30:1382–1387.

Steinhoff M, Sander S, Seeliger S, et al. Modern aspects of cutaneous neurogenic inflammation. Arch Dermatol 2003; 139:1479–1488.

Sutton-Tyrrell K, Najjar SS, Boudreau RM, et al.; Health ABC Study. Elevated aortic pulse wave velocity, a marker of arterial stiffness, predicts cardiovascular events in well-functioning older adults. Circulation 2005; 111:3384–3390.

Suzuki E, Kashiwagi A, Hidaka H, et al. 1H- and 31P-magnetic resonance spectroscopy and imaging as a new diagnostic tool to evaluate neuropathic foot ulcers in Type II diabetic patients. Diabetologia 2000; 43:165–172.

Tesfaye S, Boulton AJ, Dickenson AH. Mechanisms and management of diabetic painful distal symmetrical polyneuropathy. Diabetes Care 2013; 36:2456–2465.

Tesfaye S, Boulton AJM, Dyck PJ, et al.; Toronto Diabetic Neuropathy Expert Group. Diabetic neuropathies: update on definitions, diagnostic criteria, estimation of severity, and treatments. Diabetes Care 2010; 33:2285–2293.

Tesfaye S, Chaturvedi N, Eaton SEM, et al.; EURODIAB Prospective Complications Study Group. Vascular risk factors and diabetic neuropathy. N Engl J Med 2005; 352:341–350.

Tesfaye S, Vileikyte L, Rayman G, et al.; Toronto Expert Panel on Diabetic Neuropathy. Painful diabetic peripheral neuropathy: consensus recommendations on diagnosis, assessment and management. Diabetes Metab Res Rev 2011; 27:629–638.

Uccioli L, Giacomini PG, Pasqualetti P, et al. Contribution of central neuropathy to postural instability in IDDM patients with peripheral neuropathy. Diabetes Care 1997; 20:929–934.

van Deursen RW, Sanchez MM, Ulbrecht JS, Cavanagh PR. The role of muscle spindles in ankle movement perception in human subjects with diabetic neuropathy. Exp Brain Res 1998; 120:1–8.

van Schie CH. Neuropathy: mobility and quality of life. Diabetes Metab Res Rev 2008; 24:S45–51.

van Schie CHM, Simoneau GG, Ulbrecht JS, Derr JA, et al. Postural instability in patients with diabetic sensory neuropathy. Diabetes Care 1994; 17:1411–1421.

van Sloten TT, Savelberg HH, Duimel-Peeters IG, et al. Peripheral neuropathy, decreased muscle strength and obesity are strongly associated with walking in persons with type 2 diabetes without manifest mobility limitations. Diabetes Res Clin Pract 2011; 91:32–39.

Veves A, Murray HJ, Young MJ, Boulton AJ. The risk of foot ulceration in diabetic patients with high foot pressure: a prospective study. Diabetologia 1992; 35:660–663.

Vileikyte L, Peyrot M, Gonzalez JS, et al. Predictors of depressive symptoms in persons with diabetic peripheral neuropathy: a longitudinal study. Diabetologia 2009; 52:1265–1273.

Volpato S, Blaum C, Resnick H, et al.; Women's Health and Aging Study. Comorbidities and impairments explaining the association between diabetes and lower extremity disability: The Women's Health and Aging Study. Diabetes Care 2002; 5:678–683.

Wallace C, Reiber GE, LeMaster J, et al. Incidence of falls, risk factors for falls, and fall-related fractures in individuals with diabetes and a prior foot ulcer. Diabetes Care 2002; 25:1983–1986.

Williams DT, Harding KG, Price P. An evaluation of the efficacy of methods used in screening for lower-limb arterial disease in diabetes. Diabetes Care 2005; 28:2206–2210.

Willum-Hansen T, Staessen JA, Torp-Pedersen C, et al. Prognostic value of aortic pulse wave velocity as index of arterial stiffness in the general population. Circulation 2006; 113:664–670.

Wukich DK, McMillen RL, Lowery NJ, Frykberg RG. Surgical site infections after foot and ankle surgery: a comparison of patients with and without diabetes. Diabetes Care 2011; 34:2211–2213.

Yokoyama H, Yokota Y, Tada J, Kanno S. Diabetic neuropathy is closely associated with arterial stiffening and thickness in Type 2 diabetes. Diabet Med 2007; 24:1329–1335.

Zelman DC, Brandenburg NA, Gore M. Sleep impairment in patients with painful diabetic peripheral neuropathy. Clin J Pain 2006; 22:681–685.

Zelman DC, Gore M, Dukes E, Tai KS, Brandenburg N. Validation of a modified version of the brief pain inventory for painful diabetic peripheral neuropathy. J Pain Symptom Manage 2005; 29:401–410.

Ziegler D, Nowak H, Kempler P, Vargha P, Low PA. Treatment of symptomatic diabetic polyneuropathy with the antioxidant alpha-lipoic acid: a meta-analysis. Diabet Med 2004; 21:114–121.

Ziegler D. Current concepts in the management of diabetic polyneuropathy. Curr Diabetes Rev 2011; 7:208–220.

Zimny S, Schatz H, Pfohl M. The role of limited joint mobility in diabetic patients with an at-risk foot. Diabetes Care 2004; 27:942–946.

Chapter 22

Surgical treatment of diabetic neuropathy

A. Lee Dellon

SUMMARY

- Patients with diabetes can have chronic nerve compressions in the upper and lower extremity, and these compressions can give symptoms in a stocking and glove distribution if more than one nerve is involved

- Surgical approaches to decompress the peroneal nerve at the knee, in the leg and at the dorsum of the foot, and to decompress the tibial nerve in the four medial ankle tunnels have been developed

- These surgical procedures can be undertaken safely in the patient with diabetes as long as there is adequate circulation to the foot and the surgeon has been trained appropriately

- Chronic nerve compression in the presence of a metabolic neuropathy such as diabetes is difficult to diagnose with traditional electrodiagnostic techniques

- The physical examination must include an evaluation of the Tinel's sign at known sites of anatomic narrowing in the lower extremity to identify chronic nerve compressions

- Decompression of nerves in the patient with neuropathy may result in an economic cost–benefit improvement by prevention of neuropathy-related morbidities

INTRODUCTION

The medical management of the patient with diabetic peripheral neuropathy (DPN) is now standardized based on the research of the past four decades. For the purposes of this chapter, DPN is defined as a diffuse, symmetrical, distal polyneuropathy. For the majority of patients with DPN, there is no pain component, and the bulwark of treatment is to provide a euglycemic state, with a HbA1c in the range of <7.0%. When one reviews the extensive experience of Peter J. Dyck from 1968 (Dyck 1968) through 2005 (Sinnreich et al. 2005), it is clear that there really has been little if any change in the basic concepts of the pathophysiology of DPN. While traditional neurology reviews suggest the prevalence of painful DPN is 10%, the most recent estimate is 50% (Argoff et al. 2006). For this important subgroup, there is the established pain management approach using medications such as tricyclic antidepressants, serotonin uptake inhibitors, and finally opioids (Argoff et al. 2006, Bril et al. 2011). This is a costly approach that often leaves cognitive function impaired, the patient drug dependent and impoverished.

Despite many successful basic science models and phase I/II clinical trials, a 2005 review by the world's most respected diabetologists, led by Andrew Boulton of Manchester, England, has demonstrated that the randomized clinical trial approach has failed to identify the pharmacologic agent to reverse or prevent DPN (Boulton et al. 2005). Drug types reviewed included aldose reductase inhibitors, myoinositol, alpha lipoic acid, vasodilators, protein kinase C inhibitors, C-peptide, nerve growth factors (nerve growth factor, brain derived growth factor), acetyl-1-carnitine, gamma-linolenic acid, and others. Indeed,

Dr Boulton wrote in 2005 about DPN: 'to date no treatment that prevents or reverses its development and progression has been identified' (Rather & Boulton 2005).

CAN MEDICAL MANAGEMENT PREVENT NEUROPATHY?

Two critically important outcome studies demonstrate that regardless of achieving the best possible medical management of the underlying diabetes, symptomatic neuropathy will occur anyway in a significant percentage of patients with diabetes. In one case-control study with an 8-year follow-up, 300 patients with diabetes were included, 100 of whom had neuropathy, defined as a vibratory perception threshold (VPT) >25 volts (Coppini et al. 2006). At the onset of the study, the HbA1c was 9.1% in the neuropathy group and 8.6% in the patients without neuropathy. Despite modest improvements in glycemic control (HbA1c – 0.5% in the neuropathy and – 0.2% in the control group), the VPT increased over time in patients with neuropathy, with no change in control patients, demonstrating that diabetic neuropathy can be progressive and irreversible in many patients.

Eight years after the completion of the Diabetes Comprehensive Control Trial (DCCT), neuropathy was present in 17.8% of those patients with type 1 diabetes who had been on strict glycemic control ($n = 633$), and in 28% of the usual control group ($n = 624$) (Martin et al. 2006). The prevalence of neuropathy was based on a physical examination. This significant difference demonstrates that tight glycemic control reduces, but does not prevent neuropathy. Importantly, there were ulcerations in both groups of patients (4 vs. 11) and amputations in both groups (2 vs. 5). While this knowledge is sobering, and perhaps discouraging, it should serve as the stepping off point to ask if there is no another approach to prevent and treat the consequences of DPN then purely attempt to control blood glucose levels and mask the neuropathy symptoms with mind-altering polypharmacopia.

A PROACTIVE SURGICAL APPROACH TO SYMPTOMATIC DPN

The classic involvement of the surgeon in DPN is to debride wounds, drain infection, and amputate necrotic tissues (Rather & Boulton 2005). This comprises the majority of the literature of the surgical management of DPN. However, beginning in 1988, a theoretical editorial suggested that there was some cause for 'optimism' for diabetic neuropathy if peripheral nerve entrapments could be identified in the patient with diabetes (Dellon 1988). Since the first clinical series of patients with DPN and chronic nerve compressions in the lower extremity was reported in 1992 (Dellon 1992), there has been a continuing increase in peer-reviewed scientific publications, mostly level IV retrospective surgical series, confirming those initial clinical observations (**Table 22.1**). These studies consistently demonstrate that, when

Table 22.1 Dellon triple nerve decompression in subjects with diabetes

Study	Number of nerves	Preoperative		Results: improved		New or recurrent ulceration/ amputation
		Ulcers	Amputation	Pain	Touch	
Dellon, 1992	31	0	0	85%	72%	0%
Wieman, 1995	33	13	0	92%	72%	7%
Chaffe, 2000	58	11	6	86%	50%	0%
Aszmann, 2000	16	0	0	na	69%	0%
Wood, 2003	33	0	0	90%	67%	0%
Lee, 2004	46	0	0	92%	92%	na
Yong, 2005	90	0	0	94%	90%	0%
Rader, 2005	49	0	0	90%	75%	0%
Siemionow, 2006	36	0	0	90%	90%	0%
Yuksel, 2006	22	0	0	89%	85%	0%
Zhang, 2012	513	260	0	85%	80%	5%
Valdivia, 2013	208	0	0	88%	83%	0%

the medical approach fails to relieve the symptoms of DPN and superimposed chronic nerve compressions are present, then decompression of those nerve compressions can relieve pain and restore sensation in up to 80% of these patients (Wieman & Patel 1995, Chafee 2000, Aszmann et al. 2000, Wood & Wood 2003, Lee & Dellon 2004, Yao & Wang 2005, Rader 2005, Siemionow et al. 2006, Karagoz et al. 2008, Zhang et al. 2014, Valdivia et al. 2013). If sensation can be even partially restored, foot ulcers, amputations, hospitalization for foot infection, and falls due to loss of balance, resulting in hip and wrist fractures, can be prevented. The rest of this chapter reviews the evidence that demonstrates that by identifying and surgically releasing compressed lower-extremity peripheral nerves, the natural history of diabetic neuropathy can be reversed, and its associated morbidity can be greatly reduced.

Why is the subject of lower-extremity nerve decompression in subjects with diabetes and symptomatic neuropathy so controversial? The controversy begins with the classic teaching in medical schools that diabetic neuropathy is progressive and irreversible. Furthermore, diabetic neuropathy occurs in a stocking and glove distribution, consistent with a systemic metabolic disease. These concepts lead to the immediate conclusion that there should be no role for surgery in this debilitating condition. In patients with diabetes referred for the treatment of their carpal tunnel syndrome, the similarity of the symptoms of chronic nerve compression and those of diabetic neuropathy were very close, and identical in many patients. When the thumb, index, and middle finger felt 'normal' after carpal tunnel decompression in the patient with diabetes, but the little and ring fingers still felt numb, tingling, burning, or cold, it seemed reasonable to consider that these symptoms might represent cubital tunnel syndrome. If a positive Tinel's sign could be identified over the ulnar nerve in the postcondylar groove, then it was possible that there was nerve compression at this location. Although traditional ulnar nerve transposition has varied success depending on the degree of nerve compression, an approach to submuscular transposition of the ulnar nerve was developed that included a lengthening of the flexor/pronator muscle mass (Dellon 1991). This approach was found to give excellent relief of symptoms despite advanced degrees of nerve compression and relief of these symptoms was also found in the patient with diabetes, with restoration of strength to the hand. The patients would still have

numbness and burning over the dorsal radial aspect of their hand, which was presumed to be due, still, to their diabetic neuropathy. In 1986, compression of the radial sensory nerve in the forearm was described (Dellon & Mackinnon 1986). Thereafter, decompression of this nerve was added to my approach to the patient with diabetes and with painful upper-extremity complaints. At this point, it could be considered that three different sites of nerve compression in the arm suggested that decompression of these three peripheral nerves resulted in relief of pain symptoms that were in a glove distribution.

Patients with diabetes who found relief of upper-extremity nerve symptoms after nerve decompression might, therefore, also benefit from a similar approach in the lower limb, because the nerves should, in theory, behave the same way in the lower extremity as they do in the upper extremity. Anatomical investigation then identified the sites of compression for the nerves of the lower extremity. While compression of the common peroneal nerve at the fibular head had been described as early as 1897, decompression of this nerve is still not commonly reported. The author's research has demonstrated a fibrous band deep to the peroneus muscles that must be released to achieve nerve decompression in these patients (Dellon et al. 2002). In general, decompression of the tarsal tunnel for compression of the posterior tibial is not commonly done because it has not been reported to give excellent results. However, our work identified four separate tunnels that needed to be decompressed, not just one, in order to achieve relief of symptoms in the medial ankle (Mackinnon & Dellon 1987) (**Figure 22.1**). The relationships between the tunnels at the wrist and ankle are described in **Table 22.2**. Furthermore, our work identified a new site of distal compression of the deep peroneal nerve over the dorsum of the foot (Dellon 1990). The implication of these observations is that decompression of multiple peripheral nerves in the lower extremity can restore sensation in a stocking distribution. Technical details of these procedures were published for the upper and the lower extremities in 1989 (Mackinnon & Dellon 1988).

■ The nerve in diabetes is susceptible to compression

There is ample evidence in the medical and surgical literature that patients with diabetes have a relative high incidence of chronic nerve

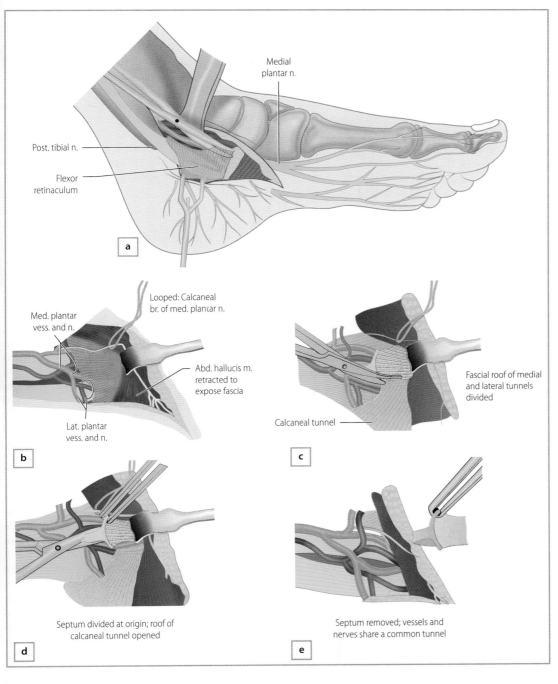

Medial plantar n.

Post. tibial n.

Flexor retinaculum

a

Med. plantar vess. and n.

Looped: Calcaneal br. of med. plantar n.

Abd. hallucis m. retracted to expose fascia

Lat. plantar vess. and n.

b

Fascial roof of medial and lateral tunnels divided

Calcaneal tunnel

c

Septum divided at origin; roof of calcaneal tunnel opened

d

Septum removed; vessels and nerves share a common tunnel

e

Figure 22.1 The medial ankle tunnels are depicted in this drawing. (a) The tarsal tunnel is illustrated with its flexor retinaculum. This is not the site of pressure causing symptoms but is necessary to open in order to identify the anatomy and its variations. (b) The abductor hallucis muscle is retracted, and the frequently present branch from the medial plantar nerve to the medial calcaneal region is identified and preserved. The roof of the medial and lateral plantar tunnels is identified. (c) The roof of the medial plantar tunnel has been incised. The roof of the lateral plantar tunnel is being incised. (d) The calcaneal tunnel has been incised, and the septum between these two tunnels is being incised longitudinally. (e) The septum is removed, completing Dellon's technique for the tarsal tunnel syndrome (http://www.dellon.com/free-booklets.html).

compressions. This has been reported to be as high as 33% by some authors, with the most common nerve compressions in the upper extremity being the median nerve at the wrist, the ulnar nerve at the elbow, and the radial sensory nerve in the forearm. In the lower extremity, the most common nerve compression is the tibial nerve in the tarsal tunnel, the common peroneal nerve at the fibular head (Vinik et al. 2004). Traditional electrodiagnostic studies cannot easily identify these entrapments in the presence of an underlying metabolic neuropathy, and therefore the physical examination is essential in identifying these compressions (Perkins et al. 2002). The presence of a positive Tinel's sign over the tibial nerve in the tarsal tunnel, e.g. had

Table 22.2 Homologies between the carpal and tarsal tunnels and sites for nerve compression (and decompression)

Ankle	Wrist
Tarsal tunnel	Distal forearm
Medial plantar tunnel	Carpal tunnel
Lateral plantar tunnel	Guyon's canal
Calcaneal tunnel	Tunnel for the palmar cutaneous branch of median nerve
Inter-tunnel septum	Hook process of hamate

a 92% positive predictive value in identifying patients with neuropathy who will have a good to excellent result from nerve decompression in the lower extremity (Lee & Dellon 2004). A prospective multicenter study confirmed these observations. For example, of 465 patients with a positive Tinel's sign over the tibial nerve in the tarsal tunnel, who then had the Dellon Triple Release Procedure in which the four medial ankle tunnels were decompressed (**Figure 22.1**), 80% had their visual analog scale score for pain drop from 8.5 to 2.0 at 6 months, and this reduced pain level remained during the 3.5-year follow-up (Dellon et al. 2012).

There are two metabolic changes in the peripheral nerves of the patient with diabetes that render the nerve susceptible to chronic compression. The most critical is the increased water content within the nerve as the result of glucose being metabolized into sorbitol (Jakobsen 1978). This increased water content causes the nerve to have an increased volume. A clinical example of the swollen, yellow tibial nerve in the patient with diabetes is seen in **Figure 22.2b**. The peripheral nerve, as it crosses a known areas of anatomic narrowing, like the carpal tunnel at the wrist, the cubital tunnel at the elbow, fibular tunnel at the outside of the knee, or the tarsal tunnel at the ankle, passes through a region of increased external pressure. Due to the increased volume, there is an increased pressure on the nerve in each of these anatomic regions in a subject with diabetes. This increased external pressure creates an increased intraneural pressure that decreases blood flow (Rydevik et al. 1981), resulting in a relative ischemia of the peripheral nerve. The neurophysiologic consequence of the decreased blood flow is the perception of paresthesias, interpreted centrally as numbness and tingling. The second metabolic change is a decrease in the slow anterograde component of axoplasmic flow that transports the lipoproteins necessary to maintain and rebuild the nerve (Jakobsen & Sidenius 1980). Due to this decreased axoplasmic flow, as in the patient with diabetes, the nerve cannot transport sufficient protein structures to rebuild itself, as has been demonstrated in a model of chronic compression in the diabetic rat (Dellon et al. 1994). It is this demyelination that is the neurophysiologic basis of the positive Tinel's sign used to localize the site of chronic nerve compression in the patient with diabetes and neuropathy.

■ Additional critical studies related to neurolysis

A retrospective study was undertaken on 50 patients with DPN who had one leg operated utilizing the Dellon Triple Release Procedure, while the other leg was not decompressed for various reasons (e.g. health condition, travel distance). After a mean of 4.5 years (range 2–7), patients were sent a questionnaire or were contacted by telephone. All patients reported that they had no new ulcerations or amputations in the extremity that had decompression, while in 15 patients, 3 amputations were performed and 12 new ulcerations had developed in the contralateral extremity (Aszmann et al. 2004). If a patient with diabetes has had successful release of the carpal tunnel to treat symptoms of nerve compression in the hand, then there was an 88% positive predictive value that decompression of nerve entrapments in the lower extremity will also result in good to excellent relief of pain and restoration of sensation to the foot in that patient (Maloney et al. 2006).

In a study presented during the Endocrinology Society's 94th annual meeting, the prevalence of a positive Tinel's sign was determined in a consecutive series of 81 patients with diabetes in an urban community-based endocrinology practice. The prevalence increased in direct proportion to the degree on neuropathy (as measured by the Michigan Neuropathy Symptom Instrument). In the patient with neuropathy, the percentage of patients with a positive Tinel's sign was at the common peroneal nerve at the fibular neck 59%, and at the tibial nerve in the tarsal tunnel 60% (Hashemi, S, Cheikh, I, Dellon, AL, unpublished observations 2012).

Finally, during a prospective, observational multicenter (38 different surgeons) study, 628 patients had a follow-up of 3.5 years (Dellon et al. 2012). The contralateral limb had a Dellon Triple Release procedure in 211 patients, and all had a positive Tinel's sign over the tibial nerve in the tarsal tunnel. During follow-up, new ulceration developed in 0.3%, the percentage of patients admitted to the hospital for foot infections was 0.6%, and amputation was performed in just 0.2%.

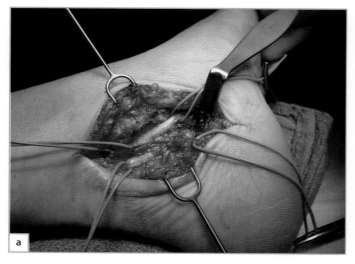 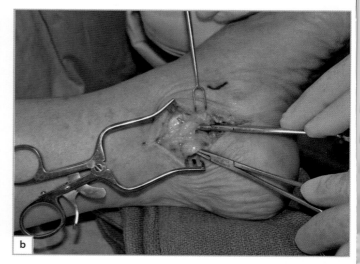

Figure 22.2 Comparison of color and size of nerves in (a) a patient without diabetes and with tarsal tunnel syndrome, and in (b) a patient with type 2 diabetes and neuropathy and tarsal tunnel syndrome. Note that in each patient, there is a high division of the tibial nerve above the ankle into the medial and lateral plantar nerves, so that each nerve may be seen over its course through the tarsal tunnel. Note that the diabetic nerve is larger in diameter and more yellow in color.

AREAS OF CONTROVERSY AND/OR FUTURE RESEARCH

- Level I studies of nerve decompression in patients with diabetes and neuropathy and superimposed nerve compressions versus control group, which could be best possible medical control in a matched population of patient with diabetes, or using the contralateral limb without surgery
- Evaluation of whether an 'inching technique' used by neurologists could identify nerve compressions in the lower extremity in the patient who also has neuropathy

IMPORTANT FURTHER READING

Dellon AL. Treatment of symptomatic diabetic neuropathy by surgical decompression of multiple peripheral nerves. Plast Reconstr Surg 1992; 89:689–697.

Dellon ES, Dellon AL, Seiler WA IV. The effect of tarsal tunnel decompression in the streptozotocin-induced diabetic rat. Microsurg 1994; 15:265–268.

Dellon AL, Muse VL, Nickerson SA. Positive Tinel sign as a predictor of pain relief or sensory recovery after decompression of chronic tibial nerve compression in patients with diabetic neuropathy, J Reconstr Microsurg 2012; 28:235–240.

Dellon AL, Muse VL, Nickerson DS. Prevention of ulceration, amputation, and reduction of hospitalization: outcomes of a prospective multi-center trial of tibial neurolysis in patients with diabetic neuropathy. J Reconstr Microsurg 2012; 28:241–246.

REFERENCES

Argoff CE, Backonja M, Belgrade MJ, et al. Consensus guidelines: treatment planning and options. Mayo Clin Proc 2006; 81:S12–25.

Aszmann O, Tassler PL, Dellon AL. Changing the natural history of diabetic neuropathy: incidence of ulcer/amputation in the contralateral limb of patients with a unilateral nerve decompression procedure. Ann Plast Surg 2004; 53:517–522.

Aszmann OA, Kress KM, Dellon AL. Results of decompression of peripheral nerves in diabetics: a prospective, blinded study. Plast Reconstr Surg 2000; 106:816–822

Boulton AJM, Vinik AI, Arezzo JC, et al. Diabetic neuropathies: a statement by the American Diabetes Association. Diabetes Care 2005; 28:956–962.

Bril V, Franklin GM, Backonja M, et al. Evidence-based guideline: treatment of painful diabetic neuropathy. Neurology 2011; 76:1758–1765.

Chafee H. Decompression of peripheral nerves for diabetic neuropathy, Plast Reconstr Surg 2000; 106:813–815.

Coppini DV, Spruce MC, Thomas P, Masding MG. Established diabetic neuropathy seems irreversible despite improvements in metabolic and vascular risk markers: a retrospective, case-control study in a hospital patient cohort. Diabet Med 2006; 23:1016–1020.

Dellon AL, Ebmer J, Swier P. Anatomic variations related to decompression of the common peroneal nerve at the fibular head. Ann Plast Surg 2002; 48:30–34.

Dellon AL, Mackinnon SE. Radial sensory nerve entrapment in the forearm. J Hand Surg 1986; 11A:199–205.

Dellon AL, Muse VL, Nickerson DS. Prevention of ulceration, amputation, and reduction of hospitalization: outcomes of a prospective multi-center trial of tibial neurolysis in patients with diabetic neuropathy. J Reconstr Microsurg 2012; 28:241–246.

Dellon AL, Muse VL, Nickerson SA. Positive Tinel sign as a predictor of pain relief or sensory recovery after decompression of chronic tibial nerve compression in patients with diabetic neuropathy. J Reconstr Microsurg 2012; 28:235–240

Dellon AL. Techniques for successful management of ulnar nerve entrapment at the elbow. Neurosurg Clin N Am 1991; 2:57–73.

Dellon AL. A cause for optimism in diabetic neuropathy. Ann Plast Surg 1988; 20:103–105.

Dellon AL. Entrapment of the deep peroneal nerve on the dorsum of the foot. Foot Ankle 1990; 11:73–80.

Dellon AL. Treatment of symptomatic diabetic neuropathy by surgical decompression of multiple peripheral nerves. Plast Reconstr Surg 1992; 89:689–697.

Dellon ES, Dellon AL, Seiler WA IV. The effect of tarsal tunnel decompression in the streptozotocin-induced diabetic rat. Microsurg 1994; 15:265–268.

Dyck PJ. Peripheral neuropathy: changing concepts, differential diagnosis, and classification. Med Clin N Amer 1968; 52:895–890.

Jakobsen J, Sidenius P. Decreased axonal transport of structural proteins in Streptozotocin diabetic rats. J Clin Invest 1980; 66:292.

Jakobsen J. Peripheral nerves in early experimental diabetes: Expansion of the endoneurial space as a cause of increased water content. Diabetologia 1978; 14:113–118.

Karagoz H, Yuksel F, Ulkur E, Celikoz B. Early and late results of nerve decompression procedures in diabetic neuropathy: a series from Turkey. J Reconstr Microsurg 2008; 24:95–101.

Lee CH, Dellon AL. Prognostic ability of Tinel sign in determining outcome for decompression surgery in diabetic and nondiabetic neuropathy. Ann Plast Surg 2004; 53:523–527.

Mackinnon SE, Dellon AL. Homologies between the tarsal and carpal tunnels: Implications for treatment of the tarsal tunnel syndrome. Contemp Orthop 1987; 14:75–79.

Mackinnon SE, Dellon AL. Surgery of the peripheral nerve. New York: Thieme, 1988.

Maloney CT Jr, Dellon AL, Heller C Jr, Olson JR. Prognostic ability of a good outcome to carpal tunnel release for decompression surgery in the lower extremity. Clin Pod Med Surg N Am 2006; 23:559–568.

Martin CL, Albers J, Herman PC, et al. Neuropathy among the diabetes control and complications trial cohort 8 years after trial completion. Diabetes Care 2006; 29:340–344.

Perkins BA, Olaleye D, Bril V. Carpal tunnel syndrome in patients with diabetic polyneuropathy. Diabetes Care 2002; 25:565–569.

Rader AJ, Surgical decompression in lower-extremity diabetic peripheral neuropathy. J Am Podiatr Med Assoc 2005; 95:446–450.

Rather HM, Boulton AJM. Recent advances in the diagnosis and management of diabetic neuropathy. J Bone Joint Surg 2005; 87B:1605–1610.

Rydevik B, Lundborg G. Effects of graded compression on intraneural blood flow. J Hand Surg 1981; 6A:3–12.

Siemionow M, Alghoul M, Molski, M, Agaoglu G. Clinical outcome of nerve decompression in diabetic and non-diabetic peripheral neuropathy. Ann Plast Surg 2006; 57:385–390.

Sinnreich M, Taylor BV, Dyck PJ. Diabetic Neuropathies, classification, clinical features and pathophysiologic basis, Neurologist 2005; 11:63–79.

Valdivia JMV, Weinand M, Maloney CT Jr, Blount AL, Dellon AL. Surgical Treatment of superimposed, lower extremity, peripheral nerve entrapment with diabetic and idiopathic neuropathy. Ann Plastic Surg 2013; 60, in press.

Vinik, AI, Mehrabyan A, Colen L, Boulton A. Focal entrapment neuropathies in diabetes. Diabetes Care 2004; 27:1783–1788.

Wieman TJ, Patel VG. Treatment of hyperesthetic neuropathic pain in diabetics; decompression of the tarsal tunnel. Ann Surg 1995; 221:660–665.

Wood WA, Wood MA. Decompression of peripheral nerves for diabetic neuropathy in the lower extremity. J Foot Ankle Surg 2003; 42:268–275.

Yao Y, Wang R-Z. Peripheral Nerve Decompression (Dellon Procedure) and Diabetic Neuropathy. Chinese J Med 2005; 10:1756–1758.

Zhang W, Li S, Zheng X. Evaluation of the clinical efficacy of multiple lower extremity nerve decompression in diabetic peripheral neuropathy. J Neurol Surg A Cent Eur Neurosurg 2013; 74:96–100.

WOUNDS AND ULCERATION

Chapter 23

Acute and chronic wound healing biology in diabetes

Michelle Griffin, Ardeshir Bayat

SUMMARY

- Normal wound healing involves a timely order of events including coagulation, inflammation, matrix synthesis and deposition, angiogenesis, epithelialization, and remodeling
- When the normal phases of wound healing are disrupted, acute wounds fail to heal and become chronic wounds
- Diabetic foot ulcers (DFUs) are one type of chronic wound caused by the failure of normal wound healing, leading to a huge social and economic health-care burden in the United Kingdom
- The molecular mechanisms and signals responsible for the abnormal healing of DFU are currently being explored to identify potential therapeutic targets
- The inflammatory phase is prolonged in DFUs due to the alteration in production of growth factors and peptides leading to delayed wound healing
- Failure of bacterial clearance, maintenance of the extracellular matrix (ECM), and collagen production during the proliferative phase have all been shown to contribute to poor DFU healing
- Inadequate angiogenesis from disruption of hypoxia-regulating pathways and decreased production of angiogenic mediating growth factors has also been linked to the abnormal wound healing of DFUs. Biomechanical overloading has been shown to act as an inflammatory stimulus, leading to poor wound healing
- Production of glycation end products has been recognized to contribute to poor wound healing of DFUs due to disruption of intracellular pathways controlling hypoxia and angiogenesis and directly through damage to the ECM
- Through a greater understanding of the altered growth factors, modified molecular pathways, and disrupted cellular function in DFUs, emerging technology will be able to target specific molecules and cells to reduce morbidity and mortality of DFUs

INTRODUCTION

A wound is the loss of the epithelial integrity of the skin, causing a disruption of the anatomic structure and function of the normal tissue (Dubay et al. 2003). Wounds vary from minor lacerations to burns and major traumatic injuries (Dubay et al. 2003). Wound healing is a response initiated by the body that begins immediately after it sustains an injury; it is the body's survival mechanism to repair itself (Li et al. 2007). The tissues, which are damaged, are removed to allow tissue integration to restore homeostasis (Li et al. 2007). Each area of the body undergoes similar stages of wound healing; however, certain specialized tissues including the liver, eye, and skeletal tissue undergo specific healing mechanisms (Robson et al. 2001). Wound healing is a complex and highly orchestrated sequence of processes including coagulation, inflammation, matrix synthesis and deposition, angiogenesis, fibroplasia, epithelialization, contraction, and remodeling (Reinke et al. 2012). When wounds progress through these

stages in a timely manner, they will achieve wound healing (Reinke et al. 2012). However, when wounds are disrupted by local and systemic factors the normal wound healing process is altered that can cause certain wounds to become chronic (Li et al. 2007). Clinically, chronic wounds can be defined as wounds that have remained unhealed for >6 weeks, and can be further classified according to their pathology, e.g. pressure ulcer, venous leg ulcers, and DFUs.

In the United Kingdom, chronic wounds present a significant burden to patients and national health services. In a recent UK study, it was estimated that a wound affected 3.55 per 1000 population, with 49% being chronic wounds (Vowden et al. 2009). Chronic wounds may need hospitalization, extensive nursing time, and regular dressing changes, causing a huge social economic burden (Vowden et al. 2009). In addition, social interaction can be affected due to the odor and drainage seen in some chronic wounds, causing considerable physiological problems for patients (McGuckin & Kerstein 1998). The impact on the patient's self-esteem, the continued pain, and reliance on others significantly affects patient's activities of daily living and working status (McGuckin & Kerstein 1998).

A common complication of diabetes is foot ulceration. In the United Kingdom, it has been estimated that there are about 64,000 individuals with active foot ulceration at one time and 2600 amputations in patients with a foot ulcer (Gordois et al. 2003). Similarly to chronic wounds, DFUs will present significant economic and social burden for the patient and health services (Gordois et al. 2003). The progression of the acute wound to the chronic DFU has been shown to be multifactorial in etiology (Gordois et al. 2003). Local factors at the wound site including the oxygen supply and presence of infection as well as systemic patients factors have been shown to be implicated in transition of an acute wound to a chronic DFU (Loots et al. 1998, Woo et al. 2007). However, more recently specific molecular mechanisms and biochemical steps have been identified that alter the normal wound healing process, and could contribute to the delayed wound healing in DFUs (Loots et al. 1998, Woo et al 2007).

This chapter will first briefly review the processes involved in normal acute soft tissue wound healing repair. Second, the specific molecular signals and mechanisms that have been linked to the progression of acute wounds to chronic DFUs will be discussed. Lastly, the importance and relevance of recognizing molecular mechanisms implicated in chronic DFU for potential treatment targets will be reviewed.

THE NORMAL WOUND HEALING PROCESS

Wound healing is a dynamic and regulated process involving several cells types, multiple cell interactions, interrelated molecular signals, and biochemical process and restoration of the ECM. Wound healing is a continuum of processes that may overlap including hemostasis, inflammation, proliferation, remodeling, and scar maturation (see **Figure 23.1**) (Baum et al. 2005). The specific cellular processes

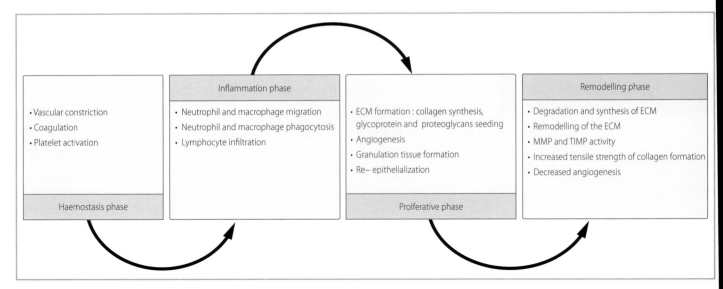

Figure 23.1 Stages of normal wound healing.

that occur in each of these stages are due to the release of molecular messengers in the form of growth factors and chemokines, which signal cell–cell and cell–matrix events to allow for wound repair (**Table 23.1**) (Baum et al. 2005).

Hemostasis

Within seconds of a wound, vessel vasoconstriction occurs to reduce blood loss and the coagulation cascade is initiated resulting in clot formation and platelet aggregation (Lawrence 1998). Vasoconstriction is initiated by the release of vasoactive amines from the damaged dermis and thromboxane from injured cells (Lawrence 1998). Platelet aggregation is stimulated by tissue factor, which is released from the damaged dermis cells (Lawrence 1998). The platelets are essential for hemostasis and to trigger the next stage of the wound healing process, the inflammatory response (Cohen et al. 1999). The platelets degranulate releasing several growth factors including platelet-derived growth factor (PDGF), insulin-like-growth factor 1 (IGF-1), epidermal growth factor (EGF), transforming growth factor beta (TGF-β), and platelet factor 4 (PF4) (Deuel et al. 1982). These growth factors cause the migration of several cell types including fibroblasts, endothelial cells (ECs), and macrophages, which initiate wound healing (Deuel et al. 1982). Furthermore, the kinin system, complement cascade, and clotting mechanism are amplified at this stage to ensure the healing process continues (Dahlback et al. 2000). The clot (containing fibronectin, von Willebrand factor, fibrin, vitronectin) is vital to support the incoming cells, providing a temporary matrix that itself is perpetuated by tissue factor (Dahlback et al. 2000, Lawrence 1998).

Inflammation

This stage is often divided into early and late phases.

EARLY PHASE OF INFLAMMATION (DAYS 1–2)

This stage is clinically characterized by edema, erythema, heat, and pain. Inflammation commences with the activation of the

body's complement cascade, leading to the migration and influx of inflammatory cells. Within the first 24–48 hours, polymorphonuclear neutrophils (granulocytes) are attracted to the wound site (Kloth et al. 1990). Several chemotactic signals enable these cells to arrive at the site including TGF-β, complement signals, ECM signals, and more importantly peptide products from bacteria (Newman et al. 1982). The neutrophils adhere to the EC via the intracellular adhesion molecules of the EC cell and integrins of the leukocytes, in a process called margination (Newman et al. 1982). The neutrophils then migrate though the endothelium in a process called diapedesis mediated by the PF4 and platelet-activating factor (Newman et al. 1982). The neutrophils start phagocytosing bacteria and foreign material by either releasing their degrading enzymes or free radicals derived from oxygen (Newman et al. 1982). Toll-like receptors (TLR), a group of highly conserved molecules, also sense molecules that are present in many classes of pathogens such as bacteria and viruses, but not the host in order to coordinate mechanisms against these pathogens (Kluwe et al. 2001). The recognition of pathogen-associated molecular patterns by TLRs provides a quick and efficient response to pathogens (Kluwe et al. 2001). Vasodilatation occurs in the inflammation stage, reversing the initial vasoconstriction in the hemostasis stage. In addition, gaps develop between ECs, allowing plasma to leak through into the extravascular compartments causing clinical edema (Glat et al. 1997, Lawrence 1998). Complement factors C3a and C5a, release of histamine, kinins, and prostaglandins are all responsible for the leakage of the capillaries (Glat et al. 1997).

LATE PHASE OF INFLAMMATION (DAYS 2–3)

Over the next couple of days, the neutrophils begin to disappear via apoptosis and the late phase of inflammation occurs (Glat et al. 1997, Kloth et al. 1990, Lawrence 1998). Monocyte cells, which have been slowly arriving at the wound bed since the start of the inflammatory phase, then continue the wound healing process. Several signals are responsible for attracting the monocyte to the site including ECM products such as collagen, tumor necrosis factor alpha (TNF-α),

Table 23.1 Growth factors and cytokines responsible for the molecular signals in the various stages of normal wound healing

Molecule	Major source	Action in acute wound healing
Growth factors		
FGF	Endothelial cells, smooth muscle cells, macrophages, fibroblasts	Proliferation of fibroblasts Extracellular matrix formation Angiogenesis Wound contraction (Dinh & Veves 2005, Mast & Schultz 1996, Pecoraro et al. 1991)
TNF-α	Neutrophils, macrophages	Proliferation, migration, adhesion, and differentiation of keratinocytes Re-epithelialization (Mast & Schultz 1996)
VEGF	Macrophages, platelets	Stimulate angiogenesis (Dinh & Veves 2005, Khoosal & Goldman 2006, Pecoraro et al. 1991)
EGF	Platelets, macrophages, keratinocytes	Proliferation, migration, adhesion, and differentiation of keratinocytes Re-epithelialization (Pecoraro et al. 1991)
TGF-β	Platelets, macrophages, fibroblasts, neutrophils, and keratinocytes	Stimulate angiogenesis and collagen synthesis Chemotaxis for macrophages Proliferation of fibroblasts (Gibran et al. 2002, Malik et al. 2013)
HGF	Fibroblasts, keratinocytes, endothelial cells	Re-epithelialization Neovascularization (Arnold & Barbul 2006, Pecoraro et al. 1991)
IGF-1	Fibroblasts	Collagen synthesis Fibroblast proliferation Re-epithelization (Baynes & Thorpe 2000, Beer et al. 1997, Bento & Pereira 2011)
PDGF	Fibroblasts, macrophages, endothelial cells, and platelets	Stimulate angiogenesis Chemotaxis of neutrophils, macrophages, and fibroblasts Fibroblast proliferation and collagen synthesis Re-epithelialization (Bauer et al. 1986)
KGF	Fibroblasts	Stimulate keratinocyte migration, differentiation, and proliferation Re-epithelialization (Guvakova 2007)
Interleukins		
IL-1β	Macrophages, neutrophils, macrophages, endothelial cells, smooth muscle cells Neutrophils, macrophages	Neutrophil chemotaxis Fibroblast proliferation (Pecoraro et al. 1991) Neutrophil chemotaxis Re-epithelialization (Arnold & Barbul 2006, Tonnesen et al. 2000)
IL-6 IL-8	Macrophages, neutrophils	Neutrophil chemotaxis Angiogenesis (Arnold & Barbul 2006, Tonnesen et al. 2000)

GF, endothelial growth factor; FGF, fibroblast growth factor; HGF, hepatocyte growth factor; IGF-1, insulin-like-growth factor 1; KGF, keratinocyte growth factor; PDGF, platelet-derived growth factor; TGF-b, transforming growth factor beta; TNF-α, tumor necrosis factor alpha; VEGF, vascular endothelial growth factor.

GF-β, PDGF, and PF4 (Wright et al. 1990). The monocytes undergo phenotype change into tissue macrophages as they are attracted to the wound by variety of molecular signals including serum factors, thrombin, fibronectin, complement molecules, and elastin (Fauci & Haynes 1994). The macrophages act with the remaining neutrophils to debride the wound by phagocytosing bacteria and foreign material.

Surface receptors allow the macrophage to recognize foreign particles (Wright et al. 1990), once bound the bacteria are digested and engulfed by oxygen radials and hydrolytic enzymes within the macrophage cell (Fauci & Haynes 1994). Other than debriding the wound, the macrophages are vital in providing signals via cytokines that mediate and permit the later stages of wound healing. TGF-β,

IGF-1, fibroblast growth factor 2 (FGF-2), and PDGF are all vital macrophage-derived cytokines allowing for a variety of processes to occur such as angiogenesis by ECs, collagen production by fibroblasts, wound contraction, smooth muscle cell proliferation (Fauci & Haynes 1994). The result of the inflammatory phase is a clean wound bed with the control of bleeding (Glat et al. 1997).

Proliferation (from day 3)

The proliferative phase is characterized by a large number of fibroblast cells migrating and arriving at the wound site, from day 3 of the acute tissue injury. The fibroblasts main role is to replace the fibrin provisional matrix from the inflammatory phase and replace it with a collagen-rich granulation tissue (Lawrence 1998). Granulation tissue is a highly vascular connective tissue, which is used to fill the wound site. In addition, the provisional fibrin–fibronectin matrix that was populated with inflammatory cells becomes replaced with endothelial and fibroblast cells (Lawrence 1998).

Fibroblast migration

Fibroplasia describes the process of fibroblast proliferation and migration into the wound site. Fibroblasts migrate from adjacent tissues approximately after day 2 (Fauci & Haynes 1994, Glat et al. 1997, Lawrence 1998). However, from day 4, as fibroblasts are the dominant cell in the wound bed, the number of fibroblasts increase due to the proliferation of the fibroblast cell within the wound bed itself. There are many molecular signals that stimulate fibroblast migration including growth factors such as PDGF, TGF-β, EGF, and IGF-1, which are secreted by fibroblasts, keratinocytes, and ECs (Gharaee-Kermani et al. 2001).

Formation of the extracellular matrix

Collagen, a triple alpha helix, is the most abundant protein in the body and a key component of the wound matrix (Nimmi et al. 1974). The collagen helix is made of a repeating tripeptide sequence of glycine-X-Y, where X is proline and Y is hydroxyproline (Nimmi et al. 1974). There are many different isoforms of collagen, being specific to different tissue types (Nimmi et al. 1974). Collagen synthesis requires hydroxylation of the lysine and proline residues (Nimmi et al. 1974). The normal dermis contains 80% of type I collagen and 20% type III collagen. In the acute wound healing setting, type III expression is greater, in the region of 30–40% (Ignotz & Massaugue 1986). The increase in type III collagen after initial injury is a consequence of the fibronectin secretion after the injury (Ignotz & Massaugue 1986). Normal collagen fibers are in a woven basket arrangement but after wound healing they are arranged parallel to wound stress lines (Ignotz & Massaugue 1986). Collagen synthesis begins 4–5 days after wound healing (Ignotz & Massaugue 1986). Fibroblasts are responsible for collagen synthesis and production of other ECM components including proteoglycans and glycoproteins during the wound healing process (Glat et al. 1997).

Angiogenesis

This process refers to new vessel formation from pre-existing vessels adjacent to the wound, which occurs from day 2 (Lawrence 1998). In response to injury, the ECs of the microvessels at the wound site initiate an angiogenic stepwise process (Dubay et al. 2003, Folkman et al. 1987, Lawrence 1998, Tonnesen et al. 2000). Due to release of cytokines, growth factors, vasoactive amines, and low oxygen tension, angiogenesis is initiated (Dubay et al. 2003, Monaco & Lawrence 2003). ECs start to sprout from intact capillaries at the wound edge (Dubay et al. 2003, Lawrence et al. 2003, Tonnesen et al. 2000). The sprouts then elongate through proliferation and migration toward the angiogenic stimulus. The ECs curve and begin to form a lumen as the ECs lengthen (Dubay et al. 2003, Lawrence et al. 2003, Tonnesen et al. 2000). Eventually an endothelial sprout comes into contact with another sprout and then interconnect to form a capillary tube (Dubay et al. 2003, Folkman et al. 1987, Lawrence et al. 2003, Tonnesen et al. 2000) The angiogenic process is regulated like other events of the healing process by cytokines and growth factors including FGF, PDGF, and vascular endothelial growth factor (VEGF) (Folkman et al. 1987). Low oxygen tension, which occurs in acute tissue injury, is a major inducer of this latter growth factor. It is also important that there is an organized ECM present to support the vascular growth by the ECs (Folkman et al. 1987). The newly formed vessels invade the newly formed ECM produced by the fibroblasts to form granulation tissue (Kloth et al. 1990). This connective tissue is pink and pale, full of proliferating fibroblasts with loops of capillaries (Kloth et al. 1990). Granulation tissue is an indicative sign of optimal healing. The density of the blood vessels decreases over time as the collagen increases in the tissue enabling scar formation (Kloth et al. 1990).

Re-epithelialization

This is the process by which the body restores its epidermis after injury to the epidermal layer (Lawrence 1998). Reconstruction of the injured epithelium is vital to provide a barrier function for the skin (Lawrence 1998). Within the first 24 hours after the initial injury, the epithelial cells start to make a layer of epithelial cells. Keratinocytes will begin to migrate from the edge of the wound to form an epithelial layer (Lawrence 1998). This process of epithelial migration is under control of various cytokines including TGF-α, EGF, and keratinocyte growth factor (KGF) (Lawrence 1998).

Wound contraction

It is desirable for the wound to contract during healing as less connective tissue is required to fill the wound, thus wound healing is shorter (Gabbianni et al. 1971). Wound contraction is taken place at 2 weeks after the initial wound injury (Gabbianni et al. 1971). It has been suggested that myofibroblasts that are modified fibroblasts generate contractile forces, which pull the wound edges together (Gabbianni et al. 1971, Hinz et al. 2007, Tomasek et al. 2002).

Remodeling and scar maturation (week 1- beyond)

During the last phase of wound healing, the interconnected process of collagen synthesis and breakdown continually remodels the newly formed ECM (Kloth et al. 1990). Collagen degradation is performed by matrix metalloproteinases (MMPs), which are secreted by fibroblasts, neutrophils, and macrophages at the wound site. Eventually, during the remodeling phase, the activity of the MMPs decreases while the activity of the tissue inhibitors of metalloproteinases (TIMPs) increases, preventing breakdown of the ECM (Brew et al. 2000). With time, there is a decrease in the blood flow to the wound by a halt in the growth of the capillaries and decrease in fibroblast activity. Over time, the granulation tissue forms avascular tissue with inactive fibroblasts, dense collagen, and ECM molecules, which lead to scar tissue formation (Kloth et al. 1990).

Inflammation phase: nitric oxide

The release of nitric oxide (NO) during the inflammatory phase has been influential in DFUs (Witte et al. 2002). NO is a free radical formed by the enzymatic combination of molecular oxygen and the amino acid L-arginine by the nitric oxide synthase (NOS) enzyme (Witte et al. 2002). Three isoforms of NOS exist in tissues that can produce NO including the constitutive enzyme system (cNOS) that are found in neuronal cells (nNOS) and endothelial cells (eNOS), and the third system is the inducible form (iNOS) formed during inflammatory processes produced by macrophages, neutrophils, and vascular smooth muscle (Witte et al. 2002). The molecule NO with its iNOS form is vital for normal wound healing and is produced at specific times during the normal healing cascade (Witte et al. 2002). NO is released by macrophages to achieve their antimicrobial activity (Witte et al. 2002). L-arginine is also used by arginase during normal wound healing (Witte et al. 2002). Therefore, when quantities of L-arginine are low due to increased arginase activity in a healing wound, NOS can generate biological toxic oxygen-free radicals such as superoxide (Witte et al. 2002). Such free radicals can then react with NO and form more potent radicals called peroxynitrite and peroxynitrous acids, which accumulate into toxic hydroxyl (OH^-) and nitrogen dioxide (NO_2) molecules (Witte et al. 2002). Such molecules can then cause destruction in the ECM and cell DNA, accumulating in delayed wound healing (Witte et al. 2002). Alternatively, L-arginine can be metabolized via the arginase pathway to form ornithine and urea. Ornithine is then converted to proline to form collagen, aiding the normal healing process. Elevated levels of NOS and arginase have been found in the diabetic ulcers compared with diabetic skin and normal skin (Witte et al. 2002). TGF-β1 has been found to regulate the production of iNOS by macrophages and epithelial cells, but the lack of this control in DFUs can lead to greater NOS in diabetic wounds (Witte et al. 2002).

Inflammatory and proliferative phase: alteration in cell prolife

The alteration in the cellular profile and function during the inflammatory phase could also be linked to the poor wound healing in diabetic ulcers. It has been showed that there is decrease in CD4+ T cells and increase in B lymphocytes (B cells) and macrophages in ulcer edges, which would disrupt the normal wound healing process (Loots et al. 1998). In addition, the direct bactericidal activity of the neutrophils in DFUs has been shown to be decreased (Wierusz-Wysocka et al. 1985). During the proliferative phase, the fibroblasts of patients with diabetes have shown to display altered characteristics including impaired migration and cytokine production, delayed response to growth factors all causing delay in wound healing (Loots et al. 1999).

Proliferative phase: formation of the extracellular matrix

The maintenance of the ECM during the proliferative phase is modified in diabetic ulcers. The normal balance of the MMPs and their inhibitors, TIMPs, is disrupted in diabetic ulcers. There is an increase in MMPs and lack of TIMPs in diabetic ulcers, resulting in the destruction in the ECM and growth factors required for normal wound healing (Lobman et al. 2002). The lack of TGF-β1 observed in DFUs has been linked to the lack of TIMPs control on MMPs from fibroblasts in DFUs (Lobman et al. 2002). The lack of TIMPs also causes decreased proliferation of keratinocytes and epithelial cells in DFUs. NO also has a role in stimulating the production of the collagen by fibroblasts during the proliferative phase that is downregulated in diabetic foot wounds (Baynes & Thorpe 2000). Furthermore, decreased production of aforementioned growth factors during the inflammatory phase such as IGF-1 and TGF-β1 by fibroblasts decreases collagen production during the proliferative phase (Blakytny et al. 2000, Galkowska et al 2006).

Inflammation and proliferation phase: mechanical damage and glycation

Biomechanical overloading of DFUS can act as a proinflammatory stimulus and contribute to the delay in wounds healing. Several studies have shown that effectively off-loading a DFU can lead to rapid healing rates (Armstrong et al. 2001, 2005, Piaggesi et al. 2003). For instance, in a prospective clinical trial of 63 patients with superficial noninfected, nonischemic diabetic plantar foot ulcers, total contact casts healed a higher proportion of wounds in a shorter amount of time than removable cast walkers and half-shoes (Armstrong et al. 2001).

High blood glucose is another factor in which the normal wound healing process can be affected in DFUs. The free glucose molecules in diabetic foot wounds attach to free amino acid groups, forming complex advanced glycation end products (AGEs) (Nishikawa et al. 2000). More than 20 AGEs have been identified in tissue proteins, and many have been found to be increased in diabetes and atherosclerosis (Nishikawa et al. 2000). Formation of AGE in intracellular tissues has been proposed to account for the altered metabolism, oxidative stress, and apoptosis in the microvasculature of patients with diabetes (Nishikawa et al. 2000). Sandu et al. illustrated that dietary AGE inhibited wound healing in diabetic mice (Sandu et al. 2005).

Extracellular AGE molecules alter normal wound healing in three ways in DFUs: (1) AGEs disrupt the normal cross-linking of ECM proteins, affecting its structure and physical properties; (2) AGEs affect the signaling molecules attached to the ECM, modifying cell–matrix interactions; and (3) AGEs stimulate the inflammatory response and oxidative stress (Amarnath et al. 2004, Stern et al. 2002). AGE molecules can also disrupt wound healing by altering intracellular signaling pathways responsible for wound healing. Tchaikovski et al. illustrated that AGEs caused the activation of VEGFR-1 related to signaling pathways and to desensitization of VEGFR-1 response in patients with diabetes mellitus (Tchaikovski et al. 2009). Furthermore, Bento et al. found that AGE prevented the hypoxia-inducible factor 1 (HIF-1) signaling pathway, which is responsible for combating hypoxia by regulating angiogenesis, metabolic reprogramming, and survival (Bento et al. 2011). There is some development in techniques to decrease the effects of AGEs including producing inhibitors of the proinflammatory AGE receptors called RAGE and using small molecules that break down pre-existing AGEs (Stern et al. 2002). A number of pharmaceutical companies are trying to develop low molecular weight inhibitors of RAGE and also a soluble form of RAGE (sRAGE). Among the AGE inhibitor to date, pyridoxamine is the most effective and least toxic against the vascular complications of diabetes in animal models (Amarnath et al. 2004). AGE breakers that cleave pre-existing AGEs in tissue protein are not so well understood; however, 3-phenacyl-4,5-dimethylthiazolium chloride was shown to be effective in a diabetic animal model (Vaitkevicius et al. 2001). High levels of glucose, in addition, cause direct wound healing effects (Ahmed et al. 2005). Proliferation of human fibroblasts, ECs, and keratinocytes is inhibited by high levels of glucose in wounds (Ahmed et al. 2005). Furthermore, the cells will produce high level of MMPs in the presence of a high level of glucose, causing direct ECM breakdown and preventing the formation of a collagen scaffold for cells to migrate and attach to (Ahmed et al. 2005).

Decreased angiogenesis

As explained previously, wound healing requires a good blood supply to allow oxygen to reach the cells to carry out wound healing processes. Blood vessel formation is disrupted in DFUs due to a variety of reasons. There are three main ways in which angiogenesis is compromised in DFUs. The initial hypoxic conditions of a normal acute wound induce expression of the transcription factor HIF-1α (Catrina et al. 2004). This normally attaches to the constitutively expressed HIF-1β to form the HIF complex (Catrina et al. 2004). The HIF complex then modulates the cell nucleus to stimulate production of angiogenic growth factors such as VEGF (Catrina et al. 2004). However, in DFUs hyperglycemia prevents the upregulation of HIF-1α and therefore the angiogenesis cascade is halted (Catrina et al. 2004). Impaired regulation of HIF-1α transcription factor has been shown to impair the wound healing in diabetic mice (Botusan et al. 2008). Second, the excessive amounts of NO seen in DFUs can be inhibitory to angiogenesis (Pipili-Synetos et al. 1994). Lastly, several of the normal growth factors that stimulate angiogenesis are decreased including TGF-β, FGF, and PDGF (Pierce et al. 1992). More recently, it has been observed that the lack of migration of bone marrow endothelial progenitor cells (EPC) in diabetic wounds could be influential in the diminished angiogenic response during DFU healing (Gallagher et al. 2007). Normal EPC mobilization to the wound healing site is stimulated by eNOS activation, a process, which is impaired in patients with diabetes (Gallagher et al. 2007). However, causing hyperoxia using hyperbaric oxygen therapy (HBOT) has shown to increase the EPC recruitment via eNOS activation in diabetic mice (Gallagher et al. 2007). The increased eNOS activation increases NO production, which stimulates EPC from the bone marrow (Gallagher et al. 2007). However, it has been shown that correct EPC recruitment to the injury site is only achieved by expression of stromal cell-derived factor 1 alpha (SDF-1α) by epithelial cells and myofibroblasts (Gallagher et al. 2007). Therefore, decreased expression of SDF-1α and eNOS activation are both involved in the reduced EPC mobilization in diabetic wounds, consequently causing decreased angiogenesis at the wound site (Gallagher et al 2007).

Re-epithelialization

This initial formation of an epithelial barrier is not completed at the correct time during diabetic ulcer formation, leaving an open wound. Growth factors, cytokines, and NPs that are responsible for normal keratinocyte proliferation and migration are compromised in DFUs including TGF-β1, IGF-1, PDGF, IL-5, IL-10, and SP (Galkowska et al. 2006, Guvakova 2007). TIMPs are normally responsible for epidermal cell migration but lose their ability in the presence of MMP molecules (Armstrong & Jude 2002). Therefore, due to the reduced level of TIMPs and high level of MMP in DFUs, epidermal cell migration is inhibited.

Vasculopathy

Another contributing factor to the progression of DFUs is vasculopathy. Patients with diabetes will have more macrovascular disease than people without diabetes and with more distal involvement including the pedal arch and metatarsal arteries that consequently can make the DFU wound site ischemic (Ferrier 1967, Dinh et al. 2005). Early studies have suggested that anatomical changes of the microcirculation may contribute to the impaired healing in DFUs (Dinh et al. 2005). These microcirculatory changes include the reduced size of the capillaries, increased capillary fragility, thickening of the basement membrane, and arteriolar hyalinosis (Dinh et al. 2005). These anatomical changes could lead to decreased cell migration, exchange of nutrients, and capacity of the capillaries to vasodilate (Dinh et al. 2005). Although these microvascular changes have the potential to interfere with the physiological processes during the normal wound healing, further clinical evidence is required to support these theories (Chakrabarti & Sima 1987, Dinh et al. 2005, Williamson et al. 1976). Endothelial dysfunction has been suggested to reduce endothelium-dependent vasodilatation in patients with diabetes, decreasing vasodilatation in periods of increased stress (Caballero et al. 1999, Dinh et al 2005). Although further understanding and clinical evidence are required, new pharmacological approaches are developed to reverse endothelial dysfunction (Sena et al. 2013).

Neuropathy

Another major contributing factor to diabetic ulceration is the prevalence of neuropathy among patients with diabetes. There are multiple proposed causes of diabetic neuropathy including metabolic insult to the nerve fibers, neurovascular insufficiency, autoimmune damage, and neurohormonal growth factor insufficiencies (Vinik et al. 1999). Motor, sensory, and autonomic fibers can all be affected. Sensory deficits cause the patient with diabetes to lose their protective mechanisms against pressure and heat. Loss of motor fiber capacity can cause physical stresses on the insensate foot, causing anatomical deformities, which allows the development of infection as bacterial growth is enhanced in areas of high force.

There are links between the vasculopathy and neuropathy in patients with diabetes that cause the progression of DFUs. For example, the normal vasodilatation response to stress from trauma and pressure is disrupted because of the impaired release of SP, calcitonin gene-related peptide, and histamine in the c-nociceptive nerve fibers and adjacent C-fibers (Veves et al. 1998). The production of SP has also been found to be important for the adhesion of ECs, chemotaxis of neutrophils and macrophages, and release of proinflammatory cytokines such as NO, histamine, and prostaglandins from macrophages. The inadequate response by the nerve fibers has also been postulated to be due to patients with diabetes having reduced cutaneous nerve terminals compared with nondiabetic controls, causing the inability to mount an appropriate wound healing response (Forst et al. 1998). This consequently leads to necrotic tissue and further risk of bacterial colonization (Forst et al. 1998). A recent study showed that addition of SP alone for a short time period can accelerate wound healing of excisional wounds in diabetic mice (Gibran et al. 2002).

MANAGEMENT STRATEGIES BASED ON MOLECULAR TARGETS

It is clear that the pathology of diabetic wounds is complex and still being investigated. However, gaining understanding into the molecular mechanisms involved in diabetic wounds has enabled technology to start target-specific molecules to alter the outcome of DFUs. Various treatments are already being used that target the molecular pathways thought to be causative of diabetic ulcers (**Table 23.2**). It is clear from this review that diabetes is based on sustained inflammation, with release of altered anti-inflammatory and proinflammatory mediators, resulting in imbalance in defense mechanisms. It has been shown that growth factors influence the normal wound healing process by binding to specific receptors in the plasma membranes of target cells activating signal transduction pathways, and therefore it has been proposed that the addition of them to diabetic wounds may act as a catalyst for wound healing (Papanas & Maltezos 2008). The main targets of interest to date include PDGF, FGF, VEGF, and EGF due to their stimulatory effects on normal wound healing processes, with some limited success in animal trials (Papanas & Maltezos 2008). More recently, recombinant PDGF produced by DNA technology has been formulated into a gel form called becaplermin and given US FDA approval, showing early success in a number of randomized control trials (Papanas & Maltezos 2008). It should be noted, however, that a recent systematic review by the International Working Group concluded that further evidence is required to determine the efficacy of becaplermin (Game et al. 2012). Experience with other growth factors remains limited, with the optimal choice, delivery mode, and concentration of growth factors remaining unknown (Papanas & Maltezos 2008).

As low oxygen at the DFU site contributes to chronic foot ulcer wounds, HBOT has been widely advocated in the treatment of foot ulceration (Tibbles et al. 1996). It has been postulated that enhanced oxygen supply will promote leukocyte action and enhance fibroblast function, which will decrease the bacterial overload and promote the deposition of ECM at the wound site (Tibbles et al. 1996). However to date, the effectiveness of HBOT is from few randomized controlled clinical trials, and questions remain on which patients might benefit the most and at which point HBOT should be implemented (Wu et al. 2010).

The identification that the proliferation phase is delayed in DFU and the ECM formation is delayed and insufficient has generated interest in developing living skin equivalents. Such wound healing techniques provide the wound with the ECM allowing for cells to migrate and adhere, and to commence proliferation, fibroplasia, and angiogenesis (Marston et al. 2003). Acellular skin substitutes have been extensively explored for the management of diabetic ulcers with a few randomized control trials performed to date (Greaves et al. 2013). In 2003, the acellular human dermal matrix called Graftjacket was developed by Wright Medical Technology Inc. (Brigido et al. 2004). Forty patients with chronic full thickness lower extremity wounds, secondary to diabetes mellitus, were assigned to either human dermal matrix grafting using Graftjacket or standard control treatment (sharp debridement followed by wound dressing) (Brigido et al. 2004). After 4 weeks of treatment, the dermal matrix wounds had significantly more healing in depth (89% vs. 25%) and area (73% vs. 34%) compared with the control treatment wounds (Brigido et al. 2004). Brigido further reported another 14 patients treated with acellular human dermal grafts and 14 with standard treatment (Brigido et al 2006). After 16 weeks, 12 of the 14 matrix grafts healed compared with only 4 of the 14 control wounds (Brigido et al. 2006). However, with few trials having controls, varying wound etiology and starting points, and lack of qualitative information, further evidence is required to support the use of acellular dermal matrix grafts for wound healing in DFUs (Greaves et al. 2013).

The use of cellular wound substitutes in DFUs has also been investigated. Dermagraft is a cryopreserved human fibroblast dermal bioresorbable substitute composed of fibroblasts and ECM (Marston et al. 2003). Human dermal fibroblasts are obtained from a monitored cell bank and then grown on the bioresorbable scaffold (Marston et al. 2003). After implantation, the fibroblasts form new granulation tissue, while the scaffold degrades over time (Marston et al. 2003). It has been shown to be effective for DFUs over 6-week duration (Marston et al. 2003).

Table 23.2 Current and future molecular targets for diabetic wound healing

Current treatment options	Targeted wound healing process
Antimicrobial agents	Decrease micro-organism number to decrease the production of growth factors/cytokine messengers, which prolong the inflammatory phase (Davis et al. 2006, Ravari et al. 2011)
Multiple debridements	Decrease micro-organism number to decrease the production of growth factors/cytokine messengers, which prolong the inflammatory phase (Davis et al. 2006)
Application of growth factors	Provide molecular signals for cells to carry out the wound healing processes in inflammation/proliferation/angiogenesis phases (Rodriguez et al. 2008)
Hyperbaric oxygen therapy	Provide oxygen for cells to produce ATP to carry out wound healing processes in inflammation/proliferation/angiogenesis phases (Tchaikovski et al. 2009)
Biological skin substitutes	Provide a fibroblast and keratinocyte scaffold for further cell attachment and migration in the inflammation and proliferation phases (Bitar 1997, Blakytny et al. 2000, Gabbianni et al. 1971)
Future targeted treatment options	
Application of stem cells	Increase fibroblast proliferation and migration, neutrophil migration, macrophage cytokine production and enhance angiogenesis (Bento & Pereira 2011)
Gene therapy	Provide growth factor signal via wound cell to stimulate the inflammation and proliferation phases of wound healing (Lobmann et al. 2002)

Due to the identification that infection is one key local factor that contributes to chronic wound healing, wound debridement has been shown to be useful in controlling bacterial load and promoting healthy granulation tissue. In addition, topical agents have been developed that reduce bacterial load such as topical antimicrobial including chlorhexidine, hydrogen peroxide, silver sulfadiazine and silver nitrate (Storm-Versloot et al. 2010), but further clinical evidence is required to determine their true efficacy to promote wound healing in DFUs (Game et al. 2012).

■ FUTURE DIRECTIONS

Despite the advancements in technology, wound healing for DFU is a slow process, taking months to heal completely in many patients (Prompers et al. 2008). Therefore, it is becoming even more important to identify molecular mechanisms that could be used as potential DFU therapies. The future of DFUs is moving at a rapid rate due to advances in other medical areas. There has been a recent interest in using stem cells as a treatment option for DFUs due to their ability to mobilize and target ischemic and wounded tissue and secrete growth factors and chemokines to promote angiogenesis and ECM formation (Blumber et al. 2012). Several diabetic animal models have shown that stem cells can regenerate dermal and subdermal tissue (Di Rocco et al. 2011, Maharlooei et al. 2011). Ravari et al. illustrated accelerated wound healing in eight subjects after topical application of bone marrow-derived stem cells. However, collagen and platelet matrix were also applied and as such it is difficult to ascertain the efficacy of stem cells alone (Ravari et al. 2011). Therefore, the applications of stem cells appear to be a promising treatment option for DFU. However, with few human trials being conducted, further studies are needed to demonstrate safety and efficacy in improving wound healing (Blumberg et al. 2012).

Due to the identification of abnormal growth factor and chemokine prolife in DFU wounds, research interest has began to emerge in the use of gene therapy for healing of DFUs. Gene therapy could overcome the obstacles of the short half-life and expensive production of topical application of growth factors by enabling the wound to over express growth factors via cell vehicles (Mulder et al. 2009). However, how to deliver these genes into the host cells and which growth factor would be of the most importance are key questions that are under current investigation (Mulder et al. 2009). To understand what molecular mechanisms are required to enhance wound healing, technology must advance to be able to identify quickly and effectively molecular therapeutic targets. RNA interference (RNAi) technology, which mimics the natural process of turning down or silencing the activity of specific genes, is one recent technological advancement that could help understand the importance of independent genes in wound healing pathways (Cullen et al. 2005). For instance, Guan et al. illustrated that primary human dermal fibroblast cells with RNAi knockdown of the endogenous Nckalpha or Nckbeta genes failed to migrate in response to PDGF-BB, the only FDA-approved growth factor for chronic wound healing in the clinic. Therefore, further understanding into the mechanism of action of Nck would be crucial to understand the PGDF-BBs mitogenic signaling pathway for dermal fibroblasts, leading to the development of effective molecular targets (Guan et al. 2009).

CONCLUSIONS

Due to the multiple intervening processes occurring during diabetic foot ulcer healing that have been highlighted in this review, it is likely that a multifactorial treatment approach is required for a successful clinical outcome. Knowledge into the pathophysiology of DFUs is currently still evolving with the determination of the roles of specific growth factors, AGEs and altered molecular pathways; also the distribution and type of microbial overload is still being explored. As we learn more about why DFUs fail to heal adequately, we will be able to use emerging technology to address these issues in order to decrease the morbidity and mortality associated with chronic DFUs.

AREAS OF CONTROVERSY AND/OR FUTURE RESEARCH

- Knowledge into the pathophysiology of DFUs has started to evolve, enabling technology to identify molecular targets as potential DFU therapies
- All stages of the wound healing process have been found to be altered in DFUs including the proliferation, inflammation, and angiogenesis
- The timing and production of a large number of growth factors during the inflammatory and angiogenesis phase are disrupted in DFUs causing abnormal wound healing
- A greater understanding into the molecular pathways is required before growth factors are utilized to promote healing of DFUs
- The maintenance of the ECM during the proliferative phase is modified in DFUs
- There is a change in the normal cell profile and growth factors production preventing the normal production of the ECM, allowing normal wound healing
- Further investigation of the importance of such molecular mechanisms is required before molecular targets can be developed
- AGEs have been shown to disrupt the normal wound healing of DFUs through disruption of the intracellular pathways controlling angiogenesis and direct damage to the ECM
- Additional evidence is needed to establish the effect of glycation products on fibroblasts, ECs, and keratinocytes before AGE inhibitors are utilized in clinical practice

IMPORTANT FURTHER READING

Baum CL, Arpey CJ. Normal cutaneous wound healing: clinical correlation with cellular and molecular events. Dermatol Surg 2005; 31:674–686; discussion 686.

Catrina SB, Okamoto K, Pereira T, Brismar K, Poellinger L. Hyperglycemia regulates hypoxia-inducible factor-1alpha protein stability and function. Diabetes 2004; 53:3226–3232.

Gallagher KA, Liu ZJ, Xiao M. Diabetic impairments in NO-mediated endothelial progenitor cell mobilization and homing are reversed by hyperoxia and SDF-1α. J Clin Invest 2007; 117:1249–1259.

Stern DM, Yan SD, Yan SF, Schmidt AM. Receptor for advanced glycation endproducts (RAGE) and the complications of diabetes. Ageing Res Rev 2002; 1:1–15.

REFERENCES

Ahmed N. Advanced glycation endproducts--role in pathology of diabetic complications. Diabetes Res Clin Pract 2005; 67:3–21.

Ahn C, Mulligan P, Salcido RS. Smoking—the bane of wound healing: biomedical interventions and social influences. Adv Skin Wound Care 2008; 21:227–238.

Amarnath V, Amarnath K, Amarnath K, Davies S, Roberts LJ II. Pyridoxamine: an extremely potent scavenger of 1,4-dicarbonyls. Chem Res Toxicol 2004; 17:410–415.

Anand P, Terenghi G, Warner G, et al. The role of endogenous nerve growth factor in human diabetic neuropathy. Nat Med 1996; 2:703–707.

Apelqvist J, Agardh CD. The association between clinical risk factors and outcome of diabetic foot ulcers. Diabetes Res Clin Pract 1992; 18:43–53.

Apelqvist J, Bakker K, van Houtum WH, Nabuurs-Franssen MH, Schaper NC, on behalf of the International Working Group on the Diabetic Foot. International consensus and practical guidelines on the management and the prevention of the diabetic foot. Diabetes Metab Res Rev 2000; 16:S84–92.

Armstrong DG, Jude EB. The role of matrix metalloproteinases in wound healing. J Am Podiatr Med Assoc 2002; 92:12–18.

Armstrong DG, Lavery LA, Wu S, Boulton AJ. Evaluation of removable and irremovable cast walkers in the healing of diabetic foot wounds: a randomized controlled trial. Diabetes Care 2005; 28:551–554.

Armstrong DG, Nguyen HC, Lavery LA, et al. Off-loading the diabetic foot wound: a randomized clinical trial. Diabetes Care 2001; 24:1019–1022.

Arnold M, Barbul A. Nutrition and wound healing. Plast Reconstr Surg 2006; 117:42S–58S.

Ballas CB, Davidson JM. Delayed wound healing in aged rats is associated with increased collagen gel remodelling and contraction by skin fibroblasts, not with differences in apoptotic or myofibroblast cell populations. Wound Repair Regen 2001; 9:223–227.

Bauer EA, Silverman N, Busiek DF, Kronberger A, Deuel TF. Diminished response of Werner's syndrome fibroblasts to growth factors PDGF and FGF. Science 1986; 234:1240–1243.

Baum CL, Arpey CJ. Normal cutaneous wound healing: clinical correlation with cellular and molecular events. Dermatol Surg 2005; 31:674–686; discussion 686.

Baynes JW, Thorpe SR. Glycoxidation and lipoxidation in atherogenesis. Free Radic Biol Med 2000; 28:1708–1716.

Beer HD, Longaker MT, Werner S. Reduced expression of PDGF and PDGF receptors during impaired wound healing. J Invest Dermatol 1997; 109:132–138.

Bento CF, Pereira P. Regulation of hypoxia-inducible factor 1 and the loss of the cellular response to hypoxia in diabetes. Diabetologia 2011;54:1946–1956.

Bishop A. Role of oxygen in wound healing. J Wound Care 2008; 17:399–402.

Bitar MS. Insulin-like growth factor-1 reverses diabetes-induced wound healing impairment in rats. Horm Metab Res 1997; 29:383–386.

Blakytny R, Jude EB, Gibson JM, Boulton AJM, Ferguson MWJ. Lack of insulin-like growth factor I (IGF I) in the basal keratinocyte layer of diabetic skin and DFUs. J Pathol 2000; 190:589–594.

Blumberg SN, Berger A, Hwang L, et al. The role of stem cells in the treatment of diabetic foot ulcers. Diabetes Res Clin Pract. 2012; 96:1–9.

Botusan IR, Sunkari VG, Savu O, et al. Stabilization of HIF-1alpha is critical to improve wound healing in diabetic mice. Proc Natl Acad Sci U S A 2008; 105:19426–19431.

Brew K, Kinakarpandian J, Nagase H. Tissue inhibitors of metalloproteinases: evolution, structure and function. Biochim Biophys Acta 2000; 1477:267–283.

Brigido SA, Boc SF, Lopez RC. Effective management of major lower extremity wounds using an acellular regenerative tissue matrix: a pilot study. Orthopedics 2004; 27:s145–149.

Brigido SA. The use of an acellular dermal regenerative tissue matrix in the treatment of lower extremity wounds: a prospective 16-week pilot study. Int Wound J 2006; 3:181–187.

Caballero AE, Arora S, Saouaf R, et al. Microvascular and macrovascular reactivity is reduced in subjects at risk for type 2 diabetes. Diabetes 1999; 48:1856–1862.

Catrina SB, Okamoto K, Pereira T, Brismar K, Poellinger L. Hyperglycemia regulates hypoxia-inducible factor- 1alpha protein stability and function. Diabetes 2004; 53:3226–3232.

Chakrabarti S, Sima AA. Pathogenetic heterogeneity in retinal capillary basement membrane thickening in the diabetic BB-rat. Diabetologia 1987; 30:966–968.

Cohen IK, Diegelman RF, Dome RY, et al. Wound care and wound healing. In: Schwartz SI, Shires GT, Spencer FC, et al. (eds). Principles of Surgery, 7th edn. New York: McGraw-Hill, 1999:263–951.

Cook N, Stephens P, Davies J, et al. Defective extracellular matrix reorganization by chronic wound fibroblasts is associated with alterations in TIMP-1, TMIP-2 and MMP-2 activity. J Invest Derm 2000; 115:225–233.

Ctercteko GC, Dhanendran M, Hutton WC, Le Quesne LP. Vertical forces acting on the feet of diabetic patients with neuropathic ulceration. Br J Surg 1981; 68:608.

Cullen LM, Arndt GM. Genome-wide screening for gene function using RNAi in mammalian cells. Immunol Cell Biol 2005; 83:217–223.

Dahlback B. Blood coagulation. Lancet 2000; 355:1627–1632.

Davis SC, Martinez L, Kirsner R. The diabetic foot: the importance of biofilms and wound bed preparation. Curr Diab Rep 2006; 6:439–445.

Dennis PA, Rifkin DB. Cellular activation of latent transforming growth factor β requires binding to the cation-independent mannose 6–phosphate/insulin-like growth factor type II receptor. Proc Natl Acad Sci USA 1991; 88:580–584.

Deuel TF, Senior RM, Huang JS, et al. Chemotaxis of monocytes and neutrophils to platelet-derived growth factor. J Clin Invest 1982; 69:1046–1049.

Di Rocco G, Gentile A, Antonini A, et al. Enhanced healing of diabetic wounds by topical administration of adipose tissue-derived stromal cells overexpressing stromal-derived factor-1: biodistribution and engraftment analysis by bioluminescent imaging. Stem Cells Int 2011; 2011:304–562.

Dinh T, Veves A. Microcirculation of the diabetic foot. Curr Pharm Des 2005; 11:2301–2309.

Dong Y-L, Fleming RYD, Yan TZ, Herndon DN, Waymack JP. Effect of ibuprofen on the inflammatory response to surgical wounds. J Trauma 1993; 35:340–343.

Doxey DL, Ng MC, Dill RE, Iacopino AM. Platelet-derived growth factor levels in wounds of diabetic rats. Life Sci 1995; 57:1111–1123.

Dubay DA, Franz MG. Acute wound healing: the biology of acute wound failure. Surg Clin North Am 2003; 83:463–481.

Edwards R, Harding KG. Bacteria and wound healing. Curr Opin Infect Dis 2004; 17:91–96.

Fantuzzi G. Adipose tissue, adipokines, and inflammation. J Allergy Clin Immunol 2005; 115:911–919; quiz 920.

Fauci AS, Haynes BF. Cellular and molecular basis of immunity. In: Issclacher K, Braunwald E, Wilson J, et al. (eds), Harrison's principles of internal medicine, 13th edn. New York: McGraw-Hill; 1994:1552.

Ferrier TM. Comparative study of arterial disease in amputated lower limbs from diabetics and non–diabetics (with special reference to feet arteries). Med J 1967; 1:5–11.

Folkman J, Klagsbrun M. Angiogenic factors. Science 1987; 235:442–447.

Forst T, Pfutzner A, Kunt T, et al. Skin microcirculation in patients with type I diabetes with and without neuropathy after neurovascular stimulation. Clin Sci (Lond) 1998; 94:255–261.

Gabbianni G, Ryan GB, Majno G. Presence of modified fibroblasts in granulation tissue and their possible role in wound contraction. Experientia 1971; 27:549–550.

Galkowska H, Olszewski WL, Wojewodzka U, Rosinski G, Karnafel W. Neurogenic factors in the impaired healing of DFUs. J Surg Res 2006; 134:252–258.

Gallagher KA, et al. Diabetic impairments in NO-mediated endothelial progenitor cell mobilization and homing are reversed by hyperoxia and SDF-1α. J Clin Invest 2007; 117:1249–1259.

Game FL, Hinchliffe RJ, Apelqvist J, et al. A systematic review of interventions to enhance the healing of chronic ulcers of the foot in diabetes. Diabetes Metab Res Rev 2012; 28:119–141.

Gharaee-Kermani M. Role of cytokines and cytokine therapy in wound healing and fibrotic disease. Curr Pharm Des 2001;7:1083– 103.

Gibran NS, Jang YC, Isik FF, et al. Diminished neuropeptide levels contribute to the impaired cutaneous healing response associated with diabetes mellitus. J Surg Res 2002; 108:122–128.

Glat PM, Longaker MT. Wound healing. In: Aston SJ, Besley RW, Thorn CH (eds), Grabb and Smith's plastic surgery, 5th edn. Philadelphia: Lippincott-Raven, 1997:3.

Gogia PP. Physiology of wound healing. In: Gogia PP (ed.), Clinical wound management. Thorofare, NJ: Slack Incorporated, 1995:8–12.

Gordois A, Scuffham P, Shearer A, Oglesby A. The healthcare costs of diabetic peripheral neuropathy in the UK. Diabet Foot 2003; 6: 62–73.

Grant M, Jerdan J, Merimee TJ. Insulin-like growth factor-1 modulates endothelial cell chemotaxis. J Clin Endocrinol Metab 1987; 65:370–371.

Greaves NS, Iqbal SA, Baguneid M, Bayat A. The role of skin substitutes in the management of chronic cutaneous wounds. Wound Repair Regen 2013; 21:194–210.

Greiffenstein P, Molina PE. Alcohol-induced alterations on host defense after traumatic injury. J Trauma 2008; 64:230–240.

Guan S, Fan J, Han A, Chen M, Woodley DT, Li W. Non-compensating roles between Nckalpha and Nckbeta in PDGF-BB signaling to promote human dermal fibroblast migration. J Invest Dermatol 2009; 129:1909–1920.

Guvakova MA. Insulin-like growth factors control cell migration in health and disease. Int J Biochem Cell Biol 2007; 39:890–909.

Hinz B. Formation and function of the myofibroblast during tissue repair. J Invest Dermatol 2007; 127:526–537.

Ignotz RA, Massaugue J. Transforming growth factor beta stimulates the expression of fibronectin and collagen and their incorporation into the extracellular matrix. J Biol Chem 1986; 261:4337–4345.

Jude EB, Blakytny R, Bulmer J, Boulton AJ, Ferguson MW. Transforming growth factor-β1, -2, -3 and receptor type I and II in DFUs. Diabet Med 2002; 19:440–447.

Khoosal D, Goldman RD. Vitamin E for treating children's scars. Does it help reduce scarring? Can Fam Physician 2006; 52:855–856.

Kloth LC, McCulloch JM, Feedar JA. Wound healing. In: Kloth LC, McCulloch JM, Feedar JA (eds), Wound healing: alternatives in management. Philadelphia: FA Davis Company, 1990:3–13.

Kluwe J, Mencin A, Schwabe RF. Toll-like receptors, wound healing, and carcinogenesis. Diabetes Care 2001; 24:1019–1022.

Lawrence WT. Physiology of the acute wound. Clin Plas Surg 1998; 25:321–340.

Levy DM, Terenghi G, Gu XH, et al. Immunohistochemical measurements of nerves and neuropeptides in diabetic skin: relationship to tests of neurological function. Diabetologia 1992; 35:889–897.

Li J, Chen J, Kirsner R. Pathophysiology of acute wound healing. Clin Dermatol 2007; 25:9–18.

Lobmann R, Ambrosch A, Schultz G, et al. Expression of matrix-metalloproteinases and their inhibitors in the wounds of diabetic and non-diabetic patients. Diabetologia 2002; 45:1011–1016.

Loots MA, Lamme EN, Zeegelaar J, et al. Differences in cellular infiltrate and extracellular matrix of chronic diabetic and venous ulcers versus acute wounds. J Invest Dermatol 1998; 11:850–857.

Loots MAM, Lamme EN, Mekkes JR, Bos JD, Middelkoop E. Cultured fibroblasts from chronic diabetic wounds on the lower extremity (non-insulin-dependent diabetes mellitus) show disturbed proliferation. Arch Dermatol Res 1999; 291:93–99.

Maharlooei MK, Bagheri M, Solhjou Z, et al. Adipose tissue derived mesenchymal stem cell (AD-MSC) promotes skin wound healing in diabetic rats. Diabetes Res Clin Pract 2011; 93:228–234.

Malik A, Mohammad Z, Ahmad J. The diabetic foot infections: biofilms and antimicrobial resistance. Diabetes Metab Syndr 2013; 7:101–107.

Marston WA, Hanft J, Norwood P, et al. The efficacy and safety of Dermagraft in improving the healing of chronic diabetic foot ulcers: results of a prospective randomized trial. Diabetes Care 2003; 26:1701–1705.

Mast BA, Schultz GS. Interactions of cytokines, growth factors, and proteases in acute and chronic wounds. Wound Rep Reg 1996; 4:411–420.

McGuckin M, Kerstein MD. Venous leg ulcers and the family physician. Adv Wound Care 1998; 11:344–346.

Monaco JL, Lawrence WT. Acute wound healing an overview. Clin Plast Surg. 2003; 30:1–12.

Mulder G, Tallis AJ, Marshall VT, et al. Treatment of nonhealing diabetic foot ulcers with a platelet-derived growth factor gene-activated matrix (GAM501): results of a phase 1/2 trial. Wound Repair Regen 2009; 17:772–779.

Newman SL, Henson JE, Henson PM. Phagocytosis of senescent neutrophils by human monocyte derived macrophages and rabbit inflammatory macrophages. J Exp Med 1982; 156:430–442.

Nimmi ME. Collagen: its structure and function in normal and pathological connective tissues. Semin Arthritis Rheum 1974; 4:95–150.

Nishikawa T, Edelstein D, Du XL, et al. Normalizing mitochondrial superoxide production blocks three pathways of hyperglycaemic damage. Nature 2000; 404:787–790.

Noble D, Mathur R, Dent T, Meds C, Greenhaigh T. Risk models and scores for type 2 diabetes: systematic review. BMJ 2011; 343:d7163.

Papanas N, Maltezos E. Becaplermin gel in the treatment of diabetic neuropathic foot ulcers. Becaplermin gel in the treatment of diabetic neuropathic foot ulcers. Clin Interv Aging 2008; 3:233–240.

Patel V, Chivukala I, Roy S, et al. Oxygen: from the benefits of inducing VEGF expression to managing the risk of hyperbaric stress. Antioxid Redox Signal 2005; 7:1377–1387.

Pecoraro RE, Ahroni JH, Boyko EJ, Stensel VL. Chronology and determinants of tissue repair in diabetic lower-extremity ulcers. Diabetes 1991; 40:1305–1313.

Piaggesi A, Viacava P, Rizzo L, et al. Semiquantitative analysis of the histopathological features of the neuropathic foot ulcer: effects of pressure relief. Diabetes Care 2003; 26:3123–3128.

Pierce GF, Tarpley JE, Yanagihara D, et al. Platelet-derived growth factor (BB homodimer), transforming growth factor-beta 1, and basic fibroblast growth factor in dermal wound healing. Neovessel and matrix formation and cessation of repair. Am J Pathol 1992; 140:1375–1388.

Pipili-Synetos E, Sakkoula E, Haralabopoulos G, et al. Evidence that nitric oxide is an endogenous antiangiogenic mediator. Br J Pharmacol 1994; 111:894–902.

Prompers L, Schaper N, Apelqvist J, et al. Prediction of outcome in individuals with diabetic foot ulcers: focus on the differences between individuals with and without peripheral arterial disease. The EURODIALE Study. Diabetologia 2008; 51:747–755.

Ranzer MJ, Chen L, DiPietro LA. Fibroblast function and wound breaking strength is impaired by acute ethanol intoxication. Alcohol Clin Exp Res 2011; 35:83–90.

Ravari H, Hamidi-Almadari D, Salimifar M, et al. Treatment of non-healing wounds with autologous bone marrow cells: platelets, fibrin glue and collagen matrix. Cytotherapy 2011; 13:705–711.

Reinke JM, Sorg H. Wound repair and regeneration. Eur Surg Res 2012; 49:35–43.

Roberts AB. Transforming growth factor-β: activity and efficacy in animal models of wound healing. Wound Rep Regen 1995; 3:408–418.

Robson M. Wound healing: biologic features and approaches to maximum healing trajectories. Curr Prob Surg 2001; 38:61–148.

Robson MC. Cytokine manipulation of the wound. Clin Plast Surg 2003; 30:57–65.

Robson MC. Pathophysiology of chronic wounds. In: Surgery in wounds Part 1. Berlin: Springer, 2004:29–40.

Rodriguez PG, Felix FN, Woodley DT, Shim EK. The role of oxygen in wound healing: a review of the literature. Dermatol Surg 2008; 34:1159–1169.

Sandu O, Song K, Cai W, et al. Insulin resistance and type 2 diabetes in high-fat-fed mice are linked to high glycotoxin intake. Diabetes 2005; 54:2314.

Schäffer M, Schier R, Napirei M, et al. Sirolimus impairs wound healing. Langenbecks Arch Surg 2007; 392:297–303.

Schreml S, Szeimies RM, Prantl L, et al. Oxygen in acute and chronic wound healing. Br J Dermatol 2010; 163:257–268.

Sena CM, Pereira AM, Seiça R. Endothelial dysfunction – a major mediator of diabetic vascular disease. Biochim Biophys Acta 2013 pii: S0925-4439(13)00271-8.

Shepherd AA. Nutrition for optimum wound healing. Nurs Stand 2003; 18:55–58.

Stern DM, Yan SD, Yan SF, Schmidt AM. Receptor for advanced glycation endproducts (RAGE) and the complications of diabetes. Ageing Res Rev 2002; 1:1–15.

Sternberg EM. Neural regulation of innate immunity: a coordinated nonspecific host response to pathogens. Nat Rev Immunol. 2006; 6:318–328.

Storm-Versloot MN, Vos CG, Ubbink DT, et al. Topical silver for preventing wound infection. Cochrane Database Syst Rev 2010; 3:CD006478.

Surwit R, Schneider M, Feinglos M. Stress and diabetes mellitus. Diabetes Care 1992; 15:1413–1422.

Swift ME, Burns AL, Gray KL, DiPietro LA. Age-related alterations in the inflammatory response to dermal injury. J Invest Dermatol 2001; 117:1027–1035.

Tchaikovski V, Olieslagers S, Böhmer FD, Waltenberger J. Diabetes mellitus activates signal transduction pathways resulting in vascular endothelial growth factor resistance of human monocytes. Circulation 2009; 120:150–159.

Tibbles P, Edelsbrg J. Hyperbaric oxygen therapy. N Engl J Med 1996; 334:1642–1648.

Tomasek JJ, Gabbiani G, Hinz B, Chaponnier C, Brown RA. Myofibroblasts and mechano-regulation of connective tissue remodelling. Nat Rev Mol Cell Biol 2002; 3:349–363.

Tonnesen MG, Feng X, Clark RA. Angiogenesis in wound healing. J Investig Dermatol Symp Proc 2000; 5:40–46.

Trengove NJ, Bielefeldt-Ohmann H, Stacey MC. Mitogenic activity and cytokine levels in non-healing and healing chronic leg ulcers. Wound Repair Regen 2000; 8:13–25.

Vaitkevicius PV, Lane M, Spurgeon H, et al. A cross-link breaker has sustained effects on arterial and ventricular properties in older rhesus monkeys. Proc Natl Acad Sci U S A 2001; 98:1171–1175.

Veves A, Akbari CM, Primavera J, et al. Endothelial dysfunction and the expression of endothelial nitric oxide synthetase in diabetic neuropathy, vascular disease, and foot ulceration. Diabetes 1998; 47:457–463.

Vinik AI. Diagnosis and management of diabetic neuropathy. Clin Geriatr Med 1999; 15:293–320.

Vowden K, Vowdewn P, Posnett J. The resource costs of wound care in Bradford and Airedale primary care trust in the UK. J Wound Care 2009; 18:93–94, 96–98.

Wierusz-Wysocka B, Wysocki H, Wykretowicz A, Szczepanik A, Siekierka H. Phagocytosis, bactericidal capacity, and superoxide anion (02–) production by polymorphonuclear neutrophils from patients with diabetes mellitus. Folia Haematol Int Mag Klin Morph Blutforsch 1985; 112:658–668.

Williamson JR, Kilo C. Basement-membrane thickening and diabetic microangiopathy. Diabetes 1976; 25:925–927.

Wilson JA, Clark JJ. Obesity: impediment to postsurgical wound healing. Adv Skin Wound Care 2004; 17:426–435.

Witte MB, Kiyama T, Barbul A. Nitric oxide enhances experimental wound healing in diabetes. Br J Surg 2002; 89:1594–1601.

Woo K, Ayello EA, Sibbald RG. The edge effect: current therapeutic options to advance the wound edge. Adv Skin Wound Care 2007; 20:99–117.

Wright SD, Ramos RA, Tobias PS, Ulevitch RJ, Matchison JC. CD14, a receptor for complexes of lipopolysaccharide (LPS) and LPS-binding protein. Science 1990; 249:1431–1433.

Wu S, Martson W, Armstrong D. Wound care: the role of advanced wound healing technologies. J Vasc Surg 2010; 52:59S–66.

Chapter 24

Scoring systems and assessment of the ulcerated foot

Fran Game

SUMMARY

- Before deciding on the use of any system for the classification of diabetic foot ulcers, the clinician must be clear about the purpose of classification; for research, audit, or clinical prognosis
- Few systems have been extensively validated, particularly in populations or countries outside those from which they were derived
- Clinicians must agree about when an ulcer is classified, as features affecting prognosis, such as infection, may change during an episode of care
- There is still a need for internationally agreed and validated classification systems for clinical care and audit to allow for comparison of treatment methods and outcomes for patients with diabetic foot ulcers

INTRODUCTION

It is well recognized that the relative importance of the pathogenic factors involved in diabetic foot lesions; neuropathy, peripheral arterial disease (PAD), and infection, for example varies from person to person and lesion to lesion (Reiber et al. 1999, Jeffcoate & Harding 2003, Boulton 2004, Singh et al. 2005). This leads to varying presentations, and may be one of the reasons why outcome has been noted to vary from country to country as well as within populations. The need to classify or 'score' and describe lesions of the foot of patients with diabetes in a manner that is agreed across all communities and is simple to use in day-to-day clinical practice would therefore seem to be of importance. Surprisingly, to date, no such system is currently in widespread use, although a number have been described. Not all have been adequately validated however, and it has not always been made clear the clinical purposes to which such scoring systems or classifications should be put to use, whether that be for research, clinical description in routine clinical care, or audit.

WHY CLASSIFY, SCORE, OR DESCRIBE?

Classification or scoring systems are used in three broad ways: as a description in routine clinical care, research, or audit. The first is concerned with an individual lesion, limb, or patient. Research and audit, however, are concerned with groups of patients, limbs, and lesions.

Clinical care

The advantage of an agreed classification, scoring system, or the description of foot lesions in routine clinical care would be to facilitate note taking in a more consistent and potentially concise fashion and may be used to follow the progress of a lesion or lesions through an episode of care. This could improve communication between the different professional members of the multidisciplinary team and facilitate the discussion of potential outcomes with the patients from early in the episode. If there was then an agreed management plan based on a particular type of lesion or lesions, then an additional benefit would be a reduction in the variation in treatment(s) offered to patients.

Clinical research

The purpose of a research classification is to identify groups of similar lesions or patients for inclusion in trials or studies. In this case, only those lesions or patients who fit pre-agreed criteria need to be identified and classified, and only those centers participating in the research need to agree the criteria and descriptions. This is very different from a classification system for clinical care or audit when all lesions and patients need to be able to be classified, and the descriptions need to be understood by all health-care professionals.

Clinical audit

The purpose of clinical audit may vary from simple event counting (e.g. number of patients with a particular type of foot disease) to seeking associations between disease and outcome. This may include seeking to explain differences in outcome between different centers. If performance between centers is to be compared, it is important to establish that the population managed by each is similar or that account is taken of the severity of presenting disease. Because the cohort studied in each case will be large and will usually be cared for by busy clinicians, any classification or scoring system must be simple, unambiguous, easily understood by all health-care professionals in every multidisciplinary team, and easily documented. Systems for audit are thus by far the most challenging to develop.

WHAT SHOULD BE CLASSIFIED OR SCORED? LESIONS, ULCERS, FEET, OR PEOPLE?

The decision to classify features of the lesion or ulcer alone as opposed to features of the limb or person depends heavily on the purpose of the classification. If the purpose is for clinical care then it may be sufficient to describe the lesion or ulcer. It is, as previously discussed, a requirement for clinical classification that it is inclusive, and all lesions should be classifiable. It is possible that a patient may be seen with a preulcerative lesion, such as hemorrhagic callous, or with infection with no clear portal of entry, or with an acute Charcot foot, and so classification systems designed solely for classifying ulcers may not be appropriate. Prior to choosing a particular classification system therefore, health-care professionals must ensure that it will capture the spectrum of presenting clinical disease that they feel is appropriate.

When a clinical classification is being used to design a treatment strategy, then features of the limb, which are known to affect outcome (Armstrong et al. 1998, Oyibo et al. 2001a, Ince et al. 2007) may also be included. For example, a classification system for diabetic foot ulcers may also include whether or not there are signs of PAD (as this may indicate the need for revascularization) or whether the ulcer is complicated by infection, and whether the infection is deep or superficial. A classification system for the purposes of audit, however, should also include the features of the lesion (usually an ulcer) and those of the limb, which affect treatment choices or outcome (e.g. the need to off-load if neuropathy is present), depending on whether the purpose of the audit is for ensuring adherence to agreed management guidelines or for comparison between different centers. If, however, audit is being done at a population level (e.g. looking at amputation rates in different regions), then it may also be necessary to include features of the person in a classification, as age, social deprivation and ethnicity have an influence on the risk of the development of foot disease in the first place.

Multiple lesions

The decision on how to handle multiple lesions on a single foot or feet is difficult and is again dependent on the purpose of the classification or scoring system. If the system of classification is used simply as an aid to clinical practice and to improve communication, then it should be applied to every lesion that exists. If, however, the intention is to use the system to link ulcer type with outcome (as in research or audit), then the issue is slightly more complex. If the chosen outcome relates to the lesion (such as healing or incidence of secondary infection), then every ulcer should be considered. If, however, the outcome is person centered (such as well-being or survival), then it will usually be invalid to classify all ulcers, and one (the largest or most relevant to the question, for instance) must be selected as the index lesion.

WHEN SHOULD CLASSIFICATION OR SCORING BE DONE?

Clinical care

If a classification or scoring system is being used to plan clinical management or for communication between health-care professionals, then it should be capable of being applied and changed as often as necessary. An ulcer that is clean and uninfected, for example, could be categorized as such, and management principles defined accordingly. If, however, it becomes infected, then its classification (or description) should change and the management should also be changed. Such a classification should therefore be simple enough to do quickly and frequently in clinical practice.

Clinical research

The question of timing presents little problem in the selection of lesions for prospective research – because the only concern is whether a lesion meets the criteria for selection at the time of recruitment to the study, and it matters little how much it has changed in the period prior to selection.

Clinical audit

Timing is more problematic, however, when a classification system is used as the basis for audit. If the aim of the exercise is to determine the outcome of all ulcers or lesions seen, then obviously each should counted only once. The time when this is done is likely to be arbitrary – perhaps when, for example, a person is first referred to the specialist unit. This dependence of audit on timing poses a special problem when the character of a foot lesion changes. Thus, a lesion may present as a clean, uncomplicated ulcer and be classified as such. If however, it becomes complicated by infection, then the prognosis changes. If the infection extends to bone then surgical debridement may be considered and the patient could then be left with a surgical wound – which is different from the first lesion, although it is the result of it. These different lesions or complications could simply be classified as complications of the original presenting lesion. They may however be subjects of audit themselves, e.g. the outcome of osteomyelitis or the healing of postsurgical wounds. Thus, there may need to be a secondary or later reclassification. One suggestion has been the adoption of the 'lesion narrative' (Jeffcoate & Game 2006). An example that describes a fictitious case is shown in **Table 24.1**. Using such a method, it is possible to flag dominant or significant events (often easier electronically) such that both individual lesions can be tracked clinically and individual conditions (e.g. osteomyelitis, amputation) can later be used on the basis of separate analysis.

CLASSIFICATION OR SCORING?

It is clear that there is a difference between classification and scoring. Classification is descriptive, organizing lesions or people into different groups depending on clinical characteristics, whereas a score is a numerical descriptor and is usually meant to give an idea of severity. It is difficult to see how a single classification system can do both of these and again the choice of descriptive or numerical depends on the clinical scenario.

Table 24.1 An example of a fictitious lesion narrative. This illustrates the possible use of a narrative classification of a fictitious patient presenting with two ulcers. The original lesions are highlighted in bold, but significant comorbidities and complications are also highlighted, which could then form the basis of other classifications, audits, or study

Date	Problem 1	Problem 2	Problem 3	Problem 4	Problem 5
13/2/2008	Ulcer of R 3rd toe tip	Ulcer of L heel	PAD: ABPI <0.7 L leg		
14/3/2008	Persists complicated by Problem 4	Persists		Osteomyelitis R 3rd toe	
15/6/2008	Healed	Persists		Healed	
18/7/2008					L Below-knee amputation

ABPI, ankle-brachial pressure index; PAD, peripheral arterial disease.

Beckert S, Witte M, Wicke C, Konigsrainer A, Coerper S. A new wound-based severity score for diabetic foot ulcers: a prospective analysis of 1000 patients. Diabetes Care 2006; 29:988–992.

Boulton AJ. The diabetic foot: from art to science. The 18th Camillo Golgi Lecture. Diabetologia 2004; 47:1343–1353.

Foster A, Edmonds M. Simple staging system: a tool for diagnosis and management. Diabetic Foot 2000; 3:56–62.

Game FL, Hinchliffe RJ, Apelqvist J, et al. A systematic review of interventions to enhance the healing of chronic ulcers of the foot in diabetes. Diabetes Metab Res Rev 2012; 28:119–141.

Hinchliffe RJ, Valk GD, Apelqvist J, et al. A systematic review of the effectiveness of interventions to enhance the healing of chronic ulcers of the foot in diabetes. Diabetes Metab Res Rev 2008; 24:1520–7552.

Ince P, Abbas ZG, Lutale JK, et al. Use of the SINBAD classification system and score in comparing outcome of foot ulcer management on three continents. Diabetes Care 2008; 31:964–967.

Ince P, Kendrick D, Game F, Jeffcoate W. The association between baseline characteristics and the outcome of foot lesions in a UK population with diabetes. Diabet Med 2007; 24:977–981.

Jeffcoate W, Game F. The description, classification and registration of diabetic foot lesions. In: Boulton AJM, Cavanagh P, Rayman G (eds), The foot in diabetes, 4th edn. London, United Kingdom: John Wiley and Sons Ltd; 2006.

Jeffcoate WJ, Harding KG. Diabetic foot ulcers. Lancet 2003; 361:1545–1551.

Karthikesalingam A, Holt PJE, Moxey P, et al. A systematic review of scoring systems for diabetic foot ulcers. Diabet Med 2010; 27: 544–549.

Knighton DR, Ciresi KF, Fiegel VD, Austin LL, Butler EL. Classification and treatment of chronic nonhealing wounds. Successful treatment with autologous platelet-derived wound healing factors (PDWHF). Ann Surg 1986; 204:322–330.

Lavery LA, Armstrong DG, Harkless LB. Classification of diabetic foot wounds. J Foot Ankle Surg 1996; 35:528–531.

Macfarlane RM, Jeffcoate WJ. Classification of diabetic foot ulcers: the S(AD) SAD system. Diabet Foot 1999; 2:123–131.

Meggitt B. Surgical management of the diabetic foot. Br J Hosp Med 1976; 16:227–232.

Oyibo SO, Jude EB, Tarawneh I, et al. The effects of ulcer size and site, patient's age, sex and type and duration of diabetes on the outcomes of diabetic foot ulcers. Diabet Med 2001a; 18:133–138.

Oyibo SO, Jude EB, Tarawneh I, et al. A comparison of two diabetic foot ulcer classification systems: the Wagner and the University of Texas wound classification systems. Diabetes Care 2001b; 24:84–88.

Parisi MCR, Zantut-Wittmann DE, Pavin EJ, et al. Comparison of three systems of classification in predicting the outcome of diabetic foot ulcers in a Brazilian population. Eur J Endocrinol 2008; 159:417–422.

Reiber GE, Vileikyte L, Boyko EJ, et al. Causal pathways for incident lower-extremity ulcers in patients with diabetes from two settings. Diabetes Care 1999; 22:157–162.

Schaper NC. Diabetic foot ulcer classification system for research purposes: a progress report on criteria for including patients in research studies. Diabetes Metab Res Rev 2004; 20:S90–S95.

Singh N, Armstrong DG, Lipsky BA. Preventing foot ulcers in patients with diabetes. JAMA 2005; 293:217–228.

Treece KA, Macfarlane RM, Pound P, Game FL, Jeffcoate WJ. Validation of a system of foot ulcer classification in diabetes mellitus. Diabet Med 2004; 21:987–991.

Van Acker K, De Block C, Abrams P, et al. The choice of diabetic foot ulcer classification in relation to the final outcome. Wounds 2002; 14:16–25.

van Battum P, Schaper N, Prompers L, et al. Differences in minor amputation rate in diabetic foot disease throughout Europe are in part explained by differences in disease severity at presentation. Diabet Med 2011; 28,199–205.

Wagner FW, Jr. The dysvascular foot: a system for diagnosis and treatment. Foot Ankle 1981; 2:64–122.

Younes NA, Albsoul AM. The DEPA scoring system and its correlation with the healing rate of diabetic foot ulcers. J Foot Ankle Surg 2004; 43:209–213.

Chapter 25 | Wound dressings and debridement

Elizabeth J. Mudge, Alastair J. Richards, Keith G. Harding

SUMMARY

- Effective use of dressings is essential to ensure optimal ulcer management
- The ideal dressing should aim to alleviate symptoms, protect damaged tissue, and enhance wound healing
- No single dressing is capable of fulfilling all of the above criteria throughout an entire episode of diabetic foot ulceration
- The choice of appropriate dressing should form part of a multidisciplinary assessment of the patient and be accompanied by a clear understanding of the process of wound healing and the concepts of wound bed preparation and moist wound healing

INTRODUCTION

The outcome for patients with diabetic foot ulcers (DFUs) is generally considered to be poor, and there remains uncertainty concerning optimal approaches to management (Game et al. 2012). The choice of wound dressing may be perceived as less crucial than other treatment modalities in achieving healing, although modern dressings may well provide significant benefits to the patient and clinician and thus form a key part of the overall management of DFU (International Working Group on the Diabetic Foot 2011). The effective use of dressings is essential to ensure the optimal care of ulceration. However, although there is a wealth of literature on the subject of DFU, there is less conclusive information on the use of dressings in the management of DFU (Jeffcoate et al. 2009).

The ideal dressing should alleviate symptoms, provide protection to the ulcerated area, and encourage wound healing. However, no single dressing is capable of fulfilling all these criteria throughout an episode of foot ulceration, nor is a single dressing capable of addressing all the requirements of a patient with DFU. Systematic reviews of dressings for DFU are restricted by the limited number of comparative studies of alternative dressings, in a field where there are several different dressing options, thus research in this area is generally of poor quality and there is a lack of evidence to support a dressing effect on increasing the rate of healing in DFU, although there may be other benefits to the patient, such as reduction of pain and odor.

The appropriate choice of dressing is an important and integral part of the management of DFU and should be made, where possible, as part of an interdisciplinary approach to the assessment and treatment of the person with a DFU (Bakker et al 2012). Fundamentally, dressing selection should take into account the clinical characteristics of the ulcer (type of wound and stage of healing), patient requirements, and costs.

The aim of this chapter is to discuss the variety of dressing types currently available and review the most recent evidence for dressings in wound healing and debridement of DFUs. Negative pressure, hyperbaric oxygen, and surgical or sharp debridement are covered in other chapters.

WOUND-HEALING AND WOUND-BED PREPARATION

Wound-healing process

Wound healing is a dynamic and complex biological process involving a number of organized phases, which include coagulation, inflammation, epithelialization, matrix deposition, angiogenesis, proliferation, cellular remodeling, and wound contraction (Enoch et al. 2006, Mast & Schultz 1996). The restoration of tissue integrity and functional healing requires complex interactions between various biological entities, such as growth factors and proteases, matrix components, and cell types, such as platelets, macrophages, fibroblasts, and endothelial cells (Hackam & Ford 2002). Although it is generally accepted that acute wounds can heal following an orderly series of events, it is clear that chronic wounds do not. Many studies, which have examined the underlying biochemistry of chronic ulcers, have noted that such wounds tend to remain stuck in the inflammatory phase of healing. Chronic wounds have also been noted to contain elevated levels of inflammatory cytokines, free radicals, and proteases, which create a hostile wound environment (Henry & Garner 2003).

Dressing development and the concept of moist wound healing

Throughout history a variety of materials, including substances such as cobwebs, dung, animal fat, and honey, have been used as wound dressings to arrest bleeding, absorb exudates, ease pain, and protect the wound from further trauma (Thomas 1990), but it was not until the mid-20th century that the possible beneficial effects of dressings that occluded the wound and created a moist wound environment began to be understood and studied.

Research conducted in the 1950s and 1960s brought about the most significant scientific discovery to impact on the evolution of wound dressings when Odland (1958) first noted that if a blister remained intact, it healed faster than if it were deroofed. This assumption was further confirmed by a small study conducted on domestic pigs (Winter 1962), which demonstrated that re-epithelialization of acute wounds occurred twice as fast if the wounds were covered with an occlusive dressing and kept moist as compared with wounds that were left exposed or treated with conventional (of the time) dressings. Winter's findings were confirmed by Hinman and Maibach (1963) who investigated the effect of occlusion on wound healing in acute human wounds. The results of these and others investigations led to the concept of 'Moist Wound Healing' which advocated completely the opposite philosophy to traditional practice, which up until that time, had promoted that wounds should be allowed to dry out and scab over in an attempt to prevent bacterial infection.

It is now a well-established view that dressings that create and maintain a moist wound environment are considered to provide the optimal conditions for wound healing (Hilton et al. 2004). Moisture under occlusive dressings not only increases the rate of epithelialization but also promotes healing through moisture itself and the presence, initially, of a low oxygen tension, which is known to promote the inflammatory phase of healing. In contrast, gauze does not exhibit these properties, and it may be disruptive to the healing wound as it dries and can cause tissue damage when it is removed, especially if adherent.

Occlusive dressings are thought to modify the wound environment by increasing cell proliferation and cell activity by retaining an optimum level of wound exudate, which contains vital proteins and cytokines produced in response to injury. These facilitate autolytic debridement of the wound and promote healing. Nevertheless, a difference in acute and chronic wound environments created by moist wound healing has been observed. When acute wounds are occluded it has been noted that there is an increase in proteolytic enzymes such as collagenase, thus facilitating wound debridement through degradation of collagen, cells and bacteria, and subsequent keratinocyte migration from the wound edge, leading to more rapid re-epithelialization (Field & Kerstein 1994). However, in people with chronic diabetic foot wounds, these processes are frequently diminished or absent (Greenhalgh 2003).

In vitro studies have demonstrated that human wound fluid taken from beneath occlusive dressings stimulates the growth of fibroblasts and endothelial cells (Katz et al. 1991) and also many growth factors, such as platelet-derived growth factor (PDGF), transforming growth factor beta (TGFβ), and epidermal growth factor (EGF), known to be involved in chemotaxis, migration, stimulation, and proliferation of cells. Conversely, in chronic wounds, fluid taken from beneath occlusive dressings has been found to be inhibitory to the proliferation of a variety of cells necessary to wound healing (Lobmann et al. 2005), although the mechanisms of action of wound fluid taken from chronic wounds under occlusive dressings are less understood.

Furthermore, although it is recognized that bacterial colonization of a wound increases under occlusive dressings (Eaglestein 2001), the potential for increased risk of infection has not been substantiated in clinical trials

■ Wound bed preparation and TIME

The concept of 'wound bed preparation' was first considered toward the end of the 20th century and has gained international recognition as a framework that can provide a structured approach to the management of chronic wounds. It aims to provide criteria for the optimal environment for wound healing by controlling exudate, bacterial load, level of necrotic tissue, and cellular dysfunction to accelerate endogenous healing or to facilitate the effectiveness of other therapeutic measures (Falanga 2000). To assist with implementing wound bed preparation, the 'TIME' acronym was developed in 2002, as a practical guide for use when managing patients with chronic wounds (Schultz et al. 2003). It aims to aid the clinician in making a systematic interpretation of the observable characteristics of a wound and to decide on the most appropriate intervention by summarizing the four main components of wound bed preparation:

- T – Tissue management: nonviable or deficient
- I – Infection and inflammation: control
- M – Moisture imbalance
- E – Edge of wound: advancement of the epithelial edge of the wound

■ DRESSING SELECTION

Dressings have a number of purposes, the choice of an appropriate dressing therefore requires careful clinical assessment and depends not only on the type of wound but also on the severity, stage of healing, the wound bed characteristics, the anatomical position of the wound, and, most importantly, an understanding of the principles of the wound healing process. However, in the absence of robust research evidence, there remains to be no systematic framework for dressing choice.

Desirable characteristics for wound dressings must incorporate the principles of moist wound healing while also controlling the growth or micro-organisms, absorbing exudates, providing debridement, allowing gaseous exchange, thermally insulating the wound, easing pain, and allowing for atraumatic dressing removal (see **Table 25.1**). A variety of different dressings may be indicated throughout the healing process; e.g. a hydrogel may be indicated to break down devitalized tissue, whereas a foam dressing may be used to absorb wound exudates. Among each of the categories of dressing, there is a wide choice of products available, with different physical characteristics and costs.

Practical issues should also be taken into account such as whether the dressing allows for simple observation of the wound and whether it provides mechanical protection and conformability. Foster et al. (1994) described the ideal dressing for DFU as one that does not take up too much room in the shoe, performs well in an enclosed environment, can withstand shear forces, does not increase the risk of infection, absorbs exudates, allows drainage, and can be changed frequently and easily.

Table 25.1 Criteria for determining choice of dressing

Wound attributes	Type of dressing	Rationale for use
Necrosis/slough	Hydrogel Hydrocolloid	Surgical or mechanical debridement Donate liquid Promote autolysis and healing Decrease risk of infection
Gangrene	Dry: low/nonadherent Wet: antimicrobial	Prevent formation of wet gangrene Bacterial control
Infection	Alginate Foam Antimicrobial	Daily dressing change Antiseptic
Low exudate	Hydrocolloid Semipermeable film Hydrogel	Maintain a moist environment
High exudate	Alginate	Prevent maceration/strike through High absorbent qualities Daily dressing change
Flat/shallow	Semipermeable film Hydrocolloid Hydrogel Foams	Promote moist environment Allow visual check Able to be left in place for several days
Cavity with sinus	Alginate Hydrogel	Daily dressing change Fill the cavity
Cavity with no sinus	Foams Hydrocolloid Hydrogel Alginate	Maintain moist environment

PROPERTIES OF THE IDEAL DRESSING

The properties of the ideal dressing are summarized in **Box 25.1**. It is important to note that conventional dressings may not withstand the high and repeated forces that are exerted on the sole of the foot and toes during the gait cycle, and such pressure and overloading may alter dressing properties if adequate provision for off-loading devices is not also provided. Furthermore, ulcer dressings may have an impact on footwear fit leading to pressure damage to other areas of the foot, and therefore alternative footwear should also be considered.

Box 25.1 Properties of the ideal dressing (Thomas 1990)
- Capable of maintaining high humidity at the wound site while removing excess exudates
- Free of particles and toxic wound contaminants
- Nontoxic and nonallergic
- Capable of protecting the wound from future trauma
- Can be removed without causing trauma to the wound
- Impermeable to bacteria
- Thermally insulating
- Will allow gaseous exchange
- Comfortable and conformable
- Requires infrequent changing
- Cost effective
- Long shelf life
- Acceptable to the patient

TYPES OF WOUND DRESSINGS

The function of wound dressings may be described as passive (i.e. simple protection), active (i.e. creating a moist wound environment), or interactive (i.e. capable of modifying the biology of the wound environment). In more recent years, there has been an abundance of interactive dressings coming onto the market. Such dressings have the capability to modulate or stimulate cell proliferation via growth factor release or by moderating protease activity (Trengove et al. 1999). Interactive dressings are designed to be left in place for several days, which may result in minimal disruption to the wound bed, reduce the risk of wound contamination, and reduce cost, although in the case of infected ulcers such action may be contraindicated. Interactive dressings include alginates, foams, hydrocolloids, hydrogels, semipermeable films, cadexomer iodine, hydrofibers, and also skin equivalents. These dressings also promote debridement and may enhance granulation and re-epithelialization.

■ Debriding agents

Debridement is the removal of nonviable tissue from the wound bed, and its role in the preparation of the wound bed is well documented (Falanga 2001, EWMA 2004, Wolcott et al. 2009). The removal of necrotic and devitalized tissue and callous is essential before the application of a dressing as chronic wounds often contain necrotic or sloughy tissue, which can harbor bacteria and act as a barrier to healing. The availability of nutrients and oxygen, and presence of ischemic tissue, makes this an ideal environment in which both aerobic and anaerobic bacteria can multiply (White & Cutting 2008), increasing the risk of malodor and infection.

A variety of debridement techniques may be employed, but the choice of technique should be determined by assessment of systemic and local factors, availability of materials and resources, the experience of the practitioner and consideration that the method of debridement selected is the most effective for the patient. Evidence defining the best method of debridement is scarce, and the most recent Cochrane review of debridement techniques for DFU (Edwards & Stapley 2010) concluded that there was insufficient evidence from randomized controlled trials (RCTs) to promote one technique over another. In clinical practice, a range of debridement techniques is used (see **Box 25.2**).

Box 25.2 Debridement techniques
- Autolytic
- Biosurgical
- Hydrosurgical
- Mechanical
- Sharp
- Surgical
- Ultrasonic

Autolytic debridement

This promotes the use of the body's own enzymes to break down devitalized tissue and separate it from healthy tissue. The central cell responsible for this process is the macrophage, which produces proteolytic enzymes to degrade the devitalized tissue. Products that can be used to facilitate autolytic debridement include hydrogels, hydrocolloids, cadexomer iodine, and honey. In choosing dressings that promote autolytic debridement, it is important to consider the moisture balance in the wound and take necessary steps to avoid maceration by the use of a suitable skin protectant or barrier film. However, it should be acknowledged that autolytic debridement tends to be a slow process and as such may lead to detrimental effects for a DFU.

Biosurgical debridement

This is performed by the application of larvae, e.g. of the green bottle fly (*Lucilia sericata*), to remove necrotic and devitalized tissue from the wound. Larvae are selective in the wound bed, and they avoid harming healthy tissue and are also thought to ingest pathogenic organisms in the wound (Pyatt 2011). Larvae therapy is also suitable for debriding gangrenous areas, thus avoiding the potential for maceration; however, provision of adequate off-loading should be exercised when applying larvae to plantar foot ulcers, to avoid crushing the larvae while weight bearing.

Hydrosurgery

Hydrosurgery systems (e.g. Versajet; Smith & Nephew, London, United Kingdom) combine lavage with sharp debridement, which has been shown to precisely target damaged and necrotic tissue (Caputo et al. 2008). Other innovative methods include low-frequency, low-dose ultrasound using either a contact (Sonica Soring, Quickborn, Germany) or noncontact device (Mist Therapy, Celleration, Minneapolis, USA). Ultrasonic-assisted debridement is a relatively painless method of removing nonviable tissue and has been shown to be effective in reducing bacterial burden, (Ennis et al. 2006).

Mechanical debridement

This is a traditional method, which involves using wet to dry gauze that dries and adheres to the top layer of the wound bed, which is 'pulled' away when the dressing is removed. However, this method is potentially harmful and requires frequent dressing changes and can be very painful for the patient. More recently, an active debridement pad (Debrisoft; Activia Healthcare - Staffordshire, UK.) has been introduced, which uses a fleece-like contact layer to mechanically remove debris, necrotic tissue, slough, and exudate (Gray et al. 2011).

Sharp and surgical methods of debridement are presented elsewhere in this book.

Low adherent dressings/wound contact layers

Low adherent dressings are cheap and widely available. They tend to be advocated as primary dressings for use on lightly exuding or granulating wounds (**Figure 25.1**). Their major function is to allow exudate to pass through into a secondary dressing while maintaining a moist wound bed (**Figure 25.2**). They are traditionally manufactured in the form of tulles, which are open weave cloth soaked in soft paraffin or chlorhexidine; textiles; or multilayered or perforated plastic films. However, more recently developed products tend to use soft silicone, or combinations of hydrocolloid particles and petroleum jelly. These dressings are designed to reduce adherence at the wound bed and are particularly useful for patients with sensitive or fragile skin, although if tulle dressings are left in place for too long they can dry out allowing granulation tissue to grow into the weave of the dressing, resulting in trauma to the wound bed. A recent RCT found no difference, in terms of healing outcome, between a nonadherent dressing and more costly dressings (Jeffcoate et al. 2009).

Semipermeable films

Semipermeable films were one of the first major advances in wound management and heralded a major change in the way wounds were treated. They consist of sterile plastic sheets of polyurethane coated with hypoallergenic acrylic adhesive and are used mainly as a transparent primary wound cover. Although they are impermeable to fluids and bacteria, they are permeable to air and water vapor, the control of which is dependent on the moisture and vapor transmission rate, which varies depending on the brand. It is through this mechanism that a moist wound environment is created thus preventing the formation of a scab. Film dressings are primarily indicated for shallow wounds (**Figure 25.3**), their impermeability to environmental liquids enables patients to bath or shower without risk of contaminating the wound (Pudner 2001). Films are very flexible and are good for wounds on 'difficult' anatomical sites, e.g. over joints; however, they do not perform well in areas exposed to high levels of friction. Furthermore, they are unable to cope with large amounts of exudate and may cause maceration of the skin surrounding the wound bed if they are used injudiciously (Sehgal et al. 2009). As semipermeable films are transparent, when used as a primary dressing it is possible to inspect the wound bed without disturbing the dressing.

Hydrocolloids

Hydrocolloids were first introduced in Europe in the 1980s. They are primarily composed of carboxymethyl cellulose, gelatin, pectin, elastomers, and adhesives, which are bonded to a carrier of semipermeable film or a foam sheet to produce a flat, occlusive, adhesive dressing that forms a gel on the wound surface. Cross-linkage of the materials used influences the viscosity of the gel under the dressing. This gel, which may be yellow and malodorous, may be mistaken for infection by the inexperienced practitioner. Hydrocolloids are virtually impermeable to water vapor and air and as a result provide a moist wound environment, which can rehydrate dry necrotic eschar and promote autolytic debridement, granulation tissue formation, and epithelialization. Hydrocolloids are suitable

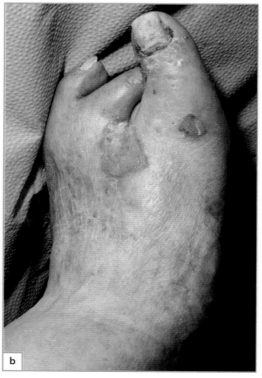

Figure 25.1
Flat, shallow wound, suitable for dressing with a semipermeable film or wound contact layer.

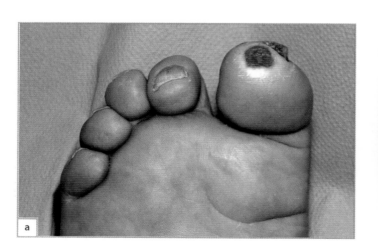

a

b

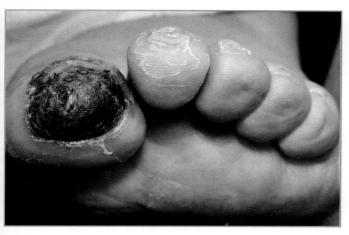

Figure 25.2 Dry gangrene, suitable for dressing with a low adherent dressing or wound contact layer.

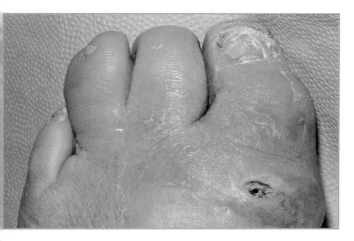

Figure 25.3 Cavity diabetic foot ulcers with no sinus, suitable for dressing with a foam, hydrocolloid, or alginate dressing.

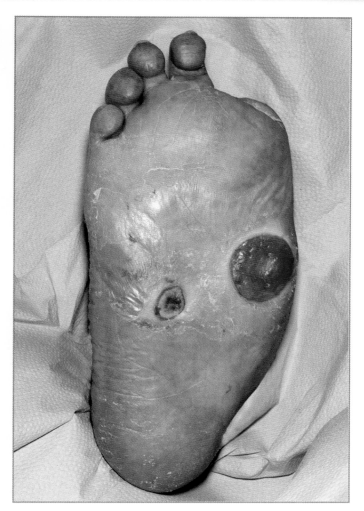

Figure 25.4 Shallow granulating diabetic foot ulcers, suitable for dressing with a semipermeable film, foam, or wound contact layer.

for clean, granulating wounds or sloughy/necrotic wounds but are principally indicated for low to moderately exuding wounds (**Figure 25.4**). They are reported to reduce wound pain, and their barrier properties allow the patient to bath or shower without disturbing or risking contamination of the wound. However, caution should be exercised when using hydrocolloids for wounds that require frequent inspection and there remains controversy as to whether they should be used on infected wounds (Hess 1999). Hydrocolloid fibers are available in the form of a hydrophilic, nonwoven flat sheet, referred to as hydrofiber dressings. On contact with exudate, fibers are converted from a dry dressing to a soft coherent gel sheet, making them suitable for wounds with large amounts of exudate. Unlike semipermeable films, their inherent conformability and adhesive properties ensure that they adhere well to areas subjected to high levels of friction.

Hydrogels

Hydrogels consist of a matrix of insoluble polymers with up to 96% water content enabling them to donate water molecules to the wound surface and to maintain a moist environment at the wound bed. As the polymers are only partially hydrated, hydrogels have the ability to absorb a degree of wound exudate, the amount varying between different brands. They transmit moisture vapor and oxygen, but their bacterial and fluid permeability is dependent on the type of secondary dressing used. Hydrogels should be changed regularly as they have a tendency to macerate the wound if left for too long. Hydrogels promote wound debridement by rehydration of nonviable tissue, thus facilitating the process of natural autolysis. Amorphous hydrogels are the most commonly used and are thick, viscous gels (Vermeulen et al. 2007). More recent developments include second-generation hydrogels, which have the capacity to absorb or donate water according to the needs of the wound (Moore 2006). Hydrogels are considered to be a standard form of management for sloughy or necrotic wounds (**Figures 25.5** and **25.6**). They are not indicated for wounds producing high levels of exudate or where there is evidence of gangrenous tissue, which should be kept dry to reduce the risk of infection. Hydrogels are also suited to the management of dry wounds but if a leathery eschar is present autolytic debridement is unlikely to occur as the protective enzymes are not delivered to the wound bed in the absence of exudates.

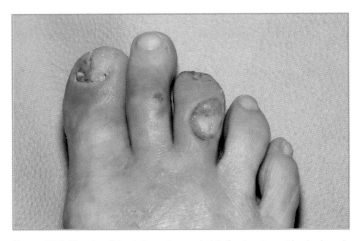

Figure 25.5 Sloughy diabetic foot ulcers, suitable for dressing with a hydrogel.

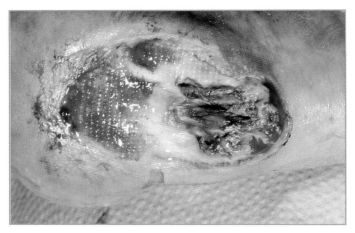

Figure 25.6 Mixed wound bed displaying areas of granulation tissue as well as sloughy/necrotic tissue, suitable for dressing with a hydrogel or hydrofiber.

Alginates

Alginates were discovered in the 1880s, when sailors would bind their wounds with seaweed to take advantage of the therapeutic properties of alginic acid. They are produced from the naturally occurring calcium and sodium salts of alginic acid found in a family of brown seaweed (Phaeophyceae). They generally fall into one of two kinds: those containing 100% calcium alginate or those that contain a combination of calcium with sodium alginate, usually in a ratio of 80:20. Alginates are rich in either mannuronic acid or guluronic acid, the relative amount of each influencing the amount of exudate absorbed and the shape the dressing will retain. Alginates partly dissolve on contact with wound fluid to form a hydrophilic gel as a result of the exchange of sodium ions in wound fluid for calcium ions in the dressing. Those high in mannuronic acid (such as Kaltostat) can be washed off the wound easily with saline, but those high in guluronic acid (such as Sorbsan) tend to retain their basic structure and should be removed from the wound bed in one piece. Alginates can absorb 15 to 20 times their weight of fluid, making them suitable for highly exuding wounds and those containing mannuronic acid also have hemolytic properties. They should not be used, however, on wounds with little or no exudate as they will adhere to the wound

surface, causing pain and damaging healthy tissue on removal. It is important that all alginate material be removed from a wound to avoid the risk of an inflammatory response (Stansfield 2000).

Foam dressings

Foam dressings are manufactured as either a polyurethane or silicone foam. They are popular due to their ease of application and capacity to satisfy many of the criteria for an ideal wound dressing. They transmit moisture vapor and oxygen and provide thermal insulation to the wound bed. Polyurethane foams consist of two or three layers, including a hydrophilic wound contact surface and a hydrophobic backing, making them highly absorbent. They facilitate uniform dispersion of exudate throughout the absorbent layer and prevent exterior leakage (strikethrough) due to the presence of a semipermeable backing. Polyurethane foam dressings are also available as cavity dressings. Silicone foams consist of a polymer of silicone elastomer derived from two liquids, which, when mixed together, form a foam while expanding to fit the wound shape forming a soft open-cell foam dressing. The major advantage of foam is the ability to contain exudate. In addition, silicone foam dressings protect the area around the wound from further damage. Foam dressings are more suited to wounds with low to moderate levels of exudate (**Figure 25.7**). Foams have a wide range of indications, they remove slough from the wound bed and can be used as secondary dressings. Other useful properties include their ability to conform to body contours, their cushioning properties, low adherence, lack of residue, and thermal insulation (Lohmann et al. 2004).

Antimicrobial dressings

The presence of bacteria in a chronic wound does not necessarily indicate that infection has occurred or that it will lead to impaired wound healing (Cooper & Lawrence 1996). Micro-organisms are present in all chronic wounds and low levels of certain bacteria can facilitate wound healing as they produce enzymes such as hyaluronidase, which contributes to wound debridement and stimulates neutrophils to release proteases (Stone 1980). However, the severe and detrimental effects that an infected DFU (**Figure 25.8**) can inflict on the patient with diabetes have resulted in a tendency for some clinicians to use antimicrobial and/or antibiotic therapy prophylactically for protracted periods of time. The increasing risk of antibiotic resistance, along with product development and education, has therefore resulted in increased interest in the topical use of antiseptics in wound care. At present the most popular topical applications are silver, iodine, polyhexamethylene biguanide (PHMB) and honey.

Silver, in ionic or nanocrystalline form, has for many years been used as an antimicrobial agent particularly in the treatment of burns (in the form of silver sulfadiazine cream). The development of dressings impregnated with silver has widened its use for many other wound types that are either colonized or infected. Much work remains to be done to establish silvers' in vivo efficacy as doubts remain about its clinical efficacy (Michaels et al. 2009); however, when used responsibly, silver has been shown to be of great clinical value.

Iodine also has the ability to lower the microbiological load in chronic wounds. Clinically, it is mainly used in one of two formats: as povidone-iodine (polyvinylpyrrolidone–iodine complex), which is an iodophor (a compound of iodine linked to a nonionic surfactant), produced as an impregnated tulle or as cadexomer iodine (a three-dimensional starch lattice containing 0.9% iodine). Cadexomer iodine has good absorptive properties; 1 g of cadexomer iodine can absorb

Game FL, Hinchcliffe RJ, Apelqvist J, et al. A systematic review of interventions to enhance the healing of chronic ulcers of the foot in diabetes. Diabetes/Metab Res Rev 2012; 28:119–141.

Gray D, Acton C, Chadwick P, et al. Consensus guidance for the use of debridement techniques in the UK. Wounds UK 2011; 7:77–84.

Greenhalgh DG. Wound healing and diabetes mellitus. Clin Plast Surg 2003; 30:37–45.

Hackam DJ, Ford HR. Cellular, biochemical and clinical aspects of wound healing. Surg Inf 2002; 3:S23–S35.

Henry G, Garner WL. Inflammatory mediators in wound healing. Surg Clin N Am 2003; 83:483–507.

Hess CT. When to use hydrocolloid dressings. Nursing 1999; 29:11,20.

Hilton JR, Williams DT, Beuker B, Miller DR, Harding KG. Wound dressings in diabetic foot disease. CID 2004; 39:S100–S103.

Hinchcliffe RJ, Valk GD, Apelquist J, et al. A systematic review of the effectiveness of interventions to enhance the healing of chronic ulcers of the foot in diabetes. Diabetes/Metabol Res Rev 2008; 24: S119–S144.

Hinman CD, Maibach H. Effect of air exposure and occlusion on experimental human skin wounds. Nature 1963; 200:377–378.

International Working Group on the Diabetic Foot (IWGDF). International Consensus on the Diabetic Foot, 2011. http://www.iwgdf.org (accessed 07 March, 2014).

Jeffcoate WJ, Price PE, Phillips CJ, et al. Randomised controlled trial of the use of three dressing preparations in the management of chronic ulceration of the foot in diabetes. Health Tech Assess 2009; 13:1–110.

Jensen JL, Seeley J, Gillin B. A controlled, randomized comparison of two moist wound healing protocols: Carrasyn hydrogel wound dressing and wet-to-moist saline gauze. Adv Wound Care 1998; 11:S1–S4.

Katz MH, Alvarez AF, Kirsner RS, et al. Human wound fluid from acute wounds stimulates fibroblasts and endothelial cell growth. J Am Acad Dermatol 1991; 25:1054–1058.

Lawrence JC. The use of iodine as an antiseptic agent. J Wound Care 1998; 7:421–425.

Lobmann R, Schultz G, Lehnert H. Proteases and the diabetic foot syndrome: mechanisms and therapeutic implications. Diabetes Care 2005; 28:461–471.

Lohmann M, Thomsen JK, Edmonds ME. Safety and performance of a new non-adhesive foam dressing for the treatment of diabetic foot ulcers. J Wound Care 2004; 13:118–120.

Mast BA, Schultz GS. Interactions of cytokines, growth factors and proteases in acute and chronic wounds. Wound Repair Regen 1996; 4:411–420.

McDonnell G, Russell AD. Antiseptics and disinfectants: activity, action and resistance. Clinical Microbiol Rev 1999; 12:147–179.

Michaels JA, Campbell B, King B, et al. Randomized controlled trial and cost-effectiveness analysis of silver-donating antimicrobial dressings for venous leg ulcers (VULCAN trial). Br J Surg 2009; 96:1147–1156.

Moore K. The interaction of a 'Second Generation' Hydrogel with the Chronic Wound Environment. Poster Presentation, EWMA, 2006. http://ewma.org/english/ewma-conferences/conference-abstracts/2006/2006-poster-abstracts.html

Odland G. The fine structure of the inter-relationship of cells in the human epidermis. J Biophys Biochem Cyto 1958; 4:529–535.

Pudner R. Vapour-permeable film dressings. J Commun Nurs 2001; 15:12.

Pyatt V. The use of larval therapy in modern wound care. Wounds Int 2011; 2(4) November. http://www.woundsinternational.com/product-reviews/the-use-of-larval-therapy-in-modern-wound-care (accessed 07 March, 2014).

Schultz G, Sibbald G, Falanga V, et al. Wound bed preparation: a systematic approach to wound management. Wound Repair Regen 2003; 11:1–28.

Sehgal PK, Sripriya R, Senthikumar M. Drug delivery dressings. In: Rajendran S (ed), Advanced textiles for wound care. Cambridge, UK: Woodhead Publishing, 2009.

Stansfield G. Managing wound exudates in the diabetic foot ulcer. Diabet Foot 2000; 3:93–98.

Stone LL. Bacterial debridement of the burn eschar: the in vivo activity of selected organisms. J Surg Res 1980; 29:83–92.

Thomas S. Wound management and dressings. London, United Kingdom: The Pharmaceutical Press, 1990.

Trengove NJ, Stacey MC, Macauley S, et al. 1999. Analysis of the acute and chronic wound environments: the role of proteases and their inhibitors. Wound Repair Regen 1980; 7:442–452.

Vandeputte J, Gryson L. Diabetic foot infection controlled by immuno-modulating hydrogel containing 65% glycerine. Presentation of a clinical trial. In: 6th European Conference on Advances in Wound Management. vol. 1997. Amsterdam, Netherlands, 1996:50–53.

Vermeulen H, Ubbink DT, de Zwart F, et al. Preferences of patients, doctors and nurses regarding wound dressing characteristics: a conjoint analysis. Wound Repair Regen 2007; 15:302–307.

White R, Cutting C. Critical colonisation of chronic wounds: microbial mechanisms. Wounds UK 2008; 4:70–78.

Winter G. Formation of the scab and the rate of epithelialisation of superficial wounds in the skin of the young domestic pig. Nature 1962; 193:293–294.

Wolcott RD, Kennedy JP, Dowd SE. Regular debridement is the main tool for maintaining a healthy wound bed in most chronic wounds. J Wound Care 2009; 18:54–56.

Woods EJ, Davis P, Barnett J, Percival SL. Wound healing immunology and biofilms. In: Percival S, Cutting K (eds), Microbiology of wounds. Boca Raton, FL: CRC Press, 2010.

Table 26.1 JADAD scoring of randomized clinical trials evaluating the effects of hyperbaric oxygen therapy in patients with diabetic foot ulcers

	Doctor et al. (1992)	Faglia et al. (1996)	Kessler (2003)	Abidia et al. (2003)	Duzgun et al. (2008)	Löndahl et al. (2010)
Randomization	Not described	Not described	Not described	Described	Described	Described
Conclusion	Number of patients in each group is not sure	Uncertain, due to high number of vascular interventions	Yes, but one patient excluded due to barotraumatic otitis	Yes, one patient in each group excluded before treatment	Yes	Yes, intention-to-treat and per-protocol
Blinding	No	Only surgeons	Blinded observer	Double-blinded	No	Double-blinded
Concomitant treatment	Unknown	Interventions post-HBO may interfere with outcome	Similar	Similar	Unknown	Similar
Baseline characteristics	Similar	Similar	Similar	Similar	Not similar	Similar
End point	Described; amputation	Described; amputation	Ulcer area reduction	Described; 1. Ulcer healing 2. Amputation	Healing without surgical intervention	Described; 1. Ulcer healing 2. Amputation
Time-frame	Unknown	Until healing or amputation	4 Weeks	1 Year	Until healing (?)	1 Year
Power	No analysis n=30	No analysis n=70	No analysis n=28	No analysis n=18	No analysis n=100	Estimation n=94
JADAD score	2	2	2	5	2	5

used normally. A Cochrane analysis concluded that this trial is at high risk of several potential confounding biases.

In 2010, Löndahl et al. published the outcome of a double-blind, controlled study comparing the effect of HBO with that of hyperbaric air (40 sessions, 90 minutes per session at 2.5 ATA) in 94 patients with diabetes and Wagner grade 2–4 foot lesions of at least 3 months duration (Löndahl et al. 2010). None of the patients were eligible for, nor had a need for, vascular surgical intervention at the time of inclusion, as assessed by a vascular surgeon. Healing rate curves diverged after only 2 months and at the 9- and 12-month follow-up visits, statistically significant differences in favor of HBO were present. At the 1-year follow-up visit, HBO doubled the number of healed ulcers compared with adjunctive treatment with hyperbaric air. In those patients fulfilling the predefined requisite of the per-protocol analysis (a complement of at least 36 out of 40 scheduled treatment sessions), 61% of all patients healed in the HBO group compared with 27% in the placebo group (P<0.01). During the first year of follow-up, vascular surgical interventions occurred in six HBO-treated and four placebo-treated patients, but these endovascular interventions could not explain the higher ulcer healing rate in the HBO group as only three ulcers, one of them in the placebo group, healed following endovascular intervention. No differences in major or minor amputations were seen between groups during the first year of follow-up. Data from RCTs suggest that HBO improves health-related quality of life in patients with chronic diabetic foot ulcers (Londahl 2013).

Health economics

Health economic data are sparsely reported in the randomized clinical trials that have been conducted to dat, but a crude analysis of the study by Abidia et al., taking only HBO and dressing costs into account, suggests a saving of approximately 3300 Euros per patient during the first year of follow-up (Abidia et al. 2003).

Recommendations

When pooling data from all randomized clinical trials, the Cochrane Collaboration could not identify any significant benefit from HBO beyond improved ulcer healing at 6 weeks (Kranke et al. 2012). However, due to differences in study designs and populations, the Cochrane Collaboration stated that this analysis should be interpreted with caution. As there is a large heterogeneity between the randomized studies and their study populations, it might be most appropriate to let every study stand for itself, and avoid data pooling. This approach is supported by the International Working Group on the Diabetic Foot which, in their latest guidelines, concluded that: 'new studies provide further evidence that the use of systemic hyperbaric oxygen therapy may increase the incidence of healing and improve the long-term outcome – even though further blinded studies are required to confirm its cost-effectiveness and identify the population most likely to benefit' (Game et al. 2012).

Indications and contraindications

Based on the inclusion criteria of the two published double-blind, randomized clinical studies, the following selection criteria for HBO treatment can be suggested:
- Diabetic full-thickness ulcers not healing despite the best available care in a multidisciplinary foot clinic setting for at least 6 weeks (Abidia et al. 2003) or 3 months (Löndahl et al. 2010)
- No need for, or unsuitable (technically) for revascularization
- Capacity and ability to complete an HBO session series
- No contraindications for HBO

The only absolute contraindications for HBO are untreated pneumothorax, ongoing treatment with some chemotherapeutic agents, and any history of treatment with bleomycin. Relative contraindications include sinusitis, severe chronic obstructive pulmonary disease, history of pneumothorax or thoracic surgery, uncontrolled high fever, claustrophobia, upper respiratory infection, and an inability to equalize pressure in the middle ear. The inability to equalize middle ear pressure could be ameliorated by tympanostomy with tube placement.

Complications

HBO has several potential side effects, but compared with many other medical therapies, HBO may be considered as a relatively safe treatment. Among the most commonly reported complications is barotrauma. Barotrauma may occur where tissues and gases interface within the body. In clinical practice, middle ear barotrauma dominates. In a large case series including >11,000 treatment sessions, 17% of patients reported ear pain or discomfort during compression (Kranke et al. 2012). However, persistent injuries visible on ear microscopy were less common with reported incidences between 0.5% and 3.8% (Löndahl et al. 2010, Plafki et al. 2000, Sheffield 2002).

Reversible myopia, due to oxygen toxicity of the lens, is a common side effect affecting up to one in five patients. Visual acuity usually returns to the pretreatment level within 2 months after the last HBO session. Patients with diabetes mellitus, especially those on insulin therapy, are at increased risk of hypoglycemia. The highest risk appears within 2–6 hours after the HBO session.

An oxygen seizure is a very rare complication, occurring in approximately 1 case per 10,000 treatments. It may be foreshadowed by other symptoms of cerebral oxygen toxicity such as nausea and vomiting, dizziness, tinnitus, tunnel vision, anxiety, and muscle twitching, but in half of cases, generalized seizures begin without any warning signs. These convulsions are self-limiting after stopping oxygen administration and do not have any long-term implications. Prolonged exposures to oxygen may cause pneumonitis and alveolitis, but the consequences of pulmonary oxygen toxicity are not present in the clinical usage of HBO. The most common fatal complication of HBO is associated with fire in the chamber.

Practical considerations

Two different kinds of hyperbaric chambers, monoplace and multiplace chambers, are clinically available. A monoplace hyperbaric chamber is generally made of acrylic material to permit direct patient observation. The cylinder is either pressurized entirely with oxygen or with air, patients breathing oxygen through a mask. Multiplace chambers are typically steel constructions in which two or more patients are pressurized. For safety reasons (fire hazards), the ambient gas is pressurized with air and patients breathe oxygen via hoods or masks.

Robust evidence is lacking for selection of the treatment regimen leading to optimal therapeutic benefit (i.e. hyperbaric pressure level, duration of treatment sessions, number of HBO sessions, and not least the timing of HBO). Patients with diabetic foot ulcers are usually treated once daily at pressures between 2.0 and 2.5 ATA (Londahl et al. 2011). A typical treatment session usually includes 80–90 minutes of oxygen breathing. Another 5–10 minutes per session is generally required for compression and decompression. If a patient experiences discomfort during a session, compression can be intermittently arrested. To minimize the risk of oxygen toxicity – a rare but severe complication of HBO – periods of breathing 100% oxygen may be separated by one or two 5-minute long intervals of air breathing. A typical treatment protocol consists of 30–40 treatment sessions (Londahl et al. 2011).

AREAS OF CONTROVERSY AND/OR FUTURE RESEARCH

- Larger and better designed RCTs (with blinding) are required to confirm the effectiveness of NPWT and HBO in patients with diabetic foot ulcers
- The most clinically effective negative pressure level and cycle required for different types of wounds (particularly ischemic vs. nonischemic) remains to be determined
- More research is required on the most appropriate and effective wound filler in patients undergoing NPWT
- More data is required to confirm the clinical effectiveness and, importantly, the cost-effectiveness of patients with diabetic foot ulcers undergoing HBO
- The group of patients with diabetic foot ulcers most likely to benefit from HBO requires identification

IMPORTANT FURTHER READING

Armstrong DG, Lavery LA, Diabetic Foot Study C. Negative pressure wound therapy after partial diabetic foot amputation: a multicentre, randomised controlled trial. Lancet 2005; 366:1704–1710.

Blume P, Walters J, Payne W, et al. Comparison of negative pressure wound therapy using vacuum-assisted closure with advanced moist wound therapy in the treatment of diabetic foot ulcers: a multicenter randomized controlled trial. Diabetes Care 2008; 31:631–636.

Game FL, Hinchliffe RJ, Apelqvist J, et al. A systematic review of interventions to enhance the healing of chronic ulcers of the foot in diabetes. Diabetes Metab Res Rev 2012; 28:119–141.

Game FL, Hinchliffe RJ, Apelqvist J, et al. Specific guidelines on wound and wound-bed management 2011. Diabetes Metab Res Rev 2012; 28:232–233.

Londahl M, Katzman P, Nilsson A, et al. Hyperbaric oxygen therapy facilitates healing of chronic foot ulcers in patients with diabetes. Diabetes Care 2010; 33:998–1003.

REFERENCES

Abidia A, Laden G, Kuhan G, et al. The role of hyperbaric oxygen therapy in ischaemic diabetic lower extremity ulcers: a double-blind randomised-controlled trial. Eur J Vasc Endovasc Surg 2003; 25:513–518.

Argenta LC, Morykwas MJ, Marks MW, et al. Vacuum-assisted closure: state of clinic art. Plast Reconstr Surg 2006; 117:127S–142S.

Armstrong DG, Lavery LA, Diabetic Foot Study C. Negative pressure wound therapy after partial diabetic foot amputation: a multicentre, randomised controlled trial. Lancet 2005; 366:1704–1710.

Birke-Sorensen H, Malmsjo M, Rome P, et al. Evidence-based recommendations for negative pressure wound therapy: Treatment variables (pressure levels, wound filler and contact layer). Steps towards an international consensus. J Plast Reconstr Aesthet Surg 2011; 64:S1–S16.

Blume P, Walters J, Payne W, et al. Comparison of negative pressure wound therapy using vacuum-assisted closure with advanced moist wound therapy in the treatment of diabetic foot ulcers: a multicenter randomized controlled trial. Diabetes Care 2008; 31:631–636.

Borgquist O, Ingemansson R, Malmsjo M. The influence of low and high pressure levels during negative-pressure wound therapy on wound contraction and fluid evacuation. Plast Reconstr Surg 2011; 127:551–559.

Chariker M, Jeter K, Tintle T, et al. Effective management of incisional and cutaneous fistulae with closed suction wound drainage. Contemp Surg 1989; 34:59–63.

Doctor N, Pandya S, Supe A. Hyperbaric oxygen therapy in diabetic foot. J Postgrad Med 1992; 38:112–114, 111.

Dumville JC, Hinchliffe RJ, Cullum N, et al. Negative pressure wound therapy for treating foot wounds in people with diabetes mellitus. Cochrane Database Syst Rev 2013; 10:CD010318.

Duzgun AP, Satir HZ, Ozozan O, et al. Effect of hyperbaric oxygen therapy on healing of diabetic foot ulcers. J Foot Ankle Surg 2008; 47:515–519.

Faglia E, Favales F, Aldeghi A, et al. Adjunctive systemic hyperbaric oxygen therapy in treatment of severe prevalently ischemic diabetic foot ulcer. A randomized study. Diabetes Care 1996; 19:1338–1343.

Game FL, Hinchliffe RJ, Apelqvist J, et al. A systematic review of interventions to enhance the healing of chronic ulcers of the foot in diabetes. Diabetes Metab Res Rev 2012; 28:119–141.

Game FL, Hinchliffe RJ, Apelqvist J, et al. Specific guidelines on wound and wound-bed management 2011. Diabetes Metab Res Rev 2012; 28:232–233.

Glass G, Nanchahal J. The methodology of negative pressure wound therapy: Separating fact from fiction. J Plast Reconstr Aesthet Surg 2012; 65:989–1001.

Glass GE, Nanchahal J. The methodology of negative pressure wound therapy: separating fact from fiction. J Plast Reconstr Aesthet Surg 2012; 65:989–1001.

Hinchliffe RJ, Valk GD, Apelqvist J, et al. A systematic review of the effectiveness of interventions to enhance the healing of chronic ulcers of the foot in diabetes. Diabetes Metab Res Rev 2008; 24:S119–144.

Hunt TK, Linsey M, Grislis H, et al. The effect of differing ambient oxygen tensions on wound infection. Ann Surg 1975; 181:35–39.

Hunt TK, Pai MP. The effect of varying ambient oxygen tensions on wound metabolism and collagen synthesis. Surg Gynecol Obstet 1972; 135:561–567.

Jadad AR, Moore RA, Carroll D, et al. Assessing the quality of reports of randomized clinical trials: is blinding necessary? Control Clin Trials 1996; 17:1–12.

Kloth LC. 5 questions-and-answers-about negative pressure wound therapy. Adv Skin Wound Care 2002; 15:226–229.

Knighton DR, Silver IA, Hunt TK. Regulation of wound-healing angiogenesis-effect of oxygen gradients and inspired oxygen concentration. Surgery 1981; 90:262–270.

Kranke P, Bennett MH, Martyn-St James M, et al. Hyperbaric oxygen therapy for chronic wounds. Cochrane Database Syst Rev 2012; 4:CD004123.

Krogh A. The number and distribution of capillaries in muscles with calculations of the oxygen pressure head necessary for supplying the tissue. J Physiol 1919; 52:409–415.

Londahl M, Fagher K, Katzman P. What is the role of hyperbaric oxygen in the management of diabetic foot disease? Curr Diab Rep 2011; 11:285–293.

Löndahl M, Katzman P, Nilsson A, et al. Hyperbaric oxygen therapy facilitates healing of chronic foot ulcers in patients with diabetes. Diabetes Care 2010; 33:998–1003.

Londahl M. Hyperbaric oxygen therapy as adjunctive treatment of diabetic foot ulcers. Med Clin North Am 2013; 97:957–980.

Morykwas MJ, Argenta LC, Shelton-Brown EI, et al. Vacuum-assisted closure: a new method for wound control and treatment: animal studies and basic foundation. Ann Plast Surg 1997; 38:553–562.

Plafki C, Peters P, Almeling M, et al. Complications and side effects of hyperbaric oxygen therapy. Aviat Space Environ Med 2000; 71:119–124.

Sheffield PJ, Smith APS. Physiological and pharmacological basis of hyperbaric oxygen therapy. In: Bakker DJ, Cramer FS (eds). Hyperbaric surgery. Flagstaff, AZ: Best Publishing Company, 2002: 63–109.

Tibbles PM, Edelsberg JS. Hyperbaric-oxygen therapy. N Engl J Med 1996; 334:1642–1648.

Chapter 27

Standardization of outcomes and end points of wound healing in everyday practice and clinical trials

Finn Gottrup

SUMMARY

- Evidence-based medicine (EBM) uses the current best evidence in making decisions about the care of individual patients and health-care procedures and technologies

- The gold standard for optimal evidence in the Cochrane system is level I – randomized controlled trials (RCTs), and meta-analyses of several RCTs. In order to achieve this level of evidence, one of the most important measures is the use of standardized outcomes/ end points

- Consistency in measuring end points/outcomes improves quality of care. To achieve such consistency, it is important to:

  - Use predefined and robust outcomes

  - Adapt outcomes to the intervention under investigation

  - Use the best evidence available

- Using complete wound closure or healing as an outcome measure is not always possible or suitable. Adopting a 'patient focus' clarifies which other end points are relevant

- 'Basic care' must be clearly defined and standardized when used as a comparative intervention in an RCT

INTRODUCTION

Nonhealing wounds are a significant problem for health-care systems all over the world. In the industrialized world, up to 1.5% of the population has a problem wound at any one time and these account for 2–4% of the health-care budget – a figure that is likely to rise in a population of increasing age and diabetes prevalence (Dale 1983, Liu et al. 1991, Gottrup 2004). For these reasons, there is an urgent need to review wound strategies and treatments in order to reduce the burden of care in an efficient and cost-effective way. A primary question is which of the available interventions, technologies, and dressing materials achieve the best outcomes for the best value? To be able to answer this question health-care professionals are expected to keep up-to-date and to apply research evidence in their daily practice. Ideally, the evidence-based practice (EBP) paradigm promotes evidence-based treatment choices in clinical practice, preferably derived from proper systematic reviews or well-performed RCTs. However, 30–40% of patients receive care that is not in accordance with best available research evidence and 20–30% of patients receive care that is contraindicated (Schuster et al. 1998). Furthermore, guideline recommendations are only followed for two-thirds of treatments (Grol 2001). Therefore, it is apparent that EBP paradigm is not routinely adopted by most health-care professionals in everyday clinical

practice (Knops et al. 2009). This is particularly the case in wound care, where confusion exists about the various treatments available (Gottrup 2009, Bell-Syer et al. 2009, Gottrup 2012). The result has been that most systematic reviews in the wound area have a substantial deficiency in the quality of clinical research. This is primarily due to a lack of high-quality primary research evidence, the studies often being based on inadequate sample size, short follow-up, nonrandom allocation to treatment arms, nonblinded assessment of outcomes, and poor description of control and concurrent intervention.

Quality of evidence in wound management is, however, important in several ways: From the clinical perspective the question is which interventions, technologies, and dressing materials are the best from the point of view of a single patient or group of patients, where the primary focus is healing and the absence of complications (as well as patient satisfaction). From the policy maker and health-care system perspectives, two issues arise: (1) whether or not a particular product or intervention is safe and effective when used as indicated – this is a question of regulatory approval and (2) whether or not the product or intervention represents a cost-effective use of funds.

Too few good quality clinical or economic studies in wound care have resulted in challenges to the reimbursement of modern dressings in favor of supposedly better value traditional products. From the industry perspective (medical device industry), the challenge is that the standard of care and evidence requirements for reimbursement are different in each country and that the large investments related to RCTs are rarely justified by the pace of innovation and size of markets of most wound care products.

The end points or outcomes of a study are the keystone when discussing the evidence of an intervention. Therefore, the European Wound Management Association (EWMA) set up a Patient Outcome Group (Gottrup 2009) to address these challenges. This group has produced a survey document, focusing on precise outcomes in both RCTs and clinical studies (Gottrup et al. 2010), and this document furthermore describes how to ensure that studies are consistent and reproducible. This chapter is a summary of the content of this survey document (Gottrup et al. 2010).

To date, the obvious outcome measure in evaluating interventions in wound healing has been complete healing. However, this may not be the only appropriate outcome in wound healing studies. Other end points including clinical, intermediate, and surrogate outcomes (such as infection rate, bacterial contamination, wound pain, resource utilization, and cost) may also need to be considered. For this reason, the aim of this chapter is to provide recommendations and guidance on how to achieve rigorous end points/outcomes in studies on wound management and to describe an approach that will enable the design of RCTs and clinical studies to be both consistent and reproducible in order to reach a higher quality of evidence in wound management. These recommendations should provide a framework for clinicians, policy makers, and industry-related research.

BACKGROUND, DEFINITIONS OF OUTCOME/END POINT, AND PRODUCING RECOMMENDATIONS

The background information, evaluations, and recommendations of the EWMA survey document are based on a large amount of available guidance for evidence collection and an analysis of recent RCTs and comparative studies (Gottrup et al. 2010). An updated status on how end points/outcome parameters were used, defined, and evaluated was achieved by a literature search of RCTs, the Cochrane Library, MEDLINE, and Embase from 2003 to 2009 studying chronic or problem wounds or ulcers. The end points used were evaluated and examined for quality of definitions and the robustness of methodology. Controlled randomized or nonrandomized clinical or preclinical studies qualified for inclusion in the analysis, if they reported a measured end point or outcome of any aspect of wound management. Reviews, opinion papers, and case reports were excluded.

An end point/outcome parameter is defined as the objective of an evaluation or study (FDA 2006, Biomarkers Definitions Working Group 2001, Matousek et al. 2007). The objectives should include a precise statement of the degree of benefit expected from the intervention and its duration; moreover, it should include clear statements on the time frame of the study (especially in relation to how quickly the benefits might start) and a definition of the patients for whom the benefit is sought. Objectives can be classified as either primary or secondary. Primary objectives provide the focus of the study. The collection and measurement of outcomes affecting the primary objective are critical and, if resources are scarce, this takes priority over any other, secondary, outcomes. An exception is the collection of safety information, which is always considered a high priority, regardless of whether or not safety is the focus of the study. It is crucial to minimize missing data relating to the primary objective. Secondary objectives allow for the investigation of subsidiary questions that, while scientifically important, do not have the same priority of clinical interest in the patient group being studied. In most randomized trials, the efficacy of the intervention or its equivalence with standard care is the primary objective, whereas safety (e.g. toxicity and side effects) is usually a secondary objective. As with objectives, the outcomes of a trial require precise description and definition.

In the past, the most commonly used clinical outcome in trials was visible reduction in wound size, particularly restoration of intact skin (full healing). The development of tests and techniques to improve tissue sampling and analysis, imaging technology, and scientific progress in cellular and molecular biology has enabled the development of more 'objective' wound outcome parameters such as transepidermal water loss for re-epithelialization (Hinman & Maibach 1963) and surrogate outcome parameters that relate to both the wound condition and the treatment intervention being assessed. Examples of objective measures of the wound condition that can be used as outcome include exudation rate (Gelfand et al. 2002), pain (Arnold et al. 1994), granulation rate (Romanelli 1997), and resolution of necrosis (Romanelli 1997) or infection (Gardner et al. 2001). Another example of an objective measure of a treatment intervention is the operational

definition of moist wound healing in terms of dressing moisture vapor transmission rate (Bolton 2007).

A surrogate end point/outcome parameter is defined as a physical sign or a laboratory measurement that can be used as a substitute for a clinically meaningful end point, measuring how a patient feels, functions, or survives (Prentice 1998, Cohn 2004). The challenge, in nonhealing wounds, is that end points/outcome parameters such as complete wound closure are difficult to achieve and maintain. If the only gold standard was total wound closure, efficacious therapies capable of hastening partial wound closure, or preparing wounds for successful grafting may never be considered. Alternative clinical or surrogate end points are therefore needed. The term 'intermediate' end point has also been used, e.g. to describe a relative change in wound area. However, the present document uses the terms surrogate and clinical end points.

The recommendations from the author panel in the survey document (Gottrup et al. 2010) addressed the following:

1. Study design to optimize wound care intervention or product safety and efficacy
2. Industry requirements to optimize product development, registration, and reimbursement
3. Operational definitions of 'standard care' including management of underlying disease

From the clinical research perspective, there is a need to be aware of the strengths and limitations of different study designs in order to effectively evaluate which health-care practices are worth considering for different patients in different health contexts. Key issues are, e.g. the use of a study protocol, problems related to heterogeneity of the study population, and underlying conditions. From an industry perspective, external evidence needs are set up by the requirements of national regulatory and reimbursement authorities, and other payers. When developing a new product, there are also internal needs for evidence, which mirror the phases of the development process. When focusing on payment or reimbursement for a new product, the key issue will often be budgetary impact and/or cost-effectiveness, rather than healing.

The EWMA survey document also discusses the importance of a generally accepted definition of 'standard care' in connection with data collection in wound management. 'Standard care' refers to generally accepted wound care procedures and the management of underlying disease outside of the investigational product/device or drug that will be used in the clinical trial/evaluation. It is essential that the standard care procedures/regimens used are consistent as this will minimize variability and enable assessment of the treatment effect.

OUTCOMES USED IN WOUND HEALING STUDIES

Studies published before 2003 are described by Matousek et al. (2007) and between 2003 and 2009 by the EWMA Patient Outcome Group (Gottrup et al. 2010). After a systematic literature search, abstracts from RCTs and comparative studies were evaluated, identifying 176 articles that qualified for analysis. Many studies measured multiple end points – in total, this analysis generated a list of 313 different end points. The most often found end points are described in **Box 27.1**.

The findings of the analysis were used as a basis for discussing and suggesting procedures for the successful measurement of each type of end point categories defined. In general, it was found that a substantial number of end points (45%) were either not predefined or insufficiently defined. As part of the analysis, the degree of

SURGICAL INTERVENTION

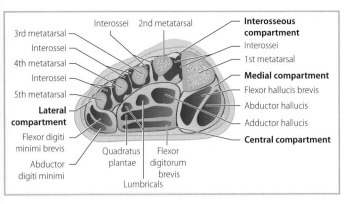

3rd metatarsal
Interossei
4th metatarsal
Interossei
5th metatarsal
Lateral compartment
Flexor digiti minimi brevis
Abductor digiti minimi
Quadratus plantae
Lumbricals
Flexor digitorum brevis
Interossei   2nd metatarsal
Interosseous compartment
Interossei
1st metatarsal
Medial compartment
Flexor hallucis brevis
Abductor hallucis
Adductor hallucis
Central compartment

Figure 28.7 The four-foot compartments and their contents.

The lateral compartment is bound by the plantar fascia superficially and laterally, an intermuscular septum medially and the 5th metatarsal dorsally. Contained in this compartment are the abductor digiti minimi and flexor digiti minimi brevis. The interosseous compartment is bound by the interosseous fascia between metatarsals. Contained within this compartment are the seven interosseous muscles.

Knowledge of these compartments is important in cases of trauma or infection where fracture and/or soft tissue injury may give rise to swelling and raised pressure within these compartments resulting in compartment syndrome. Muscle necrosis and eventually contracture can result from this and is a common complication of the diabetic foot. However, these compartments to some degree may contain and limit spread of infection, particularly if extraosseous.

LAYERS OF THE PLANTAR ASPECT OF THE FOOT

The muscles and tendons on the plantar aspect of the foot are arranged in layers. Knowledge of these layers and what is found at what depth can aid in the identification of structures when debriding plantar foot ulcers as well as when performing other surgical procedures on the foot. The contents of these individual layers are identified here from superficial to deep.

The 1st layer

Found in the most superficial layer are abductor hallucis, FDB and abductor digiti minimi. Abductor hallucis lies on the medial border of the foot covering the plantar nerves and vessels as they enter the foot. Indeed, the fascia overlying this muscle can occasionally be a cause of nerve compression and is often released as part of a tarsal tunnel decompression. This muscle arises from the medial process of the calcaneal tuberosity, laciniate ligament, plantar fascia, and intermuscular septum between it and FDB. Its tendon inserts together with the medial tendon of FHB into the plantar medial base of the hallux. Rarely, a slip to the base of the 2nd toe can be found.

The FDB occupies the middle of the foot and is found immediately deep to the central plantar fascia to which it is also attached. The lateral plantar neurovascular structures pass immediately deep to this muscle. It arises from the calcaneal tuberosity, plantar fascia, and intermuscular septae and then splits into four tendons for each of the lesser toes. At the level of the proximal phalanx, these tendons

divide to allow FDL to pass through them. The two slips insert into the sides of their corresponding middle phalanx. Rarely, the tendon to the little toe can be absent. It acts to flex the toes at the proximal IP joint.

Abductor digiti minimi makes up the lateral border of the foot. It arises from the lateral side of the calcaneal tuberosity, plantar fascia, and intermuscular septum. Its tendon inserts into the plantar lateral base of the 5th toe proximal phalanx along with flexor digiti minimi brevis tendon. It acts to plantarflex and abduct the 5th toe.

The plantar neurovascular bundles lie between the 1st and 2nd layers of the foot. Here, they are protected from the forces of ambulation and possible injury, but they are still able to reach all the structures they supply.

The 2nd layer

Flexor digitorum longus, FHL, quadratus plantae, and the lumbricals are found in the 2nd layer.

The FDL originates from the posterior surface of the tibia, passes behind the medial malleolus, and splits into four tendons just distal to the knot of Henry. These tendons insert into the bases of their respective distal phalanges of the lesser toes after passing through the bifurcation of FDB. It acts to flex the lesser toes at both IP joints.

The FHL originates from the inferior two thirds of the posterior surface of the fibula and adjacent interosseous membrane. It passes behind the medial malleolus, crosses FDL at the knot of Henry, and inserts into the base of the hallux distal phalanx. There are often commissures or slips of tendon around the knot of Henry connecting FHL and FDL. FHL acts to flex the hallux at the IP joint.

The lateral plantar vessels and nerves separate quadratus plantae from the muscles of the 1st layer. It has two heads at its origin from the calcaneus and inserts onto the lateral margin of FDL. It usually sends slips to FDL tendons travelling to the 2nd, 3rd, and 4th toes. It functions to keep tension in FDL and assists in flexion of the DIP joints of the lesser toes. It reorientates the FDL tendons and makes their pull less oblique and more longitudinal.

The lumbricals are four small muscles arising from the tendons of FDL. They become tendons inserting into the medial side of the extensor expansion of the lesser toes. Because they pass plantar to the axis of rotation of the MTP joints, they cause plantarflexion of the toes at the MTP joint and extension at the IP joints.

The 3rd layer

Flexor hallucis brevis, adductor hallucis, and flexor digiti minimi brevis are found in the 3rd layer.

The FHB has its origins from the plantar surface of the cuboid and lateral cuneiform. As it reaches the 1st MTP joint, it divides into two tendons incorporating a sesamoid bone each and inserts into the medial and lateral sides of the hallux proximal phalanx. It acts to flex the hallux at the MTP joint.

Adductor hallucis has two heads, an oblique head and a transverse head. The oblique head arises from the bases of the 2nd, 3rd, and 4th metatarsals and is a thick muscle occupying the space underneath these bones. Its tendon joins with the lateral tendon of FHB inserting into the lateral base of the hallux proximal phalanx. The transverse head originates from the plantar MTP ligaments of the 3rd, 4th, and 5th toes. Its tendon merges with that of the oblique head to insert into the lateral base proximal phalanx of the hallux. It acts to adduct and plantarflex the hallux.

Flexor digiti minimi brevis arises from the base of the 5th metatarsal and the sheath of peroneus longus. It inserts into the lateral base proximal phalanx of the 5th toe plantarflexing and abducting it.

The 4th layer

Tibialis posterior, peroneus longus, and the interossei are found in the deepest (4th) layer. Tibialis posterior arises from the posterior interosseous membrane and fibula as well as the proximal tibia. It passes behind the medial malleolus, and after crossing the spring ligament, it divides into two slips. The superficial slip inserts into the navicular tuberosity and the deeper slip inserts into the plantar aspect of the cuneiforms and lesser metatarsal bases. It acts to invert the foot and maintain the medial longitudinal arch.

Peroneus longus arises from the proximal two-thirds fibula shaft and adjacent intermuscular septum. It inserts into the plantar lateral base of the 1st metatarsal. It acts to evert the foot and plantarflex the 1st metatarsal.

The interossei are divided into two groups, plantar and dorsal. They are arranged functionally around the midline of the 2nd metatarsal. The four bipennate dorsal interossei lie between the metatarsals, arising from the adjacent sides of the metatarsals between which they are situated. The 1st and 2nd dorsal interossei insert into the medial and lateral base 2nd toe proximal phalanx, respectively. The 3rd and 4th dorsal interossei insert into the lateral bases of their respective proximal phalanges. They also have insertions into the extensor expansion of the toes. They act to abduct the lesser toes with respect to the second toe. The three plantar interossei lie beneath the 3rd, 4th, and 5th metatarsals and originate from them. Their tendons insert into the medial base proximal phalanx of the 3rd, 4th, and 5th toes adducting them with respect to the 2nd metatarsal. Like their dorsal counterparts they also have insertions into the extensor apparatus of the lesser toes. Because both sets of interossei tendons pass plantar to the axis of rotation of the MTP joints, they act to plantarflex the digits at the MTP joints and extend at the IP joints.

The interossei and lumbricals counteract the action of the long flexor and extensors. Neuropathic patients with intrinsic muscle weakness have deficiency of this action, resulting in an imbalance with relative overpowering by the long flexors and extensors. This results in dorsiflexion at the MTP joints due to the long extensors and flexion at the IP joints due to the long flexors. Over time, this results in a fixed claw toe deformity.

■ IMPORTANT FURTHER READING

Armstrong DG, Lavery LA. Clinical care of the diabetic foot, 2nd edn. Alexandria, VA: American Diabetes Association, 2010.

Garcia-Diaz JB, Pankey GA, Gentry LO. Contemporary diagnosis and management of diabetic foot infections. Longboat Key, FL: Handbooks in Health Care Company, 2006.

Kelikien AK, Sarrafian SK. Sarrafian's anatomy of the foot and ankle: descriptive topographic, functional, 3rd edn. Philadelphia, PA: Lippincott Williams & Wilkins, 2011.

Nather A. The diabetic foot. Singapore: World Scientific, 2012.

Perry J. Gait analysis: normal and pathological function. Thorofare, NJ: Slack Inc., 1992.

Zgonis T. Surgical reconstruction of the diabetic foot and ankle. Philadelphia, PA: Lippincott Williams & Wilkins, 2009.

■ REFERENCES

Rogers AW. Textbook of anatomy. London, United Kingdom: Churchill Livingstone, 1992.

Siegler S, Chen J, Schneck CD. The three dimensional kinematics and flexibility characteristics of the human ankle and subtalar joints – Part I: kinematics. J Biomech Eng 1988;110:364–373.

Simpson SL, Hertzog MS, Barja RH. The plantaris tendon graft: an ultrasound study. J Hand Surg Am 1991;16:708–711.

Wrobel JS, Najafi B. Diabetic foot biomechanics and gait dysfunction. J Diabetes Sci Technol 2010;4:833–845.

Wülker N, Stukenborg C, Savory KM, Alfke D. Hindfoot motion after isolated and combined arthrodeses: measurements in anatomic specimens. Foot Ankle Int 2000;21:921–927.

Chapter 29 | Surgical debridement

Peter Vowden, Soroush Sohrabi

SUMMARY

- Surgical debridement is an emergency in patients with severe foot sepsis and saves limbs
- A detailed knowledge of the anatomy of the foot and surgical training is required to achieve the best results
- Although surgical debridement remains the gold standard, newer debridement techniques have evolved including hydrosurgery and ultrasound
- There are few data at present to compare the effectiveness of these techniques with standard sharp surgical debridement
- The frequency of debridement any wound requires is variable and dependent upon clinical judgment and overall wound progress

INTRODUCTION

Debridement is the removal of devitalized, contaminated, or foreign material from within or adjacent to a wound, until surrounding healthy tissue is exposed. It is widely practised in diabetic foot care. Diabetic foot debridement may consist of the removal of skin, including regions with hyperkeratosis (callus), soft tissue, bone, or tendon. Furthermore, it may be part of minor amputation where a digit or ray is excised as part of the debridement procedure.

This process also removes colonizing bacteria, aids granulation tissue formation, and re-epithelialization, reduces pressure at callused sites, facilitates the collection of appropriate specimens for culture, and permits examination for the presence of deep tissue (especially bone) involvement. The goal is to enable wound healing and to remove a reservoir of potential pathogens (Lipsky et al. 2012).

Debridement can usually be undertaken as a clinic or bedside procedure and without anesthesia, although patients who do not have a loss of protective sensation may require local, regional, or general anesthesia. If the wound is extensive, there is adherent eschar, or the patient finds the procedure too painful, it may be best to conduct the debridement in a stepwise manner over several days. Wounds needing deeper or more extensive debridement, however, may require surgery in a sterile operative theater environment (Lipsky et al. 2012).

Debridement may be relatively contraindicated in wounds that are primarily ischemic. However, the decision to debride in the presence of ischemia should take into account the management of sepsis as described in the following section.

Primary debridement should aim to resect all nonviable tissue and whenever possible should be undertaken in such a way as to preserve foot function. Tissue specimens, including resected bone margins, should be sent for bacterial culture and results used to optimize subsequent antibiotic therapy. Plantar skin should be conserved wherever possible and the debrided wound designed to prevent accumulation of exudate in the wound bed, taking note of the likely foot position after surgery.

After primary debridement regular and careful wound review is required. Wound care is directed at achieving rapid cover to any exposed bone or tendon and may require integration of advanced techniques, including negative pressure wound therapy with further debridement undertaken if necessary, or the use of skin substitutes or plastic surgical procedure to restore skin cover. Careful use of off-loading both during the acute phase and during subsequent foot management is important if long-term limb salvage is to be achieved.

METHODS OF DEBRIDEMENT

Surgical sharp debridement using a scalpel or a curette is considered the optimal method for rapidly cleansing the ulcer and converting it in effect to an acute wound (see Chapter 23); however, it can be painful, and not all practitioners are trained or permitted to perform such procedures. Other mechanical forms of debridement, which include pulse lavage, ultrasound disruption of debris, and high-pressure water jet dissection of the wound surface, have been suggested as alternative methods of debridement (Cardinal et al. 2009).

TIMING

Diabetic foot management is an on-going process linked to careful monitoring of the intact and at-risk foot. Many diabetic foot infections require surgical debridement, ranging from minor procedures such as drainage and excision of infected and necrotic tissues with minor amputations to major procedures including reconstruction of soft tissue or bony defects, revascularization of the lower extremity, or even lower limb amputation.

In diabetic foot ulceration, tissue necrosis and infection frequently coincide and both can progress rapidly, tracking along fascial planes and tendons. Primary debridement and drainage should therefore be regarded as a medical emergency. Once the urgent issues relating to sepsis and the management of the systemic disease have been addressed, secondary reconstruction, revascularization, or lower limb amputation may be necessary. Clinicians should seek urgent surgical consultation for patients presenting with clinical evidence of a life- or limb-threatening infection (Table 29.1) or if the involved limb is critically ischemic.

All patients with diabetes should be assessed for unexplained persistent foot pain or tenderness or possible evidence of a deep-space infection or abscess. The absence of fever or leukocytosis should not deter the clinician from considering surgical exploration.

The most common site for a severe foot infection is the plantar surface. A plantar wound accompanied by dorsal erythema or fluctuance suggests that the infection has passed through fascial compartments and is likely to require surgical drainage. Prompt and adequate surgical debridement, including limited resections or minor amputations, may decrease the likelihood that a more extensive amputation is needed later. The progressive development of an abscess within the foot, especially in the presence of ischemia, can rapidly lead to irreparable tissue damage (Lipsky et al. 2012).

Table 29.1 Indicators of potentially immediate or long-term limb-threatening tissue damage and/or infection

Infection
Evidence of systemic inflammatory response
Worsening metabolic control
Rapid progression of infection
Spreading cellulitis or lymphangitis
Extensive ecchymoses or petechiae
Bullae, especially hemorrhagic
Failure of infection to respond to appropriate therapy

Neurological
Recent or progressive acute loss of neurological function
Onset of wound anesthesia
Pain out of proportion to clinical findings

Perfusion
Extensive necrosis or gangrene
Critical limb ischemia

Tissue
Extensive soft tissue loss
Especially, loss of weight-bearing plantar skin
Bony destruction especially if involves mid- or hindfoot
Pre-existing significant structural abnormalities within the foot including Charcot

In patients with an early and evolving infection, a trial of conservative medical management may be appropriate with delay of surgical intervention. A closed infection may, however, require urgent debridement of overlying tissues to prevent progression of a deep plantar space infection.

In those with a nonsevere infection, carefully observing the effectiveness of medical therapy and the demarcation line between necrotic and viable tissue before operating may be prudent. If clinical findings worsen, surgical intervention is usually needed. The surgeon must determine the adequacy of the blood supply to apparently viable tissues, consider common operative pitfalls (e.g. infection spreading among foot compartments, to the deep plantar space, or along the tendon sheaths), and formulate a strategy for eventual soft tissue cover (e.g. closure that is primary, delayed primary closure, by secondary intention, or by tissue transfer). It is essential that surgical debridement should optimize foot ulcer healing while attempting to preserve the foot integrity and anatomy (Lipsky et al. 2012).

Most diabetic foot ulcers occur in the plantar aspect of the foot and at the head of the metatarsal bones. Severe pain in the plantar surface is often one of the first alarming symptoms, especially in the patient with neuropathy. Several factors may lead to quick deterioration and its associated complications. Edema as a consequence to infection and cellulitis can develop in a foot compartment, resulting in a compartment syndrome. When pressure in a compartment exceeds capillary hydrostatic pressure, the microvascular circulation is impaired. Compartment pressures in patients with diabetes are higher than in those without diabetes. It has been suggested that increased sorbitol molecules and their split products in diabetes may lead to tissue edema. Furthermore, the greater affinity of glycated hemoglobin (hemoglobin A1c) to oxygen compared with normal hemoglobin may reduce tissue oxygenation. As a consequence, there is an increased capillary permeability and tissue edema, resulting in high compartment pressure.

Eventually, thrombosis of the small arteries and veins will cause tissue necrosis even in a well-vascularized foot. Hence, delayed diagnosis and surgical intervention could lead to extensive bone and soft tissue loss.

In this instance, surgery is aimed at decompression and drainage of the involved compartment, followed by radical debridement of all necrotic tissue. If soft tissue infection is accompanied by osteomyelitis of one or more metatarsal bone, a ray amputation is usually needed. It is extremely important that urgent surgical debridement should always be done prior to any diagnostic test or revascularization procedure (van Baal 2004).

Wound classification is an important factor, which predicts the need and urgency of wound debridement. Patients classified according to the International Working Group of the Diabetic Foot as PEDIS 2 can be treated as outpatients with oral antibiotics, off-loading, and appropriate wound care (**Table 29.2**) (see Chapter 24). Minor debridement may be necessary; however, in the presence of any of the criteria in **Box 29.1**, hospitalization may be required.

Box 29.1 Factors suggesting hospitalization of a patient with diabetic foot may be necessary

- Severe infection
- Metabolic instability
- Intravenous therapy required
- Inpatient diagnostic tests required
- Critical foot ischemia
- Inpatient surgical procedures are required
- Failure of outpatient management
- Inability or unwillingness of the patient to comply with outpatient treatments
- Complex dressing changes are required

In PEDIS 4, immediate surgical intervention and debridement is recommended as these wounds and patients frequently do not respond to medical and antibiotic therapy. Many of these patients will require revascularization to perfuse ischemic tissues either following or at the same time as their debridement to maximize limb salvage.

Table 29.2 Diabetic foot infection classification schemes (Lavery et al. 2007)

Clinical description	Infectious Diseases Society of America	(PEDIS grade) International Working Group on the Diabetic Foot
Wound without purulence or any manifestations of inflammation	Uninfected	1
≥2 manifestations of inflammation (purulence or erythema, pain, tenderness, warmth, or induration); any cellulitis or erythema extends ≤2 cm around ulcer, and infection is limited to skin or superficial subcutaneous tissues; no local complications or systemic illness	Mild	2
Infection in a patient who is systemically well and metabolically stable but has ≥1 of the following: cellulitis extending >2 cm; lymphangitis; spread beneath fascia; deep tissue abscess; gangrene; muscle, tendon, joint, or bone involvement	Moderate	3
Infection in a patient with systemic toxicity or metabolic instability (e.g. fever, chills, tachycardia, hypotension, confusion, vomiting, leukocytosis, acidosis, hyperglycemia, or azotemia)	Severe	4

Within the PEDIS 3 group, it is often difficult to decide when or if the patient requires surgical debridement. Although many diabetic foot infections are considered superficial because they do not extend beneath the superficial fascia, the infection will not uncommonly penetrate more deeply into underlying soft tissue and create a deep space abscess. In such cases, surgical intervention is mandated to evacuate the abscess, remove necrotic tissue, and minimize the risk for further spread. Therefore, it is advisable that the treating physicians should have a low threshold for hospitalization, and aggressive surgical, and medical treatment in patients in PEDIS 3 group (Fisher et al. 2010).

TECHNIQUE

Grodinsky (1929) identified three major plantar spaces. These included the medial, central (superficial and deep), and lateral spaces. He recommended a medial surgical approach due to potential discomfort of a plantar incision. However, Loeffler and Ballard demonstrated that a plantar-based incision careful tissue dissection and handling, a plantar incision can drain infection without a sensitive scar (Loeffler & Ballard 1980). Plantar-based incisions typically start posterior to the medial malleolus, extend distally and laterally toward the midline, and end between the heads of the first and second metatarsals.

Understanding the anatomy of the fascial compartments in diabetic foot infections is essential (**Figures 29.1** and **29.2**) (see Chapter 28). This will help the clinician to understand how infections of the first toe spread through the internal compartment. The infections of the second, third, and fourth toe spread through the central compartment and the infections of the fifth toe spread through the external compartment. In these instances it is necessary that the fascia for the relevant compartment is opened to prevent an increase in the intracompartment pressure and further tissue damage. However, it is essential to understand that the foot compartments do not contain the infection.

The current approach in most units including ours is a distal approach especially in those with a PEDIS 4 wound. The starting point coincides with the distal most area of infection or ulceration and extends proximally. The incision continues until evidence of infection has been eradicated or until viable, healthy-appearing tissue is observed. This approach eliminates the need for unnecessarily long incisions that could pose future problems, particularly in a patient with vascular insufficiency. All of the infected spaces should be inspected, and all the nonviable and necrotic tissue should be debrided.

Following incision and determination of any involved tissue planes and foot compartments, debridement of any and all nonviable tissue and bone should be completed regardless of the size and the quantity of the tissue removed. Exposed tendons should be debrided as they could act as a pathway for infection. Understanding the severity of sepsis, the anatomy of the foot and spread of infection is essential to limb salvage (**Figure 29.3**).

Tourniquet

The use of tourniquet is not encouraged as it may prevent the identification of viable tissue, potentially leading to over-debridement.

Debridement tools

The basic tools for debridement include forceps, blades, scissors, curettes, and rongeurs. Toothed forceps have a better grasp and reduce additional tissue trauma. A no. 15 blade is used for dissection around bone, whereas a no. 10 or 20 blade is used on soft tissue to slice thin

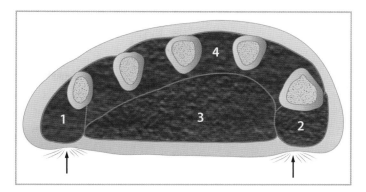

Figure 29.1 Transverse section of the foot, 1: lateral compartment; 2: central compartment; 3: medial compartment; 4: interosseous compartment. High-pressure areas at risk of ulceration are indicated with arrows.

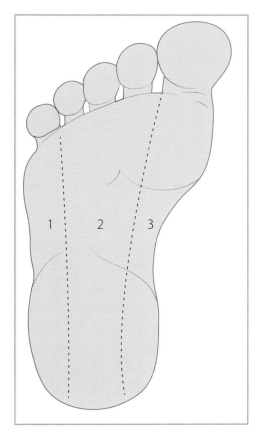

Figure 29.2 The plantar surface of the foot, 1: lateral compartment; 2: central compartment; 3: medial compartment.

layer after thin layer until healthy tissue is reached (Attinger et al. 2006). Some centers have successfully used methylene blue dye to differentiate between viable and nonviable tissues.

Curettes with sharp edges are very useful in removing the proteinaceous coagulum that accumulates; the coagulum contains proteases and bacteria that inhibit healing. Rongeurs are useful for removing hard-to-reach indurated soft tissue and for debriding bone. Electrical saw is useful for sawing off bone slices until normal cortex and marrow is reached and reduces the risk of bone fragmentation and residual bone spikes at resection margins.

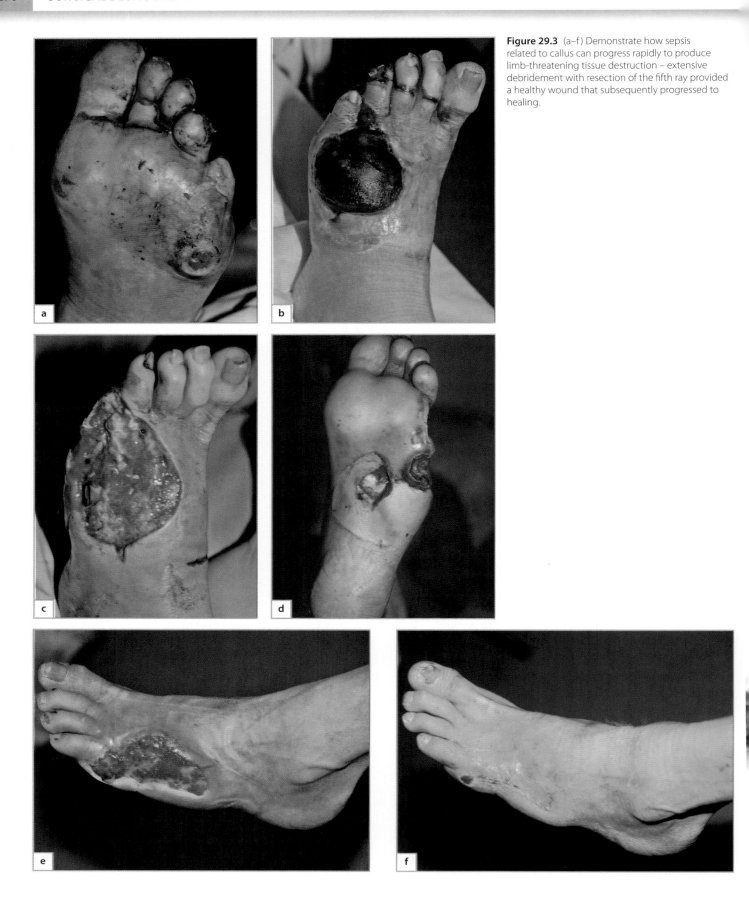

Figure 29.3 (a–f) Demonstrate how sepsis related to callus can progress rapidly to produce limb-threatening tissue destruction – extensive debridement with resection of the fifth ray provided a healthy wound that subsequently progressed to healing.

CALLUS

Callus refers to nonviable, hyperkeratotic tissue and is common to diabetic foot ulcers. The presence of callus can prevent healing and can also create increased pressure from footwear or improper gait in the neuropathic diabetic foot, ultimately leading to further ulceration. The entire callus should be resected with a sharp scalpel, and further debridement should extend to the soft tissue adjacent to the callus. The clinical margin of debridement could be confirmed by pathology and should not include epidermis with significant hyperkeratosis or parakeratosis.

SKIN

Skin debridement should consist of removing nonviable skin, which could be nonblanching, insensate, and blistered. Inadequate skin debridement could result in liquefaction necrosis in which dead skin separates from the underlying healthy tissue and may lead to functional loss, scarring, deeper tissue damage, and disseminated infection. If there is demarcation, the skin is excised along the border. If there is no demarcation, incision should start at the center of the wound and progressed until viable bleeding skin is reached. Thrombosed venules in the skin are a sign of interrupted microcirculation and mandate further debridement.

SUBCUTANEOUS TISSUE

Bleeding is not always a reliable indicator of viable subcutaneous tissue as it has decreased concentration of the blood vessels compared with the skin. Healthy subcutaneous fat has a shiny yellow color compared to gray, hard, and nonelastic nonviable tissue. Undermining should be avoided as it could affect the blood supply of the overlying skin. Diathermy should be used cautiously for bleeding control, and it may cause excessive tissue damage and result in a nidus for bacteria to proliferate. If sutures are used for bleeding control, small diameter absorbable monofilaments should be used to minimize the risk of foreign body reaction and possibly facilitating further infection. In the subcutaneous tissue, leaving exposed viable sensory nerves in a sensate patient could be very painful. If the nerve is to be preserved, it has to be kept moist until it can be covered with adequate tissue. If the nerve is to be sacrificed, under appropriate traction, the nerve should be cut proximally to allow retraction back to the normal tissue. Neuroma formation can be prevented by burying it in underlying tissue (muscle or bone) or by sowing the epineurium over the nerve fascicles with fine monofilament suture (Attinger et al. 2006).

FASCIA, MUSCLE, AND TENDON

Healthy viable fascia has a white, glistening, and hard appearance. Nonviable fascia with a soft and stringy appearance should be debrided. Care should be taken not do damage neurovascular structures under the fascia while debriding. Viable healthy muscle has a bright red and shiny appearance and contracts with diathermy or when grasped with forceps. If the viability of muscle is in question, it is advisable to debride only what is not bleeding, as unnecessary debridement could compromise surrounding tissue blood supply.

Exposed tendons should be debrided as they could act as a pathway for infection. However, excessive tendon debridement could result in loss of function and anatomy of the foot and potentially worsen the diabetic foot ulcer. Infected tendon looks dull, soft, and grainy, with parts separating and/or liquefying and should be removed. If it is decided to preserve the tendon, it should be kept moist or covered with viable tissue. In large tendons such as Achilles or anterior tibial tendons, debridement should be limited only to the infected and necrotic area. The hard and shiny tendon underneath should be left intact as there are many reconstructive options for future tendon repair.

BONE

Nonviable dead bone is soft and discolored and does not bleed at the cortex (punctuate bleeding or the 'paprika sign'). Power tools, bone cutters, and rongeurs could all be used; however, care should be taken not to cause fracture of the viable bone. It is essential to obtain cultures (tissue and bone samples) after debridement of the osteomyelitic bone.

Exposed cartilage as an avascular tissue should either be removed or covered with soft tissue as it could serve as a source for residual infection and necrotic tissue. Frequently plantar foot ulcers involve sesamoid bones; therefore, it is essential that the debridement is deep enough to assess the sesamoid bones and potentially remove them.

Wound irrigation

After debridement, wound irrigation helps reduce the bacterial count and removal of free tissue from the wound. Although saline irrigation will be effective, many centers use antibacterial solutions. Hydrogen peroxide has been found to be a useful irrigation solution by some.

Wound closure

Primary, secondary, and tertiary wound closure could be applied after foot debridement, depending on the extent of the wound debridement and severity of the infection. Negative pressure therapy or wet to dry dressing may facilitate wound granulation and assist delayed closure. The use of split-thickness skin grafts, local flaps, muscle flaps, pedicle flaps, and musculotendinous flaps is option for achieving proper wound closure. Decisions regarding closure are ultimately dependent on the volume of viable soft tissue remaining after surgery, the amount of drainage, the presence of any residual infection, and the level of correctable ischemia.

SURGICAL DEBRIDEMENT IN CHRONIC WOUNDS

The breakdown of the diabetic foot has been considered to be the result of peripheral vascular disease, peripheral neuropathy, infection, and psychological factors. Common features of chronic wounds include a prolonged or excessive inflammatory phase, persistent infections, formation of drug-resistant microbial biofilms, and the inability of dermal and/or epidermal cells to respond to reparative stimuli. A chronic wound is a wound that is arrested in one of the wound-healing stages (usually the inflammatory stage) and cannot progress further. Chronic wounds have a complex, inflammatory nature and produce substantial amounts of exudate, which interfere with the healing process and the effectiveness of advanced therapeutic agents. The normal pattern of the cellular and biochemical events is disrupted, and the wound is prevented from entering the proliferative phase of healing.

There is often a proinflammatory stimulus due to necrotic tissue, a heavy bacterial burden that causes cellular and biochemical changes in the wound bed such as increased levels of matrix metalloproteinases (MMPs), which degrade the extracellular matrix and cause in impaired cell migration and deposition of connective tissue. MMPs also degrade growth factors and their target cell receptors, preventing wound healing (Schultz et al. 2003).

Chronic wounds similar to acute wounds are treated using the same multistep approach based on contemporary knowledge of wound healing and known by the acronym 'TIME.' The nonviable tissues (T) from within and around a wound are removed using surgical debridement or debriding agents, such as bacterial collagenase. Infection and inflammation (I) are minimized with antibiotics and antimicrobial preparations. Moisture (M) imbalance is corrected, generally with carefully selected dressings. Epithelialization (E) and granulation tissue formation are promoted (sometimes by the application of specific therapies, such as growth factors) (Schultz et al. 2003).

Surgical debridement is a fast and effective way to remove debris and necrotic tissue from chronic wounds. By decreasing bacterial load and removal of old and senescent cells, surgical debridement converts a nonhealing chronic wound into a potentially healing acute wound.

In chronic wound, debrided tissue should be sent for histological analysis for diagnosis of osteomyelitis, vasculitis, or malignancy. The age of the wound is important as malignancy can develop in long-standing wounds (Marjolin's ulcer).

CONCLUSION

Effective debridement is an integral part of diabetic foot ulcer management, especially if sepsis is present. The process should be regarded as the first stage in limb salvage and as such should be integrated into a package of care involving multidisciplinary team input, which may include limb revascularization and plastic surgical reconstruction, the long-term aim being to maintain a functional foot.

AREAS OF CONTROVERSY AND/OR FUTURE RESEARCH

- The relative timings of debridement and revascularization are controversial in ischemic foot wounds
- A balance has to be struck between the need for improved perfusion of the foot and the removal of necrotic, infected tissue
- In some patients, these procedures should take place at the same time and in others a staged approach is more appropriate

IMPORTANT FURTHER READING

Attinger CE, Janis JE, Steinberg J, et al. Clinical approach to wounds: debridement and wound bed preparation including the use of dressings and wound-healing adjuvants. Plast Reconstr Surg 2006; 117:72S–109S.

Edwards J. Stapley S. Debridement of diabetic foot ulcers. Cochrane Database Syst. Rev 2010; 1:CD003556.

Gottrup F. Apelqvist J. Present and new techniques and devices in the treatment of DFU: a critical review of evidence. Diabetes Metab Res Rev 2012; 28:64–71.

Lipsky BA, Berendt AR, Cornia PB, et al. Infectious Diseases Society of America clinical practice guideline for the diagnosis and treatment of diabetic foot infections. Clin Infect Diseases 2012; 54:1679–1684.

Schultz GS, Sibbald RG, Falanga V, et al. Wound bed preparation: a systematic approach to wound management. Wound Repair Regen 2003; 11:S1–S28.

Zgonis T, Stapleton JJ, Girard-Powell VA, Hagino RT. Surgical management of diabetic foot infections and amputations. AORN J 2003; 87:935–946; quiz 947–950.

REFERENCES

Attinger CE, Janis JE, Steinberg J, et al. Clinical approach to wounds: debridement and wound bed preparation including the use of dressings and wound-healing adjuvants. Plast Reconstr Surg 2006; 117:72S–109S.

Cardinal M, Eisenbud DE, Armstrong DG, et al. Serial surgical debridement: a retrospective study on clinical outcomes in chronic lower extremity wounds. Wound Repair Regen 2009; 17:306–311.

Fisher TK, Scimeca CL, Bharara M, Mills JL, Armstrong DG. A step-wise approach for surgical management of diabetic foot infections. J Vasc Surg 2010; 52:72S–75S.

Grodinsky M. A study of fascial spaces of the feet. Surg Gynecol Obstet 1929; 49:737–751.

Lavery LA, Armstrong D G, Murdoch DP, Peters EJG,Lipsky BA. Validation of the Infectious Diseases Society of America's diabetic foot infection classification system. Clin Infect Diseases 2007; 44:562–565.

Lipsky BA, Berendt AR, Cornia PB, et al. Infectious Diseases Society of America Clinical Practice Guideline for the Diagnosis and Treatment of Diabetic Foot Infections. Clin Infect Diseases 2012; 54:1679–1684.

Loeffler RD, Jr, Ballard A. Plantar fascial spaces of the foot and a proposed surgical approach. Foot ankle 1980; 1:11–44.

Schultz GS, Sibbald RG, Falanga V., et al. Wound bed preparation: a systematic approach to wound management. Wound Repair Regen 2003; 11:S1–S28.

Van Baal JG. Surgical treatment of the infected diabetic foot. Clinical Infectious Diseases 2004; 39:S123–S128.

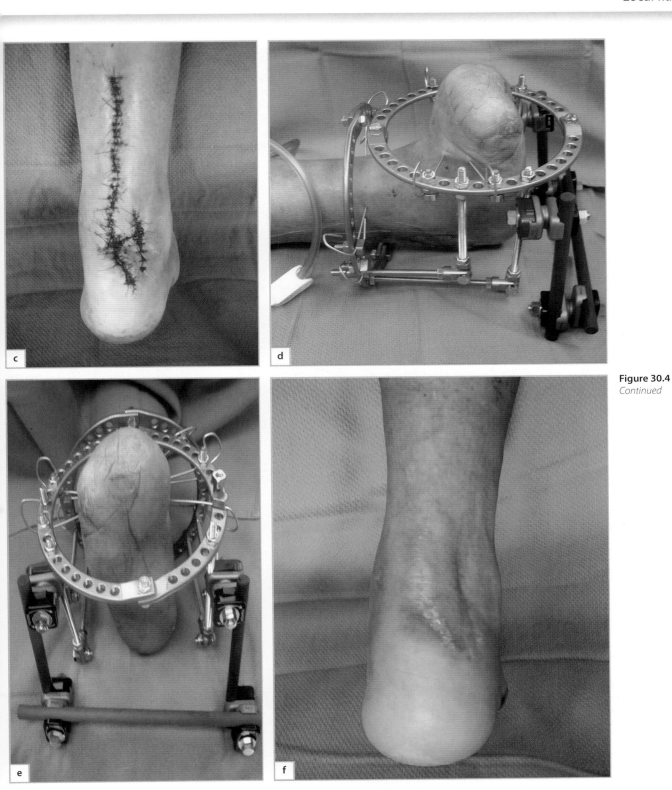

Figure 30.4
Continued

vascular pedicle. The muscle is sutured with minimal handling of the muscle to the dermis and fascia around the perimeter of the primary defect. STSG can then be applied and secured with a stent dressing or NPWT device. The extensor digitorum brevis muscle can also be used as a local axial flap for dorsal wounds in the diabetic foot and ankle.

A local axial flap may be fasciocutaneous, adipofascial, or musculocutaneous. A fasciocutaneous flap is the most common local axial flap utilized for diabetic foot and ankle wounds. The medial plantar artery and sural artery flap represent the two most common flaps used to address diabetic midfoot and rearfoot/ankle wounds, respectively. The medial plantar artery flap is typically raised with antegrade flow for ideal coverage of midfoot or distal rearfoot defects. Cohen et al. utilized the medial plantar artery flap in reconstruction of the heel, midfoot, and forefoot (Cohen et al. 1999). The sural artery flap is typically raised from the posterolateral aspect of the leg based on retrograde flow supplied by the median superficial sural artery and the arteriae nervorum of the medial sural nerve that anastomose distally with fasciocutaneous perforators of the peroneal artery (Ignatiadis et al. 2011). Venous drainage is obtained from venae comitantes to the median superficial sural artery and the lesser saphenous vein. Venous congestion because of poor outflow

is the major reason for sural artery flap failure. For this reason, the flap should be inset with minimal sutures to allow drainage. The placement of drains can facilitate further drainage preventing flap loss. Venous congestion can be treated with surgical evacuation of the hematoma and medicinal leeches. The donor sites to the medial plantar and sural artery flap are typically covered with a STSG or biological layers (**Figure 30.5**).

For diabetic soft tissue reconstruction, one possibility is to combine the concept of a local random with an axial flap. This technique focuses on creating a local random flap, most commonly a rotational flap, where the pedicle is based on a skin bridge supplied by the various

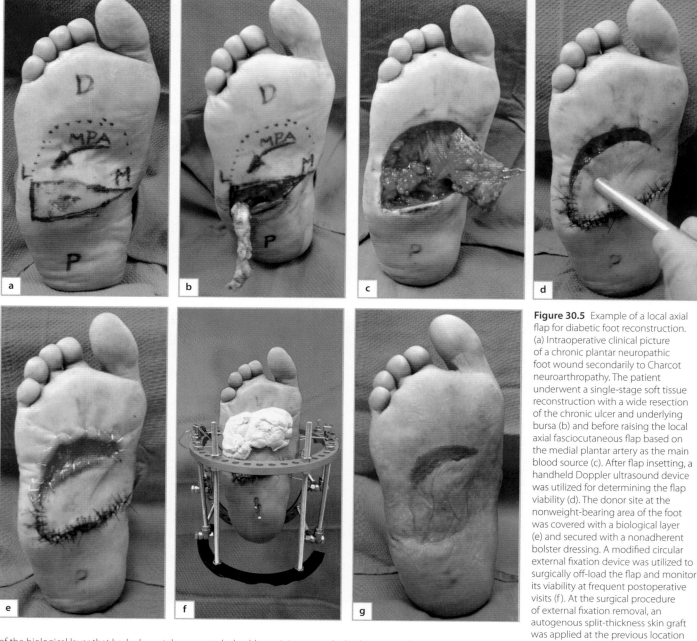

Figure 30.5 Example of a local axial flap for diabetic foot reconstruction. (a) Intraoperative clinical picture of a chronic plantar neuropathic foot wound secondarily to Charcot neuroarthropathy. The patient underwent a single-stage soft tissue reconstruction with a wide resection of the chronic ulcer and underlying bursa (b) and before raising the local axial fasciocutaneous flap based on the medial plantar artery as the main blood source (c). After flap insetting, a handheld Doppler ultrasound device was utilized for determining the flap viability (d). The donor site at the nonweight-bearing area of the foot was covered with a biological layer (e) and secured with a nonadherent bolster dressing. A modified circular external fixation device was utilized to surgically off-load the flap and monitor its viability at frequent postoperative visits (f). At the surgical procedure of external fixation removal, an autogenous split-thickness skin graft was applied at the previous location of the biological layer that had adequately promoted a healthy recipient granular bed. Note the final outcome of the patient's local axial flap closure with off-loading external fixation (g).

vascular interconnections along with identification of a patent artery within the flap. This is most commonly seen with large rotational flaps performed to cover plantar soft tissue defects associated with underlying CN deformities. The rotational flap is designed to maintain an intact skin bridge along with inclusion of an identifiable patent medial or lateral plantar artery. Identifying perforators and a source vessel with a handheld Doppler ultrasound device in conjunction with the establishment of a skin bridge with known angiosomes is the best way of preventing local flap ischemia and necrosis (Clemens & Attinger 2010).

SURGICAL OFF-LOADING OF EXTERNAL FIXATION FOR DIABETIC SOFT TISSUE RECONSTRUCTION

Off-loading of circular external fixators has become more popular over the last decade to achieve successful soft tissue coverage in the population of patient with diabetes (Clemens et al. 2008). External fixation is useful to simply off-load the extremity to protect flap coverage while allowing easy exposure for local wound care and frequent assessments (Ramanujam et al. 2011) (**Figure 30.4**). In addition, external fixation may be used to address underlying CN deformities and/or bone defects as a result of previous surgical debridement. Osseous stability and correction of deformity that led to the primary defect must be performed to prevent further soft tissue compromise when flap coverage is performed. Utilization of internal fixation is often not feasible given the presence of open wounds and history of infection and/or osteomyelitis. Various external fixation constructs and designs can be utilized to achieve osseous stabilization and off-loading of the soft tissue coverage. Finally, external fixators can easily be modified throughout the postoperative period to achieve the desired result if necessary. External fixation provides advantages since tension and compression caused by traditional casting directly against the surgical site can compromise viability of the soft tissue reconstruction; furthermore, frequent cast changes to access the site for monitoring may inadvertently cause flap damage. The specialized surgical training required for proper application and care of external fixation, in addition to the increased cost and demands of maintenance, are both important considerations in the proper patient selection for this method of off-loading.

POSTOPERATIVE MANAGEMENT

Protocols for weight-bearing status in the postoperative period depend on the location of the soft tissue reconstruction and the type of osseous procedures that may have been performed concomitantly. Graft and/or flap viability is typically evaluated in the outpatient setting at frequent intervals, along with the care of external fixation devices if utilized. Culture-specific oral or parenteral antibiotics are utilized if indicated. Hyperbaric oxygen therapy may be a useful adjunct in some patients with diabetes since it may provide improved oxygenation of the threatened margins of wounds and enhanced phagocytosis and killing of some micro-organisms (Faglia et al. 1996). Additional STSG and/or local flaps can also be performed in cases where complications have caused wound dehiscence or flap failure.

Long-term wound closure will also require appropriate accommodative footwear and bracing in the reconstructed patient with diabetes. Several prospective studies have shown a beneficial effect of the use of therapeutic footwear compared with standard footwear in preventing ulcer recurrence in patients with diabetes (Uccioli et al. 1995, Viswanathan et al. 2004). Customized footwear and multidensity insoles for specific residual deformities and partial foot amputations can address potential biomechanical imbalances and subsequently reduce risk of reulceration. Specialized bracing such as the use of double-upright ankle-foot-orthosis in diabetic CN reconstruction provides stabilization of the lower extremity during ambulation and can decrease further joint compromise.

CONCLUSION

For soft tissue coverage of complex diabetic foot and ankle wounds, various methods can be employed, among them skin grafts, local random flaps, and local axial flaps. The simplest approach that can restore the unique anatomy of the wound and fulfill the functional demands of the region represents the best option.

AREAS OF CONTROVERSY AND/OR FUTURE RESEARCH

- External fixation for diabetic soft tissue reconstruction has become an option for surgical off-loading and requires further research to determine its true efficacy

IMPORTANT FURTHER READING

Clemens MW, Attinger CE. Angiosomes and wound care in the diabetic foot. Foot Ankle Clin 2010; 15:439–464.

Shaw WW, Hidalgo DA. Anatomic basis of plantar flap design: clinical applications. Plast Reconstr Surg 1986; 78:637–649.

Blume PA, Key JJ. Local random flaps for soft tissue coverage of the diabetic foot. In: Zgonis T (ed.), Surgical reconstruction of the diabetic foot and ankle. Philadelphia: Lippincott Williams & Wilkins, 2009:140–164.

Zgonis T, Stapleton JJ, Roukis TS. Advanced plastic surgery techniques for soft tissue coverage of the diabetic foot. Clin Podiatr Med Surg 2007; 24:547–568.

Clemens MW, Parikh P, Hall MM, Attinger CE. External fixators as an adjunct to wound healing. Foot Ankle Clin 2008; 13:145–156.

Hijjawi JB, Bishop AT. Management of simple wounds: local flaps, Z Plasty, and skin graft. In: Moran SL, Coomey WP III (eds), Master techniques in orthopaedic surgery – soft tissue surgery. Philadelphia: Lippincott Williams & Wilkins, 2008:39.

REFERENCES

Aragón-Sánchez J. Treatment of diabetic foot osteomyelitis: a surgical critique. Int J Low Extrem Wounds 2010; 9:37–59.

Ashbell TS. The rhomboid excision and Limberg flap reconstruction in difficult tense-skin areas. Plast Reconstr Surg 1982; 69:724.

Belczyk R, Ramanujam CL, Capobianco CM, Zgonis T. Combined midfoot arthrodesis, muscle flap coverage, and circular external fixation for the chronic ulcerated Charcot deformity. Foot Ankle Spec 2010; 3:40–44.

Blume PA, Key JJ. Local random flaps for soft tissue coverage of the diabetic foot. In: Zgonis T (ed.), Surgical reconstruction of the diabetic foot and ankle. Philadelphia: Lippincott Williams & Wilkins, 2009:140–164.

Bouché RT, Christensen JC, Hale DS. Unilobed and bilobed skin flaps. Detailed surgical technique for plantar lesions. J Am Podiatr Med Assoc 1995; 85:41–48.

Capobianco CM, Zgonis T. Abductor hallucis muscle flap and staged medial column arthrodesis for the chronic ulcerated Charcot foot with concomitant osteomyelitis. Foot Ankle Spec 2010; 3:269–273.

Christman AL, Selvin E, Margolis DJ, et al. Hemoglobin a1c predicts healing rate in diabetic wounds. J Invest Dermatol 2011; 131:2121–2127.

Clemens MW, Attinger CE. Angiosomes and wound care in the diabetic foot. Foot Ankle Clin 2010; 15:439–464.

Clemens MW, Parikh P, Hall MM, Attinger CE. External fixators as an adjunct to wound healing. Foot Ankle Clin 2008; 13:145–156.

Cohen BK, Zabel DD, Newton ED, Catanzariti AR. Soft-tissue reconstruction for recalcitrant diabetic foot wounds. J Foot Ankle Surg 1999; 38:388–393.

Colen LB, Replogle SL, Mathes SJ. The V-Y plantar flap for reconstruction of the forefoot. Plast Reconstr Surg 1988; 81:220–228.

Faglia E, Favales F, Aldeghi A, et al. Adjunctive systemic hyperbaric oxygen therapy in treatment of severe prevalently ischemic diabetic foot ulcer: a randomized study. Diabetes Care 1996; 19:1338–1343.

Faries PL, Teodorescu VJ, Morrissey NJ, et al. The role of surgical revascularization in the management of diabetic foot wounds. Am J Surg 2004; 187:34S–37S.

Ha Van G, Siney H, Danan JP, et al. Treatment of osteomyelitis in the diabetic foot. Contribution of conservative surgery. Diabetes Care 1996; 19:1257–1260.

Hijjawi JB, Bishop AT. Management of simple wounds: local flaps, Z plasty, and skin graft. In: Moran SL, Coomey WP III (eds), Master techniques in orthopaedic surgery – soft tissue surgery. Philadelphia: Lippincott Williams & Wilkins, 2008:39.

Ignatiadis IA, Tsiampa VA, Galanakos SP, et al. The reverse sural fasciocutaneous flap for the treatment of traumatic, infectious or diabetic foot and ankle wounds: a retrospective review of 16 patients. Diabet Foot Ankle 2011; 2.

Kim BS, Choi WJ, Baek MK, et al. Limb salvage in severe diabetic foot infection. Foot Ankle Int 2011; 32:31–37.

Levin LS. Foot and ankle soft-tissue deficiencies: who needs a flap? Am J Orthop 2006; 35:11–19.

Lipsky BA, Berendt AR, Cornia PB, et al. 2012 Infectious Diseases Society of America clinical practice guideline for the diagnosis and treatment of diabetic foot infections. Clin Infect Dis 2012; 54:e132–173.

Mader JT, Ortiz M, Calhoun JH. Update of the diagnosis and management of osteomyelitis. Clin Podiatr Med Surg 1996; 13:701–724.

Ramanujam CL, Facaros Z, Zgonis T. External fixation for surgical off-loading of diabetic soft tissue reconstruction. Clin Podiatr Med Surg 2011; 28:211–216.

Ramanujam CL, Stapleton JJ, Kilpadi KL, et al. Split-thickness skin grafts for closure of diabetic foot and ankle wounds: a retrospective review of 83 patients. Foot Ankle Spec 2010; 3:231–240.

Ramanujam CL, Zgonis T. Salvage of Charcot foot neuropathy superimposed with osteomyelitis: a case report. J Wound Care 2010; 19:485–487.

Ramanujam CL, Zgonis T. Primary arthrodesis and sural artery flap coverage for subtalar joint osteomyelitis in a diabetic patient. Clin Podiatr Med Surg 2011; 28:421–427.

Rosenblum BI, Giurini JM, Miller LB, et al. Neuropathic ulcerations plantar to the lateral column in patients with Charcot foot deformity: a flexible approach to limb salvage. J Foot Ankle Surg 1997; 36:360–363.

Roukis TS, Schweinberger MH, Schade VL. V-Y fasciocutaneous advancement flap coverage of soft tissue defects of the foot in the patient at high risk. J Foot Ankle Surg 2010; 49:71–74.

Saap LJ, Falanga V. Debridement performance index and its correlation with complete closure of diabetic foot ulcers. Wound Repair Regen 2002; 10:354–359.

Schade VL, Roukis TS. The role of polymethylmethacrylate antibiotic-loaded cement in addition to debridement for the treatment of soft tissue and osseous infections of the foot and ankle. J Foot Ankle Surg 2010; 49:55–62.

Schintler MV. Negative pressure therapy: theory and practice. Diabetes Metab Res Rev 2012; 28S:72–77.

Shaw WW, Hidalgo DA. Anatomic basis of plantar flap design: clinical applications. Plast Reconstr Surg 1986; 78:637–649.

Steed DL, Donohoe D, Webster MW, Lindsley L. Effect of extensive debridement and treatment on the healing of diabetic foot ulcers. Diabetic Ulcer Study Group. J Am Coll Surg 1996; 183:61–64.

Sumpio BE, Aruny J, Blume PA. The multidisciplinary approach to limb salvage. Acta Chir Belg 2004; 104:647–653.

Uccioli L, Faglia E, Monticone G, et al. Manufactured shoes in the prevention of diabetic foot ulcers. Diabetes Care 1995; 18:1376–1378.

Viswanathan V, Madhavan S, Gnanasundaram S, et al. Effectiveness of different types of footwear insoles for the diabetic neuropathic foot: a follow-up study. Diabetes Care 2004; 27:474–477.

Yetkin H, Kanatli U, Oztürk AM, Ozalay M. Bilobed flaps for nonhealing ulcer treatment. Foot Ankle Int 2003; 24:685–689.

Zgonis T, Orphanos J, Roukis TS, Cromack DT. Use of a muscle flap and a split-thickness skin graft for a calcaneal osteomyelitis after an open reduction and internal fixation. J Am Podiatr Med Assoc 2008; 98:139–142.

Zgonis T, Roukis TS, Stapleton JJ, Cromack DT. Combined lateral column arthrodesis, medial plantar artery flap, and circular external fixation for Charcot midfoot collapse with chronic plantar ulceration. Adv Skin Wound Care 2008; 21:521–525.

Zgonis T, Stapleton JJ, Roukis TS. Advanced plastic surgery techniques for soft tissue coverage of the diabetic foot. Clin Podiatr Med Surg 2007; 24:547–568.

Table 31.1 A review of risk factors involved in free flap reconstruction

Risk factor	Odds ratio	95% CI Lower limit	95% CI Upper limit	P
CT angiography				
1 vessel‡	2.114	0.216	20.725	0.560
2 vessel	2.041	0.512	8.140	0.052
3 vessel	Reference			0.312
Angioplasty				
None	Reference			
Angioplasty	17.590	4.040	76.582	<0.001
Peripheral arterial disease				
None	Reference			
Peripheral arterial disease	10.212	2.874	19.231	0.032
Heart problem				
None	Reference			
Heart problem	0.913	0.243	3.425	0.893
Chronic renal failure				
None	Reference			
Chronic renal failure	1.707	0.466	6.253	0.419
Immunosuppressive agent				
None	Reference			
Immunosuppressive agent	4.857	1.068	22.086	0.041
ASA score†				
4	2.453	0.524	5.342	0.915
3	1.031	0.251	4.241	0.872
2	Reference			0.966
Smoking				
None	Reference			
Smoking	1.231	0.328	4.625	0.759
Osteomyelitis				
None	Reference			
Osteomyelitis	1.056	0.289	3.851	0.935
Body mass index	1.034	0.848	1.260	0.743
HBA1c	0.736	0.479	1.130	0.161
Lymphocyte count	1.000	0.998	1.001	0.527
CRP level	1.054	0.934	1.190	0.393
Ankle brachial index	1.420	0.285	7.088	0.669

*Shown are the odds ratio and its 95% confidence interval (CI) and p values yielded by univariate logistic regression analysis of 14 preoperative risk factors for total flap loss ($p < 0.05$).
**Number of intact vessels on computed tomography angiography.
†American Society of Anesthesiologists physical status classification system.
CRP, C-reactive protein.

distal flow. An alternative anastomosis may be the T-style anastomosis, where a bypassing artery segment with a branch to the flap is interanastomosed between the proximal and distal recipient artery. The possibility of using the end vessels located superficially beneath the skin or small digital arteries according to the supermicrosurgery concept is now being explored. Knowing that these end vessels or small perforators will be supplied not only from major vessels but also from multiple collateral vessels; these small vessels will often have good perfusion flow (Hong 2009, Hong & Koshima 2010). Using these small vessels with a good pulsatile flow can be a viable option, especially when major vessels are in doubt as a recipient vessel.

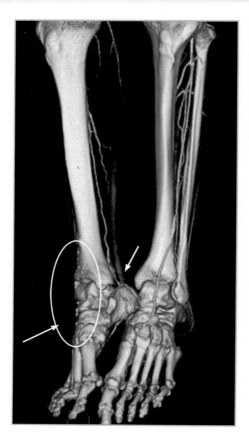

Figure 31.5
Angiogram prior to reconstruction. Note the spared and calcified segment of the peripheral artery. One should find a segment free from calcification to use as recipient artery in end-to-side manner.

Selection of flaps

The flap for reconstruction of the diabetic foot should provide a well-vascularized tissue to control infection, an adequate contour for footwear, durability, and a solid anchorage point to resist shearing forces. Controversy still remains as to which flap (muscle flaps with skin grafts, fasciocutaneous flaps, or recently added perforator flaps) offers the optimal solution to reconstruct the foot, in particular the weight-bearing surface (Colen et al. 1990, Ducic & Attinger 2011).

Muscle flaps with skin grafts have been advocated to be more stable than fasciocutaneous flaps because of their ability to conform to the irregular contours of the foot (Ferreira et al. 1994). The abundant vascular supply to the muscle may provide better infection control against wounds and osteomyelitis. The bulk was assumed to provide a cushioning effect, but the lack of sensitivity was thought to lead to frequent breakdown of the flap (Sonmez et al. 2003). Clinical experience with muscle flaps led to frequent breakdown and recurrence of ulceration due to a lack of resistance to pressure, and furthermore, it took a longer time to heal and allow weight bearing. Muscle flaps may also require secondary debulking procedures in this region to allow the patient to use normal footwear.

Studies regarding fasciocutaneous flaps to reconstruct the foot with or without diabetes have also demonstrated excellent results. A consensus has developed that a thin fasciocutaneous flap may be advantageous to reduce shearing, provide better contouring, and increase the chance of reinnervation (Noever et al. 1986). However, clinical experience with fasciocutaneous flap to reconstruct the foot has shown that the layer between the skin and fascia may not be anatomically sufficient enough to prevent gliding of the skin when pressure is applied. A similar phenomenon is seen when

reconstruction is undertaken with a thick muscle flap. This is most likely due to the lack of mimicking of the fibrous septa found in the normal heel and sole of the foot.

It has been shown that the control of infection is more closely related to debridement than to the selection of flap types. And as long as the defect is covered with any well-vascularized tissue, it will provide an independent and well-nourished vascular supply to eradicate infection, increase local oxygen tension, enhancing antibiotic activity, and neovascularization to the adjacent ischemic tissue (Chang & Mathes 1982, Shestak et al. 1990). Now the focus of the question to be addressed in the reconstruction of diabetic foot is shifting toward function, such as solid anchorage and durability. We all know that any reconstruction is best served with a like-for-like tissue, but reconstruction using similar tissue, especially in the plantar surface of the foot, is limited. Finding a tissue that adequately mimics the thin plantar skin with fibrous septa tightly adhering to the surface of the aponeurosis would be ideal.

In the author's clinical experience, there is a shift toward using perforator flaps such as the anterolateral thigh (ALT) perforator and superficial circumflex iliac perforator flap as they provide a thin flap to minimize shearing, can take only the superficial fat to imitate the fibrous septa of the sole to adhere tightly, enhance neovascularization of the subdermal plexus with adjacent tissue, and provide an adequate blood supply to fight infection (Hong 2006).

Anterolateral thigh perforator

Isolation of the pedicle is first performed to confirm patency of the recipient pedicle. Aggressive debridement of foot wounds is then performed including removal of non-viable bone. Bone abnormalities are corrected if necessary. After noting brisk bleeding from the wound bed, flap harvesting is performed. A line is drawn between the anterior superior iliac spine (ASIS) and the superior lateral border of the patella on the donor thigh. The perforator branches are identified with Doppler near the midpoint of this line. According to our clinical experience, about 90% of perforators are found within a 3-cm diameter drawn at the midpoint of the line. The skin flap is designed to include the perforator and then elevated from either the medial or lateral border. The incision can be made through the deep fascia or above the deep fascia. When elevating beneath the deep fascia, elevate until the intermuscular septum between the rectus femoris and vastus lateralis muscle is reached. At that point, the descending branch of the lateral femoral circumflex is explored along with the perforator to the skin flap. The flap can be harvested either as a perforator flap including only the perforator branch to the skin or combined with the vastus lateralis muscle as a musculocutaneous flap. The skin paddle may be defatted according to need up to 3 to 4 mm thickness except for the portion in which the perforator branch enters. When elevating above the deep fascia, raise the flap until a perforator piercing the deep fascia is encountered. It is possible to isolate multiple perforators and choose the best one or multiple perforators. Open the deep fascia and trace the perforator until an adequate length is achieved. In either approach, the motor branch of the femoral nerve running medial to the descending branch of the lateral circumflex femoral artery should be preserved. To elevate as a sensate flap, a branch of the lateral femoral cutaneous nerve should be included. The donor site can be primarily closed depending on the laxity of the skin. Reconstruction using an ALT perforator flap is seen in **Figure 31.6**.

A study using the ALT flap has shown that the majority of patients (69 of 71) achieved a full walking gait. The advantage of this flap is that it consists of well-vascularized tissue to control infection, is a thin enough to provide one-stage contouring and minimize shearing, and has a skin paddle to resist pressure and improve durability. It can

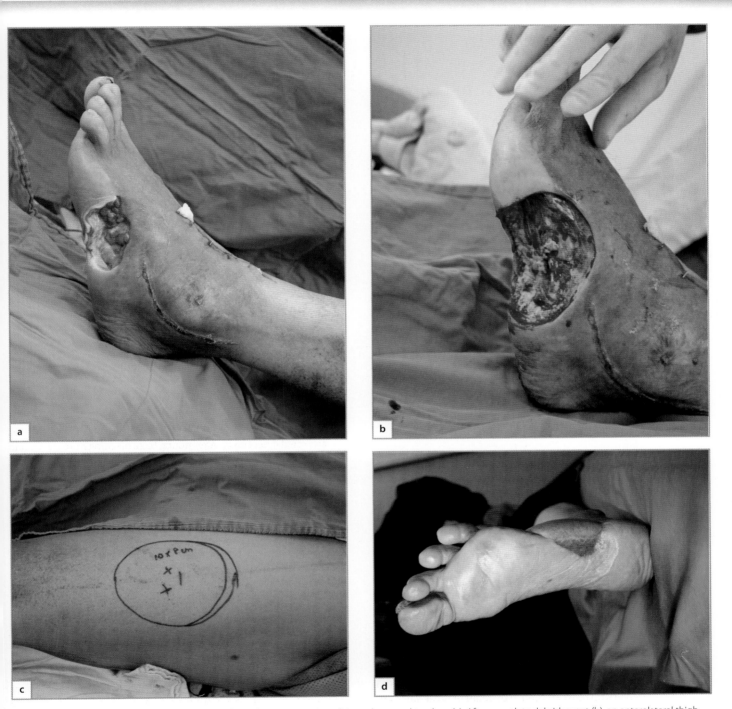

Figure 31.6 A 57-year-old man with diabetes with foot ulceration, osteomyelitis, and exposed tendons (a). After complete debridement (b), an anterolateral thigh flap of 10 × 8 cm is elevated (c). A branch from the dorsalis pedis artery was used as a recipient artery along with accompanying veins. The flap after 2 years is well maintained with good contour (d).

also be combined with the vastus lateralis muscle to increase bulk and blood supply against large dead spaces and chronic infections (Hong 2006).

Superficial circumflex iliac artery perforator (SCIP)

An SCIP flap is an evolved form of groin flap. While preserving the advantage of a well-hidden donor scar, modifications have allowed

elevation of this flap as a very thin flap that is able to provide excellent contouring in the reconstruction of the diabetic foot (Hong et al. 2012) (**Figure 31.7**).

Preoperative angiography using CT angiography or digital subtraction angiography is helpful to evaluate the vascular anatomy and presence of PAD. Preoperative Doppler ultrasound is used to mark the potential recipient perforators around the soft tissue defect. During the tracing of the recipient perforator, the intensity of the sound from the Doppler monitor is observed and marked.

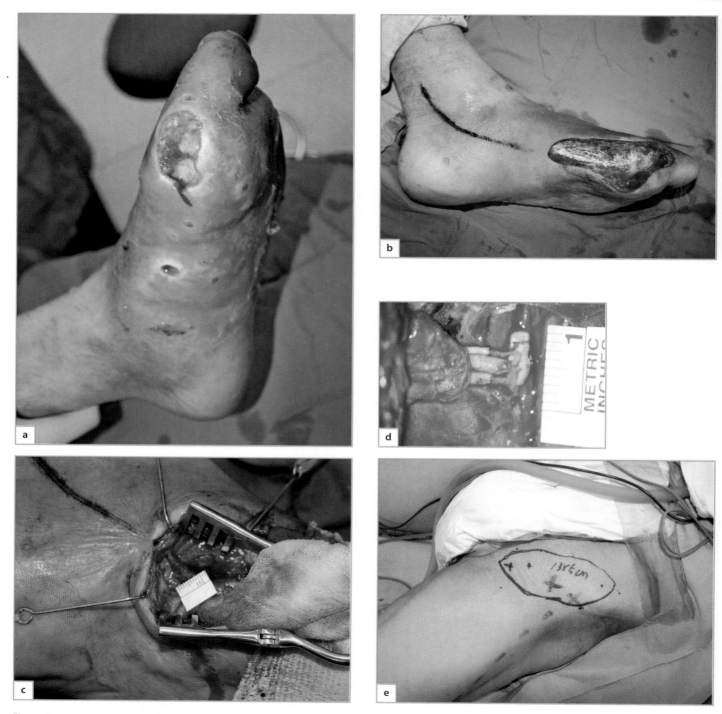

Figure 31.7 A 63-year-old man with severe swelling, and osteomyelitis was referred for treatment (a). After multiple debridements and metabolic/infection control, the patient underwent final debridement (b). Small end vessels were exposed adjacent to the defect and used as a recipient pedicle preserving all other distal flow to the feet (c, d). Elevation of superficial circumflex iliac artery perforator flap was performed with a dimension of 13 x 5 cm (e). Note the great contour after surgery without any additional debulking procedures (f, g).

Prior to any reconstructive procedure, complete debridement is performed, extending to the bone when needed. In cases where bone fixation is needed externally or internally, it is performed prior to a soft tissue reconstruction procedure. The recipient perforators are identified using loupe magnification and upon location, further dissection is carried out under the microscope to prevent damaging

to the perforator. A strong visible pulse of the perforator is a useful clinical marker. When the diameter is too narrow, dissection can extend beneath the fascia. The required pedicle length of the flap is then predicted, and the SCIP flap elevation is performed. A line is drawn from the inguinal crease to the ASIS, marking the topographical pathway of the perforator. An acoustic Doppler scan is then used to

CHARCOT

Chapter 32

The causes and diagnosis of acute Charcot foot in diabetes

William Jeffcoate

SUMMARY

- The acute Charcot foot is an uncommon complication of diabetes and is often missed by nonspecialists
- Delays in the diagnosis of acute Charcot foot can result in such major changes to the structure and function of the foot that it leads to amputation of the limb
- The pivotal abnormality in the pathogenesis of Charcot foot is an uncontrolled cycle of inflammation, which is itself facilitated by distal symmetrical neuropathy, but it is likely that any of a number other facilitatory processes are likely to be involved
- Diagnosis relies on pattern recognition and is confirmed by visible fracture and dislocation on plain X-ray, and/or evidence of marrow edema on magnetic resonance imaging (MRI)
- The occurrence of an acute Charcot foot is associated with a marked reduction in life expectancy

DEFINITION

The acute Charcot foot has no definition, and no single clinical feature is diagnostic. It is more of a syndrome complex, comprising unexplained inflammation of one or more bones of the foot or ankle, associated with varying degrees of fracture, dislocation and foot deformity, and without other obvious cause.

HISTORY

The condition described by Jean-Martin Charcot in 1868 was of inflammation leading to painless and sometimes gross fracture and deformity of the long bones and larger joints of the lower half of the body, but he made no reference to the foot. The cases he described were in people with syphilis complicated by tabes dorsalis. The first report of the disease affecting the foot was by an English surgeon, Herbert W. Page, in 1881 (Sanders et al. 2013).

PRESENTATION

The condition occurs as a complication of neuropathy and is seen most often in people in their sixth decade, with no gender difference (Rogers et al. 2011). There is also no apparent difference between people with type 1 and type 2 diabetes, in either incidence or clinical presentation – although those with type 1 disease obviously tend to have a longer duration of known disease. It is often suggested that the condition is more likely in those who are obese, but this has never been conclusively demonstrated.

The acute Charcot foot typically affects the mid- and hindfoot. The affected person may present with a relatively short history – usually of inflammation of the foot, which cannot be explained by any significant trauma or other episode. Alternatively, they may give a history of inflammation that has continued for several weeks or months and is associated with varying degrees of deformity. In some cases, the deformity is gross, and in others, it is minimal. Part of this variability may result from varying time to presentation, but it is otherwise unexplained.

CAUSES

The role of inflammation

The likely central role of unrestrained inflammation was first proposed in 2005 (Jeffcoate et al. 2005). The essence of the hypothesis is that although trauma-induced inflammation is normally curtailed because the injury is painful and the person protects the inflamed part by limiting movement, this will not happen in the presence of sensory loss and relative painlessness. In the absence of splinting, the inflammation will continue, and this allows a vicious cycle of local inflammation to be established. Continuing inflammation results in bone breakdown through activation of the receptor activator of NF-kappaB ligand (RANKL)–nuclear factor-kappaB (NFκB) signaling pathway (see below) and the bone thinning predisposes to further fracture and to dislocation, which, in turn, increases local inflammation. This hypothesis has been generally accepted, although scientific data to support it currently remain thin.

RANKL–NFκB

Proinflammatory cytokines – predominantly tumor necrosis factor (TNF)-α and interleukin-1β (IL-1β) – mediate the process of inflammation through a complex interaction with signaling pathways that include the RANKL–NFκB pathway. RANKL is a polypeptide that is released from a variety of tissue cell types and acts by triggering the expression of the nuclear transcription factor, NFκB. NFκB has many roles and these include the activation of immature osteoclasts, leading to bone breakdown. NFκB also triggers the release of the glycoprotein, osteoprotegerin (OPG), which acts as a decoy receptor – and this helps moderate the effect of RANKL by competing with the receptors through which it activates NFκB expression. Both RANKL and OPG are believed to be generally released at the same time, although they have opposing actions. OPG has been technically easier to measure than RANKL, and hence circulating concentrations of OPG are used as a measure of activation of the whole pathway. OPG concentrations are elevated in diabetes and especially in diabetes affected by both microvascular and macrovascular complications.

■ PREDISPOSITION TO THE DEVELOPMENT OF THE ACUTE CHARCOT FOOT

One of the unexplained features of the Charcot foot syndrome is its rarity. For this reason, associations have been sought with various clinical features.

■ Neuropathy

Some degree of denervation of the affected part is believed to be invariable, although the type and extent of deficit is very variable. The original cases were described in tabes dorsalis – in which there is loss of deep pain sensation and loss of proprioception, but other peripheral sensation is intact. The most common cause of the Charcot foot today is the distal symmetrical neuropathy of diabetes, and it has been shown that deep pain sensation is to a large extent preserved in such cases (Chantelau et al. 2012), although the distal lower limb may be otherwise insensate. The acute phase is often not entirely painless in diabetes.

Attempts to associate the Charcot foot of diabetes with particular patterns of distal denervation have yielded conflicting results and, with the exception of data on vasomotor dysfunction associated with distal neuropathy (see below), no clear pattern has emerged. In the absence of evidence to suggest any one particular clinical type of neuropathy, it seems likely that any of a number of defects of peripheral nerve function may predispose to the development of the condition, either alone or in combination.

Loss of protective sensation

Loss of protective sensation is likely to be a key part of the process, which allows the vicious cycle of inflammation to become established. Thus, the person with incipient disease may worsen the damage by failing to protect the inflamed (and possibly fractured or dislocated) foot by continuing to walk on it. When the loss of pain sensation is caused by tabes dorsalis (i.e. affecting the spinal cord and with loss of sensation of deep pain), it is the more proximal, and larger, bones and joints that are involved. When, on the other hand, the disease is associated with peripheral neuropathy (with reduced sensation of pain conducted via the spinothalamic pathway), it is the foot that is most likely to be affected.

Motor neuropathy

Impaired innervation of the small muscles of the foot is known to be associated with widespread atrophy of the small muscles of the foot. This is associated with abnormal transfer of forces during walking, and the resultant increase in local forces may trigger the onset of microfracture or microdislocation; these could be factors triggering the onset of the inflammatory process.

Vasomotor neuropathy

Charcot himself speculated about the role of neuropathy on local blood flow, with particular reference to lack of nutrient blood flow to affected bones. Nowadays, it is thought that the ability to mount, and maintain, an inflammatory response requires a vascular system that can respond by vasodilatation. Three groups have separately examined the capacity of the small arteries and arterioles to vasodilate (primarily in response to local warming) and showed that whereas vasodilatation was observed in people with a history of an acute Charcot foot, it was not observed in neuropathic controls (Shapiro et al. 1998, Veves

et al. 1998, Baker et al. 2007). It is possible that this retention of the capacity for vasodilatation is necessary for uncontrolled inflammation to occur, and if the preservation of this capacity is relatively rare, it may explain why the acute Charcot foot is so uncommon – when distal neuropathy is generally thought to affect approximately 30% of people with diabetes.

Vasomotor neuropathy may also cause altered distal limb blood flow through loss of the capacity for arteriolar constriction. This effectively creates arteriovenous anastomoses with reduced peripheral resistance and widened pulse pressure. This explains the fact that in people with neuropathy (with or without an acute Charcot foot), the pedal pulses are often not only easy to feel but are also abnormally easy to feel. These changes to foot blood flow could have an impact on the nature of the inflammatory response that accompanies local injury and could play a part in the development of the acute Charcot foot.

Neuropathy-induced arterial calcification and altered blood flow

Neuropathy is known to be associated with calcification of the tunica media of the arterial wall: medial arterial calcification (MAC) (Jeffcoate et al. 2009, Ndip et al. 2011). Strictly, the process, first described by the German pathologist, Mönckeberg, should be referred to as ossification, because it is new bone that is synthesized in the media and not simply calcium deposition. MAC is, however, most marked in the distal vasculature and is more common in those with neuropathy. When the arterial walls are stiffened, it reduces compliance and the result is widening of the pulse pressure.

It now seems that the process occurs, because the RANKL–NFκB pathway that mediates bone loss in response to inflammation is also involved in the deposition of new bone in the arterial cell wall.

Loss of neuropeptides

Loss of nerve terminals will be associated with reduced availability of the various peptide hormones that are normally released from nerve terminals. Included among these are peptides that modulate the activity of the RANKL–NFκB pathway, and of these, most attention hitherto has been paid to calcitonin gene-related peptide (CGRP). CGRP tends to suppress the expression of RANKL, and hence, its loss would augment activation of NFkappaB induced by proinflammatory cytokines.

■ Genetic predisposition

Two groups have explored the possibility that people with an acute Charcot foot may have a genetic predisposition and have reported an increased prevalence of a number of OPG gene-related candidate genes, and one of these (T245G) was common to the two studies (Pitocco et al. 2009, Korzon-Burakowska et al. 2012). A genome-wide association study has not yet been performed.

■ Diabetes and the chronic inflammatory state

If the role of proinflammatory cytokines and of the RANKL–NFkappaB pathway is central to disease development, as is currently believed, then it should be noted that elevation of circulating concentrations of OPG, which is a marker of pathway activation, has been a consistent observation in diabetes (**Figure 32.1**). Type 2 diabetes is associated with elevated expression of other inflammatory markers, although the Charcot foot is equally likely in type 1 and type 2 diseases. Other

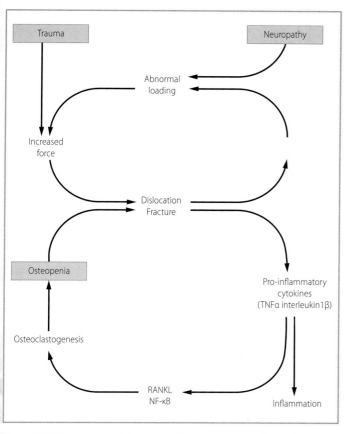

Figure 32.1 Two separate vicious cycles that we suggest are integral to development of the acute Charcot foot. Items in boxes = predispose to and trigger onset. Upper cycle = essence of well accepted 'neurotraumatic' theory. Lower cycle = topic of our hypothesis, indicating how development of condition depends on exaggerated expression of proinflammatory cytokines. With permission from Jeffcoate et al. (2005). ©2005, with permission from Elsevier.

accompaniments of poor glycemic control (including hyperlipidemia, reactive oxygen species, and advanced glycation end products) have both also been observed to lead to activation of the RANKL–NFκB pathway.

Nephropathy

The acute Charcot foot may be especially likely in people with established renal failure, provided any peripheral arterial disease (PAD) that they have is not sufficient to minimize the capacity for a distal inflammatory response. Nephropathy is also associated with increased MAC of the smaller arteries of the leg and foot, as well as many of the metabolic changes that occur in diabetes. People with renal failure will also have renal bone disease, and the bone damage induced by an acute inflammatory lesion is therefore probably more likely.

It is possible, however, that much of the association with nephropathy is not directly related to renal dysfunction but may be to a large extent the result of two confounding factors. The first is that the key predisposing abnormality that predisposes to the acute Charcot foot is neuropathy, and neuropathy and nephropathy are both microvascular complications and hence are inevitably associated. The other factor is the occurrence of the acute Charcot foot with a particular subset of people with nephropathy: those that have a kidney

transplant, and perhaps especially those undergoing combined kidney pancreas transplantation.

Combined kidney pancreas transplantation

The increased incidence of an acute Charcot foot has long been suspected in this group and has been reported in 4.6% of 130 patients in one series (Rangel et al. 2012). Valabhji (2011) also suggested that the use of immunosuppressants may mask the clinical signs, with little increased warmth accompanying the inflammation in the affected foot. If the condition is more common in this group, it could relate to the fact that the populations that undergo a combined transplant are highly selected. They will almost all be younger, with established distal neuropathy but without evidence of atherosclerotic macrovascular disease. Pre-existing renal bone disease may also have led to reduced bone strength. Similarly, the use of corticosteroids to reduce rejection may also be important because despite being immunosuppressant, they also increase expression of RANKL with resultant osteoclast activation and evidence for this has been provided by the recent observations of Rangel et al. (2012).

In the light of current knowledge, however, patients undergoing combined kidney pancreas transplant should be regarded as being at very high risk and should receive relevant education and consideration of long-term surveillance by an appropriate expert with an interest in disease of the foot in diabetes – even if the patient no longer has diabetes after the operation.

◼ Other disease of the foot in diabetes

There is abundant evidence from case and cohort observation that the acute Charcot foot may be triggered by any cause of inflammation in the foot, and this is highly relevant because this population is at risk of ulceration, and of infection. Both of these will result in local inflammation, as well as any surgery used in their management (Game et al. 2012). Revascularization procedures in the lower limb have also been associated with the onset of the disease.

Pre-existing ulceration with or without osteomyelitis

If a person with a pre-existing (usually neuropathic) ulcer develops local inflammation, this may be caused by secondary infection. However, it is also possible that the ulcer itself has triggered the onset of an acute Charcot foot. If an X-ray reveals new fracture or dislocation at a site anatomically distant from the ulcer, the possibility of an acute Charcot foot should be seriously considered.

The same is true in cases being treated for osteomyelitis of the foot. If they develop an exacerbation of inflammation during, or following, a course of antibiotic treatment, then one possibility is the occurrence of superinfection by bacteria that are resistant to the chosen antibiotics but another is that the inflammation (and any coincidental new bone change) is the result of a secondary Charcot process.

It can be very difficult to determine whether such new inflammation is the result of infection or of a new Charcot process: there is no imaging or other test, which can reliably make the distinction. Strongly supportive evidence for a new Charcot process is, however, provided by the provision of new off-loading to reduce weight bearing – without any change in antibiotic treatment. In cases of new Charcot foot, effective off-loading will lead to a prompt (within 3–4 days) reduction in the inflammation.

Other complications of diabetes

Impaired vision, unsteadiness through reduced proprioception and the consequences of comorbidities, may all increase the likelihood of an acute Charcot foot being triggered by an accident and minor injury.

INCOMPATIBILITY BETWEEN KNOWN CAUSATIVE FACTORS AND THE CLINICAL PRESENTATION

Given that the known causative factors are generally systemic, symmetrical, and irreversible, three features are unexplained. The first of these is that the condition is so rare – with an estimated lifetime cumulative incidence of approximately 3 per thousand people with diabetes, and affecting perhaps only 1% of people with neuropathy. This might suggest that other, much less common, factors play an important permissive role. These might include genetic factors or the retained capacity of the peripheral vasculature to vasodilate (see above).

The second surprising feature is that the disease is generally unilateral, with only some 20–30% being reported to have bilateral disease, either concurrently or sequentially. Given that distal neuropathy is generally symmetrical, each limb must have been exposed to identical predisposing factors at the time the disease occurs in one foot. The fact that the disease is usually unilateral might suggest that the exposure of the affected limb to a particular trigger of local inflammation, such as trauma, is important.

The third feature is that once the condition has resolved, recurrence is rare – even though the circumstances thought to have predisposed to it are unaltered. Some early recurrences (within 12 months, perhaps) may be the result of off-loading (see Chapter 36) being discontinued before the disease was truly in remission, but late recurrences of the acute inflammatory episode are exceptional. This may be because some predisposing factors are not permanent. Such factors might include progression of the extent of any neuropathy or of any associated PAD – such that the capacity to mount a continuing inflammatory response is lost.

DIAGNOSIS OF THE ACUTE CHARCOT FOOT IN DIABETES

Clinical

Diagnosis depends on awareness of the possibility, combined with pattern recognition. Unfortunately, most health-care professionals will not even consider the diagnosis of the acute Charcot foot when a person with distal neuropathy presents with unexplained inflammation. It is commonplace for someone with an acute Charcot foot to have had a deep vein thrombosis excluded and then been treated for cellulitis, sprain, gout – or all three in some cases. This failure to make the diagnosis with the necessary promptness is the main factor leading to the delay in the institution of early treatment and thereby worsening the eventual outcome. One way to try to combat this is to ensure that all people diagnosed with distal symmetrical neuropathy are informed about the possibility (however unlikely) that they may get an acute Charcot foot and advised (repeatedly) that if they ever develop unexplained inflammation of the foot, to ask their professional career if it may be a Charcot foot.

The diagnosis is primarily clinical, and there are no biochemical markers that are specific to the disease. It should be noted that elevation of C-reactive protein (CRP) may also occur in the acute Charcot foot and cannot therefore used to make a confident diagnosis of infection.

Clinical diagnosis is not, however, sufficient on its own and confirmation is required through the use of imaging. While awaiting the result of such imaging, some form of off-loading (weight-sparing, casting, orthotic walker) should be strongly considered, and the case should be reviewed as soon as the result of imaging is available.

Imaging
Plain X-ray

A plain X-ray will usually be indicated in every case, using anteroposterior (dorsal–plantar), oblique, and lateral weight-bearing views. The aim may be to seek radiological signs to confirm the clinical suspicion: fracture, dislocation, or both. However, it is also usual to do an X-ray even if the diagnosis is in little doubt, and the result of the X-ray will not affect management. The result will, however, serve as a baseline.

MRI

If the X-ray shows no diagnostic features in a suspected case, the principal requirement is to demonstrate signs of marrow inflammation by seeking signs of marrow edema, and MRI is generally regarded as the test of choice. If present, marrow edema is not specific but it is confirmatory. The degree of signal intensity derived from combining MRI with gadolinium enhancement in dynamic MRI (D-MRI) has recently been described as correlating with time to resolution, but this needs to be confirmed (Zampa et al. 2011).

Evidence of marrow inflammation may also be obtained by three-phase bone scanning using, e.g. a bisphosphonate-tagged marker. It is as sensitive as MRI but less specific.

Computed tomography (CT)

The CT scanning may detect fractures that were not apparent on either plain X-ray or MRI.

PET and SPECT–CT

The value of newer imaging modalities, such as scanning using positron emission tomography (PET) and single-photon emission CT (SPECT–CT), has not yet been established.

When the diagnosis is not confirmed by imaging, a decision on management has to be based on clinical grounds. The opinion of a rheumatologist or orthopedic surgeon may be sought. Off-loading may be continued or not, depending on circumstances. Repeat imaging may be considered if the inflammation does not settle.

MONITORING DISEASE ACTIVITY AND THE DIAGNOSIS OF REMISSION

Difference in skin temperature between the two feet

Skin temperature is most easily and reliably documented with an infrared skin surface probe. Assuming that any inflammatory process is confined to one foot, it has become accepted practice to suggest that if the difference in temperature between the skin over the affected part and an equivalent site on the other foot is ≤2°C, then it can be assumed that the disease has gone into remission. In practice, the test is not 100% reliable – partly because there is considerable variation in the difference in temperature between feet from week to week – depending perhaps on ambient temperature, how long they have waited with their cast off, posture (legs horizontal or dependent), and observer technique. Moreover a difference of 2°C is quite appreciable and must reflect some continuing inflammation. Nevertheless, there are some recent data to substantiate the use of skin temperature in this way (Moura-Neto et al. 2012), and it at least provides some sort of objective marker. Patients also become very interested in the result of skin temperature measurement, and it helps involve them in decisions made regarding management.

Imaging

Imaging may be used to establish that the condition of the foot has not deteriorated, especially when the foot is ulcerated and there is a possibility of the Charcot foot being complicated by bone infection. The place of routine re-examination by MRI to determine residual activity of the Charcot process is not established and most clinicians rely on clinical grounds. There is no published evidence to demonstrate that MRI imaging can be reliably used to demonstrate that disease has entered remission.

Venous sampling

There has been no report of a systematic study of the use of measurement of circulating proinflammatory cytokines to document disease progress. As the circulatory concentrations of these, as well as of markers of inflammatory response (such as CRP), are only inconsistently elevated in acute disease, it is unlikely that their measurement will add much to clinical assessment.

OTHER OUTCOME MEASURES

The rarity of the acute Charcot foot means that it may be impossible to conduct randomized trials of sufficient size to document the benefit of interventions unless the effect size is very great. This means that improved understanding of the benefit of different treatments requires the comparison of outcome between cohorts and centers, and this requires agreement on the use of outcome measures. At the moment, such consensus is nonexistent, and yet it is essential. Effective comparison will require careful documentation of the study population (defining both people and the extent of foot disease) and agreed measures of disease activity as well as long-term outcome measures.

Outcome measures might be undertaken during the course of management, as well as at, say, 12 and 24 months.

Function

Measures are required of function and mood. Specific scales can be used but the easiest to implement in routine clinical practice would be Euroqol 5D (EQ-5D), because it is easy to administer and has been validated in many languages.

The adverse effect of this disabling condition on mood is seriously underestimated by clinicians: depression being very common. Its main cause seems to be the restriction in lifestyle, which continues for so many months.

Radiology

The degree of ultimate skeletal deformity can be documented using standard foot alignment measures (Hastings et al. 2011).

Mortality

Life expectancy of people with an acute Charcot foot (just as of neuropathic ulceration) has been shown in the United Kingdom to be reduced by an average of 14 years, when compared with an unselected UK population, and median survival after presentation was just (van Baal et al. 2010). The cause of death is presumed to be cardiovascular, probably made more likely by the circulatory strain imposed by decreased peripheral resistance caused by vasomotor neuropathy as well as MAC.

AREAS OF CONTROVERSY AND/OR FUTURE RESEARCH

- Although the acute Charcot foot is likely to be mediated through a process of uncontrolled local inflammation, its causes are multiple with different factors likely to dominate in different people. It is best regarded as a syndrome complex
- There is no obvious reason why the disease is most commonly unilateral
- As the predisposing factors are largely persistent, it is not clear why recurrence is relatively uncommon
- If the acute Charcot foot is a syndrome that is mediated by uncontrolled inflammation, then the use of anti-inflammatory agents may be beneficial. To date, however, there has been no systematic assessment of the therapeutic benefit of any anti-inflammatory preparations
- One group of people appears to be at particular risk of developing an acute Charcot foot, and this is the population undergoing kidney transplantation. Transplant teams should alert potential recipients to the possibility of the condition occurring and the need for urgent diagnosis and treatment if it does

IMPORTANT FURTHER READING

Jeffcoate WJ, Game F, Cavanagh PR. The role of pro-inflammatory cytokines in the cause of neuropathic osteoarthropathy (acute Charcot foot) in diabetes. Lancet 2005; 366:2058–2061.

Milne TE, Rogers JR, Kinnear EM, et al. Developing an evidence-based clinical pathway for the assessment, diagnosis and management of acute Charcot Neuro-Arthropathy: a systematic review. J Foot Ankle Res 2013; 6:30.

Rogers LC, Frykberg RG, Armstrong DG, et al. The Charcot foot in diabetes. ADA Consensus statement. Diab Care 2011; 34:2123–2139. Reprinted in J Am Podiatr Med Assoc 101:437–446.

■ REFERENCES

Baker N, Green A, Krishnan S, Rayman G. Microvascular and C-fiber function in diabetic Charcot neuroarthropathy and diabetic peripheral neuropathy. Diabetes Care 2007; 30:3077–3079.

Chantelau E, Wienemann T, Richter A. Pressure pain thresholds at the diabetic Charcot-foot: an exploratory study. J Musculoskel Neuronal Interact 2012; 12:95–101.

Game FL, Callow R, Jones GR, et al. Audit of acute Charcot's disease in the UK: the CDUK study. Diabetologia 2012; 55:32–35.

Hastings MK, Sinacore DR, Mercer-Bolton N, et al. Precision of foot alignment measures in Charcot arthropathy. Foot Ankle Int 2011; 32:867–872.

Jeffcoate WJ, Game F, Cavanagh PR. The role of pro-inflammatory cytokines in the cause of neuropathic osteoarthropathy (acute Charcot foot) in diabetes. Lancet 2005; 366:2058–2061.

Jeffcoate WJ, Rasmussen LM, Hofbauer LC, Game FL. Medial arterial calcification in diabetes and its relationship to neuropathy. Diabetologia 2009; 52:2478–2488.

Korzon-Burakowska A, Jakóbkiewicz-Banecka J, Fiedosiuk A, et al. Osteoprotegerin gene polymorphism in diabetic Charcot neuroarthropathy. Diabet Med 2012; 29:771–775.

Moura-Neto A, Fernandes TD, Zantutt Wittmann DE, et al. Charcot foot: skin temperature as a good clinical parameter for predicting disease outcome. Diabet Res Clin Pract 2012; 96:e11–e14.

Ndip A, Williams A, Jude EB, et al. The RANKL/RANK/OPG signalling pathway mediates arterial calcification in diabetic Charcot neuroarthropathy. Diabetes 2011; 60:2187–2196.

Pitocco D, Zelano G, Gioffrè G, et al. Association between osteoprotegerin G1181C and T245G polymorphisms and diabetic Charcot neuroarthropathy: a case-control study. Diabetes Care 2009; 32:1694–1697.

Rangel ÉB, Sá JR, Gomes SA, et al. Charcot neuroarthropathy after simultaneous pancreas-kidney transplant. Transplantation 2012; 27:642–645.

Rogers LC, Frykberg RG, Armstrong DG, et al. The Charcot foot in diabetes. ADA Consensus statement. Diabetes Care 2011; 34: 2123–2139. Reprinted in J Am Podiatr Med Assoc 101: 437–446.

Sanders LJ, Edmonds ME, Jeffcoate WJ. Who was first to diagnose and report neuropathic arthropathy of the foot and ankle: Jean-Martin Charcot or Herbert William Page? Diabetologia 2013; 56:1873–1877.

Shapiro SA, Stansberry KB, Hill MA, et al. Normal blood flow response and vasomotion in the diabetic Charcot foot. J Diabetes Complications 1998; 12:147–153.

Valabhji J. Immunosuppression therapy posttransplantation can be associated with a difference clinical phenotype for diabetic Charcot foot neuroarthropathy. Diabetes Care 2011; 34:e135.

van Baal J, Hubbard R, Game F, Jeffcoate W. Mortality associated with acute Charcot foot and neuropathic foot ulceration. Diabetes Care 2010; 33:1086–1089.

Veves A, Akbari CM, Primavera J, et al. Endothelial dysfunction and the expression of endothelial nitric oxide synthetase in diabetic neuropathy, vascular disease, and foot ulceration. Diabetes 1998; 47:457–463.

Zampa V, Bargellini I, Rizzo L, et al. Role of dynamic MRI in the follow-up of acute Charcot foot in patients with diabetes mellitus. Skeletal Radiol 2011; 40:991–999.

Chapter 33 | Charcot osteoarthropathy: medical management and off-loading

Valeria Ruotolo, Luigi Uccioli

SUMMARY

- The mainstay of treatment in stage 0 and 1 disease remains immobilization and off-loading of the affected foot
- Immobilization and off-loading is recommended even if there is no evidence of bone abnormality on plain radiograph
- The total contact cast (TCC) is considered widely to be the therapeutic modality of choice to treat the acute Charcot foot
- An alternative to the TCC is the instant TTC (iTTC)
- The follow-up of patients with diabetes and acute Charcot osteoarthropathy (CO) undergoing treatment has traditionally been based on clinical signs
- The role of drugs to heal neuro-osteoarthropathy of the foot remains unproven

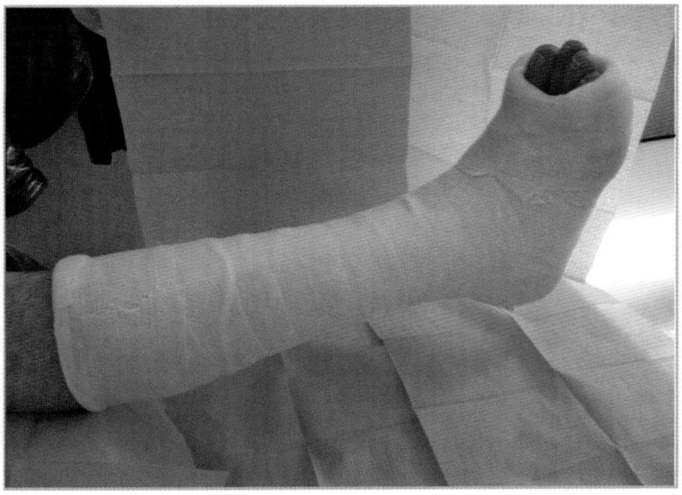

Figure 33.1 Total contact cast.

INTRODUCTION

The treatment of CO depends on many factors, including the course or stage of CO, location(s) of involvement (Sinacore 1998, Sanders & Frykberg 2007), presence of ulcers (Saltzman et al. 2005), and ability to achieve a stable and plantigrade foot. Other factors that could affect treatment options are comorbidities, such as morbid obesity, cardiovascular disease, nephropathy, or infected ulcer (Armstrong et al. 1997b, Saltzman et al. 2005). The aims for every patient undergoing treatment should be to stop and control the progression of bones and soft tissues inflammation and to protect the foot from the destructive stage; to achieve or maintain the architecture of the foot and/or ankle to stabilize the foot in a position of minimum deformity that can ultimately be accommodated in a shoe or an appropriate orthosis, and finally, to prevent deformity, ulceration, and involvement of the contralateral, nonaffected limb. The goal of CO treatment is to achieve a foot that supports the functional goals of the patient, which may be different for a young and active patient versus a patient who already uses a wheelchair.

At present, the mainstay of treatment in stage 0 and 1 disease remains immobilization and off-loading of the affected foot to limit the inflammatory process that accompanies the beginning of the acute phase. Mechanical protection to treat active CO is the most 'natural' way to stop abnormal weight bearing and inflammation in the injured bone. The TCC is the most widely used and accessible modality for maintaining stability and decreasing edema (Armstrong et al. 1997b, Sinacore 1998, Chantelau 2005, Edmonds et al. 2005, Chantelau & Poll 2006) (**Figure 33.1**). Although TCC is considered widely to be the therapeutic modality of choice to treat the bone injuries of patients with insensate feet, it is important to consider that these patients cannot report symptoms due to iatrogenic injury from casting.

RATIONALE FOR IMMOBILIZATION AND OFF-LOADING

In the acute phase, the clinical picture is characterized by nonspecific inflammatory signs; in the very early stage of CO (stage 0 in the Eichenholtz/Shibata staging) (see Chapter 34), the bone appearance is still normal on plain radiograph (X-ray) and this often causes a delay in diagnosis, with a progressive, dangerous weight-bearing, and repeat traumatization on an insensate foot; therefore, the foot is at risk to develop severe deformity and structural instability. Thereafter, in stage 0, only magnetic resonance imaging (MRI) can reveal, in great detail, the extent of the bony damage and evidence of inflammation in the bone as well as in the adjacent soft tissue (Chantelau 2005, Chantelau et al. 2006, Edmonds et al. 2005). The MRI findings in stage 0 are exactly the same as those in other cases of bone stress injury and respond equally well to cessation of the trauma-like bone injuries in feet with a preserved sensation, consistent with a cause–effect relationship between trauma and bone marrow edema in both conditions. This has induced many authors to recommend immobilization and off-loading even if there is no evidence of bone abnormality on plain radiograph (Giurini 1991, Sella & Barrette 1999, Yu & Hudson 2002).

Currently, the signs of acute nonfracture bone injuries (such as bone marrow edema), which can be visualized by MRI rather than plain radiographs, must be taken as criterion to off-load and immobilize a swollen pain-insensitive foot, because persistent weight bearing in this condition will cause the progression of the disease and the appearance of fractures and deformities. Chantelau (2005) has shown that, with persistent weight bearing, these MRI abnormalities progress to radiographically visible bone and joint pathology and deformities feet, which are insensate. In a series of 24 subjects, the early detection of incipient CO permitted an immediate off-loading of the affected foot, and therefore, a significant reduction of fractures and deformities. In another study, Edmonds et al. (2006) showed that off-loading in the early stage stopped the progression of the acute phase in 12 subjects with bone marrow edema on MRI and any abnormalities on plain radiography and scintigraphy.

Charcot osteoarthropathy is probably triggered by an initial traumatic lesion of bone, capsule, cartilage, ligament, and tendon insertion in an insensitive foot. However, the injury is necessary but not sufficient to develop the CO; in fact, the persistent foot loading is required to produce the picture of the disease with its typical devastating bone and joint destruction.

A total of 34 patients with diabetes and foot bone injuries and bone marrow edema on MRI were evaluated retrospectively in a study. All of them were treated with TCC. The authors investigated the relationship between the intensity of unrestrained weight bearing after a nonfracture injury and the development of deformities of the foot (Kimmerle & Chantelau 2007). Cumulative load forces after the onset of symptoms until treatment were estimated using the product of body weight and number of weeks of ambulation (kg x weeks).

This study provides evidence of a dose–response relationship between unrestrained weight bearing (and then trauma) and development of CO deformities in patients with nonfracture foot bone injuries. The data support the concept that the extent of the bone damage is due to the intensity of repeat traumatization (which is usually extensive in an insensate foot) (Kimmerle & Chantelau 2007).

In the literature, many studies consider trauma as a trigger for CO (Thompson et al. 1983, Armstrong et al. 1997b). Armstrong et al. reported that 26% of 55 patients with CO were able to recall an episode of foot trauma as the preceding event. However, in neither of these studies was there an objective confirmation of the patient-reported positive or negative trauma history by concurrent MRI. This imaging would have been necessary, considering the imprecision of trauma perception and the low reliability of self-reporting due to pain insensitivity of the feet. In conclusion, when there is an early diagnosis at stage 0, the off-loading and immobilization start immediately, and the treatment lasts until the foot inflammatory process ends, no bone fractures and foot deformities develop and progression to stage I is avoided (Chantelau 2005, Edmonds et al. 2005, Chantelau et al. 2007b).

PUTATIVE MECHANISM OF ACTION OF OFF-LOADING AND IMMOBILIZATION

Putting at rest a foot with acute CO invariably decreases swelling and inflammation (McGill et al. 2000).

McGill et al. studied the relationship between activity of CO and clinical variables over 12 months during which 17 patients received standard treatment of rest and TCC using scintigraphy for the qualitative assessment of the activity of CO. Although the clinical course of CO has often been described in the literature, it is difficult to document it in quantitative terms, due to a lack of objective indices. Likewise, it has been difficult to study the responses to various treatment modalities. McGill et al. proved that the ratio of isotope uptake, and then the inflammatory process, decreased after immobilization in an average period of 6 months, by comparing clinical parameters (such as the skin temperature difference) and quantitative data (three-phase quantitative bone scan). There was a strong correlation (statistically significant) between temperature difference and the ratio of isotope uptake in the affected–nonaffected feet. Twelve months later, the affected foot still had 30% more isotope uptake (McGill et al. 2000).

Such observations have encouraged the use of immobilization and off-loading that not only mitigate the fatigue processes, that inevitably occur in a damaged foot skeleton during everyday unprotected ambulation, but also reduce the inflammatory activity in an acute CO, which otherwise would be amplified.

CRITERIA FOR IMMOBILIZATION AND OFF-LOADING

Previously, only the acute fracture state of CO that could be visualized by plain radiographs (stage I and II according to Eichenholtz's classification) was taken as a criterion to off-load and immobilize a swollen insensate foot (Armstrong et al. 1997b, Chantelau 2005, Saltzman et al. 2005). Acute nonfracture bone injuries (i.e. bone marrow edema) that can be visualized only by MRI (rather than plain radiographs) must be taken as criterion to off-load and immobilize a swollen insensate foot, because persistent weight bearing in this condition will cause CO with progression and fracture (Kimmerle et al. 2007). Therefore, some authors (Edmonds et al. 2006, Chantelau et al. 2007b, Kimmerle et al. 2007) have recommended the use of MRI rather than plain radiographic examination for patients with sudden onset of edema and erythema in a neuropathic foot. They agree with Thompson's suggestion that, even where there is no fracture identified, the patient should be given a cast as initial treatment (Thompson et al. 1983). Chantelau has shown that in 12 subjects with bone marrow edema on MRI without abnormalities on standard radiographs, the off-loading leads to complete resolution of the bone marrow edema in 17 weeks without any foot deformity and/or fracture. MRI of bone marrow edema in stage 0 CO suggests a stress injury as pathogenic mechanism in a neuropathic foot. A cause–effect relationship between trauma and these MRI abnormalities is further supported by the reversal of these abnormalities by the standard treatment of stress bone injuries – nonweight bearing and immobilization – which is curative, in general, in 3–6 months (Chantelau et al. 2007b). As Giurini et al. postulated in 1991, CO can be effectively be cured if it is treated in stage 0, before bone dissolution has occurred, by off-loading and immobilization for months.

METHODS OF NONSURGICAL IMMOBILIZATION/OFF-LOADING

The TCC is considered the gold standard initial therapy for the treatment of acute CO. A TCC uses a well-molded, minimally padded cast, which maintains contact with the entire plantar surface of the foot and the lower leg; by maintaining contact with the entire plantar surface and the whole lower leg, the cast disperses pressure across the entire foot, thereby minimizing isolated areas of high pressure of the foot. The goal is to protect and rest the foot through the inflammatory and destructive stages until the foot stabilizes in a position of minimum deformity that may ultimately be accommodated in a shoe or in an appropriate orthosis. TCC has an ability to 'force compliance': the patient has little choice other than to adhere to the off-loading regimen prescribed by the clinician, because the device is nonremovable. The TCC also tends to reduce and controls edema.

Many authors strongly recommend that patients with stage 0 and I CO, although in a TCC, remain nonweight bearing (Onvlee 1998, Chantelau et al. 2007a). Chantelau has shown that rigid rather than soft or semirigid immobilization is advisable for bone healing, because it reduces peak contact stresses, decreases shear forces, and interfragmentary movements (the exact strain environment of a partially loaded foot remains unknown). However, many patients with CO tended to be noncompliant with the nonweight-bearing regimens. In many cases, it is difficult to be completely nonweight bearing, because the patient has multiple comorbidities, such as postural hypotension, high body mass index, loss of proprioception, and, in some cases, neuropathy of the upper limbs, all of which can make it difficult for him to use crutches. Furthermore, a wheelchair existence is often impractical in many home environments. Total immobility also has the disadvantage of loss of muscle tone, reduction in bone density, and loss of body fitness. Finally, fracture of the contralateral limb was reported in 72% of patients in a high-risk population (Pinzur et al. 2006). Prophylactic immobilization of the unaffected limb was recommended to reduce the risk of contralateral fracture. Therefore, based on these considerations as well as the lack of documented evidence to support a nonweight-bearing treatment plan, some investigators have suggested allowing weight bearing in the early stages of CO (Armstrong et al. 1997b, Sinacore 1998, Pinzur et al. 2006, De Souza 2008). Sinacore retrospectively reviewed the outcomes of 30 subjects with an acute CO who were allowed to partial weight bear using assistive devices; in this study, the average healing time was 3 months, with results comparable with those of a nonweight-bearing protocol (Sinacore 1998). Armstrong et al. followed 55 acute CO patients treated with a TCC and allowed them to walk without crutches; all subjects healed without deformity, although the average healing time was 6.5 weeks longer than in the non-weight bearing study.

Pinzur et al. reported on 10 patients with stage I CO of the midfoot who underwent biweekly TCC changes and were allowed full weight bearing. The average cast duration was 6 weeks, with progression to therapeutic footwear at 12 weeks. All patients in this group progressed to healing with a stable foot (Pinzur et al. 2006). TCC should be performed by a cast technician with training or experience to safely apply a TCC. Whether or not weight bearing, cast changes every 2 weeks are needed to accommodate edema reduction. The cast should be regularly checked and a change in treatment plan may be required if progressive deformity occurs despite casting. Immobilization for approximately 5–6 months is not uncommon (19 ± 11 weeks) (Armstrong et al. 2007b); however, patients with bilateral involvement required a longer duration of TCC treatment (28 ± 15 weeks); duration of TCC treatment or time to return to footwear is independent of the anatomic site of involvement (Armstrong et al. 1997b).

The absence of a clear definition of 'healing' for CO hampers the definition of the necessary duration of treatment. Healing could be defined as no recurrence after treatment, but 'recurrence' is poorly defined. The average duration of cast treatment to heal nonfracture injuries has ranged from 3 to 6 months (Chantelau 2005, Edmonds et al. 2006a, Pinzur et al. 2006, Chantelau et al. 2007a); the difference in healing time could be attributed to differences in the definition of 'healing' used by different clinicians. Apparently, the duration of off-loading and immobilization varies with the physician's treatment objectives, the patient's compliance with the TCC, and the extent of bone injury. Sinacore found that CO of the hindfoot, midfoot, and ankle took significantly longer to heal in TCC than CO of the forefoot (Sinacore 1998). The average duration of cast treatment to heal fracture injuries is about 20 months (Armstrong et al. 1997b, Chantelau 2005, Saltzman 2005, Edmonds et al. 2006). Retrospectively, Sinacore showed that 23% of limbs required bracing for >18 months, and the overall prevalence of bilateral CO was 10% in that cohort. None of the following factors influenced the likelihood of requiring long-term bracing: age, type of diabetes, location of Charcot deformity, or presence of nephropathy. The likelihood of a patient requiring an amputation depended mostly on the ability to maintain a closed skin envelope. The presence of open ulcers at presentation or recurrent ulcers increased the risk of eventual limb amputation (Sinacore 1998).

Although TCC is considered the gold standard treatment for acute CO, in clinical practice the standard care is not always applicable especially in those patients with prior major amputation, who are blind or overweight. Some even refuse a TCC. In addition, many patients experience problems with activities of daily living with the TCC, such as bathing and sleeping. For some a TCC exacerbates postural instability.

An alternative and successful alternative to the TCC in the management of acute CO is a prefabricated removable cast walker (RCW). They have the benefit of being instantly applicable without specialist skills; moreover, they are comfortable to use and may be removed at night so they tend to be more acceptable to patients than the TCC. Adjustments may be required to accommodate changes in foot shape and size due to deformity and swelling. The walker boot may be padded with a protective insole molded from materials commonly used in footwear (such as polypropylene terephthalate) (Petrova & Edmonds 2008). An example of a widely used RCW is the Aircast Pneumatic Walker: its key elements include a semirigid plastic shell surrounding the limb, a removable front panel, four individual internal air cells inflated with a manometer to 20–30 mmHg to hold

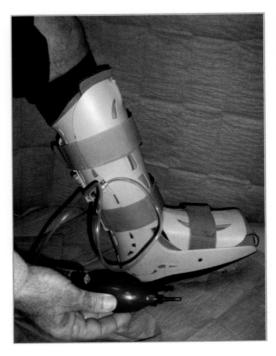

Figure 33.2 An example of a removable cast walker: pneumatic walker.

the limb, a specifically designed rocker sole for improved off-loading and a dual-intensity insole (**Figure 33.2**).

An alternative RCW is the Optima Diab, which consists of a rigid rocker sole with an innovative design, a modular insole composed of three layers of different stiffness that can be adapted and a posterior rigid brace to block the ankle high to the upper leg.

The Charcot Restraint Orthotic Walker (CROW) is a custom, bivalve, total contact foot–ankle orthosis with full foot enclosure, rigid rocker sole, and custom insole. Disadvantages of the CROW include the high costs of fabrication and maintenance (Armstrong et al. 2005).

The Stabil-D device is composed of a specifically designed rigid, boat-shaped and fully rocker-bottom sole: its rounded extremities (at the heel and tiptoe) facilitate gate and its middle section improves the mid-stance phase. The insole height (24 mm) avoids excessive lifting of the contralateral limb during walk, thus lowering the barycenter and favoring more stable walking. At the ankle, the cast is provided with removable, lateral stabilizer inserts, which ensure stability to the tibiotarsal joint and/or adequate support during gait. A rigid brace properly supports the Achilles tendon and contributes to stability during rolling steps. The cast has modular insole made of multiple layers of different stiffness.

The TCC and the RCW are similar in many aspects, and earlier studies did not show a difference in pressure relief between these two modalities (Lavery et al. 1996, Baumhauer 1997, Wukich & Motko 2004, Armstrong et al. 2005). However, for the treatment of CO, RCWs have not proven to be as effective as traditional TCC. In addition, there is an unfortunate downside: the patients can remove the RCW, and therefore their adherence to the use of removable device seems to be poor. The Charcot in Diabetes in the UK (CDUK) study compared removable versus nonremovable devices and found a slight but statistically significant difference in healing (as determined by clinicians), with healing occurring sooner when nonremovable devices were used.

To address these issues, an alternative to the TCC is the iTTC, which simply consists of a commercial RCW rendered irremovable by a layer of cohesive bandage or a plastic lace that can be removed only by cutting it with a specific tool, thus rendering it nonremovable by the patients. In a randomized study, Armstrong compared the efficacy of RCW versus the same device wrapped entirely in a cohesive bandage (iTCC) in healing neuropathic foot ulcers and reported a significantly higher proportion of patients healed at 12 weeks in the iTCC group than in the RCW group (Armstrong et al. 2002). According to these data, it is the removability of the device that makes the difference in terms of wound healing time (Armstrong et al. 2003).

Although RCW show similar plantar pressures compared with a TCC in healthy subjects, they have yet to be evaluated in the treatment of acute CO. If a RCW is used during stage 0 or 1 of CO, we highly recommend that it be rendered irremovable to limit structural damage. Hindfoot CO is probably best treated in a TCC.

HOW CAN THE RESPONSE TO IMMOBILIZATION THERAPY BE MONITORED?

The follow-up of patients with diabetes and acute CO under treatment has traditionally been based on clinical signs, such as swelling, erythema, edema, pain resolution, and a drop of the skin temperature difference (ΔT) between the affected foot and the contralateral one, determined by an infrared thermometer, stably below 2°C for at least 1 month, and on repeated plain radiographs (signs of coalescence and bone consolidation/remodeling) (Lavery et al. 1996, Armstrong et al. 1997a, McGill et al. 2000). The Consensus of the American Diabetes Association about the Charcot foot in diabetes published in 2011 emphasizes that duration and aggressiveness of off-loading are guided by clinical assessment of healing of CO based on edema, erythema, and skin temperature changes. Actually, treatment duration according to the normalization of foot temperature, the resolution of foot edema, or bone remineralization on plain radiograph is associated with a considerable rate of fracture relapse (Armstrong et al. 1997a). In fact, clinical criteria alone can be misleading. The skin temperature is not only related to the presence of inflammation, but it can also be altered by several conditions, such as peripheral arterial disease, neuropathy, and external factors. The clinical signs alone would not be sufficient to evaluate the initial response to limb off-loading, since they may lack specificity. Early weight bearing must be avoided because it may cause acute early exacerbations as reported by Sinacore in 13% of cases (Sinacore 1998). In fact, early weight bearing may favor an increase of the inflammatory process and induce an incorrect diagnosis of a relapse; indeed, that inflammatory process is a 'false relapse' and, actually, the expression of the same, long disease process that has never cleared up.

McGill et al. (2000) reported an interesting experience using scintigraphy for the qualitative assessment of the activity of CO. Scintigraphy has been proposed as a valid tool in assessing the phase of activity of CO and in monitoring the treatment outcome. In a series of eight patients studied over a 12-month follow-up period, the authors proved that the ratio of isotope uptake decreased during the follow-up period after limb immobilization. However, scintigraphic images lack anatomical detail. A more refined method of follow-up that should be applied, particularly in cases of nonfracture injuries, would be based on repeated MRI. In fact, during the return to weight-bearing activity, follow-up MRI sometimes discloses residual bone marrow edema that is not accompanied by relevant clinical symptoms. Accordingly, we argue that the duration of immobilization and off-loading should be determined in relation to MRI improvement and should probably be longer than might be suggested by clinical improvement (Chantelau et al. 2007a). Likewise, the return and monitoring to weight bearing should be based on the more sensitive MRI findings rather than on crude temperature or plain radiographic findings as has been tradition.

We evaluated the use of positron emission tomography (PET)/computed tomography (CT) scan in patients with diabetes and a clinical suspicion of an acute Charcot foot (Ruotolo et al. 2012). Both MRI and PET/CT scan confirmed the presence of an acute CO. In addition, the maximum standard uptake value (SUV) max was utilized to follow up these patients: SUV max values decreased only in patients in which the inflammatory process was damped, but no changes were observed in patients in which the disease process was still ongoing. We found signs of inflammation on PET/CT scan for an average time of 15 months, which is a longer period of time of disease duration in comparison with the data of the literature. In this study, our clinical decision was driven by PET/CT scan, but we cannot exclude that, due to its high sensitivity, this method reveals a persisting inflammatory condition that could not influence the final outcome. It is important to underline that PET/CT scan does not replace MRI; instead, it provides additional clinical information. PET/CT scanning, in conjunction with MRI, may be useful to diagnose acute Charcot foot. In addition, PET/CT scanning provides visualization of the location of the disease process and its extension, visual information of the evolution of the original localization, and eventual new localizations at follow-up. Further PET/CT provides an objective measure, SUV max values, for monitoring disease progress (Ruotolo et al. 2012).

MEDICAL THERAPY

Pharmacological agents able to inhibit pathological bone resorption are logical treatment options for disease associated with excessive bone turnover. Bisphosphonates are popular as antiresorptive drugs in the treatment of osteoporosis, Paget's disease and other diseases with increased bone turnover. There have been reports on the possibility of using this pharmacological approach in the management of CO. One study infused the bisphosphonate pamidronate intravenously in CO patients while comparing its effects to placebo. The authors performed a randomized double-blinded placebo-controlled study in 39 patients with acute CO; they received a single infusion of either 90-mg pamidronate or saline (placebo) at baseline in addition to standard care of foot immobilization. Clinical and biochemical markers of disease activity were measured over the 12-month study period. Foot temperatures fell significantly in both groups at 2 weeks, with a further fall at 4 weeks in the treatment group only, which did not reach statistical significance in comparison with the placebo group. Deoxypyridinoline (a marker of bone resorption and osteoclastic activity) was significantly decreased in the treatment group at 2–6 weeks, with a gradual return to baseline values in the following 18 weeks. Bone-specific alkaline phosphatase levels followed a similar pattern: it was significantly reduced from 4 to 12 weeks, with a gradual return to baseline over the subsequent 40 weeks (Jude et al. 2001). In another study, oral alendronate (70 mg weekly) was used in a randomized controlled trial in 11 patients and compared with placebo in 9 control patients with acute CO. Study assessments took place at baseline and again at 6 months. A significantly greater reduction in foot temperature was seen in the treatment group at 6 months. Pain scores on a visual analog scale improved significantly only in the treatment group at the follow-up assessment. Serum collagen COOH-terminal telopeptide of type I collagen (1CTP) and hydroxyproline decreased significantly in the treatment group after 6 months, and a similar trend was seen in alkaline phosphatase levels. Bone mineral density assessed by dual-energy X-ray absorptiometry demonstrated significantly improved mineralization for the total foot and distal phalanges in the treatment group (Pitocco et al. 2005). Treatment by antiresorptive drugs has been proposed because bone turnover in patients with acute Charcot foot is excessive. However, there is little evidence to support their use, but both oral and intravenous bisphosphonates have been studied in the treatment of CO in small randomized, double-blind, controlled trials (Jude et al. 2001, Pitocco et al. 2005). Moreover, many patients cannot tolerate oral bisphosphonates. At present, there is no conclusive evidence for using bisphosphonates in acute CO, and our understanding is evolving as more trials are currently underway.

Calcitonin has been used to a lesser extent than bisphosphonates for the treatment of osteoporosis, partly because of the need for parenteral administration (subcutaneously or nasally). Calcitonin is a 32-amino acid peptide synthesized in thyroid medullary cells that has a direct inhibitory effect on osteoclasts via calcitonin receptors. Long-term administration of supraphysiological doses is known to result in receptor downregulation and an escape phenomenon. The main effect of calcitonin on osteoclast activity appears to be exerted via inhibition of cytoplasmic motility, secretory activity, and a reduction in the number of osteoclasts. Calcitonin was given to 16 patients with CO and diabetes over 6 months with some effect on foot temperature and bone turnover markers but without any clinical benefits (Bem et al. 2006).

Other potential therapies include tumor necrosis factor-alpha-blockers (e.g. etanercept and infliximab) as well as high-dose corticosteroids (which decrease nuclear factor [NF]-kappa B expression), but clinical experience is as yet lacking. Future medical anti-inflammatory therapy may also include inhibitors of RANK-L (denosumab), NF-kappaB, and IL-1β, which have been used in animal studies to attenuate inflammatory arthritis (Jostel & Jude 2008).

Other adjunct therapies have also been offered to help manage CO. Electric bone growth (EBG) stimulators have been experimentally applied and clinically tested to promote healing of fractures in the acute phase. Grady et al. (2000) found that when their EBG stimulator was used during the initial period of immobilization, there was a clinical decrease in CO symptoms. A series of case reports has described the use of adjunct low-intensity ultrasound for CO treatment (Strauss & Gonya 1998).

The role of drugs to heal neuro-osteoarthropathy of the foot, including the Charcot foot, remains unproven. Whether drug treatment has a role in terms of prevention or healing of osteoarticular destructions remains to be demonstrated.

CLINICAL MANAGEMENT OF THE CHRONIC, QUIESCENT PHASE OF CO

The aims of treating the chronic phase are to reduce and redistribute plantar pressures over a greater surface area, avoid skin break down (ulceration), and provide a stable foot. The presence of CO increases the risk of foot ulceration 3.5-fold (Boyko et al. 1999); thereafter, prevention of foot ulceration is a major objective in chronic CO. Subjects should be treated with a standard protocol involving serial TCC with progression to RCW (when the skin ΔT is stably below 1°C for at least 2 weeks) and finally to prescription therapeutic shoe gear, consisting of extradepth shoes with rigid soles. RCWs are used to ease the transition from total contact casting to full, unprotected weight bearing in prescription footwear. The transition from an RCW to a prescription therapeutic footwear is permitted when the skin ΔT between the feet is stable for at least 1 month. In this phase, the focus of care transitions from minimizing skeletal structure remodeling to prevention of deformity-instigated ulceration. Foot ulcers develop in response to excessive pressure and shear forces applied to the foot. Ulceration is common beneath the cuboid and cuneiform bones. In patients with minor deformity (e.g. little or no depression of the longitudinal arch), industrially fabricated 'diabetic' shoes with a stiff walking sole and rocker bottom may be sufficient. These shoes, when furnished with custom-molded, full-contact, rigid insoles to provide arch support, will adequately minimize load bearing and mobility of the transmetatarsal and tarsophalangeal joints during walking (Frykberg & Kozak 1995). In cases of severe deformities, custom-made shoes are necessary, requiring individualized lasts; severe foot deformities or remodeled ankles may require an ankle–foot orthosis (AFO) or CROW. The rocker-bottom foot with plantar bony prominence is a site of very high pressure. Hindfoot CO may be difficult to stabilize; continued use of the cast will help achieve stability. Alternatively, a CROW may be used, followed by an AFO with bespoke footwear.

AREAS OF CONTROVERSY AND/OR FUTURE RESEARCH

- Early diagnosis with off-loading and casting are central to the management of patients with Charcot disease

- Total contact casting and the use of 'instant' TCCs are both useful methods for off-loading patients with Charcot disease and ensuring treatment
- Uncontrolled inflammation is central in etiopathogenesis of Charcot disease and therapies directed to deal with the inflammation are likely to be pivotal in the future

- The duration and aggressiveness of off-loading in acute Charcot foot remains an imprecise science, which requires further research
- The clinical effectiveness of antiresorptive drugs in altering the natural history of Charcot disease remains to be established

■ IMPORTANT FURTHER READING

Armstrong DG, Lavery LA, Wu S, Boulton AJ. Evaluation of removable and irremovable cast walkers in the healing of diabetic foot wounds: a randomized controlled trials. Diabetes Care 2005; 28:551–554.

Armstrong DG, Todd WF, Lavery LA, Harkless LB, Bushman TR. The natural history of acute Charcot's arthropathy in a diabetic foot speciality clinic. Diabet Med 1997; 14:357–363.

Chantelau E. The perils of procrastination: effects of early vs delayed detection and treatment of incipient Charcot fracture. Diabetic Med 2005; 22:1707–1712.

Frykberg RG, Kozak GP. The diabetic Charcot foot. In: Kozak GP, Campbell DR, Fryberg RG, Haberwshaw GM (eds), Management of diabetic foot problems, 2nd edn. Philadelphia, PA: WB Saunders, 1995:88–97.

McGill M, Molyneaux L, Bolton T, et al. Response of Charcot's arthropathy to contact casting: assessment by quantitative techniques. Diabetologia 2000; 43:481–484.

Rogers LC, Frykberg RG, Armstrong DG, et al. The Charcot foot in diabetes. Diabetes Care 2011; 34:2123–2129.

■ REFERENCES

Armstrong DG, Lavery LA, Kimbriel HR, Nixon BP, Boulton AJ. Activity patterns of patients with diabetic foot ulceration: patients with active ulceration may not adhere to a standard pressure off-loading regimen. Diabetes Care 2003; 26:2595–2597.

Armstrong DG, Lavery LA, Liswood PL, et al. Infrared dermal thermometry for the high-risk diabetic foot. Phys Ther 1997a; 77:169–177.

Armstrong DG, Lavery LA, Wu S, Boulton AJ. Evaluation of removable and irremovable cast walkers in the healing of diabetic foot wounds: a randomized controlled trials. Diabetes Care 2005; 28:551–554.

Armstrong DG, Short B, Nixon BO, et al. Technique for fabrication of an "instant" total contact cast for treatment of neuropathic diabetic foot ulcers J Am Podiatr Med Assoc 2002; 92:405–408.

Armstrong DG, Todd WF, Lavery LA, Harkless LB, Bushman TR. The natural history of acute Charcot's arthropathy in a diabetic foot speciality clinic. Diabet Med 1997b; 14:357–363.

Baumhauer JF, Wervey R, McWilliams J, Harris GF, Shereff MJ. A comparison study of plantar foot pressure in a standardized shoe, total contact cast, and prefabricated pneumatic walking brace. Foot Ankle Int 1997; 18:26–33.

Bem R, Jirkovska A, Fejfarova V, et al. Intranasal calcitonin in the treatment of acute Charcot neuroosteoarthropathy: a randomized controlled trial. Diabetes Care 2006; 29:1392–1394.

Boyko EJ, Ahroni JH, Stensel V, et al. A prospective study of the risk factors for diabetic foot ulcer. The Seattle Diabetic Foot study. Diabetes Care 1999; 22:1036–1042.

Chantelau E. The perils of procrastination: effects of early vs delayed detection and treatment of incipient Charcot fracture. Diabetic Med 2005; 22:1707–1712.

Chantelau E, Kimmerle R, Ludger WP. Nonoperative treatment of neuro-osteoarthropathy of the foot: do we need new criteria? Clin Podaitr Med Surg 2007a; 24:483–503.

Chantelau E, Poll L. Evaluation of the diabetic Charcot foot by RM imaging or plain radiography – an observational study. Exp Clin Endocrinol Diabetes 2006; 114:428–431.

Chantelau E, Richter A, Ghassem-Zadeh N, et al. "Silent" bone stress injuries in the feet of diabetic patients with polyneuropathy — a report of 12 cases. Arch Orthop Trauma Surg 2007b; 127:171–177.

Chantelau E, Richter A, Schmidt-Grigoriadis P, et al. The diabetic Charcot foot: MRI discloses bone stress injuries as trigger mechanism of neuroarthropathy. Exp Clin Endocrinol Diabetes 2006; 114:118–123.

De Souza LJ. Charcot arthropathy and immobilization in a weight-bearing total contact cast. J Bone Joint Surg Am 2008; 90:754–759.

Edmonds ME, Petrova N, Edmonds A, et al. Early identification of bone marrow oedema in Charcot foot on MRI allows rapid intervention to prevent deformity [abstract]. Diabet Med 2006a; 23:70.

Edmonds ME, Petrova NL, Edmonds A, et al. What happens to the initial bone marrow oedema in the natural history of Charcot osteoarthropathy (abstract)? Diabetologia 2006b; 49:684.

Edmonds ME, Petrova N, Elias D. The earliest magnetic resonance imaging sign of mid-foot Charcot osteoarthropathy is oedema of the subcondral (subarticular) bone marrow which needs prompt therapeutic offloading [abstract]. Diabet Med 2005; 22:93.

Frykberg RG, Kozak GP. The diabetic Charcot foot. In: Kozak GP, Campbell DR, Fryberg RG, Haberwshaw GM (eds), Management of diabetic foot problems, 2nd edn. Philadelphia, PA: WB Saunders, 1995:88–97.

Giurini JM, Chrzan JS, Gibbons GW, Habershaw GM. Charcot's disease in diabetic patients. Correct diagnosis can prevent progressive deformity. Postgrad Med 1991; 89:163–169.

Grady JF, O'Connor KJ, Axe TM, et al. Use of electrostimulation in the treatment of diabetic neuroarthropathy. J Am Podiatr Med Assoc 2000; 90:287–294.

Jostel A, Jude EB. Medical treatment of Charcot neuroosteoarthropathy. Clin Podiatr Med Surg 2008; 25:63–69.

Jude EB, Selby PL, Burgess J, et al. Bisphosphonates: in the treatment of Charcot neuroarthropathy: a double-blind randomised controlled trial. Diabetologia 2001; 44:2032–2037.

Kimmerle R, Chantelau E. Weight-bearing intensity produces Charcot deformity in injured neuropathic feet in diabetes. Exp Clin Endocrinol Diabetes 2007; 115:360–364.

Lavery LA, Vela SA, Lavery DC, Quebedeaux TL. Reducing dynamic foot pressures in high-risk diabetic subjects with foot ulcerations: a comparison of treatments. Diabetes Care 1996; 19:818–821.

McGill M, Molyneaux L, Bolton T, et al. Response of Charcot's arthropathy to contact casting: assessment by quantitative techniques. Diabetologia 2000; 43:481–484.

Onvlee GJ. The Charcot foot: a critical review and an observational study of a group of 60 patients. The Netherlands: Medical Faculty, University of Leiden, 1998.

Petrova NL, Edmonds ME. Charcot neuro-osteoarthropathy-current standards. Diabetes Metab Res Rev 2008; 24:S58–S61.

Pinzur MS, Lio T, Posner M. Treatment of Eichenholtz stage I Charcot foot arthropathy with a weightbearing total contact cast. Foot Ankle Int 2006; 27:324–329.

Pitocco D, Ruotolo V, Caputo S, et al. Six-month treatment with alendronate in acute Charcot neuroarthropathy: a randomized controlled trial. Diabetes Care 2005; 28:1214–1215.

Ruotolo V, Di Pietro B, Giurato L, et al. A new natural history of Charcot foot: clinical evolution and final outcome of Stage 0 Charcot's Neuroarthropathy in a tertiary referral diabetic foot clinic. Clin Nucl Med 2013 Jul;38:506-509. doi: 10.1097/RLU.0b013e318292eecb.

Saltzman CL, Hagy ML, Zimmerman B, Estin M, Cooper R. How effective is intensive nonoperative initial treatment of patients with diabetes and Charcot arthropathy of the feet? Clin Orthop Relat Res 2005; 435:185–190.

Sanders L, Frykberg R. The Charcot foot (Pied de Charcot). In: Bowker JH, Pfeifer MA (eds), Levin and O'Neal's the diabetic foot, 7th edn. Philadelphia, MA: Mosby Elsevier, 2007:257–283.

Sella EJ, Barrette C. Staging of Charcot neuroarthropathy along the medial column of the foot in the diabetic patient. J Foot Ankle Surg 1999; 38:34–40.

Sinacore DR. Acute Charcot arthropathy in patients with diabetes mellitus: healing times by foot location. J Diabetes Complications 1998; 12:287–293.

Strauss E, Gonya G. Adjunct low-intensity ultrasound in Charcot neuroarthropathy. Clin Orthop 1998; 349:132–138.

Thompson RC, Havel P, Goetz F. Presumed neurotrophic skeletal disease in diabetic kidney transplant recipients. JAMA 1983; 249:1317–1319.

Wukich DK, Motko J. Safety of total contact casting in high risk patients with diabetic foot ulcers. Foot ankle Int 2004; 25:556–560.

Yu GV, Hudson JR. Evaluation and treatment of stage 0 Charcot's neuroarthropathy of the foot and ankle. J Am Podiatr Med Assoc 2002; 94:210–220.

Chapter 34

Charcot osteoarthropathy: surgical management and off-loading

Katherine M. Raspovic, Dane K. Wukich

SUMMARY

- Currently, evidence to support optimal timing of surgical reconstruction is based on uncontrolled case studies and expert opinion

- Preoperative medical optimization is paramount before attempting Charcot reconstruction

- The most common location requiring reconstruction due to Charcot deformity is the midfoot region, and approximately 60% of Charcot surgical interventions involve the midfoot

- Patients with complications of diabetes have higher rates of infectious and noninfectious complications after surgery

- Postoperatively, patients should be keep nonweight bearing for a minimum of 3 months or until osseous healing is evident radiographically

- Appropriate off-loading is key in both nonsurgical and postsurgical management of Charcot osteoarthropathy (CO)

INTRODUCTION

Charcot osteoarthropathy is a complex and destructive pathological process that currently is most prevalent in people with diabetes. It is thought that Sir William Musgrave recorded the first descriptions of neuropathic arthritis resulting from venereal disease complications in 1703 (Wukich & Sung 2009). Jean Martin Charcot originally published his report of this destructive process in 1868, after observing a group of patients with tertiary syphilis (Pinzur 2007a). Multiple conditions have been associated with CO, including poliomyelitis, leprosy, multiple sclerosis, as well as trauma-induced neuropathy, to name only several (Pinzur 2007, Wukich et al. 2008). In more recent years, the manifestations of CO have primarily been found in those with peripheral neuropathy due to the manifestations of diabetes mellitus (DM) (Pinzur 2007a).

Multiple theories have been presented to explain the pathologic pathway that leads to the development of CO. Typically, some sort of obvious or even subtle injury to a neuropathic lower extremity initiates this destructive process. Because these patients have profound peripheral neuropathy, they are frequently unaware that they have injured their foot or ankle and continue with their usual activity. Continued ambulation or weight bearing on an injured, unstable, and insensate extremity leads to progressive collapse of osseous structures and joints of the foot and ankle, resulting in significant deformity. Deformity may then lead to ulceration, putting these patients at high risk for developing cellulitis or an abscess. Soft tissue infections may progress to osteomyelitis that may ultimately lead to

an amputation. Early recognition of Charcot-in-situ is associated with fewer complications and less risk of progression into the destructive stages (Wukich et al. 2011).

Initial treatment of the Charcot patient consists of clinical and radiographic evaluation, aggressive off-loading for an extended period of time in the early phases to allow for bony consolidation, and most importantly, prevention of ulceration. Historically, a period of non weight bearing was recommended to prevent progression of the deformity with off-loading devices such as removable boots, bracing, or casting. Two recent case series have called into question the need for complete nonweight bearing during the developmental stage (Eichenholtz stage 1) of CO. Studies by Pinzur et al. and de Sousa have demonstrated successful treatment of Eichenholtz stage 1 patients with weight bearing as tolerated in a total contact cast (Pinzur et al. 2006, de Souza 2008). Surgical intervention should be considered when these modalities fail to prevent progressive deformity, control 'pain,' and prevent healing of ulceration. Although patients with CO are profoundly neuropathic, a small subset of patients will complain of pain despite having neuropathy. Most likely, this neuropathic pain is due to destructive arthritis and instability at the site of the deformity. The goals of surgical intervention in patients with CO are to provide a stable, plantigrade foot and ankle, to prevent recurrent ulceration, and to reduce pain. In those patients with concurrent infection, eradication of soft tissue or osseous infection is also a major goal. Surgical intervention in this patient population requires a thorough understanding of CO to include proper staging as well as the associated comorbidities, such as profound neuropathy, metabolic bone disease, and deformity. Surgeons who embark on Charcot reconstruction should be experienced with both internal and external fixation techniques since each patient's deformity is unique.

CLASSIFICATION REVIEW (TABLE 34.1)

Multiple classification systems have been described to categorize and understand the various stages as well as the anatomic locations of CO. Understanding these classifications is helpful in planning the course of treatment and monitoring progression of the pathology. In 1966, Eichenholtz segregated the chronological order of the disease process into three separate stages: developmental (stage 1), coalescence (stage 2), and remodeling (stage 3) (Eichenholtz 1966). Stage 1 consists of increased warmth, edema, redness, and deformity on clinical examination and radiographic findings of fracture, subluxation or dislocation, osseous debris, and fragmentation. Stage 2 clinically demonstrates decreased warmth, edema, and redness. Stage 2 radiographs show new osseous formation, bony absorption, sclerosis,

Table 34.1 Charcot classification systems

Eichenholtz		
Stage 0	Initial Injury	
Stage 1	Developmental	
Stage 2	Coalescence	
Stage 3	Remodeling	
Anatomic classifications		
Sanders and Frykberg	**Anatomic location**	**Frequency (%)**
Pattern 1	Forefoot	15
Pattern 2	Tarsometatarsal joints	40
Pattern 3	Naviculocuneiform, talonavicular, calcaneocuboid joints	30
Pattern 4	Ankle, subtalar joint	10
Pattern 5	Calcaneus	5
Brodsky		
Type 1	Midfoot	60
Type 2	Hindfoot	30–35
Type 3A and 3B	Ankle and posterior calcaneus	9

and coalescence of fragments. Stage 3 is generally characterized clinically by lack of warmth, edema, or redness, fixed deformity, and on radiographs it shows remodeled bony structures. Stage 3 CO may result in a stable or unstable deformity, depending on the amount and quality of bone healing. Shibata later modified the Eichenholtz classification in 1990 by adding stage 0, which is characterized clinically by local pain and swelling without radiographic changes (Shibata et al. 1990). Stage 0 has also been referred to as Charcot-in-situ and may be identified by magnetic resonance imaging or nuclear medicine scans prior to demonstrating radiographic changes.

Several anatomic classifications have also been developed to describe CO. Sanders and Frykberg classified the foot into five pathological zones and identified the frequency of Charcot complications in each of these zones. Pattern 1 (forefoot) had a 15% frequency of a Charcot event, pattern 2 (tarsometatarsal joints) 40% frequency, pattern 3 (naviculocuneiform, talonavicular joint, and calcaneocuboid joint) had a 30% frequency, pattern 4 (ankle and subtalar joint) had a 10% frequency, and pattern 5 (calcaneus) had a 5% frequency of a Charcot event. Brodsky also described an alternative anatomic classification system. He described the midfoot as type 1 and also noted this was the most common area of involvement, at a rate of 60%. Type 2 involves the hindfoot (subtalar, talonavicular, and calcaneocuboid joints) and is the second most common location at 30–35%. Type 3A occurs in the ankle and 3B involves the posterior calcaneus, representing 9% of Charcot events. The forefoot was not included in Brodsky's original classification system. Other classification systems have been described such as midfoot classification of Schon et al. (1998); however, the modified Eichenholtz, Sanders and Frykberg, and Brodsky classifications tend to be the most frequently cited in the Charcot literature. Regardless of which anatomic classification is utilized, the midfoot is the most commonly involved anatomic region.

SURGICAL INTERVENTION

Charcot osteoarthropathy reconstructions are complex limb salvage procedures and complications are frequent. In addition to DM, many patients with CO also have multiple medical comorbidities such as renal insufficiency, coronary artery disease, hypertension, and peripheral arterial disease (PAD). Patients with poorly controlled DM and peripheral neuropathy are particularly prone to develop postoperative complications such as nonunion, wound dehiscence, postoperative infection, and the need for further surgery or revision. Multiple studies on patients with DM have demonstrated the negative impact of neuropathy in patients undergoing foot and ankle reconstruction or ankle fracture repair (Wukich et al. 2011, Myers et al. 2012).

The ideal timing of surgical intervention in the patient with CO has not been clearly defined in the literature. Traditionally, surgical reconstruction was not generally recommended during the acute, inflammatory stage, although two small noncontrolled retrospective case series have demonstrated encouraging results with early intervention (Simon et al. 2000, Mittlemeier 2010). Most authors recommend delaying surgical reconstruction until the edema has subsided and temperature has decreased; however, the evidence to support optimal timing of surgical reconstruction is based on uncontrolled case studies and expert opinion (Lowery et al. 2012) (**Figure 34.1**).

Preoperative medical optimization is key before attempting Charcot reconstruction. Comorbidities must be addressed such as glycemic control, vitamin D deficiency, anemia, cardiac disease, and PAD. Studies have demonstrated that poor glycemic control may affect postoperative outcomes and healing in those who undergo ankle or hindfoot fusion (Myers et al. 2012). Patients with an abnormal vascular examination should have further evaluation with

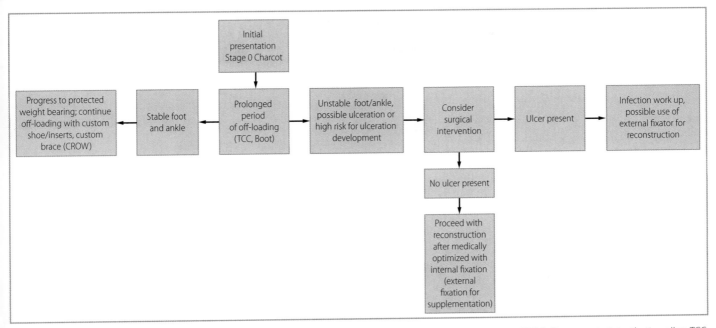

Figure 34.1 Surgical algorithm. This flowchart demonstrates the steps from initial presentation to surgical intervention. CROW, Charcot restraint orthotic walker; TCC, total contact casting.

noninvasive testing prior to major surgery. If noninvasive tests are indicative of PAD, referral to an appropriate specialist who performs interventional peripheral vascular surgery is indicated.

■ SURGICAL APPROACH TO THE FOREFOOT/MIDFOOT

The most common location requiring reconstruction due to Charcot deformity is the midfoot region, and approximately 60% of CO surgical interventions involve the midfoot (Lowery et al. 2012). The primary goal when attempting surgical correction of the forefoot/midfoot region is to reconstruct a stable, plantigrade foot without bony prominences. Midfoot CO presents with loss of the longitudinal arch and/or a rocker bottom deformity that may have sagittal and/or frontal deformity (**Figure 34.2**). Concurrently, the ankle/hindfoot is usually plantarflexed, manifested by a reduction in the calcaneal inclination angle. The presence and location of hyperkeratotic lesions or ulceration should be noted as well. In patients with ulceration, the presence or absence of infection must be determined. Preoperative radiographs should always be weight bearing, and both the foot and ankle should be assessed. Standard views should include anteroposterior, medial oblique, and lateral views. Key radiographic findings when evaluating the foot include midfoot collapse, decreased calcaneal inclination, increased forefoot abduction, and an increase in the lateral tarsal–first metatarsal angle. An increase in the lateral talar–first metatarsal angle on weight-bearing radiographic evaluation has been shown to be associated with an increased risk of ulceration (Bevan & Tomlinson 2008). Patients with diabetes and midfoot CO and a lateral talar–first metatarsal angle of > 27° were more likely to ulcerate than patients with less severe deformity (**Figure 34.3**).

The surgical plan should determine which deformities will be addressed as well as the optimal fixation that will be required. It is also

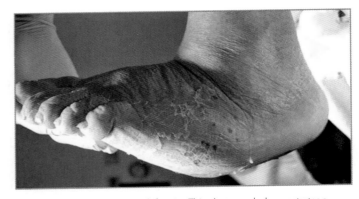

Figure 34.2 Midfoot Charcot deformity. This photograph demonstrates a midfoot Charcot 'rocker-bottom' deformity.

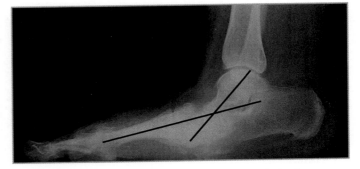

Figure 34.3 Lateral radiograph demonstrating an abnormal talar–first metatarsal angle (or Meary's angle) of about –40°. This is found by measuring the lines bisecting the talus and first metatarsal on a lateral view. These lines normally should be colinear or 180°.

important for the surgeon to prepare for the possible use of external fixation if it is decided intraoperatively that the patient has infection present or if internal fixation is not adequate and more fixation is needed to ensure stability. Adequate fixation is key in maintaining surgical correction during the prolonged healing phase. Screws, plates, bolts, and external fixation can be used to maintain correction depending on the reconstruction.

Midfoot CO reconstruction typically consists of correcting midfoot collapse or rocker bottom deformity with fusions and osteotomies as needed to construct a stable, plantigrade foot. In select cases, a simple exostectomy of a plantar bony prominence is enough to allow healing of a plantar ulceration. Healing of medial column ulceration is more predictable after exostectomy than lateral column ulceration (Brodsky & Rouse. 1993, Catanzariti et al. 2000, Laurinaviciene et al. 2008). Care must be taken during ostectomy to avoid iatrogenic instability. Most reconstructions include open or percutaneous lengthening of the Achilles tendon or gastrocnemius muscle. Internal fixation for midfoot fusion traditionally has utilized orthopedic plates and screws. The type of fixation should be stable enough to withstand the stresses that patients unknowingly will apply. Recently, solid or cannulated intramedullary screws (i.e. midfoot beaming) have become popular in CO midfoot fixation. The advantages of intramedullary fixation of the foot include restoration of anatomic realignment, minimally invasive fixation, and fixation of bone beyond the area of the Charcot collapse (Lamm et al. 2012) (**Figure 34.4**). A disadvantage of this technique is hardware failure due to the forces across the midfoot. In a recent study by Sammarco et al. (2010), multiple axial screws were placed across the midfoot in either an antegrade or retrograde manner in 22 patients. All patients maintained improved alignment radiographically; however, there were eight hardware failures in their study.

■ SURGICAL APPROACH TO THE HINDFOOT

According to Lowery et al. (2012), 11% of CO surgical intervention occurs at the hindfoot. Posterior muscle group lengthening should be addressed as well if equinus is present, as previously described for midfoot reconstruction. Surgical correction in this region usually involves a triple arthrodesis (subtalar, talonavicular, and calcaneocuboid joints) and may require adjacent midfoot fusion or

ankle fusion to achieve reduction and stability. Laterally, the subtalar and calcaneocuboid joints are accessed by an incision extending from the distal fibula to the bases of the 4th and 5th metatarsals. Medially, a utilitarian type incision can be made between the anterior and posterior tibial tendons to access the talonavicular and medial column joints. It is important to remember that due to the Charcot deformity, osseous structures and joints may not be recognizable due to bone dissolution and deformity, so the liberal use of fluoroscopy is recommended. Once the joints are prepared for fusion, restoration of the alignment between the hindfoot and adjacent joints is undertaken. We prefer to restore ankle to hindfoot alignment first by improving the calcaneal inclination angle by posterior muscle group lengthening. Usually, this angle cannot be normalized, but improving a negative inclination to neutral or slightly positive will reduce plantar pressure at the site of deformity. We have found that a half pin can be driven into the calcaneus and utilized as a temporary 'joystick' to manually restore the calcaneal inclination after posterior muscle group lengthening. A Steinman pin can be driven from the plantar aspect of the calcaneus, across both the ankle and subtalar joints to maintain correction. The temporary 'joystick' is then removed and the transarticular pin is left intact maintaining correction while the midfoot is realigned in reference to the hindfoot. This supplementary fixation can be left percutaneously out of the plantar skin and removed at a later date postoperatively. Once all arthrodesis sites have been prepared and deformity is corrected with temporary fixation, permanent fixation is placed.

■ SURGICAL APPROACH TO THE ANKLE

The ankle and hindfoot are commonly jointly involved secondary to deformity of the talus. Varus or valgus malalignment of the ankle is poorly tolerated due to prominent malleoli, and reconstruction is usually necessary to avoid ulceration or to permit healing. Very little soft tissue protects the malleoli, particularly medially, and ulceration frequently leads to osteomyelitis of the ankle if untreated. In addition to varus or valgus malalignment, deficiency of the talus is often associated with collapse, fracture, or osteonecrosis. Consequently, limb length is reduced and the malleoli rub against the sides of shoe wear leading to ulceration.

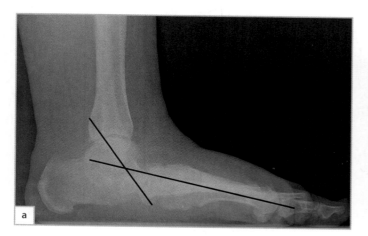

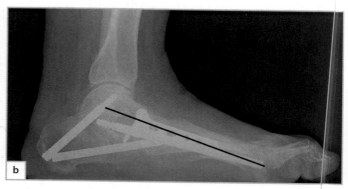

Figure 34.4 (a) Preoperative lateral radiograph demonstrating a severe break in the talar–first metatarsal or Meary's angle of about −48°. (b) Postoperative correction of this angle. The line bisecting the lateral talus and first metatarsal is now 180° or colinear. A 'beaming' technique was utilized for fixation.

Usually, the ankle and hindfoot are addressed together as a unit and a tibiotalocalcaneal (TTC) or pantalar arthrodesis is performed (**Figure 34.5**). Reconstructive surgeons should be experienced in various surgical approaches (medial, lateral, anterior, or posterior) since patients often have undergone multiple previous surgical procedures and skin integrity is often compromised. In severe varus/valgus deformity, partial or complete talectomy may be necessary to correct the deformity and restore a plantigrade foot. If the talus is still viable after talectomy, it can be reshaped and reimplanted as an autograft to maintain limb length. Preservation of the talar height also facilitates placement of hardware since it adds another point of osseous fixation. If the talus is severely diseased and nonviable, a femoral head allograft may be utilized to preserve length. In selected cases, the tibia can be fused directly to the calcaneus.

In patients with severe ankle deformity, soft tissues contractures are inevitably present, and skin closure may be difficult if limb length is preserved. Surgeons should anticipate this and advise patients that negative pressure wound therapy, skin grafting, or even flaps may be necessary to achieve wound healing. If severe valgus deformity is present (apex medial angulation), a medial incisional approach to the ankle and subtalar joints may be preferred since the lateral soft tissues are shortened and contracted. Conversely, severe varus deformity (apex lateral angulation) is associated with contracture and shortening of the medial soft tissues, and a lateral approach may minimize soft

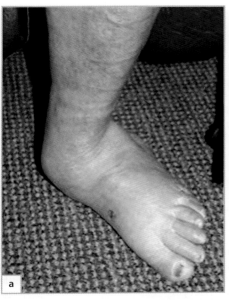
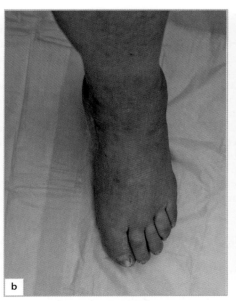
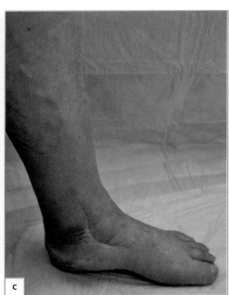

a   b   c

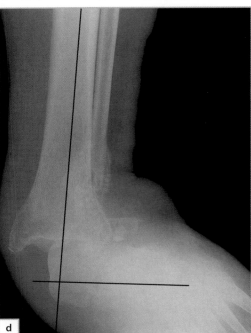
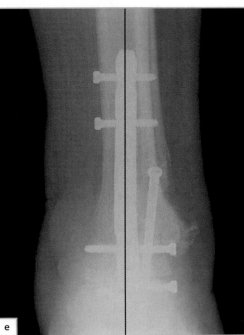

d   e

Figure 34.5 (a) Preoperative clinical photo of Charcot involving the ankle. (b) The same patient's postoperative clinical anteroposterior (AP) picture. (c) A postoperative lateral clinical picture of the patient. (d) Preoperative AP radiograph demonstrating the same patient's ankle dislocation due to Charcot at initial presentation. The bisection of the tibia and calcaneus is at 90°. These lines should be colinear. (e) The same patient's postoperative AP radiograph: note the bisections of the tibia and calcaneus are now colinear.

tissue complications. Both medial and lateral approaches to the ankle usually require an osteotomy for exposure (medial malleolar osteotomy for medial approach and fibular osteotomy for a lateral approach).

Internal fixation options for TTC or pantalar fusion include plates, screws, and intramedullary nail fixation. In selected cases, external fixation may be combined with internal fixation to provide increased stability.

The use of internal fixation in patients with grossly infected CO is generally not recommended. In the setting of chronic ulceration and osteomyelitis, external fixation with or without supplemental pins is recommended after correction of the deformity and resection of the infected bone. Charcot deformities, which present with foot ulcers, are challenging limb salvage cases since 28% of these patients may require transtibial amputation (Saltzman et al. 2005). Others have reported higher rates of limb salvage utilizing external fixation with an algorithm that includes Achilles tendon lengthening, excision of infected bone, correction of the multiplanar deformity, and culture-specific parenteral antibiotic therapy (Pinzur 2007b). After 1 year of follow-up, 24 of 26 patients were ulcer and infection free and able to ambulate with commercially available depth-inlay shoes and custom accommodative foot orthoses.

The use of external fixation in patients with diabetes is not without complications and includes superficial pin site/tract infection, fine wire failure, deep infection, and tibia fracture (Wukich et al. 2008). Careful attention to detail and knowledge of anatomic 'safe zones' is key to avoid neurovascular damage and minimizing soft tissue complications. A recent study demonstrated that patients with diabetes undergoing external fixation had significantly higher complication rates compared patients without diabetes (Wukich et al. 2008).

■ POSTOPERATIVE COMPLICATIONS

Reconstruction of a CO deformity is technically challenging not only intraoperatively, but also postoperatively. Many complications may arise in the postoperative period such as surgical site infection, wound dehiscence, hardware failure, or nonunion. Patients with complications of diabetes have higher rates of infectious and noninfectious complications after surgery (Wukich et al. 2010, Myers et al. 2012). In a recent retrospective study of patients undergoing arthrodesis surgery, 74 patients with diabetes were matched with a group of 74 without diabetes. Adverse outcomes were significantly more likely in patients with diabetes, especially those who used tobacco, who had neuropathy, and those with poor glycemic control (Myers et al. 2012).

These recent studies and our personal experience have helped us better select and prepare patients for elective Charcot reconstruction. We no longer do elective reconstruction on patients who actively use tobacco or have a hemoglobin A1c > 8%. Noninvasive arterial testing is routinely used to detect asymptomatic vascular disease, and any abnormality prompts a consultation with a vascular surgeon. The presence of diabetes and neuropathy are not modifiable in this patient group, but other contributing factors are potentially modifiable such as tobacco use, glycemic control, and lymphedema. Our complication rate has decreased with these simple, but important observations regarding tobacco use, PAD, and glycemic control.

■ OFF-LOADING

Appropriate off-loading is the cornerstone of nonsurgical and postsurgical management of CO. In patients treated nonsurgically,

the goals of off-loading are to prevent ulceration, prevent progression of deformity, and allow osseous consolidation. Multiple forms of off-loading are available such as custom inserts and shoes, custom bracing, boots, Charcot restraint orthotic walkers (CROWs), and total contact casting (TCC).

Off-loading with a boot or TCC can be utilized, especially if a plantar ulceration is present. A surgical boot can be made nonremovable by applying a roll of fiberglass around the top of the boot. A TCC is an effective modality; however, great care must be taken to avoid new ulceration from the TCC itself. TCC is effective by more evenly distributing forces during weight-bearing, decreasing edema, decreasing shear forces and causing a reduction in the number of steps a patient takes in a given day (Wukich 2010). Studies have proven the safety and efficacy of the TCC. Armstrong et al. (2001) performed a randomized prospective study comparing TCC, removable devices, and half-shoes for the treatment of plantar ulcerations. Over a 12-week course it was shown that plantar ulceration treated with a TCC had a significantly higher rate in size reduction compared with the ulcerations off-loaded with the other two devices. Wukich and Motko (2004) evaluated TCC in 13 patients with diabetes and neuropathy, who had 18 ulcerations. A total of 14 skin complications occurred in their series of 82 casts. Fifteen of the 18 wounds healed with TCC alone, demonstrating that it is a safe technique that can be utilized in these high-risk patients. Careful cast application, close follow-up, and patient education are essential for good outcomes.

Although the TCC has been considered the 'gold standard' for off-loading of diabetic ulcerations and treating CO, a recent study demonstrated that most practicing clinicians do not utilize this modality very frequently. Wu et al. (2008) conducted a survey regarding the management of diabetic foot ulcers of various physicians practicing at foot clinics in every state across the United States. A total of 895 clinicians responded and TCC was utilized by only 1.7% of the centers that responded. The majority of centers utilized shoe modifications most often (41.2%). The authors suggested that while clinicians understood the benefits of the TCC, factors such as cost/reimbursement, large patient volume, and lack of staff trained to apply the TCC may likely be reasons why this modality is used less frequently.

After surgical intervention, maintenance of correction is critical. Ideally, patients should be kept nonweight bearing in a below knee cast for a minimum of 3 months or until osseous healing is seen on radiographs. During the period of nonweight bearing, some patients may require admission to a skilled nursing facility if they are unable to function independently at home with nonweight-bearing restrictions. Patients should utilize crutches, walkers, or a wheelchair to avoid weight bearing. After this time period, progression to full weight bearing in a graded fashion is recommended transitioning to removable boots, CROW or braces. A CROW is ideal because it is removable, custom fabricated for the patient and provides a total contact orthosis. This allows for protected ambulation for an indefinite period during the recovery process, which may take 12–18 months.

■ CONCLUSION

Surgical management of CO requires a thorough understanding of all aspects of this destructive disease process. The prevalence of diabetes is increasing throughout the world, and this will translate into an increase in the prevalence of CO. Early recognition of CO, especially during stage 0, is mandatory if the morbidity associated with this disease is to be reduced. Understanding the various phases of CO allows for proper diagnosis and appropriate treatment. Appropriate off-loading is necessary until the symptoms of edema, redness, warmth, and pain subside. When off-loading, bracing and shoe wear fail to prevent deformity or ulceration, surgical intervention must be considered. Medical optimization is critical to ensure that the patient is able to tolerate reconstructive surgery and the postoperative course. The surgeon must be experienced with various fixation techniques and should be prepared for postoperative complications as they arise. Surgical management of CO is challenging and associated with many complications; however, successful outcomes result in limb salvage and high patient satisfaction. The optimal method of surgical reconstruction has not been demonstrated as of this time, but surgical techniques to enhance our outcomes will only continue to improve in the years to come.

■ AREAS OF CONTROVERSY AND/OR FUTURE RESEARCH

- The optimal timing of surgical reconstruction (i.e. during the active or chronic stage) is controversial, and current recommendations are based on small case series and expert opinion
- There are no prospective, comparative studies supporting the use of internal fixation, external fixation or hybrid (combined) fixation in the surgical management
- Prospective studies are needed to compare the outcomes of surgical reconstruction versus nonsurgical management
- Further research is needed to investigate long-term reconstructive outcomes as well as the appropriate timing of these interventions

■ IMPORTANT FURTHER READING

Crim BE, Lowery NJ, Wukich DK. Internal fixation techniques for midfoot Charcot neuroarthropathy. Clin Podiatr Med Surg 2011; 28:673–685.

Grant WP, Garcia-Levin SE, Sabo RT, Tam HS, Jerlin E. A retrospective analysis of 50 consecutive Charcot diabetic salvage reconstructions. J Foot Ankle Surg 2009; 48:30–38.

Kim PJ, Chang TJ. Equinus deformity and the diabetic foot. In: Zigonis T (ed), Surgical reconstruction of the diabetic foot and ankle, 1st edn. Philadephia, PA: Lippincott Williams &Wilkins, 2009: 205–212, Chapter 16.

Landsman AS. Preoperative and perioperative management of the High-risk patient with diabetes mellitus. In: Zigonis T (ed), Surgical reconstruction of

the diabetic foot and ankle, 1st edn. Philadelphia, PA: Lippincott Williams & Wilkins, 2009:7–11, Chapter 2.

Mendicino RW, Catanzariti AR, Saltrick KR, et al.. Tibiotalocalcaneal arthrodesis with retrograde intramedullary nailing. J Foot Ankle Surg 2004; 43:82–86.

Stapleton JJ, Polyzois VD, Zgonis T. Stepwise approach to static circular external fixation. In: Cooper PS, Polyzois VD, Zgonis T (eds), External fixators of the foot and ankle, 1st edn. Philadelphia, PA: Lippincott Williams & Wilkins, 2013:92–118, Chapter 8.

■ REFERENCES

Armstrong, DG, Nguyen, HC, Lavery, LA, et al. Off-loading the diabetic foot wound: a randomized clinical trial. Diabetes Care 2001; 24:1019–1022.

Bevan WP, Tomlinson MP. Radiographic measures as a predictor of ulcer formation in diabetic Charcot midfoot. Foot Ankle Int 2008; 29:568–573.

Brodsky, JW. Surgery of the foot and ankle. Philadelphia, PA: Mosby Elsevier, 2007: 1281–1368.

Brodsky JW, Rouse AM. Exostectomy for symptomatic bony prominences in diabetic Charcot feet. Clin Orthop Relat Res 1993; 296:21–26.

Catanzariti AR, Mendicino R, Haverstock, B. Ostectomy for diabetic neuroarthropathy involving the midfoot. J Foot Ankle Surg 2000; 39:291–300.

de Souza LJ. Charcot arthropathy and immobilization in a weight-bearing total contact cast. J Bone Joint Surg Am 2008; 90:754–759.

Eichenholtz SN (ed). Charcot joints. Springfield, IL: Charles C. Thomas, 1966:3–8.

Lamm BM, Siddiqui NA, Nair AK, LaPorta G. Intramedullary foot fixation for midfoot Charcot neuroarthropathy. J Foot Ankle Surg 2012; 51:531–536.

Laurinaviciene, R, Kirketerp-Moeller K, Holstein, PE. Exostectomy for chronic midfoot plantar ulcer in Charcot deformity. J Wound Care 2008; 17:53–55, 57–58.

Lowery NJ, Woods JB, Armstrong DG, Wukich DK. Surgical management of Charcot arthropathy of the foot and ankle: a systematic review. Foot Ankle Int 2012; 33: 113–121.

Mittlmeier T, Klaue K, Haar P, Beck M. Should one consider primary surgical reconstruction in Charcot arthropathy of the feet? Clin Orthop Relat Res 2010; 468:1002–1011.

Myers TG, Lowery NJ, Frykberg RG, Wukich DK. Ankle and hindfoot fusions: comparison of outcomes in patients with and without diabetes. Foot Ankle Int 2012; 33:20–28.

Pinzur MS. Current concepts review: Charcot arthropathy of the foot and ankle. Foot Ankle Int 2007a; 28:952–959.

Pinzur MS. Neutral ring fixation for high-risk nonplantigrade Charcot midfoot deformity. Foot Ankle Int 2007b; 28:961–966.

Pinzur MS, Lio T, Posner M. Treatment of Eichenholtz stage I Charcot foot arthropathy with a weightbearing total contact cast. Foot Ankle Int 2006; 27:324–329.

Saltzman CL, Hagy ML, Zimmerman B, Estin M, Cooper R. How effective is intensive nonoperative initial treatment of patients with diabetes and Charcot arthropathy of the feet? Clin Orthop Relat Res 2005; 435:185–190.

Sammarco VJ, Sammarco GJ, Walker EW, Guiao RP. Midtarsal in the treatment of Charcot midfoot arthropathy, surgical technique. J Bone Joint Surg 2010; 92:1–19.

Sanders LJ, Frykberg RG. Diabetic neuropathic osteoarthropathy: the Charcot foot. The high risk foot in diabetes mellitus. New York: Churchill Livingstone,1991:297–338.

Schon LC, Weinfeld SB, Horton GA, Resch S. Radiographic and clinical classification of acquired midtarsus deformities. Foot Ankle Int 1998; 19:394–404.

Shibata T, Tada K, Hashizume C. The results of arthrodesis of the ankle for leprotic neuroarthropathy. J Bone Joint Surg Am 1990; 72:749–756.

Simon SR, Tejwani, SG, Wilson, DL, et al. Arthrodesis as an early alternative to nonoperative management of Charcot arthropathy of the diabetic foot. J Bone Joint Surg Am 2000; 82-A:939–950.

Wu SC, Jensen JL, Weber AK, et al. Use of pressure offloading devices in diabetic foot ulcers. Do we practice what we preach? Diabetes Care 2008; 31:2118–2119.

Wukich, DK. Current concepts review: diabetic foot ulcers. Foot Ankle Int 2010; 31:460–467.

Wukich DK, Belczyk RJ, Burns PR, Frykberg RG. Complications encountered with circular ring fixation in persons with diabetes mellitus. Foot Ankle Int 2008; 29:994–1000.

Wukich DK, Lowery NJ, McMillen RL, Frykberg RG. Postoperative infection rates in foot and ankle surgery: a comparison of patients with and without diabetes mellitus. J Bone Joint Surg Am 2010; 92:287–295.

Wukich DK, Motko J. Safety of total contact casting in high-risk patients with neuropathic foot ulcers. Foot Ankle Int 2004; 25:556–560.

Wukich DK, Sung W. Charcot arthropathy of the foot and ankle: modern concepts and management review. J Diabetes Complications 2009; 23:409–426.

Wukich, DK, Sung W, Wipf SA, Armstrong DG. The consequences of complacency: managing the effects of unrecognized Charcot feet. Diabet Med 2011; 28:195–198.

AMPUTATION

Chapter 35

Minor amputation and major amputation

Yiu-Che Chan, Stephen W. Cheng

SUMMARY

- The incidence of lower limb amputation is eight times higher in patients with diabetes than in those without diabetes
- Perioperative and postoperative mortality after major lower limb amputations remains high
- To help ensure success in wound healing after amputation, it is essential to ensure good blood flow, control infection, and create a stable soft tissue envelope around the bone
- The energy expenditure for walking is inversely proportional to the length of the remaining limb
- All options of foot amputation should be exhausted before consideration for major amputation
- Expert surgical technique, sometimes with involvement of dedicated foot surgeons, is important

INTRODUCTION

Lower limb amputation is usually the result of deep ulceration with uncontrolled infection in patients with diabetes and is often complicated by delayed presentation or diagnosis (**Figure 35.1**). There are only a few population-based studies estimating the incidence of lower limb amputation in the general diabetes population, but the incidence rate of initial unilateral lower limb amputation at or proximal to the transmetatarsal level in the general population aged > 45 years was > eight times higher among individuals with diabetes than among those without diabetes (Johannesson et al. 2009).

Despite calls by the World Health Organisation to reduce limb amputation rates worldwide, it has remained a major burden on health-care resources with high postoperative mortality, high rate of secondary amputation, and prolonged inpatient stay (World Health Organization 1990). Jaar et al. (2004) found that amputations due to diabetes have more often involved younger individuals, with >82,000 limb amputations performed per year worldwide (Brem et al. 2006). Lower extremity amputation is an option for patients seeking to gain maximal functional recovery, when conservative measures have failed in treating these conditions. In a study of a total of 685 people admitted at a multidisciplinary diabetic foot care center, the amputation rate was 11.4%. Minor amputation and major amputations were required in 5.4% and 6.0%, respectively (Fei et al. 2012).

Lower limb sensory neuropathy in diabetics statistically has a 10-fold lifetime increased risk of amputation in patients with diabetes mellitus compared with their nondiabetic counterparts (Diabetes statistics). These patients are more likely to have a combination of risk factors for developing tissue loss such as nephropathy, neuropathy, retinopathy, peripheral artery disease, and cardiovascular disease (Davis et al. 2006). In a series of 57 patients who had a total of 62 transmetatarsal amputations, Landry et al. found that only 33 transmetatarsal wounds healed completely. Twenty-two transmetatarsal amputations (35%) proceeded to below-knee amputations and seven transmetatarsal amputations (11%) did not heal until the patients' demise. In this study, significant predictors of mortality were dialysis-dependent renal failure, nonindependent living, and need for preoperative revascularization (Landry et al. 2011).

Peri- and postoperative mortality after major lower limb amputations remains high, and the long-term survival of these patients is poor. Wong (2006) reported intraoperative mortality of 10.6% after major lower limb amputation, with female gender, high-level amputation, cerebrovascular accident, congestive heart failure, noncommunity ambulation, and institutionalization before amputation associated with an increased risk for long-term mortality. In a cohort of 577 patients in 16 operative units in Finland, with 50% being above-knee amputations for peripheral arterial diseases and diabetes, Pohjolainen et al. (1989) reported that 26% of patients with major lower limb amputations died within 2 months of the amputation and nearly 40% within 1 year. Tentolouris et al. (2004) reported a mortality of 17% within 1 year and 37% within 3 years. Similar results were described by Izumi et al. (2009) with a longer follow-up period, and mortality after major lower extremity amputations remained high: 18% within 10 months and 36% within 10 years. Rosati et al. (2012) also found that below-knee amputations took a longer time to complete wound healing (average 34 days) compared with above-knee amputations (average 25 days).

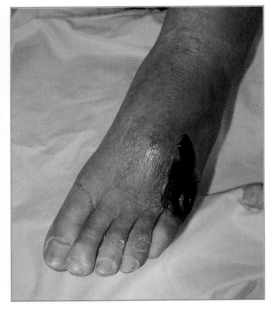

Figure 35.1
Infected diabetic foot with extensive infection and gangrene.

PREOPERATIVE PLANNING

A complete preoperative workup includes assessment of healing potential and preoperative ambulatory status, control or optimization of comorbidities when possible, and determination of amputation level using modern diagnostic modalities (Garg et al. 2011, Pino et al. 2011). The walking distance is associated with the degree of impairment in the affected leg as measured by the ankle-brachial pressure index and the time to onset of claudication pain (Gardner et al. 2008). The Prosthesis Evaluation Questionnaire exists, in part, to predict (preoperatively) whether patients will adapt to walking with a prosthesis. It also assesses patients' quality of life (QoL) and comprises 10 variables. There are four prosthesis function scales (Usefulness, Residual Limb Health, Appearance, and Sounds), two mobility scales (Ambulation and Transfers), three psychosocial scales (Perceived Responses, Frustration, and Social Burden), and one well-being scale (Legro et al. 1998). Other objective assessment scales included the Special Interest Group in Amputee Medicine self-report questionnaire, which is a clinically validated measure of amputee mobility (Ryall et al. 2003). SF-36 and the Sickness Impact Profile are useful generic tools. Preoperative independence and ambulation appear to best predictor of postoperative independence and ambulation after limb-salvage revascularization or amputation. However, the expected return to normalilty may take longer than 6 months.

Preoperative assessment should involve a multidisciplinary approach with input from physiotherapists, occupational therapists, prosthetists, rehabilitation medicine specialists, psychologists, microbiologists, dieticians, nursing staff, surgical, and anesthetic teams (Zayed et al. 2009). This is to address the multifactorial causation of the presenting pathology present in the diabetic foot, and it has been estimated that for hospitalized patients with diabetic foot complications, <14% receive adequate lower limb evaluations (Edelson et al. 1996). The decision on the level of amputation is important to assess the likelihood of flap healing.

To help ensure success, both amputation and limb salvage start with some important principles:

1. To ensure good blood flow
2. To control infection involvement of microbiologists
3. To create a stable soft tissue envelope, so that bony protuberances are well protected, not only to present pressure effect on the overlying tissues, but also to provide a stable base for future prosthesis (Attinger et al. 2006)

Ensuring a good blood supply is critical to salvaging a limb. Doppler pulses, ankle and toe pressures, and ankle brachial indices all provide information regarding the arterial flow to an extremity (Venermo et al. 2012). Some authors advocate that preoperative measurement of skin perfusion pressure and transcutaneous tissue oxygen tension (TcPO2) is a valid predictor of primary healing after amputation (Holstein 1982, Ameli et al. 1989), with a TcPO2 < 34 mmHg indicated the need for revascularization (Castronuovo et al. 1997). In a study of 211 patients with 403 limbs, Yamada et al. (2008) showed that a skin perfusion pressure > 40 mmHg, as measured by laser Doppler, was associated with a healing rate of 69%, whereas a skin perfusion pressure >50 mmHg is associated with a 100% healing rate, and suggested that skin perfusion pressure may be an objective method for assessing the severity of peripheral arterial disease or for predicting wound healing.

An understanding of the angiosomes of the foot and ankle as well as the arterial–arterial connections between the main arteries of the foot is also important in planning revascularization and in deciding the surgical incisions in the foot (Attinger et al. 2006) (see Chapter 16). There are many clinical and radiological tests to aid in the decision to amputate, in choosing the levels of amputation, and in the selection of the type of procedure that are available. The key to any amputation is to be at a level that is definitive. The patients are often very old, frail, and have multiple comorbidities. Attention to detail by a multidisciplinary multimodal pre- and postoperative program is also very important in ensuring good outcome (Kristensen et al. 2012).

INDICATIONS FOR AMPUTATION

Amputations are indicated if the patient has osteomyelitis, gangrene, or sepsis not responding to antibiotics treatment, has unreconstructable peripheral arterial disease, a large wound unresponsive to therapy and interfering with QoL or intractable pain (Wallace 2005). Critical limb ischemia requires revascularization by angioplasty or bypass surgery, to relieve rest pain and to facilitate wound healing after the amputation. In a self-assessment postal questionnaire containing scales measuring emotional disorder, social functioning and mobility sent to 112 patients who had previously undergone femorodistal bypass or primary limb amputation, Thompson et al. (1995) showed that the QoL after successful femorodistal bypass was higher than after primary or secondary amputation. Therefore, to attain the maximum QoL in patients with critical ischemia, femorodistal bypass should be performed wherever feasible (Thompson et al. 1995). Unreconstructable vascular disease is one of the most common indications for secondary amputation, accounting for >60% of patients with diabetic feet; amputation is indicated when vascular intervention is no longer possible, or when the limb continues to deteriorate despite the presence of patent vessels after revascularization (Setacci et al. 2012). Persistent sepsis is the most common cause of amputation despite successful revascularization, and many amputations can be prevented through proper patient education and frequent diligent feet inspection, together with a dedicated multidisciplinary team specializing in revascularization, staged wound closure, or even microvascular muscle flaps to cover major tissue defects.

Nonambulatory elderly patients may have fixed flexion deformity of the hips and knees. If tissue loss is extensive, then even prolonged revascularization procedures will not offer the patient a stable or useful limb, and primary amputation is a reasonable alternative. If the patients are unable to tolerate the planned procedure or unlikely to have a functional extremity despite restoration of distal flow, they should be considered for primary amputation that eliminates the source of rest pain and all necrotic tissue. Although morbidity and mortality of major amputation continues to be significant, advances in prosthetic development and amputation technique can lead to preserved ambulatory ability and improved QoL starting with early postoperative physiotherapy and rehabilitation aids (Sottiurai & White 2007). The extent of underlying sepsis in diabetic foot is often more extensive than is externally apparent, and the infection can progress rapidly and have devastating consequences if not managed appropriately. There are many cases of primary amputation worldwide for sepsis, especially if the diagnosis and antibiotic treatment is delayed. The goal of primary amputation is resolution of complete healing, preservation of the ambulatory ability postoperatively, and sometimes pain. The Trans-Atlantic Inter-Society Consensus Working Group guidelines recommend primary amputation for those patients who have had significant tissue loss of the weight-bearing areas of the foot, fixed and unremediable flexion contracture, or a very limited life expectancy (Dormandy & Rutherford 2000).

There is a lack of prospective randomized studies to compare the mortality and morbidity of the patients who had revascularization versus those with primary amputation. Indirect evident from the

Veteran Affair National Surgery Quality Improvement Plan showed that the 30-day mortality in the femorodistal revascularization patients was 2.1% versus 6.3% and 13.3% in below-knee primary amputation and above-knee primary amputation, respectively (Feinglass et al. 2001). The morbidity in revascularization was related to surgical wound complications, wound breakdown predisposed to graft infection, mortality from multiple medical comorbidities, and limb loss.

LEVEL OF AMPUTATION

Amputations can be divided into minor and major: the former where toe(s) or part of the foot is removed and latter where part of the leg is removed (usually below-, through-, or above- the knee). Arbitrarily, a minor amputation occurs below the ankle and a major amputation occurs above the ankle.

The key consideration in deciding the level of major lower limb amputation is to note that the energy expenditure for walking is inversely proportional to the length of the remaining limb (Rhim et al. 2009). Physiological energy expenditure measurement has proven to be a reliable method of quantitatively assessing the penalties imposed by gait disability. Proximal amputations and shorter stumps, accompanied by the removal of more joints, decrease the subsequent mobility and may have a profound effect on the patients' independent life as the functional outcome increases with the length of the residual limb. Gait analysis in prosthetics also allows better knowledge and insights in the different adaptive strategies to walk as normally as possible with prosthesis (Rietman et al. 2002).

In cases of ulcers or gangrene with septic component, debridement (which may be multiple and staged) is critical to prepare a wound for closure. Debridement is the medical removal of dead, nonviable, or infected tissues to improve the healing potential of the remaining viable healthy tissues. Attinger & Brown (2012) suggested that when carried out with a knife, the surgeon should make thin tangential slices until viable tissue is reached. Postdebridement culture is a useful tool to assess the adequacy of the debridement and to guide antibiotic therapy. The reconstruction can be carried out immediately or at a later stage when the infection is under control (Fisher et al. 1988). If the leg has been revascularized by either bypass or angioplasty, it takes time for the affected tissue to feel the full effect of the new blood flow.

Cochrane Database Systemic Reviews showed that hydrogel increases the healing rate of diabetic foot ulcers compared with simple dressings alone (Smith 2002, Edwards & Stapley 2010). Enzymatic debridement using streptokinase, or bacterial-derived collagenases, can be used on any wound with a large amount of necrotic debris. Maggot therapy debridement uses the larvae of *Lucilia sericata* (greenbottle fly) to digest necrotic tissue and pathogens. In the randomized controlled trial of Markevich et al. (2000), 140 patients were randomized to either maggot therapy for 72 hours or hydrogel treatment. The outcome parameter was complete healing with no significant difference between the groups.

Negative-pressure wound therapy (NPWT) is now widely available and much used worldwide (**Figure 35.2**) Argenta & Morykwas 1997, McCallon et al. 2000, Chan et al. 2006). Eginton et al. (2003) enrolled 10 patients with 11 wounds and showed that the NPWT decreased the wound volume (59% vs 0%) and depth (49% vs 8%) significantly more than moist gauze dressings. However, the cost of NPWT treatment is not insignificant (£45 per day per patient is the estimated cost), although if it reduces hospital stay and amputation rates there will be associated cost savings (Chan et al. 2006). Webster et al. (2012) showed in a Cochrane Database Systematic Review that NPWT is effective in healing wounds expected to heal by primary intention, but this study is not specific for diabetic foot wound closure.

The salvage of a limb is a challenging task that demonstrates fine balance between healing and function, and the operating surgeon has to have sufficient knowledge and expertise to create a foot that will hold up over time. An adequate protective soft tissue envelope must be created to protect the bony prominences and the pressure areas to prevent further ulceration. Equinovarus deformity and its complications, especially in midfoot and proximal-foot amputations, should be minimized by rebalancing tendons and performing tendo-Achilles lengthening when indicated. Redundant long tendons should be trimmed, but all viable tissue should be preserved during debridement to leave the foot with enough viable soft tissue for primary closure. It is essential to prepare the wound bed well to facilitate amputation wound closure.

Toe amputation

Hukill first described partial amputation of the distal phalanx of the big toe in 1874 (Rhim et al. 2009). Lapidu later revived this procedure in 1933 with surgical excision of the entire nail bed, matrix, and resection of the distal half of the distal phalanx with skin closure using the plantar skin flap from end of the toe (Lapidu 1933). This was used essentially for recurrent painful ingrown toenail with chronic paronychia, osteomyelitis, chronic nonhealing, or infected distal tuft ulcerations. Although a toe amputation is a relatively minor procedure, it may signify underlying risk factors, which may eventually lead to future limb loss.

Single-digit amputation for infection, trauma, or ulceration can be performed at the distal or proximal interphalangeal joints. Pinzur et al. (1999) stated that in big toe amputation, preservation of the metatarsophalangeal joint results in a better gait and foot stability. If the first ray with its powerful toe is to be deprived of its function, be it through muscular fatigue, infection, or through surgery, the second metatarsal bone will also fail. Myerson et al. (1994) stated that it is necessary to understand the pathomechanics and physiological function of the foot: to maintain the equilibrium and stability in push-off and in the late-stance phase of gait, the big toe amputation should be 1 cm proximal to the base of the proximal phalanx distal to the insertion of the flexor hallucis brevis tendons, plantar fascia, and sesamoid bones. The flexor hallucis longus and brevis tendons exert about 52% and 36% body weight, respectively and the peroneus longus muscle exerts > 58% body weight. The resultant force on the first metatarsal head amounts to about 119% body weight. The second metatarsal bone is subjected to a high bending moment with a resultant force of about 45% body weight acting on its head (Jacob 2001).

The preferred incision for partial or full toe amputation is fish-mouth or racquet-shaped equal flaps. There are two alternatives with regard to the orientation of the skin incisions, either medial/lateral and dorsal/plantar. Rhim et al. (2009) stated that the former allows for ambulation on a more durable plantar skin, the latter allows for easier visualization of proximal tissues during the operation, and the wound may cause more pain on walking. The bone should be shortened sufficiently for a tension-free closure. This may involve disarticulation of the metatarsophalangeal joint. It is generally accepted that the articulate cartilage should be removed, as it is avascular, and may lead to necrosis and delayed healing.

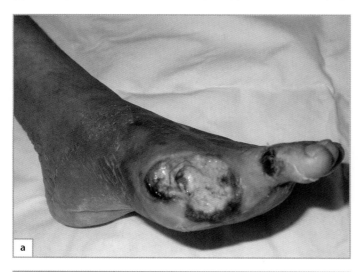

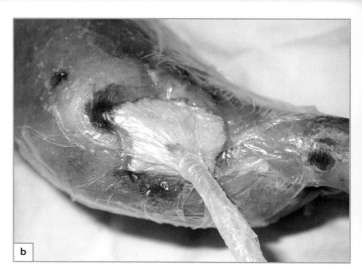

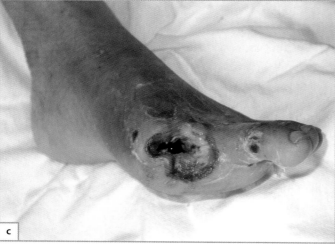

Figure 35.2 Vacuum-assisted closure device to facilitate healing.

■ Ray and transmetatarsal amputation

If the sepsis or tissue loss extends beyond the toe, then a transmetatarsal or ray amputation may be necessary. A ray is the unit involving the metatarsal and its corresponding toe, with those of the first and the fifth as the most commonly performed. The most common indication is the plantar erosion of prominent metatarsal head with osteomyelitis on plain radiograph, or with necrosis or sepsis extending to the level of the metatarsophalangeal joint.

Strict definition of a ray amputation refers to excision of the entire metatarsal and its corresponding toe, in contrast to a transmetatarsal amputation, which divides the metatarsal, usually at the neck or shaft of the metatarsal during the excision of the toe. Atnip advocated a ray resection over a disarticulation at the metatarsophalangeal joint, as he believed that leaving the head and neck of the metatarsal may produce a potential pressure point (so called 'transfer ulceration' to the remaining rays), which may ulcerate or be subjected to infection over time. Skin and soft tissue closure may be difficult with the bulk of the articulate cartilage or metatarsal head remain (Atnip 2005). However, while performing a ray amputation of the fifth metatarsal, it is important to leave the base of the metatarsal intact if possible because this is the insertion

site of the peroneus brevis. It is also important to retain the base of the second metatarsal while performing ray amputation of the second, third, or fourth toes, as the second metatarsal is important in maintaining a balanced gait.

Using a robotic gait simulator simulated physiologic tibial motion, tendon loading, and ground reaction forces on the cadaveric feet, and with measurements of peak pressure and pressure–time integral under the second metatarsophalangeal joints during gait, Weber et al. (2012) found that the second metatarsal peak pressure and pressure–time integral were positively correlated with an increase in second metatarsal length, and that the first metatarsal peak pressure and pressure–time integral were significantly negatively associated with second metatarsal length. If the second ray is excised, the patient may end up with a severe hallux valgus because of the lack of buttressing support provided by the second toe. If three lesser rays are performed, the foot will be very narrow, and the remaining two toes (such as the big toe and the fourth or fifth) are prone to deformity or ulceration and the foot is unsteady for gait. In such cases, it is generally recommended (and technically easier) to perform a transmetatarsal or more proximal foot amputation (Myerson et al. 1994).

Before performing a transmetatarsal amputation, the surgeon must ensure adequate perfusion of the plantar and dorsal tissue and preserve the connection between the dorsalis pedis and lateral plantar arteries when necessary. Hamilton et al. advocated recreation of a parabola by making the second metatarsal osteotomy the most distal, which may even involve the transfer of the peroneus longus tendon to the peroneus brevis tendon, and resection of the second through fifth metatarsal heads may provide surgeons with an alternative to solitary ray resection, transmetatarsal amputation, or panmetatarsal head resection in the salvage of the unbalanced, ulcerated forefoot of a patient with neuropathy (Hamilton et al. 2005). It is very common for patients who have had a transmetatarsal amputation to ultimately develop an equinovarus deformity because of the loss of toe extensors that formerly contributed to ankle extension and eversion. Lengthening the tendo-Achilles may redistribute the weight and lead to a more efficient healing rate.

Pure neuropathic diabetic ulcers may be the result of joint deformity and abnormally high foot pressures present over the metatarsophalangeal joint on the plantar aspect of metatarsal heads (Grimm et al. 2004). They will usually heal if pressure is relieved, infection is treated, and arterial circulation is sufficient. The conventional ray amputation may have to sacrifice healthy tissue at the expense of a small area of ulceration next to the infected metatarsophalangeal joint. Chan et al. (2007) described a technique where a skin incision is made on the dorsum of the foot overlying the osteomyelitic metatarsus and metatarsophalangeal joint remote from inflammation. The operation is very similar to Keller's excision arthroplasty for hallux valgus (Ferrari et al. 2004), but it is important to dissect close to the metatarsal bone to avoid damage to the digital neurovascular bundle. The infected bones are excised and all septic tissue carefully debrided, and then the skin closed with interrupted sutures over a corrugated drain (**Figure 35.3**) (Chan et al. 2007). This technique saves the toe and heals rapidly. The mobile flail joint created quickly fills up with granulation and fibrous tissue, allowing a reasonable range of movement. Other toe preservation procedures can also be adopted, if the involved sepsis or inflammation is not too extensive. Roukis presented a technique of lesser toe salvage with external fixation and delayed autogenous bone grafting for the treatment of osteomyelitis of metatarsal heads. Each patient underwent initial resection of involved soft tissue ulceration and underlying osseous components of the lesser toe with application of external fixation and polymethylmethacrylate antibiotic-loaded bone cement spacer. Once osteomyelitis was eradicated, the spacer was removed, and delayed insertion of autogenous bone graft harvested from the ipsilateral calcaneus was performed. The external fixation device was maintained until complete osseous integration was verified, and all the patients had complete osseous incorporation of the proximal and distal graft–host bone interfaces and no recurrent soft tissue ulcerations (Roukis 2010).

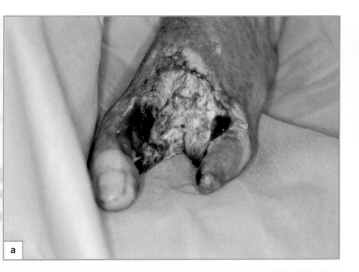

a

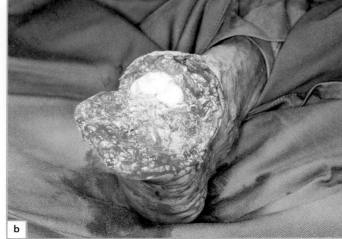

b

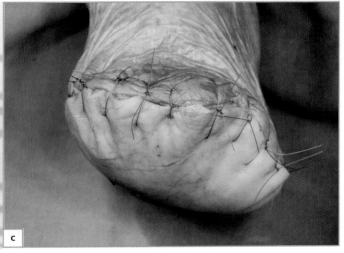

c

Figure 35.3 Nonhealing wounds require revascularization and further debridement.

Despite the careful considerations above, the chance of healing depends on the degree of tissue loss and sepsis. Hematoma within the dead space or skin tension from inadequate bone resection frequently leads to wound breakdown, recurrent sepsis, or delayed healing. Control of edema is also important, and the foot should be elevated for at least a few days before mobilization. Transfer ulcers due to redistribution of weight on mobilization are also common after multiple metatarsal resections. In a systematic review of peer-reviewed literature by Borkosky and Roukis (2012) involving a total of 435 patients with a mean follow-up of 26 months, the incidence of reamputation after partial first ray amputation associated with diabetes mellitus and peripheral neuropathy was determined to be 20%.

Midfoot and hindfoot amputation

The midfoot and hindfoot amputation should only be performed by experienced surgeons, or at least by those with sound knowledge of anatomy and biomechanics of the foot. There is often a need for good posterior tibial arterial supply for these amputations. These are difficult procedures that are usually performed for patients who have extensive tissue loss or where transmetatarsal amputations have failed

and should only be considered after eradication of sepsis or ischemia. The inevitable detachment of tendons and the loss of the forefoot in Lisfranc and Chopart amputations result in varus and equinus of the residual foot, because of the unopposed pull of the calf muscles and the lack of anterior static and dynamic counterbalance. Equinus leads to increased pressure and ulceration at the plantar distal aspect of the stump, whereas the varus deformity will cause ulceration at the lateral malleolus and at the plantar lateral border of the foot. The technique was first introduced by French surgeons Jacques Lisfranc de St. Martin and Francois Chopart, and these procedures now bear their names. Advantages are superior function with retention of ankle motion and equal limb length, increased sensory perception, greater surface for weight bearing, better cosmesis, and less disturbance of self-confidence (Krause et al. 2007).

The Lisfranc amputation is a partial amputation of the foot through the tarsometatarsal joint. The patient is able to mobilize with a modified shoe rather than a prosthesis. Every attempt should be made to maintain as much pedal length as possible to increase biomechanical function and ambulatory power with the Lisfranc amputation considered as a limb-salvage procedure (**Figures 35.3** and **35.4**). A fish-mouth incision is used with disarticulation performed at the tarsometatarsal joints. Decotiis (2005) advised leaving the bases

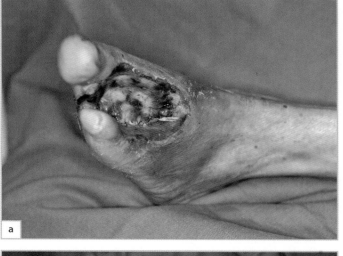
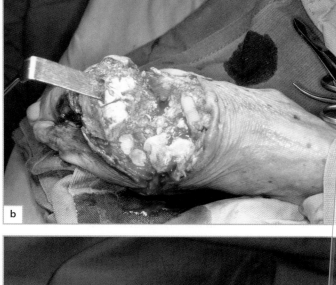
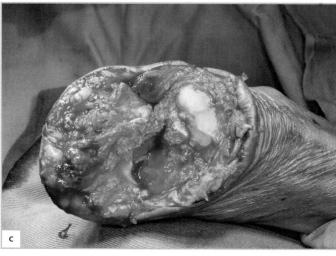
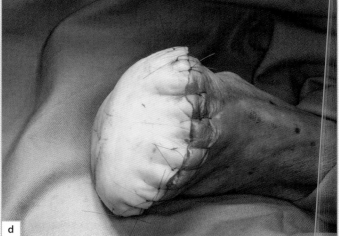

Figure 35.4 Tarsometatarsal amputation after failed transmetatarsal amputation.

of the second (for balance medially) and fifth metatarsal bones (for balance laterally) because the peroneus brevis, peroneus tertius attach to the base of the fifth metatarsal. The tendon of the tibialis anterior should be sutured onto the cuboid if possible, to allow some eversion control of the foot. The base of the second metatarsal bone is important as it provides stability to the medial cuneiform through the network of plantar ligaments (Early 1999). It is also important to remove as much articulate cartilage as possible from the cuneiforms and cuboid surfaces to prevent necrosis of the cartilages.

Chopart's amputation is a foot amputation performed with disarticulation of the talonavicular and calcaneocuboid joints. After this amputation, only the talus and calcaneus remain in the foot. The main disadvantages of the Chopart amputation is the loss of considerable foot length, interruption of tendinous attachment, leaving unopposed plantar flexors, and thus equinous and equinovarus deformity as consequence (Reyzelman et al. 1999). The gait is unsteady, and pressure ulcers on the stump are common. Appropriate tendon balancing is necessary, which generally includes anterior tibial tendon transfer to the neck of talus. This is done through a hole drilled in the neck of talus. The tendon is then sutured upon itself and the extensor tendons are carefully sutured to the fascia and soft tissues of the sole. Chopart's amputation eliminates the cuboid and obviates the potential varus deformity present in Lisfranc's amputation. Foot surgeons recommend using the durable and plantar skin to creatively cover the anterior aspect of the amputation (Attinger & Brown 2012). Resecting 1–2 cm of the distal Achilles tendon to avoid equinovarus deformity is also necessary unless one uses a calcaneal tibial pin to fuse the ankle in neutral (Stone et al. 2005).

Proper prosthetic fitting for large and bulbous stumps after Lisfranc and Chopart amputations is difficult. Krause designed a 'flap-shaft' prosthesis for primary or secondary prosthetic fitting of Chopart-level and Lisfranc-level amputees with insensate feet (Krause et al. 2007). The prosthesis consists of a soft socket and a rigid shaft up to the knee, with the thermoplastic polyethylene foam socket custom-made to corrected valgus and dorsiflexion. The access into the soft socket is posterior to protect the skin of the lower leg and foot from catching while closing the lateral flap. The hinge of the flap is obliquely oriented, from posterior distal to anterior proximal. While the mobile flap supports a large area of soft tissue around and above the lateral malleolus, the fixed shaft supports the heel and the calf medially. The sole of the foot is embedded in as much dorsiflexion as is possible (Krause et al. 2007). Without this prosthesis, these stumps are probably only useful for short distance walking or weight transfer, and psychologically better to the patient than a below-knee amputation.

Heel amputation

Amputation of the heel, partial or complete calcanectomy, demands orthopedic expertise, as the heel (calcaneum) is vital for weight-bearing gait. Eradication of osteomyelitis is important in calcanectomy, and it is also preferable to revascularize the posteriotibial and peroneal arteries, as they supply nutrient branches to the calcaneum. The decision for partial versus total calcanectomy is based on advanced imaging such as magnetic resonance imaging as radiographs usually underestimate the degree of osteomyelitis. Combined findings of low signal intensity in marrow on T1-weighted images, high signal intensity in marrow on T2-weighted images, and marrow enhancement after the administration of contrast material are indicative of osteomyelitis. Secondary signs of osteomyelitis include periosteal reaction, sinus tract, cellulitis, and abscess formation (Donovan & Schweitzer 2010).

Intraoperatively, the patient is ideally placed in the prone position, and the incision started 2-cm cranial to the insertion of tendo-Achilles and extends distally to the level of the calcaneocuboid joint (Rhim et al. 2009). The dissection continues deep down to bone to create a full-thickness soft tissue flap with preservation of the blood supply. Medially and laterally, the neurovascular bundles should be identified and preserved intact. If the tendo-Achilles is infected, then that should also be debrided. Sharp dissection is required to separate the periostium from the bone, and all infected bone should be removed. In cases of severe sepsis, the wound can be packed with interval debridement 24–48 hours later. For total calcanectomy, the subtalar and calcaneocuboid joints are entered with resection of all the ligaments around these joints, followed by excision of the articular cartilages of the inferior surface of the talus and posterior aspect of the cuboid (Baumhauer et al. 1998).

Crandall and Wagner reviewed 20 partial and 11 total calcanectomies in 29 patients from 1968 to 1978, 18 of whom had diabetes in association with ulceration of the heel. In about one half of the patients with diabetes, immediate failure of the procedure led to amputation. Primary wound healing occurred in only 4 of the 18 patients with diabetes, but in the patients without diabetes 10 of the 13 heels showed primary healing. Late failure also occurred in three patients with diabetes. The overall rate of failure in those with diabetes was 65% (Crandall & Wagner 1981). In a review of 50 patients who had partial calcanectomies, Cook et al. (2007) found that on average these wounds were difficult to heal, with a closure rate of 71% at 1 year. Although the procedure itself was fairly straightforward, the course of recovery was complex with a fairly high failure and/or recurrence rate. Furthermore, preoperative infections with methicillin-resistant *Staphylococcus aureus*, ongoing vascular disease, poor nutrition, and preoperative ulcer grade had a significant bearing on the outcomes. In a systematic review on 16 studies involving 100 patients (76 partial and 28 total calcanectomies) for the treatment of calcaneal osteomyelitis with a mean follow-up of 12 months or longer, Schade showed that minor complications with subsequent healing occurred in <24% of patients. Most major complications were related to residual soft tissue infection and osteomyelitis, and about 10% of patients required a major amputation eventually, with diabetes being a major risk factor (Schade 2012). Eighty-five percent of the patients had improved ambulatory status postoperatively, and the authors concluded that in properly selected patients, partial or total calcanectomy is a viable option for limb salvage.

Syme's amputation

The Syme's amputation is one of the most difficult operations to perform well, and it is named after James Syme, a professor of surgery in Edinburgh, in 1843. It is an amputation of the foot through the articulation of the ankle with removal of the malleoli of the tibia and fibula and leaves a long end-bearing stump for better leverage. The normal tough skin of the heel is brought forward directly underneath the end of the tibia, where the weight of the entire body is transmitted into the socket of the prosthesis.

The skin incision starts across the front of the ankle joint on a line connecting the two most prominent points of the malleoli and continues across the sole of the foot in a line at right angles to the long axis of the foot (Alldredge & Thompson 1946). The ankle is then dislocated, with removal of the calcaneus while preserving the heel pad. Both malleoli are then removed with a saw, and the long tendons and nerves are divided, with careful ligation of arteries (especially posteriotibial) to preserve perfusion of the heel pad. The stump is then closed, drained, and dressed (Alldredge & Thompson 1946). Since this is a technically difficult operation, various modifications (such as Pirogoff 1854, Elmslie 1924, Boyd 1939, Sarmiento 1972, and Wagner 1977) have been described. The Syme's operation can also be performed one-stage or two-stage, the latter popularized by Wagner (1977).

Francis et al. made a deliberate attempt to perform the Syme's amputation in 26 patients with forefoot necrosis who had palpable posteriotibial pulses, including 17 patients with diabetes requiring insulin and a further three controlled by diet. Three patients underwent a one-stage and 23 underwent a two-stage Syme's amputation. Overall, 20 patients (77%) had successful Syme's amputations. With a mean follow-up of all patients to 23 months, only one patient required revision to the below-knee level (Francis et al. 1990). Pinzur et al. performed a prospective randomized trial comparing a Syme ankle disarticulation using a one-stage versus Wagner's two-stage technique. Initially, 21 patients were randomized into one-stage and two-stage surgery. The randomization was stopped when the results of both procedures appeared to be similar. The next 22 consecutive patients underwent 23 Syme ankle disarticulations in one-stage surgery. As a total group, 31 of 44 amputations healed and progressed to prosthetic limb fitting. In all, 26 of 36 one-stage and 5 of 8 two-stage operations healed successfully, and the authors concluded that the Syme's amputation could be performed as safely in one stage as in two stages in properly selected patients (Pinzur et al. 1995).

■ Below-knee amputation

It is noteworthy to remember that the energy expenditure of ambulation increases as the level of amputation rises from calf to thigh. Preservation of the knee joint permits the use of lightweight prosthesis, minimizes the energy of ambulation, and enables elderly frail patients to walk independently. However, long-term rehabilitation is rarely successful in elderly, frail patients who receive above- or below-knee amputation: only 5% of these patients can use prosthesis to walk outside the home, and most patients remain wheelchair-bound after 5 years. Despite the poor outcome, return to ambulatory existence postoperatively should be the ultimate goal for all patients who have a below-knee amputation. Keeping the knee joint gives a better chance of walking using an artificial leg or prosthesis and social independence after the amputation. The bone and deep tissues are generally treated in a similar way, but the type of skin incision varies between techniques (**Figure 35.5**).

When performing a below-knee amputation, the gastrocnemius, soleus, and plantaris muscles are usually supplied by the sural arteries. These sural arteries, also known as inferior muscular arteries, are large branches arising from the popliteal artery, with a distribution to the muscles and integument of the calf, and they anastomose to the posterior tibial, medial, and lateral inferior genicular arteries. The sural arteries are often spared from peripheral arterial disease, allowing the use of a long posterior myocutaneous flap (consisting of majority of gastrocnemius and minority of soleus muscle bulk) to close the below-knee amputation (Aligne et al. 1990). The minimal level permitted for successful limb fitting after a below-knee amputation is 7 cm below the joint line. The tibial osteotomy should be about 11–18 cm (usually about 12 cm) distal to the tibial tubercle and the fibula osteotomy 1–2 cm proximal to the tibial osteotomy (Marshall & Stansby 2010). Below-knee amputations may be carried out using either a long posterior flap or skewed flaps mainly due to surgeons'

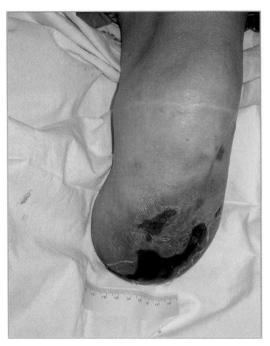

Figure 35.5 Failed below-knee amputation stump due to pressure effects from the prosthesis, requiring revision to above-knee amputation.

preferences. In a series of 90 patients in the group aged ≥70 years, 22% had above-knee amputations and 75% had below-knee amputations, 69% of the latter were discharged home walking (Robinson 1976). The patients with below-knee amputations had the Burgess long posterior flap technique, and below-knee amputation gives the elderly patient a better chance of walking because of the use of the patellar tendon bearing prosthesis, and 36% of those patients with below-knee amputation were fully independent for periods exceeding 6 months. The Burgess flap may have several technical problems: the stump may be wide and bulbous in transverse diameter, causing delays or difficulties in limb fitting, and the scar crossing the tibia may break down with prosthetic use.

When the posterior calfskin or subcutaneous tissue is of poor quality or very edematous, the Robinson's skewed flap technique may be favored, thus producing a cylindrical stump well suited for limb fitting. Using thermography and skin blood flows measurements with intradermal radioisotope clearance technique, McCollum et al. (1985) showed that there was a significant medial to lateral thermal gradient in many cases and concluded that a more medially based posterior below-knee amputation skin flap may be of more value in some patients. In the skew flap technique, the bone section is selected 10 to 15 cm below the tibial plateau, and equal anteromedial and posterolateral skew flaps are fashioned. The original paper by Robinson described the surgical technique most eloquently (McCollum et al. 1985). This paper also gave the results of 131 skew-flap below-knee amputations, of which 109 patients had peripheral arterial disease and 54 had diabetes. Ninety-five percent of the patients were rehabilitated to independent walking, and only nine patients (6.8%) required reamputation to a higher level (Robinson 1991). Although Robinson reported that the skew flap amputation was easy to learn and produced satisfactory stump shape, a lot of surgeons who looked at skew flap amputation versus the long posterior flap technique were new to the skew flap operation and so were on a learning curve. Factors that might have influenced the findings include previous experience

SUMMARY

- The perioperative mortality after major amputation in the United Kingdom is currently 17% and shows poor long-term survival
- A transtibial (below-knee) amputation is preferable to a transfemoral (above-knee) amputation, because it is associated with increased mobility
- A transtibial amputee consumes about 25% and a transfemoral amputee about 60% additional energy compared with normal walking
- Patients who have had a midfoot amputation are at high risk of developing an equinovarus deformity and may require a muscle balancing procedure of the hindfoot to prevent this complication
- Patient rehabilitation should be considered as soon as the decision to perform an amputation has been taken
- Rehabilitation occurs in phases from preamputation assessment and preparation through early postoperative phases and training to long-term follow-up
- Rehabilitation programs require interdisciplinary coordination between a group of well-trained health-care professionals
- Despite assessment, some patients (about 25%) will be unsuitable for prosthetic limb fitting
- All patients who have a prosthetic limb will require a wheelchair and modifications to their dwelling to accommodate one

INTRODUCTION
Incidence, risk factors, and prevention of amputation

Diabetes is now widely recognized as a significant cause of both minor and major lower extremity amputation. The risk of a person with diabetes undergoing amputation during their lifetime is estimated as eight times higher than in individuals without diabetes. One in four amputees with diabetes may require reamputation or contralateral limb amputation.

An aggressive-coordinated approach to diabetic foot care is both cost-effective and clinically efficient in reducing the burden of foot-related complications in a diabetic population (Nason et al. 2013, Rogers et al. 2010). Amputation rates have declined after implementation of a multidisciplinary team work, and amputation should not be considered inevitable in those with ulceration (Moxey et al. 2011).

All-cause mortality is high after an amputation in both patients with and without diabetes. Mortality rate, hospital stay, and postoperative complications are similar between amputees with and without diabetes. No modifiable factors, with the exception of nephropathy, were found to improve survival in amputees (Tentolouris et al. 2004).

Recent studies have demonstrated that the major amputation rate in England is 5.1/100,000 population and that has not changed over a 5-year period. The mortality rate for major leg amputation was 16.8% (21.4% for above-knee amputation (AKA) and 11.6% for below-knee amputation (BKA), and this mortality has decreased significantly over time ($p < 0.001$). There was a significant difference in amputation rate, mortality rate, and BKA:AKA ratio between different areas of England between 2003 and 2008, accompanied by a significant reduction in perioperative mortality (Moxey et al.). The variation in incidence of both major and total amputations between different parts of England was recently reported to be up to 10-fold (Moxey et al).

In the USA, reports on primary amputation incidence rates vary between 12 and 50 per 100,000 per year. Increasing revascularization rates have been associated with a reduction in amputation rates in the United States, with a 50% decrease in amputation rates during a 10-year-study period with a corresponding increase in surgical and endovascular revascularization (Paulus et al. 2012).

The role of amputation in limb salvage is often poorly defined because the surgeon and the patient often attempt to save all limbs at all costs. The difficulty lies in selecting the appropriate patient on whom to attempt limb salvage versus early amputation. For the sedentary patient, a poorly functional salvaged limb can provide him/her with a higher quality of life (QoL) than he/she would have with an amputation. For the active patient, early major amputation may offer the best functional outcome (Attinger & Brown 2012).

The recent trend in the incidence of nontraumatic amputations in individuals with and without diabetes has been estimated. A nationwide study in England has suggested that the overall population burden of amputations increased in people with diabetes at a time when the number and incidence of amputations decreased in the aging population without diabetes (Vamos et al. 2010).

AMPUTATION OF THE FOOT

In the forefoot, amputations may be performed either transversely or longitudinally (ray) according to the degree of tissue damage with minimal disturbance of normal biomechanics of foot. Necessary support is provided by shaped foam filler in a supportive shoe with a reinforced sole and possibly a 'rocker' profile if needed. Supply of silicone-made forefoot replacement provides improved cosmesis when worn with open shoes or sandals. Minor foot amputations commonly require revision or more proximal amputation. One out of every five patients undergoing any version of a partial first ray amputation will eventually require more proximal reamputation (Borkosy & Roukis 2012) as do transmetatarsal amputations (Dudkiewicz et al. 2009) (**Figure 36.1**).

In midfoot (tarsometatarsal or Lisfranc and midtarsal or Chopart) amputations, it is important to carry out a muscle balancing procedure to maintain balance of power in the hindfoot and avoid the complication of equinovarus deformity. If the residual foot is balanced to be plantar grade, then the patient may be able to manage with an ortholene back splint incorporating a sole plate and toe filler. The advantage of this level of amputation is the ease of mobilizing indoors without the need of prosthetic support and proprioceptive and sensory feedback, particularly in the elderly. Partial foot amputations have the advantage of being an end-bearing limb and require less energy expenditure for the patient to walk, theoretically suggesting improved functional outcome.

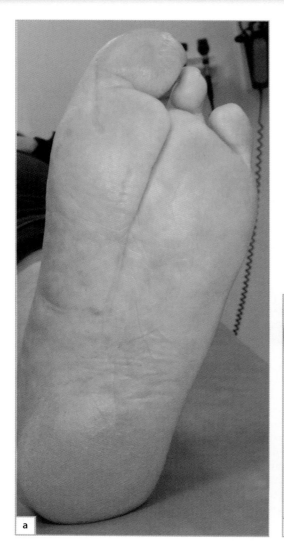

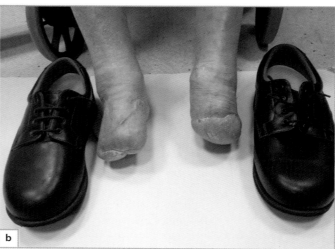

Figure 36.1 A middle ray (a) and transmetatarsal (b) amputation.

At the level of mid- and hindfoot, bone and joint involvement is quite common in diabetes. The relationship between infection, necrosis, and poorly perfused tissue is very strong in this part of the foot. A Boyd amputation consists of talectomy, excision of articular surfaces of the tibia, and calcaneum and tibiocalcaneal arthrodesis. It can be performed as a one- or two-staged operation. It is claimed to be superior to other partial midfoot and hindfoot amputations in terms of anatomy and function (Altindas & Kilic 2008).

Syme's ankle disarticulation is often overlooked as an alternative to BKA in cases of life- and limb-threatening foot infections and gangrene (Frykberg et al. 2011). Syme's amputation can provide a reliable alternative to more proximal amputations, but they are not without their occasional complication. Varus heel pad migration has been well documented as a complication as well as poor flap healing (especially when the posterior tibial artery is diseased or occluded) (Smith et al. 2012).

TRANSTIBIAL AMPUTATION

Amputation below the knee allows natural extension and flexion of the knee joint but requires a prosthetic ankle and foot. A long BKA has no advantage and compromises fitting of a functional prosthesis. Utilizing modern prosthetic techniques, a residuum as short as 7 cm may be fitted successfully. The functional mobility outcome of a short below-knee segment with an intact extensor mechanism compared with knee disarticulation or transfemoral amputation is significant. Incorporating a thigh corset to a below-knee prosthesis for partial weight distribution and knee stability is more favorable to sacrificing the natural knee and performing a proximal amputation. An optimal average length for transtibial amputation would be 16 cm from the knee joint axis. A BKA transects all four muscle compartments, tibia and fibula. Beveling of the tibial crest, chamfering sharp bone edges and myodesis are recommended to produce a well-contoured pain-free residual limb (Robinson 1991) (**Figure 36.2**). Patellar tendon bearing prostheses have become the prosthesis of choice throughout the world for this level of amputation.

Advances in prosthetic technology have allowed below-knee amputees an efficient and functional return to their premorbid level of activity (**Figure 36.3**). In selected patients, BKA can be a more functional option to limb salvage. Difficulty remains in patient selection (Brown et al. 2012).

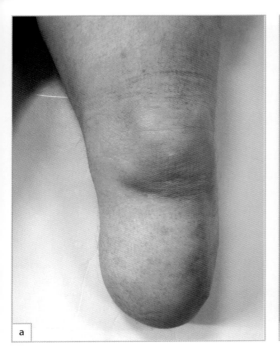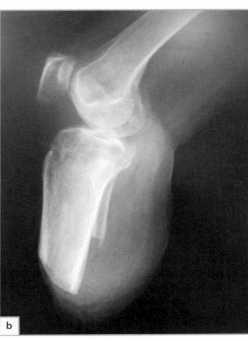

Figure 36.2 Transtibial residual limb (a) and corresponding X-ray (b).

The long-term outcome of 100 consecutive lower limb amputations in 96 patients was monitored by annual review for 5 years. The ratio of primary BKA to AKA was 2:1, with 9% of BKA undergoing revision to a higher level. At 2 years after amputation only 26% of patients were successfully walking out of doors, whereas 40% had died. By 5 years, 67% were dead and only 9% continued to walk out of doors with an artificial limb, although an additional 8% continued to use the limb within the confines of their own homes. In a previous audit of 193 amputations performed during 3.5 years to December 1984, stump healing was a problem in 45% of primary BKAs, compared with 25% in the present study. Although the BKA to AKA ratio in 1984 was only 1:2, the overall rehabilitation rate, as determined by the proportion of patients able to walk at 2 years, was 34%. These authors concluded that increasing the proportion of BKAs for peripheral arterial disease does not necessarily improve effective rehabilitation rates, although this is not a widely held view (McWhinnie et al. 1994).

◼ TRANSFEMORAL AMPUTATION

To lose the knee joint is a grave disadvantage to any patient and transfemoral amputation should not be performed where there is a possibility of an amputation at a lower level being successful. The longer the residual limb (within certain limits) the better the leverage. The recommendation is to section the bone 13 cm above knee joint line to provide adequate room to fit a prosthetic knee in the prosthesis. Equal anterior and posterior skin flaps are advocated. The muscles separated into four quadrants. The best functional outcome may be achieved by performing myodesis. The adductor muscle and iliotibial tract are sutured to the bone end through drill holes (myodesis). The quadriceps and hamstrings are sutured to each other in physiologic tension (myoplasty) (**Figure 36.4**).

The sockets of the AKA prostheses are traditionally proximal bearing and ischial bearing, although an element of more distal loading and total surface bearing is now a common approach. There are number of shapes, which have evolved from different researchers. The shaped brim has to accommodate the adductor longus tendon at its origin, the ischial tuberosity, and the greater trochanter. The soft tissues may be distorted to meet the mechanical requirements. The type of suspension depends on hip stability and residual limb length. For those with hip instability, a metal hip joint with pelvic belt is provided to control the prosthesis. A modified form of Silesian belt is an alternative in patients whose residual limb fluctuates in volume and cannot use a suction type socket. Self-suspension with locking liner or vacuum suction is the preferred option. The Silicone Seal-In Liner rolls over the residual limb and is in direct contact with the skin. A rubber hypobaric sealing membrane is situated around the circumference of the liner. Once in contact with the socket, a seal is created providing a suction suspension system. A valve is incorporated within the socket, and to remove the socket, the valve is opened letting air into the system (Smith et al. 2004) (**Figure 36.5**).

◼ THROUGH HIP AND HINDQUARTER AMPUTATIONS

In hip disarticulation, the femur is detached at the hip joint and all muscles controlling the lower limb are severed. The bony pelvis remains stable, which is capable of weight bearing on the ischial tuberosity. In hindquarter amputation, the lower extremity including the hip joint and the related hemipelvis is ablated. Success of mobilizing with such a full-length relatively heavy prosthesis at this level of amputation would depend on the patient's age, fitness, and motivation.

A prosthesis for these amputations comprises the socket embracing the whole pelvis and goes above the iliac crest over which it is closely molded. This provides the needed suspension. The prosthetic hip joint is placed anteriorly, giving stability on standing. Most patients would be fitted with a stable knee joint, and the rest of the components would be decided according to the patient's mobility potential.

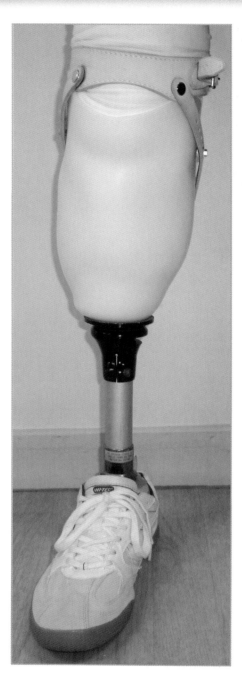

Figure 36.3 Modular transtibial prosthesis.

BILATERAL LOWER LIMB AMPUTEES

The percentage of bilateral lower limb amputees who continue to use prostheses is 37% (18% among those with peripheral arterial disease and 64% without peripheral arterial disease). In one study, diabetes mellitus, hypertension, depression, visual deficit, obesity, number of complications, etiology of amputation, amputation level, and age were found to be associated with patients abandoning prostheses. However, after multivariate regression was performed, only age and the number of residual limb complications were correlated with the use of prostheses. Younger individuals, with less residual limb complications,

were more likely to continue using prostheses (Guarita et al. 2012). Patients undergoing bilateral BKA continue to do well at long-term follow-up and survive on average for >4 years after discharge (MacNeil et al. 2008) (**Figure 36.6**).

■ REHABILITATION PROGRAM AND MOBILITY OUTCOME

■ Phases of lower limb rehabilitation
Preamputation stage

In the case of elective amputations, patients benefit from a preamputation consultation with the prosthetic team to understand the details of the relevant prosthesis, realistic potential/rehabilitation outcome, and possible complications related to amputation and the use of a prosthesis. This gives an opportunity for the patient to be introduced to other age and amputation level matched established amputees. The physiotherapist should assess general strength, mobility, specific joint weakness, and deformities and recommend appropriate preamputation exercise programs. Patient's home conditions, employment, driving status, hobbies, etc. are assessed and appropriate advice given. Adequate preamputation pain control for 48 hours and continued a few days postoperatively reduce the incidence of severe phantom limb pain (PLP).

Postamputation preprosthetic stage

The patient returns from theater with a drain and light dressing over the suture line, held in place with light crepe bandage. Preprosthetic physiotherapy should commence within a few days of amputation, depending on adequate wound healing. Early postoperative pain and PLP should be adequately controlled to enable the patient to participate in physiotherapy, bed mobility, regain independence for personal hygiene, and wheelchair mobility. The patient is encouraged to look and handle the residual limb. The drain is removed by the third postoperative day, the wound dressing changed, and patient dressed in his clothes to attend the physiotherapy department. An otherwise fit patient should be able to weight bear and mobilize between rails in the physiotherapy department using a pneumatic postamputation mobility (PPAM) aid within 10 days from amputation (**Figure 36.7**). PPAM aid is a partial weight-bearing prosthesis to be used within parallel bars or with crutches if the patient's balance is good. Active joint exercises and re-education of balance and core stability are commenced. Postoperative edema is avoided by using special elasticated socks.

Prosthetic gait training

The prosthetic clinics within the UK National Health Service (NHS) setting provide prostheses for all amputees when clinically appropriate. Once the swelling on the residual limb is sufficiently resolved and wound healing is satisfactory, measurements or a cast is taken and the first prosthesis is supplied to be used in the physiotherapy department within 3 weeks of amputation. The gait training starts in the parallel bars, and once a good gait pattern is achieved a walking aid is supplied (**Figure 36.8**). During this period, the patient learns the mechanics and maintenance of the prosthesis, to put on and take off the prosthesis independently, to sit and stand safely, to walk correctly, and to manage stairs, kerbs, and slopes. If the patient is fit enough to manage transport, he should be escorted on a journey and taught to get in and out of car. As it is possible that the patient might at some time have a fall, he must be taught how to

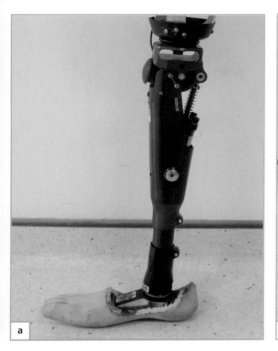

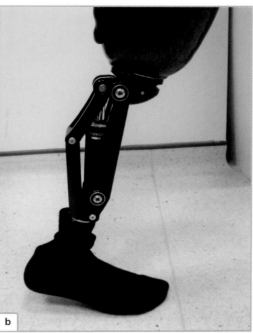

Figure 36.4 (a) Polyaxial and (b) single-axis knee joints.

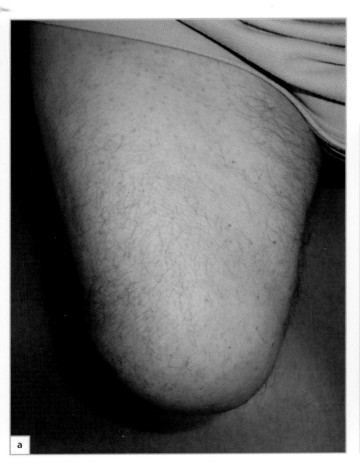

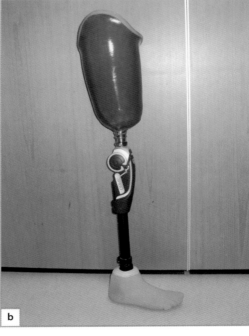

Figure 36.5 (a) Transfemoral residual limb and (b) prosthesis.

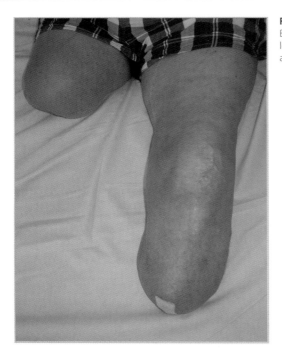

Figure 36.6 Bilateral lower limb amputation.

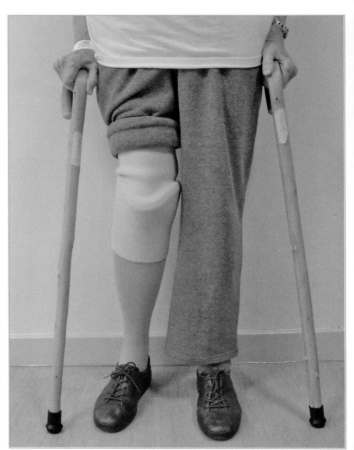

Figure 36.8 Prosthetic gait training.

Follow-up

Patient's early recovery is then monitored at 4- to 6-week intervals, gradually reducing in frequency to once in 3 to 4 months by the end of the first year and less frequently there afterward. Appropriate adjustments of prosthesis are made to match any changes in the residual limb. Patients may warrant a refresher course of physiotherapy when major changes are made in prosthetic components or when bad gait habits are detected. Higher level amputation and multiple limb amputations take longer periods to complete gait training programs. The younger amputee should make greater efforts to walk with as normal a gait as possible.

Requirements of prostheses to fulfill daily walking, hobbies, sports, and employment are taken into account in prescribing prostheses. The aim is to provide the range of prostheses and appropriate components to restore as near normal a life as possible in the long term.

At the early stages, most amputees depend on crutches or a wheelchair until completing prosthetic fitting and training. They often revert to using wheelchair when they are not able to use a prosthesis at a later stage. Higher level or multiple limb amputees may consistently resort to a wheelchair in addition to walking with prostheses. A suitable model wheelchair is prescribed by an occupational therapist in the United Kingdom (**Figure 36.9**). If the NHS is unable to provide an appropriate model, the patient may have to part fund it using a voucher scheme or purchase it privately.

The normal human gait is extremely efficient, and any inefficiency, which is any alteration in the normal pattern of gait,

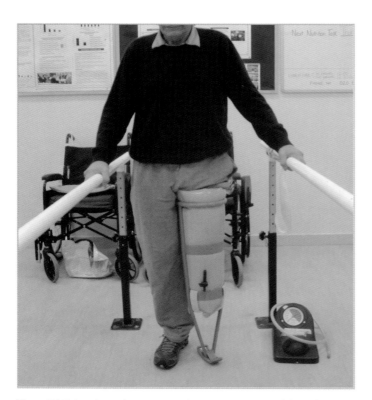

Figure 36.7 A patient using a pneumatic postamputation mobility aid.

get up from lying. The prosthesis may or may not be completed with a cosmetic cover depending on the patient's wishes. At discharge, further therapy from colleagues in the community is arranged as needed.

BIOMECHANICS AND PREVENTION

Chapter 37 — Off-loading

Martin C. Berli, Thomas Böni

SUMMARY

- Off-loading is one of the central elements in the treatment of the diabetic foot, whether the problem consists of an ulcer or neuro-osteo-arthropathy (Charcot disease)
- In addition to off-loading, a patient with an ulcer needs assessment and management by an interdisciplinary team
- The ideal off-loading device is a custom-made cast, which is changed regularly and produced by well-trained cast specialists
- Prefabricated devices are less expensive and easier to deliver. For patients who have difficulties getting to the hospital to have their cast changed regularly, they might be a better solution
- Prefabricated devices carry a significant risk of creating new ulcers, particularly in patients with diabetic polyneuropathy
- In a custom-made cast it is crucial to use no artificial material, to avoid allergic reactions
- Special casts, such as a combination of a plaster of Paris cast and Scotch cast, can be used in patients with secreting wounds
- A significant problem with off-loading is patient compliance, which can be increased by using a closed instead of a removable total contact cast (TCC)
- Once off-loading treatment is finished, the patient needs adapted orthopedic shoes

INTRODUCTION

The main orthopedic problem of the foot in diabetes consists of complications caused by long-term hyperglycemia. Part of the problem is micro- and macroangiopathy as well as polyneuropathy. Together, they lead not only to the loss of sensitivity in the foot – which may lead to impressive wounds via unnoticed injuries – but also to an impaired healing of the wounds because of the reduced blood supply. Patients also have an impaired infection defense, which both predisposes them to and accelerates the spread of infection. Therefore, every effort needs to be made not only to heal ulcers as quickly as possible, but also to prevent their occurrence in the first place (Howard et al. 2009).

The impairment of the sensory nervous system, which is responsible for the perception of pain, and the autonomic nervous system, which is responsible for sweat production and capillary perfusion (arteriovenous shunting), leads to a reduced physical stress tolerance of the sole of the foot. Decreased sweat production causes the skin to become brittle and cracked, causing fissures and ulcers. This tendency appears in the areas of increased pressure at the heel and the ball of the foot. In this situation, repetitive trauma, which is instinctively avoided by healthy patients with intact sensation, can cause pressure spots, hyperkeratosis, and finally ulcers.

In addition, the shape of the foot can change due to neuropathy of the motor nerves, which leads to increased pressure on the foot. The cause of the deformities may be due to rupture of the plantar fascia, or contractures of the ligaments (Myerson & Shereff 1989, Taylor et al. 1998). Others have suggested it is due to muscle imbalance. The intrinsic muscles atrophy due to (unopposed extrinsic musculature)

neuropathy leading to malposition of the toes (Delbridge 1985, Boulton 1996).

Diminished elasticity of the tissues (Stucke et al. 2012) in diabetic feet results in a reduced tolerance to shearing forces, which are difficult to evaluate and measure clinically. Typically, the following toe deformities are found in the context of a diabetic foot (Mansour et al. 2008): claw toe (hyperextension in the metatarsophalangeal joint), hammertoe, mallet toe, digitus flexus, and crossover toe. All of these deformities may lead to dorsal pressure problems (in addition to the more common plantar disease), which can develop further to ulcers and open joints. In addition, the deformities with a flexion contracture in an articulation can lead to ulcers of the tips of the toes, which frequently develop osteomyelitis of the distal phalanges.

Typical deformities affecting the hallux (Boffeli et al. 2002) include hallux valgus, valgus interphalangeus, varus, flexus, or the bunion deformity. These deformities often cause ulcers of the medial margin of the foot and, due to their need for space, present a challenge for an adequate shoe fitting. Hallux valgus can develop up to a maximum valgus angle of 90°. The resulting pressure on the second and third toe causes limited perfusion and may lead to a need for amputation to reduce the risk of infection brought on by chronic pressure ulcers.

With the little toe, the following deformities are frequent: digitus quintus varus, tailor's bunion. If pressure ulcers appear on the little toe, they can usually be removed with a small surgical intervention and without amputation. If the effect of the neuropathy is not limited to individual toes but affects the entire foot (Lavery et al. 2002), technical orthopedic care will be more difficult and corrective surgical interventions may have to be considered.

One should not forget that pressure ulcers may not only be precipitated by deformities, but by a reduced range of motion of individual joints (Fernando et al. 1991). The principal example of this is hallux rigidus. Due to the limited dorsiflexion, the hallux cannot avoid the pressure during ambulation, which increases the risk of ulceration. These are difficult to eliminate with orthopedic footwear. One approach is the shift and stiffening of the rocker in the sole of the shoe.

Amputations lead to an alteration of the foot skeleton and have an important influence on the distribution of pressure in the foot, since they result in a deformation of the original shape of the foot and reduce the footprint. Patients with Charcot disease often have the most severe deformities (see Chapters 32, 33, and 34).

OFF-LOADING DEVICES

If, during a regular check-up, pressure marks on the feet are noticed with or without callus (hyperkeratosis), patients should be offered an appropriate off-loading device to reduce the risk of ulceration. For this purpose, numerous means are available:

1. Socks
2. Insoles
3. Shoe modifications
   i. Rocker
   ii. Roller
4. Walker (walking aid or frame)

5. Ankle foot orthoses (AFO):
   i. patellar tendon bearing (PTB)
   ii. non-PTB
6. Non-removable TCC or removable (rTCC)

The simplest measure is the avoidance of walking barefoot at home by wearing seamless socks, which can be adequately padded and help prevent slipping with integrated rubber nipples. Veves et al. (1990) have shown that simple socks can reduce pressure peaks up to 10%.

In addition, plantar pressure peaks can be reduced up to 25% by wearing shoes with an adapted insole because of cushioning and pressure redistribution (Cavanagh & Owings 2006, Illgner et al. 2009). Interestingly, Drerup et al. (2004) have found that these measures provide less pressure reduction in patients with diabetes compared with those without diabetes.

The principal methods of mechanical prophylaxis include custom-made insoles, which can be inserted into ready-made shoes, orthopedic serial shoes with a custom-made foot bed (nonremovable), and finally orthopedic custom-made shoes, which are built and adapted to a shoe last corresponding to the shape of the foot and the needs of the individual patient. In addition, there are diverse means of shoe modifications available, e.g. rocker and roller. For patients with diabetes, normal ready-made shoes – even well-cushioned sneakers – must not be used, as they do not take into account the pathological pressure distribution and the patients cannot perceive pressure spots because of their polyneuropathy (Drerup et al. 2004, Erdemir et al. 2005, Cavanagh et al. 2006).

As an orientation guide, a table with the prescription criteria for orthopedic footwear to treat the diabetic foot and analogous neuroangioarthropathies was established in Germany. This guide is considered the national standard in Germany and has been composed by the country's most prominent medical boards (**Table 37.1**). In Switzerland, the orientation paper of the interdisciplinary workgroup diabetic foot of the Diabetes Education Study Group provides information on the different risk levels and their supply (Furrer et al. 2001).

As a further off-loading measure, the use of a walking aid, such as a walking frame, a rollator, or crutches, can be prescribed. Use of a walker transfers part of the plantar pressure during the gait via the upper extremities to the walking aid.

If ulcers appear on the feet despite all footwear precautions, more aggressive unloading is required. Depending on the causes, either a surgical or a nonsurgical (conservative) approach may be considered. As conservative methods, off-loading with an AFO or TCC is available as valuable treatment options (Armstrong et al. 2008).

The AFO exists in diverse forms and is continuously refined along with the development of new materials (synthetics, carbon fibre, etc). Its purpose is to achieve off-loading of the lower leg but especially in the discharging of the foot. In the case of diabetic feet, the AFO is mostly built in a closed version as a boot, but can also be produced as an open version in the form of a posterior splint with a foot base. The percentage amount of pressure to be off-loaded can be individually determined. The pressure of the AFO is either transferred on to the insertion of the patellar tendon (PTB) or more proximally as non-PTB.

The most sophisticated device, which is best adapted to the individual and changing needs of the patient, is the TCC, which is described in detail in the next section. The TCC is the core element of off-loading treatment in diabetes and, if administered correctly, also the most efficient one (Boulton 2012, Jeffcoate 2008).

THE TOTAL CONTACT CAST

Historically, it was thought that patients with diabetes and neuropathy suffering from an ulcer should continue to put weight on it normally, to accelerate healing of the wound. This theory was proven to be incorrect by the pioneering work of Brand (1983). In patients with leprosy and other neuropathic conditions in India, treatment with off-loading in a cast was, for the first time, shown to be associated with good outcomes (Brand et al. 1983, Boulton et al. 1990, Rathur 2007, Brem et al. 2004).

Several studies have analyzed off-loading treatment with a cast and demonstrated accelerated wound healing in a higher percentage of patients compared with patients who were treated without pressure relief (Mueller et al. 1989, Lavery et al. 1996, Armstrong et al. 2003). Currently, TCC treatment is considered the 'gold standard' therapy in off-loading treatment of diabetic foot ulcers (Jeffcoate 2008, Wu SC, et al. 2008). Experience has shown that the irremovable TCC is clearly superior to the rTCC due to generally poor compliance. Patients, who are equipped with an rTCC only wear it during 28% of their daily

Table 37.1 Prescription criteria for off-loading diabetic footwear

Class of prescription		Explanation	Supply
0	Diabetes mellitus (DM) without PN/PAD	Education and advice	Ready-made comfortable shoes without orthopedic adaptation
I	Like 0 with foot deformity	Elevated risk	Orthopedic adapted shoe
II	DM with loss of sensitivity due to PN/ clinically significant PAD	PN with loss of sensitivity, PAD	Protective diabetic shoe with removable ready-made soft padded insole, if applicable with orthopedic shoe modification, e.g. fat pad atrophy or early deformity
III	After plantar ulcer	Significantly elevated risk for recurrent ulcer compared with group II	Protective diabetic shoe generally with diabetes adapted foot bedding (DAFB), if applicable with orthopedic shoe modification
IV	Like II with deformities, respectively, disproportions	Not treatable with ready-made shoe last	Custom-made orthopedic shoe with DAFB
V	Charcot disease, (Charcot: Sanders type II–V, LEVIN stadium III)	Orthoses generally with DNOAP (Diabetic Neuroosteoarthropathy) Sanders type IV–V or with severe perpendicular deviation	Ankle-deep orthopedic custom-made shoe with DAFB, inner shoe, orthoses
VI	Like II with partial amputation of the foot	At least transmetatarsal or inner amputation (e.g. PIP joint resection leaving toe in place)	Supply like IV plus prostheses
VII	Acute lesion/acute/active Charcot disease	Always as a temporary supply	Off-loading shoes, dressing shoes, interim shoe, orthoses, TCC if applicable with DAFB and orthopedic modifications

DNOAP, diabetic neuroosteoarthropathy (Charcot disease); PAD, peripheral arterial disease; PIP, proximal interphalangeal joint; PN, peripheral neuropathy; TCC, total contact cast.

activities (Armstrong et al. 2003). This fact could explain the poor outcome of many auxiliary devices, which were designed to speed up the healing process. Many patients wear their rTCC only outside the house but spend most of their time at home without adequate off-loading.

To offload the forefoot, there are several products available that dorsally incline the position of the foot. In these shoes (e.g. OrthoWedge®, Darco International, Huntington WV, USA), the foot takes up a 10° dorsiflexed angle compared with the ground with an unloaded forefoot. However, many patients with diabetes have a shortened gastrocnemius complex, which results in a reduction in dorsiflexion in the talocalcaneal joint. Together with the 10° dorsiflexed position of the foot, this leads to an additionally increased load in the forefoot, which may paradoxically increase the pressure and reduce wound healing (Baumgartner et al. 2011).

Our approach is to avoid prefabricated lower leg braces (e.g. VACO®ped-shoe; OPED, Valley/Oberlaindern, Germany) in our clinic. The main reasons are that patients with a polyneuropathy are unable to perceive pressure spots, that perspiration is increased due to the materials used (which may give rise to new skin lesions), and perhaps most importantly, that the foot base can only insufficiently be adapted to the needs of the patient. These risks are much lower when an expertly made and individually fitted TCC is used.

For the following reasons, the TCC has a positive biomechanical effect on the healing of the wound: during gait, the highest pressure loads are located under the calcaneus and the metatarsal heads and shift accordingly during roll-over. Important factors influencing this process are body weight, strength, and acceleration. With the shift of the load, the longitudinal and transverse arches of the foot are spread, which generates shearing forces. In off-loading, the auxiliary means minimize this effect by altering the mechanics of the gait. The better the device fits the patient's limb, the more this effect is increased.

Furthermore, with the TCC applied, patients are less active because of the limitation of their mobility and take smaller steps. This leads to a reduced load in the area of the ulcer. As a result, edema regresses in the TCC, which improves the oxygen supply and accelerates healing of the wound (Apelqvist 2012).

There are some disadvantages of the TCC. It is costly, requires appropriately trained health-care professionals to apply and is associated with low levels of patient comfort. The patient needs to be able to move around securely with an irremovable TCC. There is a distinct risk with a TTC if improperly applied of worsening the situation of the diabetic foot through the development of focal areas of pressure, which increase the risk of ulceration. However, when well applied by properly trained health-care professionals, these risks appear very low (Wukich & Motko 2004, Guyton 2005). Other risks of the TCC include osteopenia and venous thromboembolism (functional limitation of the venous calf muscle pump). For this reason, some centers advocate the use of venous thromboembolic prophylaxis during the entire duration of treatment with a TCC.

Another difficulty is muscular atrophy caused by the immobilization. Muscles need to be rebuilt after prolonged treatment with a TCC. Depending on the medical condition and the age of the patient, this may take considerable time (**Table 37.2**).

There remains controversy about the use of TCC in patients with peripheral arterial disease and/or infection. For some clinicians, these remain absolute contraindications to TCC (Nabuurs et al. 2005, Ali et al. 2008, Maderal et al. 2012, Malhotra et al. 2012). However, we believe that under close supervision, TCC may actually be beneficial in the management of these patients. In contrast to others, we consider marked edema of the lower leg to be an indication rather than a contraindication for TCC. The reason for our opinion lies in an

Table 37.2 Pros and cons of total contact cast (TCC) treatment

Pros
• Positive healing effect via off-loading
• Maintains the patient as ambulatory instead of on bed rest
• Protects from further trauma and prevents reulceration
• Edema reduction
• Supports infection control
• Requires minimal patient compliance (nonremovable)

Cons
• Alters gait (balance, coordination, low back pain)
• Risk of thromboembolism
• Joint stiffness, muscle atrophy, and inactivity osteopenia with long-term immobilization
• Weight of the TCC
• Limited wound care possible without removing TCC
• Expensive long-term treatment
• Need for specialized staff (to keep complications low and achieve the maximum effect)
• Compliance (keep TCC dry, no instruments use to scratch, etc.)

Risks
• Falls
• Thromboembolism
• New ulcers caused by pressure spots of the cast

improved vascular perfusion because of the regression of the edema, which helps accelerate wound healing (Apelqvist 2012). With regard to infections, it is well known that immobilization contributes to the healing process with or without an antibiotic treatment. Osteomyelitis needs to be considered separately but does not in our experience represent an absolute contraindication for TCC.

Although undisputed in its clinical efficacy, in the USA TCC treatment is only applied in 1.7% of medical centers in which patients with diabetic foot problems are treated. An rTCC is applied in only 15.2% of diabetic foot centers (Wu et al. 2008). Included in this study were 895 specialized centers. The reason for the infrequent application of TCC is explained in part by the time required to apply the cast and the potential financial impact of the duration of each treatment. Furthermore, trained and specialized staff are required and there remain (largely unsubstantiated) concerns about their potential to precipitate falls and iatrogenic ulceration. There have been a number of approaches made to simplify and reduce the cost of the application of TCC (Katz et al. 2005). These consist of a prefabricated off-loading boot (VACO®ped; OPED, Valley/Oberlaindern, Germany), which is adaptable to the shape of the foot of the patient and is removable. This boot can easily be transformed to an irremovable TCC – e.g. with the wrapping of a plaster bandage – to improve a patient's compliance (Katz et al. 2005).

TCC MANUFACTURE

To apply a TCC, the patient is positioned in a semisitting position or on their back. The knee joint of the relevant limb is bent at a 45° angle, which relaxes the gastrocnemius complex and allows a 90° flexion in the ankle joint. The cast can be outfitted with additional padding in the heel to achieve an even, horizontal contact surface if the patient is unable to bend their ankle joint at 90° due to a shortened gastrocnemius muscle group and a slight pes equinus as a result.

Patients tend to contract their toes during the application of the cast. If this is not taken into account, it leads to the foot part of the TCC being too short. The toes will then abut against or extend beyond the cast.

A TCC may be made from plaster of Paris or a synthetic material. The advantages of plaster of Paris are that it can be formed to fit more precisely, has a good wicking effect on secreting wounds, and can be disposed of in an environmentally friendly fashion. The disadvantages lie in its comparatively heavy weight, its brittleness, and its lack of water resistance. Casts should not be allowed to get wet as the padding will soak up fluids, causing skin maceration and potentially soft tissue infections. As explained below, there is also the possibility of combining both cast varieties: plaster of Paris and synthetic material.

The actual cast is applied as follows: first, after wound cleansing and debridement, a wound dressing is applied. The dressing should be thin and covered by thin compresses (cotton pads) to avoid compromising the desired support through excessive padding and thereby exposing the foot to detrimental shear forces. Second, if necessary, cream is applied to the lower leg (not the foot) to avoid the skin drying out. Now, padding and bracing is applied directly to the foot of the patient to provide foot support when walking and relieve ulcerated skin patches (**Figure 37.1**). This measure enlarges the contact surface and channels pressure to the areas able to support it (Eldor et al. 2004). Furthermore, it protects the sole against injuries. As padding, so-called Cellona®-pads (Synthetic pads, Lohmann & Rauscher, St Gallen, Switzerland) may be used, which are adhesive and are able to absorb some moisture.

The contour of the foot can be drawn with the patient standing on the pads, to ensure correct sizing of the TCC. Afterward, the padded dressings are marked and cut out in the areas of the ulcers. The padded dressings have the advantage of being able to absorb exudate to a limited degree. This enables the cast to be left intact for several days and changed less frequently depending on the amount of exudate.

Now, a thin textile padded dressing of the Stockinette™ (Mölnlycke Health Care, Dietikon, Switzerland) type is pulled over the whole padding and the lower leg. On top of this, more padding is applied to protect the rim of the tibia, the malleoli, and the arch of the foot. Adhesive foil may be used on the sole without problems to avoid

displacement of the pads during cast confection. However, skin reactions are likely to occur when the foil is placed on the lower limb, especially in dry, delicate skin. For this reason, the padding on the lower limb is applied on top of the Stockinette. Dry, delicate skin can be additionally protected against injuries and irritations by applying thin, nonadhesive dressings, such as siliconized Mepilex® (Mölnlycke Health Care, Dietikon, Switzerland). A thin layer of cotton wool padding protects the lower limb from cast-saw injuries.

Now, a second textile stocking is applied to ensure that all components fit snugly and to add compression. Attention needs to be paid to avoiding any creasing or bunching of the stocking, which could cause pressure sores. The stocking is made of pure cotton to prevent allergic skin reactions. It is important that a breathable fabric such as pure cotton is used, as such materials do not cause the patient to sweat unduly inside the cast.

It is important to differentiate between a Stockinette™, a Tubigrip™ cylindrical elastic bandage (Mölnlycke Health Care, Dietikon, Switzerland) and a tube made from towelling cloth. These materials differ in weaves and density and therefore have different characteristics. Fluids can evaporate better through a Stockinette™ than through a tube made from toweling cloth, which tends to retain moisture.

Where there is a high volume of exudate from ulcers, there is the option of fashioning a cast of the foot from plaster of Paris including the malleoli (**Figure 37.2**). As mentioned above, plaster of Paris has a good wicking effect and can siphon off fluids from secreting wounds. In this way, skin macerations can be avoided. The dressing tube is thin enough not to reduce the wicking effect. If the exudate from the wound is so heavy as to cause maceration of the skin, the cast boot needs to be changed more frequently. Historically, some practitioners have used plaster of Paris applied directly to the wound due to its disinfecting properties.

Next, a rigid longuette is dorsally applied along the entire length of the cast (**Figure 37.3**). Under the sole, the longuette is applied in double layers, strengthening the cast in this area. We recommend applying the double layers on the outside, to avoid causing a hole in the heel area through application of a retrograde layer, which is too short.

In the proximal area, the cast is now wrapped in a semirigid synthetic cast roll (3M™ Soft-Cast casting tape, 3M, St Paul, MN, USA) to its full extent. The advantage of the semirigid cast is its elasticity. It

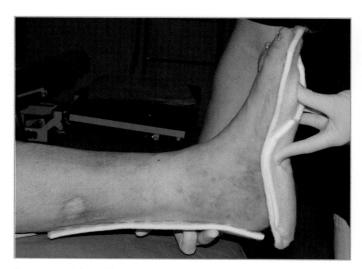

Figure 37.1 Adapted footpad off-loading a plantar ulcer under the metatarsophalangeal joint.

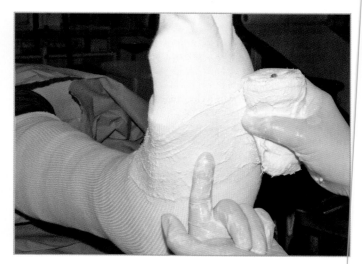

Figure 37.2 Special cast with plaster of Paris cast for draining ulcers over a Stockinette combination.

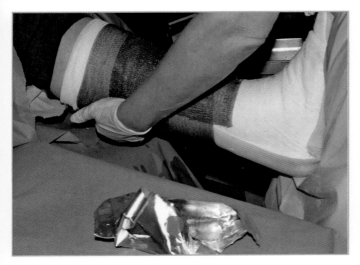

Figure 37.3 Casting with soft cast over a longuette.

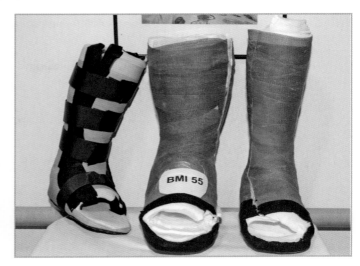

Figure 37.4 The final form of the total contact cast.

does not grate on the thigh or the lower leg if the patient assumes a sitting position and still affords good support.

As a further step, the cast is wrapped in synthetic cast (3M™ Scotchcast™ casting tape 3M, St Paul, MN, USA). The cast is wrapped with one finger to spare below or a maximum of two fingers extending beyond the head of the fibula, to provide the necessary stability (**Figure 37.4**). A side effect of the stability achieved may be soft tissue edema proximal to the end of the cast. This can be very pronounced in patients with severe leg edema und can strongly restrict the function of the knee joint.

With the cast thus prepared, the hardening process is initiated by wrapping the cast in a wet elastic dressing. Subsequently, the cast boot is shaped without any dents being created. To this end, pressure points on the sole and on the heel need to be shaped with great accuracy.

As soon as the cast is solid enough, the Stockinette™ tubes are turned back in the toe area. We apply the cast to extend one finger beyond the extended toes to avoid the toes abutting against the edge of the foot part. At the same time, this protection should not extend too far beyond the toes in order to not create a tripping hazard.

Finally, the foot of the cast is formed and rounded using a rigid synthetic cast. In the case of significant edema in the toes, thin compresses may be placed between the toes as a protection against friction. During the entire process, it is important to focus on the correct positioning of the foot. The foot needs to be in an approximate 90° angle to the upper ankle joint to enable the patient to walk with the cast. If this angle is incorrect, the patient runs a higher risk of falling.

After the cast is complete, it needs to be outfitted with a slip-resistant sole. In the past, material from old car tires was used for this purpose, but today, the following methods are preferred: as a slip-resistant sole, a removable cast shoe can be applied to the cast. This provides the patient with the hygienic advantage of being able to remove the shoe when going to bed. However, due to the height added to the cast by the cast shoe, the risk of tripping and falling is increased. Another solution is to fix a sole directly to the cast. This method provides the advantage of the sole adhering directly to the cast and reducing the danger of tripping when walking. For patients with a reduced range of mobility, this solution is easier to apply as it does not require manipulation with a separate cast shoe. The fixed sole, however, does have the drawback of having to be replaced with

every change of the cast. Furthermore, this method is less hygienic than the removable cast shoe.

If, as in most TCC treatments, a long duration of treatment is necessary, it is advisable to consider correcting the difference in leg lengths caused by the TCC, to prevent back pains. This can be done by way of augmenting the shoe sole on the opposite side.

It is very important to alert patients to the risks and guidelines relating to TCC treatment. For instance, it should be made clear that the cast must not get wet inside to avoid skin maceration and infection. Patients should sit down when showering and protect the cast with a plastic bag, which needs to be closed tightly with suitable adhesive tape. If water gets into the cast despite all efforts to prevent it, the cast immediately needs to be checked by a qualified specialist and replaced if necessary.

Early on in the treatment, the cast should be changed more frequently than in the later stages of treatment. Changes should occur at least once a week due to the significant reduction in the volume of the limb as swelling subsides. Later on, the cast can be changed every 2 weeks depending on wound condition and compliance.

It is important to note that Charcot foot requires treatment with a different TCC than those used for the treatment of ulcers. The same applies to TCC treatment after off-loading surgery. In our hospital, we prescribe subcutaneous low molecular weight heparin venous thromboembolism prophylaxis to all patients who undergo TCC or rTCC treatment for the duration of the treatment, if patients are not otherwise treated with anticoagulants.

◼ SURGICAL OFF-LOADING

If conservative treatment as outlined above fails to reduce pressure on the foot to a level that permits healing of ulcers or prevents recurrence of ulceration, the option of surgical off-loading is available. In surgical off-loading, it is crucial to thoroughly assess tissue perfusion, to avoid postoperative-delayed wound healing. This will usually entail noninvasive vascular investigations and an assessment by a vascular specialist. The following may be regarded as indications for surgical off-loading in the diabetic foot:

1. A nontreatable (unshoeable, uncastable, unbraceable) deformity
2. An osteomyelitis of the adjacent prominent bone (to reduce contact with the infected bone)

3. Failure to heal despite adequate treatment of the wound and exhaustion of conservative treatment options (off-loading, redistribution of pressure, TCC)
4. An ulcer recurrence despite adequate treatment with orthopedic shoes or braces

The following surgical options are available:
1. Procedures on tendons: lengthening of the Achilles tendon (Armstrong et al. 1999, Mueller et al. 2003, Maderal et al. 2012), tenotomies, tendon transfers, release of the joint capsule
2. Osteotomies: dorsiflexion osteotomy of the metatarsals (Fleischli et al. 1999)
3. 'Exostosectomy' of pseudoexostoses, joint resection (= 'inner resection') or entire foot rays
4. Correcting arthrodesis
5. External off-loading with an external fixator or an Ilizarov frame (Clemens et al. 2008)
6. Amputation: complete or partial

Furthermore, there is the option of silicone injections (Maderal et al. 2012), which are, however, only offered in a small number of centers and have very little published data to support their use. Tendon surgery aims to heal pressure ulcers caused by toe deformities and to preventing their recurrence. Flexor tendons are significant players in regard to claw toe and toe tip ulcers. Where tenotomy of the flexor tendons is not sufficient, or a balance needs to be established, tendon transfers may be affected. Long-term misalignment of the toes often causes tightening and adherence of the joint capsule, which can be surgically released.

The lengthening of the Achilles tendon retains a potentially key role in relieving pressure on the forefoot (Armstrong et al. 1999, Mueller et al. 2003, Maderal et al. 2012). Many patients with diabetes suffer from a shortening of the gastrocnemius complex and thus mobilize in the equinus position of the foot. In addition, the inversion effect of the Achilles tendon intensifies the pressure on the lateral margin of the foot (an area prone to ulceration).

In cases of toe misalignment, which can lead to pressure ulcers, corrective osteotomies may be performed, such as a dorsiflexion osteotomy of the metatarsals. This surgery provides for pressure reduction under the respective metatarsal heads and redistributes the pressure toward the remaining ones, without causing a shortening of the foot rays.

An exostosectomy for removing pseudoexostoses is predominantly applied in Charcot foot deformities. Through deformation of the foot skeleton, bony prominences are surgically removed to reduce the deformity and pressure and permit ulcer healing.

Joint resection ('inner resection') and the resection of an entire foot ray are applied most frequently in joint infections or osteomyelitis. Correcting arthrodeses lead to an adjustment of the bone positions and are mostly applied to correct a significant rigid misalignment in the area of the hind foot. In general, the use of metalwork such as plates and screws should be avoided in the diabetic foot where ulcers significantly increase the risk of infection.

For external off-loading and stabilization, an external fixator or an Ilizarov frame may be applied. The Ilizarov frame may be associated with shorter healing times, decrease pin track infections, and allow early weight bearing by the addition of a protective plantar plate. A downside is that the frame reduces the soft tissue reconstruction options because the pins limit access for flap dissection or microsurgical anastomosis (Mc Kee et al. 1998). Aside from stabilization, both fixators – particularly the Ilizarov – have the advantage of being able to align

a limb and compress a joint, providing for a tight pseudarthrosis, and thus simplifying a subsequent shoe or orthotic treatment.

If none of these means leads to a satisfactory situation, amputation remains as a last resort. The amputation can be carried out as a partial amputation of a toe or a foot, or as a complete amputation of the entire lower leg. Amputations in selected groups of patients are a straightforward and rapid solution to complex wounds that can have the patient ambulating again in short order (Clemens et al. 2010).

However, at present, no conclusive statement can be made regarding the effectiveness and safety of preventive surgical off-loading procedures due to a shortage of reliable data. Broad application of these procedures can therefore not be recommended, although amputations can be successful in individual cases (Bus et al. 2008) (see Chapter 38).

As off-loading treatment with a TCC is only prescribed for a limited amount of time, it is important to know how the patient will be treated after the conclusion of the successful off-loading treatment. In most cases the patient will receive treatment with a custom-made shoe (**Figure 37.5**). Six to eight weeks may pass until the shoe is completed by specialized orthopedic shoemakers. During this period, the patient can be treated with a removable off-loading cast. The course of the treatment will determine the success of the latter treatment with the orthopedic custom-made shoe. First, the foot of the patient is protected in a less stable fashion than in the nonremovable off-loading cast and therefore exposed to more pressure and shear forces. Second, the compliance of the patient plays a part, as the patient can also mobilize the limb without the cast boot. For these reasons, a decrease in treatment success can often be observed at this stage. Sometimes patients even develop a recurrent or new ulcer. For this reason, it is very important to monitor the patient closely and perform frequent follow-up visits.

It is essential to inform the patient that they may not wear noncustom shoes, even briefly, as the danger of recurrence is significantly higher, particularly in the months after the closing of the wound (National supply guidelines, Germany, 2006). One of the major problems worldwide is the variation in cost (and reimbursement

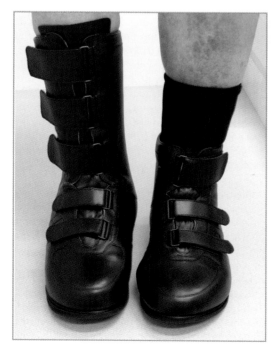

Figure 37.5
Custom-made orthopedic shoes.

schemes) and the availability (or otherwise) of expertise in the manfacture of orthopedic shoes. In Switzerland, for example, health insurers currently pay up to $6000 for an elaborate custom-made shoe, but in the United States, the compensation afforded is just $150 (Medicare Therapeutic Shoe Bill 2011).

CONCLUSION

Off-loading is a principal component of successful and enduring ulcer treatment. The treatment can be administered by applying a TCC, through surgery or through prevention by way of the use of orthopedic footwear. It must be kept in mind that off-loading is a dynamic process in the course of which a patient's feet will keep changing in form. Regular follow-ups and consistent patient management therefore remain essential.

AREAS OF CONTROVERSY AND/OR FUTURE RESEARCH

- Further research is required to identify methods to improve patient compliance with off-loading devices

- Greater awareness is needed of the importance of and training in delivering appropriate off-loading devices among health-care professionals managing patients with a diabetic foot
- There remains some controversy about the most effective method to off-load any foot ulcer, particularly comparing prefabricated and custom-made devices (specifically with respect to training issues, cost, and compliance)
- The use of prefabricated devices can help to control costs. With the increased risk of additional damage in the feet of patients with polyneuropathy, the pros and cons need to be pondered. In addition, the need for well-trained specialists limits the availability of custom-made casts
- Future research is required to identify new materials and improved prefabricated devices, as well as the precise duration of treatment necessary to heal ulcers

ACKNOWLEDGMENT

The authors would like to thank our two casting specialists Karin Hochhard and Oscar Nanlohy for their excellent work and valuable input in this article. Furthermore, we would like to thank Prof. Dr. med. Beat Ruettimann for his continuous enthusiasm and support in our training.

IMPORTANT FURTHER READING

Armstrong DG, Lavery LA, et al. Activity patterns of patients with diabetic foot ulcers: patients with active ulcers may not adhere to a standard pressure offloading regimen. Diabetes Care 2003; 26:2595–2597.

Boulton AJ. The pathogenesis of diabetic foot problems: an overview. Diabet Med 1996; 13:12–16.

Bus SA, Valk GD, van Deursen RW, et al. Specific guidelines on footwear and offloading. Diabetes Metab Res Rev 2008; 24:S192– S193.

Cavanagh PR, Owings TM. Nonsurgical strategies for healing and preventing recurrence of diabetic foot ulcers. Foot Ankle Clin 2006; 11:735–743.

Jeffcoate WJ, International Working Group on the Diabetic Foot. Unresolved issues in the management of ulcers of the foot in diabetes. Diabet Med 2008; 25:1380–1389.

Lavery LA, Vela SA, Lavery DC, et al. Reducing dynamic foot pressures in high-risk diabetic subjects with foot ulcerations: a comparison of treatments. Diabetes Care 1996; 19:818–821.

Mueller MJ, Diamond JE, Sinacore DR, et al. Total contact casting in the treatment of diabetic plantar ulcers: controlled clinical trial. Diabetes Care 1989; 12:384–388.

REFERENCES

Ali R, Oureshi A, Yagoob MY, et al. Total contact cast for neuropathic diabetic foot ulcers. J Coll Physicians Surg Pak 2008; 18:695–698.

Armstrong DG, Lavery LA, et al. Activity patterns of patients with diabetic foot ulcers: patients with active ulcers may not adhere to a standard pressure offloading regimen. Diabetes Care 2003; 26:2595–2597.

Armstrong DG, Lavery LA, Wrobel JS, et al. Quality of life in healing diabetic wounds: does the end justify the means? J Foot Ankle Surg 2008; 47:278–282.

Armstrong DG, Stacpoole-Shea S, Nguyen H, Harkless LB. Lengthening of the Achilles tendon in diabetic patients who are at high risk for ulceration of the foot. J Bone Joint Surg Am 1999; 81: 535–538. Erratum in: J Bone and Joint Surg Am. 2000; 82-A: 1510.

Apelqvist J. Diagnostics and treatment of the diabetic foot. Endocrine 2012; 41:384–397.

Baumgartner R, Moeller M, Stinus H. Orthopädie-Schuhtechnik, 1st edn. Geilsingen (Steige): C Maurer Print and Publisher, 2011. (Book in German).

Boffeli TJ, Bean JK, Natwick JR. Biomechanical abnormalities and ulcers of the great toe in patients with diabetes. J Foot Ankle Surg 2002; 41:359–364.

Boulton AJ. Lawrence Lecture: the diabetic foot: neuropathic in aetiology? Diabet Med 1990; 7:852–858.

Boulton AJ. The pathogenesis of diabetic foot problems: an overview. Diabet Med 1996; 13:12–16.

Boulton AJ. Diabetic neuropathy: is pain god's greatest gift to mankind? Semin Vasc Surg 2012; 25:61–5.

Brand PW. The diabetic foot. In: Ellenberg M, Rifkin H, (eds), Diabetes mellitus: theory and practice, 3rd edn. New York: Medical Examination Publishing Co, 1983:829–849.

Brem H, Sheehan P. Protocol for treatment of diabetic foot ulcers. Am J Surg 2004; 187:1S–10S. Review.

Bus SA, Valk GD, van Deursen RW, et al. Specific guidelines on footwear and offloading. Diabetes Metab Res Rev 2008; 24: S192– S193.

Cavanagh PR, Owings TM. Nonsurgical strategies for healing and preventing recurrence of diabetic foot ulcers. Foot Ankle Clin 2006; 11:735–743.

Clemens MW, Attinger CE. Functional reconstruction of the diabetic foot. Semin Plast Surg 2010; 24:43–56.

Clemens MW, Parikh P, Hall MM, et al. External fixators as an adjunct to wound healing. Foot Ankle Clin 2008; 13:145–156.

Delbridge L, Ctercteko G, Fowler C, et al. The aetiology of diabetic neuropathic ulceration of the foot. Br Surg 1985; 72:1–6.

Drerup B, Kolling Ch, Koller A, et al. Reduction of plantar peak pressure by limiting stride length in diabetic patients. Orthopade 2004; 33:1013–109. (Article in German).

Eldor R, Raz I, Ben Yehuda A, et al. Experimental approaches to treatment of diabetic foot ulcers: a comprehensive review of emerging treatment strategies. Diabet Med 2004; 21:1161–1673.

Erdemir A, Saucerman JJ, Lemmon D, et al. Local plantar pressure relief in therapeutic footwear: Design guidelines form finite element models. J Biomech 2005; 38:1798–1806.

Fleischli JE, Anderson RB, Davis WH. Dorsiflexion metatarsal osteotomy for treatment of recalcitrant diabetic neuropathic ulcers. Foot Ankle Int 1999; 20:80–85.

Fernando DJ, Masson EA, Veves A, et al. Relationship of limited joint mobility to abnormal foot pressures and diabetic foot ulceration. Diabetes Care 1991; 14:8–11.

Furrer J, Haerdi R, et al. Die sechs Risikostufen am Fuss des Diabetikers aus der Sicht der Orthopädie-Schuhtechnik. Interdisziplinäre Arbeitsgruppe Diabetischer Fuss der Diabetes Educations Study Group (DESG) Deutschschweiz, 2001. (Article in German) Booklet, 2nd edition, Lucerne, 2002.

Guyton GP. An analysis of iatrogenic complications from the total contact cast. Foot Ankle Int 2005; 26:903–907.

Howard IM. The prevention of foot ulceration in diabetic patients. Phys Med Rehabil Clin N Am 2009; 20:595–609.

Illgner U, Wühr J, Rümmler M, et al. Orthopedic made-to-measure shoes for diabetics. Long-term 5-year outcome. Orthopade 2009; 38:1209–1214. (Article in German).

Jeffcoate WJ, International Working Group on the Diabetic Foot. Unresolved issues in the management of ulcers of the foot in diabetes. Diabet Med 2008; 25:1380–1309.

Katz LA, Harlan A, Miranda-Palma B, et al. A randomized trial of two irremovable offloading devices in the management of plantar neuropathic diabetic foot ulcers. Diabetes Care 2005; 28:555–559.

Lavery LA, Armstrong DG, Boulton AJ, Diabetex Research Group. Ankle equinus deformity and its relationship to high plantar pressure in a large population with diabetes mellitus. J Am Podiatr Med Assoc 2002; 92:479–482.

Lavery LA, Vela SA, Lavery DC, et al. Reducing dynamic foot pressures in high-risk diabetic subjects with foot ulcerations: a comparison of treatments. Diabetes Care 1996; 19:818–8121.

Maderal AD, Vivas AC, Zwick DG, et al. Diabetic foot ulcers: evaluation and management. Hosp Pract (Minneap) 2012; 40:102–115.

Malhotra S, Bello E, Kominsky S. Diabetic foot ulcerations: biomechanics, Charcot foot, and total contact cast. Semin Vasc Surg 2012; 25:66–69.

Mansour AA, Dahyak SG. Are foot abnormalities more common in adults with diabetes? A cross-sectional study in Basrah, Iraq. Perm J 2008; 12:25–30.

Mc Kee MD, Yoo D, Schemitsch EH. Health status after Ilizarov reconstruction of posttraumatic lower-limb deformity. J Bone Joint Surg Br 1998; 80:360–364.

Mueller MJ, Sinacore DR, Hastings MK, et al. Effect of Achilles tendon lengthening on neuropathic plantar ulcers. A randomized clinical trial. J Bone Joint Surg Am. 2003 Aug; 85-A(8):1436–1445.

Mueller MJ, Diamond JE, Sinacore DR, et al. Total contact casting in the treatment of diabetic plantar ulcers: controlled clinical trial. Diabetes Care 1989; 12:384–388.

Myerson MS, Shereff MJ. The pathological anatomy of claw and hammer toes. J Bone Joint Surg Am 1989; 71:45–49.

Nabuurs-Fransen MH, Sleegers R, Huijberts MS, et al. Total contact casting of the diabetic foot in daily practice: a prospective study. Diabetes Care 2005; 28:243–247.

National supply guidelines concerning type-2-diabetes, prevention and treatment strategies for foot complications. Germany. http://www.diabetes.versorgungsleitlinien.de [in German] (accessed 07 March, 2014).

Rathur HM. The diabetic foot. Clin Dermatol 2007; 25:109–120.

Stucke S, McFarland D, Goss L, et al. Spatial relationships between shearing stresses and pressure on the plantar skin surface during gait. J Biomech 2012; 45:619–622.

Taylor R, Stainsby GD, Richardson DL. Rupture of the plantar fascia in the diabetic foot leads to toe dorsiflexion deformity. Diabetologia 1998; 41:A277.

Veves A, Msson EA, Fernando DJ, et al. Studies of experimental hosiery in diabetic neuropathic patients with high foot pressures. Diabet Med 1990; 7:324–326.

Wu SC, Jensen JL, Weber AK, et al. Use of pressure offloading devices in diabetic foot ulcers: do we practice what we preach? Diabetes Care 2008; 31:2118–2119.

Wukich DK, Motko J. Safety of total contact casting in high-risk patients with neuropathic foot ulcers. Foot Ankle Int 2004; 25:556–560.

Chapter 38 Prevention of ulcer recurrence

Sicco A. Bus

SUMMARY

- Foot ulcer recurrence is common in diabetes and a major burden for the patient and the health-care system
- The risk factors for ulcer recurrence are not well understood because few studies have focused specifically on recurrence
- Recent RCTs have greatly improved our understanding on the effect of therapeutic footwear to prevent ulcer recurrence in diabetes: Footwear that properly off-loads the foot significantly reduces the risk of ulcer recurrence, provided the footwear is worn as recommended
- No definitive statements can yet be made about the efficacy of preventive surgery. Studies have shown that surgical off-loading can effectively reduce risk for ulcer recurrence, but most studies have been small and performed in highly selected patient groups
- More high-quality RCTs should be performed to better inform clinicians about effective treatment to prevent foot ulcer recurrence in diabetes

INTRODUCTION

When a patient with diabetes mellitus has healed from a foot ulcer, a new challenge arises for both the patient and the health-care professional to keep the ulcer healed. Preventing ulcer recurrence proves to be a major challenge (Boulton et al. 2004). This is because, in most cases, the risk factors that were present to cause the first ulcer (e.g. peripheral neuropathy, arterial disease, foot deformity) remain present after healing of the ulcer.

Recurrent foot ulcers are associated with deterioration of the patient's health status and quality of life and they increase the long-term costs for ulcer management, especially if they require home care services or result in an amputation (Apelqvist et al. 1995, Peikes et al. 2009). Nearly all studies on risk factors for foot ulceration demonstrate that a history of foot ulceration is one of the strongest predictors (Pham et al. 2000, Boyko et al. 2006). Furthermore, repetitive stress on the foot is significantly associated with ulceration (Pham et al. 2000). Because peripheral neuropathy as a precursor for ulcer development cannot yet be resolved, most efforts to prevent recurrence are focused on providing therapeutic footwear to accommodate the deformity present and providing frequent follow-up of these high-risk patients.

This chapter gives an overview of the evidence available on the prevention of ulcer recurrence in diabetes, viewed from a biomechanical perspective. The chapter first describes the epidemiology and risk factors of foot ulcer recurrence in diabetes. Then, the literature on the effect of conservative treatment to prevent ulcer recurrence is discussed, followed by an overview of the studies on the effect of surgical off-loading. This is followed by a description of current guidelines and recommendations on ulcer recurrence prevention, which is principally based on the work of the International Working Group on the Diabetic Foot (Bus et al. 2008). Ways to improve footwear quality and adherence to wearing prescription footwear as contributors to prevention are also discussed.

EPIDEMIOLOGY AND RISK FACTORS

Foot ulceration is an important risk factor for foot infection and lower extremity amputation (Boulton et al. 2004). Therefore, not only prevention of first ulceration but of subsequent ulcers is of paramount importance. But how good are we at preventing ulcer recurrence? **Table 38.1** gives an overview of the prospective and retrospective, noncontrolled studies that assessed the incidence of ulcer recurrence in diabetes. As the table shows, recurrence percentages vary greatly and could be the result of the specific patient groups studied, the assessment of only plantar or only dorsal foot ulcers as outcome measures, and the type and quality of preventive foot care provided in the centers where data were collected. From the table, it is clear that ulcers frequently recur and pose a major challenge to diabetic foot care.

Few studies have examined the factors that are associated with ulcer recurrence. The annual risk of developing a foot ulcer in the general population with diabetes is approximately 2% (Abbott et al. 2002, Crawford et al. 2011), but the risk of ulcer recurrence in patients who healed from a previous foot ulcer is 17–60% in the 3 years after healing (Apelqvist et al. 1993). Therefore, the International Guideline on the Diabetic Foot recommends that these patients have their feet inspected by a specialist every 1–3 months (Bakker et al. 2012). Dubsky et al. showed in a subgroup analysis of patients from the Eurodiale study who were treated for foot ulcer and were followed for 3 years after healing, that previous plantar ulcer location, HbA1C > 7.5%, presence of osteomyelitis, and C-reactive protein > 5 mg/L at entry into the Eurodiale study were significantly associated with ulcer recurrence (Dubsky et al. 2012). Previous plantar ulcer location was the strongest predictor, which corresponds to earlier findings (Peters et al. 2007) and may be explained by the higher pressures to which ulcers on the plantar foot surface were exposed compared with ulcers located elsewhere. Saltzman et al. (2005) showed in their retrospective review of patients with Charcot osteoarthropathy that ulcer recurrence was more common in patients with more severe foot deformity suggesting that deformity was another risk factor for ulcer recurrence. Most recently, Waaijman et al showed that the presence of pre-ulcerative lesions such as hemorrage, abundant callus, or blister is by far the strongest predictor of ulcer recurrence in neuropathic diabetic patients (Waaijman et al. 2014). Furthermore, these authors showed that elevated barefoot and in-shoe plantar pressures are risk factors for repetitive-stress-related foot ulcer recurrence.

TREATMENT EFFICACY
Methods

To assess the effect of conservative and surgical treatment options on ulcer recurrence in diabetes, the MEDLINE database was searched for original research papers with population of interest being patients with type 1 or type 2 diabetes mellitus and the clinical problem

Table 38.1 Noncontrolled retrospective or prospective studies on incidence of ulcer recurrence in diabetes

Study	Country	Study design	Patients enrolled	Ulcer recurrence	Comments
Dubsky et al. (2012)	Czech Republic	Prospective Single center	73 of 93 patients with healed diabetic foot ulceration	42 (57.5%) at 3-year FU	Recurrence rate significantly higher in 1st year (39.7%) than in 2nd (18.1%) or 3rd year (12.8%)
Widatalla et al. (2012)	Sudan	Prospective (2005–2010) Single center	1808 patients with a foot ulcer (87% ≤Wagner 2) without diagnosis of osteomyelitis, of which in 96% limb salvage was achieved 955 ulcers involved toes of which 355 were amputated.	218 (12.1%) at 1-year FU	Lack of information on number of healed patients included in analysis of recurrence
Aragon-Sanchez et al. (2012)	Spain	Prospective (2007–2010) Single center	65 of 81 patients with osteomyelitis, of which 48 underwent conservative surgery, 32 minor amputation, and 1 major amputation	28 (43%) after a median 46.5 weeks	Most recurrences (24 of 28) at new sites (probably due to large rate of minor amputation)
Richard et al. (2011)	France	Prospective (2007–2009) Multicenter	150 patients who healed or wound improved, from a total 291 hospitalized patients with an infected diabetic ulcer, of which 35% had major amputation. 189 patients were scheduled for 1-year FU	At 1-year FU (n = 189): 18 died 21 lost to FU 28 had amputation 96 healed with no relapse 2 infection recurrence 23 wounds remained open	There was a 0% ulcer recurrence at 1 year in this group
Winkley et al. (2009)	London	Prospective (2001–2003) Multicenter	253 patients with a first foot ulcer	18 months after first ulcer: 40 deaths (15.8%) 36 amputations (15.5%) 99 (43.2%) recurrences 52 nonhealing (21.9%)	Outcomes were after ulcer occurrence. Ulcer healing without recurrence likely occurred in the remaining 26 patients (10%)
Kloos et al. (2009)	Germany	Prospective (2003–2004) Single center	56 nondeceased of 59 patients with history of ulceration	27 (46%) at 1-year FU	78% of reulceration was superficial
Faglia et al. (2009)	Italy	Prospective (1999–2007) Single center	442 healed patients of 554 patients hospitalized for critical limb ischemia of which nearly all were revascularized	71 (16%) in a mean 5.93 ± 1.28 years FU	Data not very clear on ulcer healing. Recurrence was mainly Wagner 1
Ghanassia et al. (2008)	France	Prospective (1998–2005) Single center	69 healed without major amputation out of 89 successfully followed-up patients of a group of 94 hospitalized patients with ulcer	42 (60.9%) in a mean 79.5-month FU	Very long FU
Monami et al. (2008)	Italy	Prospective (2002–2003) Single center	63 patients who healed in 6 months of an initial 80 patients with chronic foot ulcer (>3 months)	Of 54 patients who did not die (n = 4) or refuse (n = 5): 32 (59.3%) recurrence in mean 8.5 ± 3.1 months FU	At FU, only 20 patients (31.7%) still wore prescribed therapeutic footwear
Peters et al. (2007)	USA	Prospective Single center	58 patients who healed from a group of 81 patients with a foot ulcer	35 (60.5%) in mean 31-month FU	
Pound et al. (2005)	United Kingdom	Prospective (2000–2003) Single center	226 nonamputated patients of a total 231 of 370 admitted patients (with a total 1031 ulcers) who healed	91 (40.3%) in median 126 days	Outcome was unknown in 18 of 226 patients
Saltzman et al. (2005)	USA	Retrospective (1983–2003) Single center	127 limbs of 115 patients with neuro-osteoarthropathy	62 (49%) in a median 3.8-year FU	Not clear who many patients or limbs had an ulcer
LeMaster et al. (2003)	USA	Prospective (1997–2000) Multicenter	400 patients with a prior history of foot ulceration	62 (15.5%) at 2-year FU	Data from footwear trial from Reiber et al. (2002)
Dalla et al. (2003)	Italy	Prospective (2000–2001) Single center	89 patients healed from Wagner 2 to 4 first ray lesions treated with first ray amputation and put on intensive secondary prevention	15 (16.9%) in a mean 16.4 ± 6.8 months	All ulcers were amputated, which may explain the relatively low recurrence rate
Diouri et al. (2002)	Morocco	Prospective (1997–2000) Single center	90 patients who attended FU consultations of 110 patients treated for foot ulcer	42 (46.6%) at 2-year FU	Follow-up time not known
Apelqvist et al. (1993)	Sweden	Prospective (1983–1990)	468 patients who healed from a group of 558 patients with foot ulcers	34% after 1-year FU 61% after 3-year FU 70% after 5-year FU	
Helm et al. (1991)	USA	Retrospective Single center	102 patients as random sample drawn from larger population of patients healed in TCC	20 (19.6%) in a mean 21.6 weeks	Reported causes for recurrence were nonadherence, abnormal biomechanics, osteophyte or bone fragment, osteomyelitis, or Charcot

FU, follow-up; TCC, total contact cast.

addressed being foot ulcer recurrence. The interventions considered were treatment options with an intended pressure mitigating effect on the foot. The following search string that included search terms on patient group (diabetes) and outcome (ulcer recurrence) was used to obtain references in MEDLINE: (('diabetes mellitus'[MeSH]) OR (diabetes) OR (diabetic)) and (ulcer recur* or re-ulcer* or reulcer* or ulcer-free survival or ulcer relap* or wound recur* or wound relap* or wound-free survival).

Studies on healthy subjects or patients with other diseases than diabetes were not considered. The search, performed on 14 May 2014, covered references in all languages and was not limited by date. Tracking of references in included articles was not performed. A total of 165 articles were identified in the search. All references were assessed by title and abstract to determine eligibility for full-paper review on patient group, outcome, and off-loading intervention. Full-paper copies of eligible articles were assessed for study design and outcome.

▓ Conservative treatment

Therapeutic footwear has been the most commonly studied intervention with respect to efficacy in preventing ulcer recurrence in diabetes. Other options, such as hosiery, callus removal, or other podiatric treatment that may affect foot biomechanics, have not yet been assessed for efficacy in controlled studies.

The vast majority of footwear efficacy studies have focused on ulcer recurrence, and include several RCTs. A small RCT found a significantly lower proportion of patients with ulcer recurrence over a 1-year period in those who wore therapeutic shoes than those who continued to wear their own shoes (Uccioli et al. 1995). A larger RCT, however, found no significant difference in the proportion of ulcer recurrences over a 2-year period between patients who wore therapeutic shoes and those who wore control shoes (Reiber et al. 2002).

More recently, Rizzo et al. showed that a more structured approach to footwear prescription using published prescription recommendations (Dahmen et al. 2001) can result in a significantly lower risk of ulcer recurrence compared with non-structured prescription as was performed in a historical cohort of patients (Rizzo et al. 2012). In their study, Rizzo et al. showed 1-, 3-, and 5-year incidence rates of 12%, 18%, and 24%, respectively, for the new prescription algorithm compared with 39%, 61%, and 72%, respectively, for the historical control group. Part of this difference will probably be explained by the effect of time, with improvements in foot screening and care. Nevertheless, these data provide interesting information on the potential value of using a more structured approach to footwear prescription. A non-randomized study compared treatment that included patient education and therapeutic footwear with treatment at a different clinic, which did not include therapeutic footwear (Dargis et al. 1999). A significant difference in ulcer occurrence in favor of the therapeutic footwear intervention was found over 2 years (30.4% versus 58.4%). Another non-randomized but controlled study of 93 patients with diabetes showed that the use of a rocker-soled stock diabetes shoe significantly reduced the incidence of ulcer relapse when compared with normal shoes (15% versus 60% at 1 year) (Busch & Chantelau 2003). Finally, one prospective controlled study of 57 patients with a history of foot ulceration provided support for the positive effect of special diabetes footwear on ulcer prevention, with 8 of 30 patients (27%) wearing protective shoes > 8 hours per day relapsing in 1 year, compared with 18 of 27 patients (67%) wearing normal shoes >8 hours per day (Striesow 1998).

The main drawback of the studies discussed above is that none measured the efficacy of the tested footwear to off-load the foot, nor did any measure adherence to wearing the footwear. These are two factors that are considered of primary importance in preventing foot ulcers in diabetic patients. Two recent RCTs on the topic have greatly improved our understanding on the contributing role of pressure relief and adherence in ulcer prevention (Bus et al. 2013, Ulbrecht et al. 2014). In a multicenter trial of 171 neuropathic patients with a recently healed plantar foot ulcer, our own group assessed the efficacy of off-loading-improved custom-made footwear to prevent ulcer recurrence in comparison with custom-made footwear that did not undergo such improvement (Bus et al. 2013). An average 20% pressure improvement in the intervention footwear did not lead to a significant reduction of ulcer recurrence risk in 18 months compared with the non-improved footwear (39% versus 44%). However, analysis of the subgroup of patients that were adherent to wearing the footwear showed that the off-loading-improved footwear significantly reduced ulcer recurrence risk by 46% (26% recurrence versus 48% in the non-improved footwear group). Thus, it is the combination of optimized pressure conditions and the guarantee that patients wear the shoes as recommended that leads to a significantly improved clinical outcome. In the RCT by Ulbrecht et al, 130 patients with a recently healed plantar forefoot ulcer were randomized to wear shape- and pressure-based orthoses (experimental) or to wear more traditional shape-based-only orthoses (control). The shape- and pressure-based insoles were designed using barefoot dynamic plantar pressure distribution measures of the patient (Owings et al. 2008). There was a marked difference between groups in ulcer recurrence at the metatarsal head (MTH) region after 15 months follow-up: 9.1% of patients in the experimental group had an ulcer, versus 25.0% of patients in the control group ($P = 0.007$). Both of these trials show the need for adequate pressure-relieving footwear based on plantar pressure measurements to prevent recurrence of ulceration in high-risk diabetic patients.

▓ Surgical off-loading

Most studies on surgical off-loading deal with the effects of Achilles tendon lengthening (ATL) on ulcer recurrence. An RCT by Mueller et al. compared treatment with ATL + total contact cast (TCC) with TCC alone in patients affected by forefoot neuropathic plantar ulceration (Mueller et al. 2003). The percentage of plantar ulcer recurrences was significantly lower in the ATL+TCC group than in the TCC alone group at follow-up periods of 7 months (15% vs 59%, respectively) and 2 years (38% vs 81%, respectively). In a recent observational study, Colen et al. compared the effect of ATL as an additional procedure to wound closure surgery (i.e. soft tissue reconstruction) to an earlier practice involving only wound closure surgery in patients with plantar forefoot or midfoot ulcers (Colen et al. 2013). Twenty-five percent of patients in the 'early group' and only 2% of patients in the 'later group' developed recurrent ulcers requiring reoperation. In addition, the proportion of transfer ulcers was significantly lower in the latter group (4%) than in the early group (12%). An observational study by Batista et al. (2011) showed that of 52 patients with plantar forefoot ulceration treated with ATL, 4 patients (8%) had ulcer recurrence during post-operative follow-up of 12 weeks.

In a case–control study by Armstrong et al., 92 patients with Texas 1A or 2A ulcers at the plantar forefoot were treated with either MTH resection or with standard nonsurgical care, and both groups received standard off-loading (Armstrong et al. 2012). Patients treated with surgery had significantly fewer recurrent ulcers than the control group:

15.2% versus 39.1%. An earlier cohort study by the same authors of 40 patients with neuropathic fifth MTH ulcers treated with MTH resection confirmed these findings: 4.5% recurrence compared with 27.8% in conservatively treated patients (Armstrong et al. 2005). A small retrospective study by Hamilton et al. of 10 patients with chronic nonhealing and recurrent foot ulcers demonstrated that all patients healed from a combination of gastrocnemius recession, peroneus longus to brevis tendon transfer, and resection of the second through fifth MTHs, and none of the patients recurred in a mean 14.2 months follow-up (Hamilton et al. 2005). An observational study by Widatalla et al. (2012) showed that of 330 ulcer patients with a diagnosis of osteomyelitis who were treated with either surgical debridement, sequestrectomy, resections of metatarsal and digital bones, or toe amputation, along with antibiotic treatment, 12.1% developed ulcer recurrence in 1 year. Another observational study assessed the effect of plantar fascia release on ulcer recurrence in 60 patients treated for plantar forefoot ulcers and showed that none of the 56% of patients who healed within 6 weeks had ulcer recurrence at the original wound location in a mean 23.5-month follow-up (Kim et al. 2012). Furthermore, no complications were reported. In a case–control study, Armstrong et al. showed positive effects of metatarsophalangeal (MTP) joint arthroplasty of the great toe in combination with TCC on ulcer recurrence rate at 6 months in 41 patients with Texas 1A or 2A ulcers at the plantar hallux: 4.8% recurrence when compared with TCC treatment alone (35% recurrence) (Armstrong et al. 2003). An RCT by Piaggesi et al. showed that the combination of surgical excision, debridement, removal of bone segments underlying the lesion, and surgical closure was significantly more effective than conservative off-loading treatment in preventing ulcer recurrence in 42 patients who healed from plantar ulceration: 14% versus 33% after 6 months (Piaggesi et al. 1998).

The above summary shows that ATL, surgical excision of bony prominences, joint arthroplasty, and MTH resection all appear to significantly reduce the risk of ulcer recurrence in selected patients with diabetes and forefoot neuropathic plantar ulceration when compared with conservative off-loading treatment. However, these surgical interventions may come with some disadvantages and potential complications, which should be taken into consideration. For ATL, e.g. possible negative effects on locomotion and other functional tasks and the risk of heel ulceration should be considered (Holstein et al. 2004, Mueller et al. 2004, Salsich et al. 2005). To some extent, these side effects limit the recommendations that can be made for safe and effective surgical intervention to prevent ulcer recurrence.

Clinical guideline recommendations

Guideline development has been limited in the area of prevention of ulcer recurrence. The International Working Group on the Diabetic Foot developed in 2007 an evidence-based and specific guideline on the use of footwear and off-loading to prevent ulceration in diabetes (Bus et al. 2007). These guidelines do not focus specifically on ulcer recurrence, but because of the limited data on prevention of the first ulcer, they mostly apply to prevention of recurrence.

Conservative treatment

- Regular callus removal should be performed on people with diabetes and neuropathy by a skilled health-care provider
- Patients with an at-risk diabetic foot should be urged not to walk barefoot but to wear protective footwear both at home and outside

- Although no evidence exists, it is often clinically apparent that even extra depth footwear may not accommodate a foot with a significant deformity. In such cases, custom footwear is recommended
- Therapeutic shoes can be used for preventing plantar ulceration in the at-risk diabetic foot
- To achieve maximal reduction of peak plantar pressures in footwear prescription, custom-molded insoles should be incorporated in the therapeutic footwear as long as sufficient space exists

Surgical off-loading

- Given the paucity of data, no definitive statement can be made about the effectiveness and safety of preventive surgery
- ATL may be considered in selected patients, but this procedure carries the risk of heel ulceration. More information, including high-quality studies, is needed before the procedure can be recommended for widespread use
- There are few high-quality studies on MTP joint arthroplasty and MTH resection. These approaches may be beneficial but cannot be recommended for widespread use before further evidence is available
- One should also be aware of the disadvantages of applying surgical techniques for the prevention of plantar ulcers in the diabetic foot, which can include postoperative wound infection, induction of acute neuro-osteoarthropathy (Charcot), and development of ulcers at other sites (transfer ulcers)

These clinical guidline recommendations are from the year 2007. New data on footwear and off-loading have provided additional support for the use of pressure-relieving footwear to prevent ulcer recurrence. An update of these guidelines is expected in 2015

FOOTWEAR QUALITY AND ADHERENCE

Although several aspects of footwear design and manufacturing are still more of an art than a science, the field is developing towards a more scientific base for prescription and evaluation. The lack of [use of] clear design rules shows that prescription footwear may not be optimal for its pressure-relieving properties (Arts et al. 2012). In-shoe plantar pressure measurements show that peak pressure is often above the threshold level that is indicated to be potentially protective against ulceration (Owings et al. 2009). However, pressure relief can be improved by using in-shoe plantar pressure measurements as a tool to guide the modification of footwear. Two studies from our group show that applying this approach in an iterative process of footwear modifications and pressure evaluation can result in a 17–52% decrease in in-shoe peak pressure at high-pressure regions in the foot (Bus et al. 2011, Waaijman et al. 2012). The footwear is modified by systematically incorporating pressure-relief elements that have proven to be effective, such as metatarsal bars or pads, rocker bars, and custom-made insoles (Praet & Louwerens 2003, Bus et al. 2004, Guldemond et al. 2007). Another approach to improve footwear off-loading efficacy is the use of barefoot dynamic plantar pressure measurements together with three-dimensional foot shape data in the computer-assisted design and manufacturing of customized insoles. This approach results in insoles that can reduce in-shoe peak pressures by about 30% compared with more traditionally-designed shape-based-only inserts (Owings et al. 2008).

Off-loading footwear will only be effective when it is worn. In an observational study of patients with healed foot ulcers who were prescribed with diabetic off-loading footwear and prospectively followed, Chantelau et al. showed allready in 1994 the importance of adherence. Risk for ulcer recurrence was reduced by 50% in patients who wore their footwear > 60% of the day compared with patients using their footwear less than that (Chantelau & Haage 1994). Our own prospective footwear trial has confirmed these results and thus the importance of adherence (Bus et al. 2013; Waaijman et al. 2014) However, adherence to footwear use in patients with diabetes is generally much lower: 24–38% of patients use their footwear > 80% of the time (Knowles & Boulton 1996, Macfarlane & Jensen 2003). Considering this low adherence and its undermining effect on footwear efficacy, it is surprising that only very few of the clinical studies on therapeutic footwear efficacy have assessed footwear adherence (in an appropriate manner). A reason may be that, until recently, objective means to assess footwear use were unavailable. Subjective data may lack accuracy and reliability and is therefore of limited use. We have developed a method with which footwear adherence can be measured objectively using a shoe-worn sensor (Bus et al. 2012). Using this approach, we showed that neuropathic patients with diabetes and a high prevalence of foot deformity, who recently healed from plantar foot ulceration, wear their prescription footwear on average 71% of the steps that they take (Waaijman et al. 2013). Expressed as total time per day this equals about 60% of the daytime. Although this is higher than reported in most previous studies on adherence, it is still too low for effective ulcer prevention (Waaijman et al. 2014).

More investigations are needed on the role of adherence in the prevention of ulcer recurrence. Furthermore, studies are needed on interventions that aim to improve adherence in these patients. In our recent study on adherence in high-risk patients, we found that patients are much less adherent when they are at home than when they are away from home, whereas they are much more active inside the house than outside the house (Waaijman et al. 2013). This increases the risk for ulcer recurrence. Therefore, we suggest that prescription of specific off-loading footwear for use indoors may be an approach with which overall footwear adherence can be improved. The effect of patient education on footwear adherence has not been assessed to date, and therefore requires further investigation before conclusions can be drawn on how we can effectively improve adherence.

SUMMARY AND CONCLUSION

This chapter demonstrates that the evidence base to support the use of therapeutic footwear to off-load the foot with the goal to prevent diabetic foot ulcer recurrence has improved through several high-quality trials. Future high-quality investigations should confirm these findings. In terms of the effect of surgical off-loading, promising results have been reported, but the evidence base for the prevention of ulcer recurrence is still small. Only with evidence from robust well-controlled studies, which incorporate measures on off-loading efficacy, adherence, safety, and complications, can clinicians be properly informed about effective prevention of ulcer recurrence in diabetes, and the likelihood of these modalities being widely accepted and implemented in diabetic foot practice.

AREAS OF CONTROVERSY/ FURTHER RESEARCH

- There is a paucity of high-quality studies in the sub-domains of treatment for the prevention of ulcer recurrence in diabetes
- A much larger focus on research into ulcer prevention is needed to better inform clinicians about effective treatment options
- Future studies on the prevention of ulcer recurrence should include measures of off-loading efficacy, adherence, safety and complications to improve the interpretation of the findings
- Future research should focus on interventions that aim to improve adherence to wearing prescription footwear, since adherence is an important contributor to effectiveness
- There is a paucity of data on the effect of conservative treatment options other than therapeutic footwear on ulcer recurrence in patients with diabetes
- There is still some controversy about the role of surgical off-loading in preventing foot ulcer recurrence in diabetes due to the risk of complications. These controversies should be resolved before recommendations can be widely adopted in foot care

IMPORTANT FURTHER READING

Bus SA, Valk GD, van Deursen RW, et al. The effectiveness of footwear and offloading interventions to prevent and heal foot ulcers and reduce plantar pressure in diabetes: a systematic review. Diabetes Metab Res Rev 2008; 24:S162–S180.

Bus SA, Waaijman R, Arts M, de Haart M, Busch-Westbroek T, van Baal J, Nollet F. Effect of custom-made footwear on foot ulcer recurrence in diabetes: a multicenter randomized controlled trial. Diabetes Care 2013; 36:4109–4116.

Dubsky M, Jirkovska A, Bem R, et al. Risk factors for recurrence of diabetic foot ulcers: prospective follow-up analysis of a Eurodiale subgroup. Int Wound J 2013; 10:555-561.

Ulbrecht JS, Hurley T, Mauger DT, Cavanagh PR. Prevention of recurrent foot ulcers with plantar pressure-based in-shoe orthoses: The careFUL prevention multicenter randomized controlled trial. Diabetes Care 2014. DOI: 10.2337/dc13-2956.

REFERENCES

Abbott CA, Carrington AL, Ashe H, et al. The North-West Diabetes Foot Care Study: incidence of, and risk factors for, new diabetic foot ulceration in a community-based patient cohort. Diabet Med 2002; 19:377–384.

Apelqvist J, Larsson J, Agardh CD. Long-term prognosis for diabetic patients with foot ulcers. J Intern Med 1993; 233:485–491.

Apelqvist J, Ragnarson-Tennvall G, Larsson J, Persson U. Long-term costs for foot ulcers in diabetic patients in a multidisciplinary setting. Foot Ankle Int 1995; 16:388–394.

Aragon-Sanchez J, Lazaro-Martinez JL, Hernandez-Herrero C, et al. Does osteomyelitis in the feet of patients with diabetes really recur after surgical treatment? Natural history of a surgical series. Diabet Med 2012; 29:813–818.

Armstrong DG, Fiorito JL, Leykum BJ, Mills JL. Clinical efficacy of the pan metatarsal head resection as a curative procedure in patients with diabetes mellitus and neuropathic forefoot wounds. Foot Ankle Spec 2012; 5:235–240.

Armstrong DG, Lavery LA, Vazquez JR, et al. Clinical efficacy of the first metatarsophalangeal joint arthroplasty as a curative procedure for hallux interphalangeal joint wounds in patients with diabetes. Diabetes Care 2003; 26:3284–3287.

Armstrong DG, Rosales MA, Gashi A. Efficacy of fifth metatarsal head resection for treatment of chronic diabetic foot ulceration. J Am Podiatr Med Assoc 2005; 95:353–356.

Arts ML, Waaijman R, de Haart M, et al. Offloading effect of therapeutic footwear in patients with diabetic neuropathy at high risk for plantar foot ulceration. Diabet Med 2012; doi: 10.1111/j.1464-5491.2012.03770.x:

Bakker K, Apelqvist J, Schaper NC. Practical guidelines on the management and prevention of the diabetic foot 2011. Diabetes Metab Res Rev 2012; 28:225–231.

Batista F, Magalhaes AA, Nery C, et al. Minimally invasive surgery for diabetic plantar foot ulcerations. Diabet Foot Ankle 2011; doi: 10.3402/dfa.v2i0.10358.

Boulton AJ, Kirsner RS, Vileikyte L. Clinical practice. Neuropathic diabetic foot ulcers. N Engl J Med 2004; 351:48–55.

Boyko EJ, Ahroni JH, Cohen V, Nelson KM, Heagerty PJ. Prediction of diabetic foot ulcer occurrence using commonly available clinical information: the Seattle Diabetic Foot Study. Diabetes Care 2006; 29:1202–1207.

Bus SA, Haspels R, Busch-Westbroek TE. Evaluation and optimization of therapeutic footwear for neuropathic diabetic foot patients using in-shoe plantar pressure analysis. Diabetes Care 2011; 34:1595–1600.

Bus SA, Ulbrecht JS, Cavanagh PR. Pressure relief and load redistribution by custom-made insoles in diabetic patients with neuropathy and foot deformity. Clin Biomech 2004; 19:629–38.

Bus SA, Valk GD, van Deursen RW, et al. The effectiveness of footwear and offloading interventions to prevent and heal foot ulcers and reduce plantar pressure in diabetes: a systematic review. Diabetes Metab Res Rev 2008; 24:S162–S180.

Bus SA, van Deursen RWM, Valk GD, et al. Evidence-based Guideline on Footwear and Offloading for the Diabetic Foot. International Working Group on the Diabetic Foot. 2007 [DVD]

Bus SA, Waaijman R, Nollet F. New monitoring technology to objectively assess adherence to prescribed footwear and assistive devices during ambulatory activity. Arch Phys Med Rehabil 2012; 93:2075–2079.

Bus SA, Waaijman R, Arts M, et al. Effect of custom-made footwear on foot ulcer recurrence in diabetes: a multicenter randomized controlled trial. Diabetes Care 2013; 36:4109–4116.

Busch K, Chantelau E. Effectiveness of a new brand of stock 'diabetic' shoes to protect against diabetic foot ulcer relapse. A prospective cohort study. Diabet Med 2003; 20:665–669.

Chantelau E, Haage P. An audit of cushioned diabetic footwear: relation to patient compliance. Diabet Med 1994; 11:114–116.

Colen LB, Kim CJ, Grant WP, Yeh JT, Hind B. Achilles tendon lengthening: friend or foe in the diabetic foot? Plast Reconstr Surg 2013; 131:37e–43e.

Crawford F, McCowan C, Dimitrov BD, et al. The risk of foot ulceration in people with diabetes screened in community settings: findings from a cohort study. QJM 2011; 104:403–410.

Dahmen R, Haspels R, Koomen B, Hoeksma AF. Therapeutic footwear for the neuropathic foot: an algorithm. Diabetes Care 2001; 24:705–709.

Dalla PL, Faglia E, Caminiti M, et al. Ulcer recurrence following first ray amputation in diabetic patients: a cohort prospective study. Diabetes Care 2003; 26:1874–1878.

Dargis V, Pantelejeva O, Jonushaite A, Vileikyte L, Boulton AJ. Benefits of a multidisciplinary approach in the management of recurrent diabetic foot ulceration in Lithuania: a prospective study. Diabetes Care 1999; 22:1428–1431.

Diouri A, Slaoui Z, Chadli A, et al. [Incidence of factors favoring recurrent foot ulcers in diabetic patients]. Ann Endocrinol (Paris) 2002; 63:491–496.

Dubsky M, Jirkovska A, Bem R, et al. Risk factors for recurrence of diabetic foot ulcers: prospective follow-up analysis of a Eurodiale subgroup. Int Wound J 2013; 10:555–561.

Faglia E, Clerici G, Clerissi J, et al. Long-term prognosis of diabetic patients with critical limb ischemia: a population-based cohort study. Diabetes Care 2009; 32:822–827.

Ghanassia E, Villon L, Thuan Dit Dieudonne JF, et al. Long-term outcome and disability of diabetic patients hospitalized for diabetic foot ulcers: a 6.5-year follow-up study. Diabetes Care 2008; 31:1288–1292.

Guldemond NA, Leffers P, Schaper NC, et al. The effects of insole configurations on forefoot plantar pressure and walking convenience in diabetic patients with neuropathic feet. Clin Biomech 2007; 22:81–87.

Hamilton GA, Ford LA, Perez H, Rush SM. Salvage of the neuropathic foot by using bone resection and tendon balancing: a retrospective review of 10 patients. J Foot Ankle Surg 2005; 44:37–43.

Helm PA, Walker SC, Pullium GF. Recurrence of neuropathic ulceration following healing in a total contact cast. Arch Phys Med Rehabil 1991; 72:967–970.

Holstein P, Lohmann M, Bitsch M, Jorgensen B. Achilles tendon lengthening, the panacea for plantar forefoot ulceration? Diabetes Metab Res Rev 2004; 20:S37–S40.

Kim JY, Hwang S, Lee Y. Selective plantar fascia release for nonhealing diabetic plantar ulcerations. J Bone Joint Surg Am 2012; 94:1297–1302.

Kloos C, Hagen F, Lindloh C, et al. Cognitive function is not associated with recurrent foot ulcers in patients with diabetes and neuropathy. Diabetes Care 2009; 32:894–896.

Knowles EA, Boulton AJ. Do people with diabetes wear their prescribed footwear? Diabet Med 1996; 13:1064–1068.

LeMaster JW, Reiber GE, Smith DG, Heagerty PJ, Wallace C. Daily weight-bearing activity does not increase the risk of diabetic foot ulcers. Med Sci Sports Exerc 2003; 35:1093–1099.

Macfarlane DJ, Jensen JL. Factors in diabetic footwear compliance. J Am Podiatr Med Assoc 2003; 93:485–491.

Monami M, Longo R, Desideri CM, et al. The diabetic person beyond a foot ulcer: healing, recurrence, and depressive symptoms. J Am Podiatr Med Assoc 2008; 98:130–136.

Mueller MJ, Sinacore DR, Hastings MK, et al. Impact of Achilles tendon lengthening on functional limitations and perceived disability in people with a neuropathic plantar ulcer. Diabetes Care 2004; 27:1559–1564.

Mueller MJ, Sinacore DR, Hastings MK, Strube MJ, Johnson JE. Effect of Achilles tendon lengthening on neuropathic plantar ulcers. A randomized clinical trial. J Bone Joint Surg Am 2003; 85-A:1436–1445.

Owings TM, Apelqvist J, Stenstrom A, et al. Plantar pressures in diabetic patients with foot ulcers which have remained healed. Diabet Med 2009; 26:1141–1146.

Owings TM, Woerner JL, Frampton JD, Cavanagh PR, Botek G. Custom therapeutic insoles based on both foot shape and plantar pressure measurement provide enhanced pressure relief. Diabetes Care 2008; 31:839–844.

Peikes D, Chen A, Schore J, Brown R. Effects of care coordination on hospitalization, quality of care, and health care expenditures among Medicare beneficiaries: 15 randomized trials. JAMA 2009; 301:603–618.

Peters EJ, Armstrong DG, Lavery LA. Risk factors for recurrent diabetic foot ulcers: site matters. Diabetes Care 2007; 30:2077–2079.

Pham H, Armstrong DA, Harvey C, et al. Screening techniques to identify people at high risk for diabetic foot ulceration. Diabetes Care 2000; 23:606–611.

Piaggesi A, Schipani E, Campi F, et al. Conservative surgical approach versus non-surgical management for diabetic neuropathic foot ulcers: a randomized trial. Diabet Med 1998; 15:412–417.

Pound N, Chipchase S, Treece K, Game F, Jeffcoate W. Ulcer-free survival following management of foot ulcers in diabetes. Diabet Med 2005; 22:1306–1309.

Praet SF, Louwerens JW The influence of shoe design on plantar pressures in neuropathic feet. Diabetes Care 2003; 26:441–445.

Reiber GE, Smith DG, Wallace C, et al. Effect of therapeutic footwear on foot reulceration in patients with diabetes: a randomized controlled trial. JAMA 2002; 287:2552–2558.

Richard JL, Lavigne JP, Got I, et al. Management of patients hospitalized for diabetic foot infection: results of the French OPIDIA study. Diabetes Metab 2011; 37:208–215.

Rizzo L, Tedeschi A, Fallani E, et al. Custom-made orthesis and shoes in a structured follow-up program reduces the incidence of neuropathic ulcers in high-risk diabetic foot patients. Int J Low Extrem Wounds 2012; 11:59–64.

Salsich GB, Mueller MJ, Hastings MK, et al. Effect of Achilles tendon lengthening on ankle muscle performance in people with diabetes mellitus and a neuropathic plantar ulcer. Phys Ther 2005; 85:34–43.

Saltzman CL, Hagy ML, Zimmerman B, Estin M, Cooper R. How effective is intensive nonoperative initial treatment of patients with diabetes and Charcot arthropathy of the feet? Clin Orthop Relat Res 2005; 185–190.

Striesow F. [Special manufactured shoes for prevention of recurrent ulcer in diabetic foot syndrome]. Med Klin (Munich) 1998; 93:695–700.

Uccioli L, Faglia E, Monticone G, et al. Manufactured shoes in the prevention of diabetic foot ulcers. Diabetes Care 1995; 18:1376–1378.

Ulbrecht JS, Hurley T, Mauger DT, Cavanagh PR. Prevention of recurrent foot ulcers with plantar pressure-based in-shoe orthoses: The careFUL prevention multicenter randomized controlled trial. Diabetes Care 2014. DOI: 10.2337/dc13-2956.

Waaijman R, Arts ML, Haspels R, et al. Pressure-reduction and preservation in custom-made footwear of patients with diabetes and a history of plantar ulceration. Diabet Med 2012; 29:1542–1549.

Waaijman R, Keukenkamp R, de HM, et al. Adherence to wearing prescription custom-made footwear in patients with diabetes at high risk for plantar foot ulceration. Diabetes Care 2013; 36:1613–1618.

Waaijman R, de Haart M, Arts ML, et al. Risk factors for plantar foot ulcer recurrence in neuropathic diabetic patients. Diabetes Care 2014. DOI: 10.2337/dc13-2470.

Widatalla AH, Mahadi SE, Shawer MA, et al. Diabetic foot infections with osteomyelitis: efficacy of combined surgical and medical treatment. Diabet Foot Ankle 2012; 3.

Winkley K, Stahl D, Chalder T, Edmonds ME, Ismail K. Quality of life in people with their first diabetic foot ulcer: a prospective cohort study. J Am Podiatr Med Assoc 2009; 99:406–414.

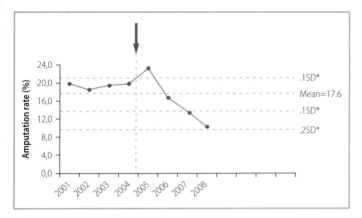

Figure 39.2 Step-by-Step Program: temporal trends in amputation rates among diabetic foot ulcer referrals to Muhimbili National Hospital, Dar es Salaam, Tanzania, 2000–2008. The denominator is the total annual number of foot referrals to MNH. With permission from Abbas et al. (2011).
*SD = standard deviation; arrow shows point of introduction of Step-by-Step program.

the same basic and advanced courses were conducted. In 2010, during the advanced course for private hospitals, cobblers were also invited from the respected centers to participate as a part of an effort to extend the multidisciplinary profile of care-giving teams beyond medicines and nursing (Abbas et al. 2011) (**Table 39.4**). After targeting doctors and nurses it was decided to target surgeons from the same center where doctors and nurses have been trained and surgical facilities are available. So in 2009, the first Step-by-Step diabetic foot training project specifically aimed at surgeons from selected centers in 20 regions were held in Tanzania; the focus was largely on optimizing surgical practice to salvage diabetic feet and reduce rates of amputation (Abbas et al. 2011).

■ MULTIDISCIPLINARY TEAM APPROACH

The principles of structured diabetic foot management include not only management of infection, aggressive angioplasty or distal revascularization, application of off-loading principles, surgical debridement, and stage-adapted local wound care, but also optimization of metabolic and glycemic control and treatment of relevant comorbidities. If diabetic foot lesions are managed

on a model based on this systematic approach, the incidence of amputation potentially could be reduced significantly or amputations, when unavoidable, could be carried out to a degree that carries a lower morbidity risk to patients – the ultimate desired outcome in treating diabetic foot problems. Clear evidence of the success of a multidisciplinary approach should lead to a wider adoption than is currently the case. Ideally, multidisciplinary foot clinics should involve the following clinical professions: podiatrist, diabetes nurse, diabetologist, angiologist/interventional radiologist, vascular surgeon, microbiologist, orthopedic surgeon, orthotist, and shoemaker. Individuals (e.g. physiotherapists, psychologists, and rehabilitation physicians) who do not work regularly within the foot clinic often have input into the management process, as deemed appropriate.

■ Western perspective of diabetic foot care

In a 1994 comparative study of patients with diabetes attending teaching hospital out-patient clinics in various European states, researchers found no major differences in the risk factors for foot ulceration; on the basis of these findings, they concluded that similar strategies for the prevention of foot problems, theoretically, should be equally successful in different European countries (Veves et al. 1994). In fact, the multidisciplinary foot care model is indeed considered the most effective approach for the management of the ulcerated diabetic foot in Europe and health-care systems across the continent have tried to implement such multifactorial approaches to diabetic foot care with varying successes and some failures. In truth, however, because there are remarkable differences among the various health-care systems, there is no common program for diabetic foot care across Europe.

In Denmark, the rate of leg amputations in patients with diabetes has decreased to an incidence of about 0.3%, which has remained stable over the last 10 years. Danish patients are reimbursed for most of the outgoing costs for special shoes, insoles, and their visits to the podiatrist (Ebskov & Ebskov 1996). The number of diabetic foot clinics or wound healing centers has increased over the years, and it is estimated that adequate treatment in multidisciplinary settings are now available for up to 75% of patients (Ebskov & Ebskov 1996). In The Netherlands, a nationwide study of all hospital admissions in which a lower extremity amputation occurred documented a 40% decrease in the incidence of diabetes-related lower-extremity amputation in both women and men (van Houtum et al. 2004).

In France, general practitioners generally serve as care managers for patients, including persons with diabetes. Moreover, there is little

Table 39.4 Outcomes of the Step-by-Step Foot Project for the 30 centers that aggregated data during 2009–2011 in Tanzania's private hospitals

	Before Jan 2009	Jan–Dec 2009	Jan–June 2010	Jan–Dec 2011	Total
Total diabetes	2253 (19%)	4042 (34%)	2974 (25%)	2675 (24%)	11,944
High risk	210 (24%)	228 (26%)	209 (23%)	244 (27%)	791
Foot ulcers	141 (35%)	107 (28%)	56 (15%)	6 (20%)	380
Total amputation	68 (52%)	24 (18%)	17 (15%)	20 (15%)	129
Referred patients	105 (57%)	36 (19%)	17 (15%)	33 (18%)	184
Trained doctors	0	88	46	30	164
Trained nurse	0	140	59	51	250
Education session	0	289	150	182	621
Death	0	6	5	2	13

opportunity for patients to contact diabetic foot specialists directly. Fifteen foot clinics (primarily in association with university hospitals) offer a multidisciplinary approach, but, overall, the organization of diabetic foot management in France is far from clear-cut. A program currently in development for screening patients and treating preulcerative conditions through a special health network will provide free care to those at increased risk for diabetic foot lesions (Morbach 2006).

In Italy, diabetic foot guidelines endorsed by all the scientific societies have been published. This document proposes a three-level structured network of diabetic foot centers to manage the different cases according to their severity. Regional health authorities have received the document and now have to implement it. A decrease in the total number of hospitalizations for diabetic foot lesions and the incidence of major amputations following the implementation of the International Consensus on the Diabetic Foot has been reported (Anichini et al. 2007). Similar types of reports have been published in Germany (Müller et al. 2006). In conclusion, shared care in a specialist network might be the best way to reduce negative outcomes and high treatment costs caused by diabetic foot disease, and availability of such services for all patients with diabetes at risk should be a major goal.

In the United States, Ileana and colleagues studied interventions that involved the modification of the risk factors that lead to an ulcer in patients with diabetes. Identified risk factors for amputation included the consequences or sequelae of peripheral neuropathy and peripheral arterial disease (e.g. callus formation, onychomycosis, structural foot deformities, circulatory disturbances, wounds, inappropriate footwear). It follows that annual screening foot examinations should, at the very least, include evaluations for peripheral neuropathy, peripheral arterial disease, and the aforementioned sequelae. Given that abnormal plantar pressure distribution is a known risk factor for ulceration, monitoring and quantification of plantar pressures have been investigated as a means of identifying patients at risk of ulceration and monitoring the effects of pressure-reducing interventions (Howard 2009).

Diabetic foot education programs generally include instruction on daily foot self-inspection, trauma avoidance (e.g. barefoot walking), and encouragement for patients to contact their physician should any new symptoms or abnormality appear. In addition to educating patients on foot care and self-examination, several studies have highlighted the importance of provider education. The American Diabetes Association guidelines recommend that providers, at a minimum, gain competency in performing a basic screening examination of the foot that includes assessment of the neurological, vascular, dermatologic, and musculoskeletal systems. Another recently investigated intervention for monitoring diabetic foot health and detecting areas at risk for development of diabetic foot ulcers is skin temperature monitoring (Mayfield et al. 2004).

Diabetic foot care in less-developed countries

Although development of diabetic foot structures in the industrialized world gradually seems to be moving in the right direction, the need for knowledgeable specialists appears to be even greater in economically less-developed countries, where the scarcity of resources (human and financial) aggravates an already difficult situation. It is postulated that by 2025 approximately 80% of the newly diagnosed cases of diabetes mellitus and two thirds of all cases will be seen in developing and newly industrialized countries (International Diabetes Federation 2013). At the same time, cultural, religious, behavioral, and climatic factors all play a role in the pathogenesis,

course, and management of diabetes and its complications in these countries, creating particular conditions that influence outcomes (Abbas et al. 2002a, 2002b, Abbas & Archibald 2005, 20007a, 2007b, Abbas & Viswanathan 2007).

As described above, the implementation of programs to educate doctors and nurses in less-developed countries, using structured programs in diabetic foot care, has resulted in the training of numerous doctors with their paramedics in India and Tanzania (Bakker et al. 2006, McGill 2006, Pendsey & Abbas 2007, Abbas et al. 2011). Using the same model in the Step-by-Step Program, health-care providers in 15 centers in Tanzania received structured education and training. The project was carried out in two phases: a basic course component followed by advanced courses. Foot care clinics were launched in different parts of India and Tanzania. Published data look promising, and the team responsible for this pilot study feels that this project is ready to be exported and implemented in other less-developed countries (Bakker et al. 2006, McGill 2006, Pendsey & Abbas 2007, Abbas et al. 2011).

■ CONCLUSION

A targeted foot care education program can allow a diabetes care system with limited resources to be more efficient and effective. In low-income settings, already limited resources should not be wasted on inappropriate education and treatment programs, especially for patients already deemed to be at low risk for foot disease. All providers of foot care should participate in ongoing professional education development programs to obtain skills aimed at assisting people to adopt a more positive attitude and pragmatism toward their condition and the importance of self-care behavior modification. A reduction in the amputation rate is feasible and can be achieved through a trained diabetes workforce working in an effective system of care that focuses on education of both health-care provider and patient. For example, institution of the Step-by-Step Foot Project in Tanzania improved foot ulcer management for persons with diabetes, enhanced the sharing of knowledge and skills among doctors and nurses, and resulted in permanent, operational foot clinics across the country. The program also showed the feasibility of managing high-risk feet at the regional level through a program of education aimed at both health-care providers and patients allied with dissemination of information to other health-care professionals involved in patient care, and empowerment of persons with diabetes to take better care of their feet on their own volition, detect problems earlier, and seek timely help when problems arise. Early detection and treatment of diabetic foot complications through sustained education and targeted screening programs, such as the Step-by-Step Program, serves as a working model to reduce morbidity and mortality and improve patient outcomes in less-developed countries.

It is hoped that the successful establishment of this model of diabetic foot care in Tanzania will encourage other countries to do likewise. To date, the model has been exported to various other countries in Africa (Democratic Republic of Cong, Guinea, Botswana, Malawi, Kenya, S. Africa, Ethiopia, and Egypt), Pakistan, Saudi Arabia, and the Caribbean (Barbados, St Lucia, St Maarten, St Kitts, and the British Virgin Islands). In December 2012, a Step-by-Step foot care workshop was successfully conducted in Brazil with participants from all 14 countries in continental South America. More recently, in July 2013, a course was conducted in Tobago, where 57 participants from 22 countries were trained. Finally, one of the least visible but important upshots of the Step-by-Step Program has been the highlighting of the importance of epidemiology and surveillance activities for characterizing foot complications in persons with diabetes, and for monitoring disease progression and outcomes, such as temporal trends of amputation rates and mortality.

ACKNOWLEDGEMENTS

The author would like to acknowledge the World Diabetes Foundation for funding Step-by-Step foot training projects, in particular in Africa, and the support of Step-by-Step project members all over the world. The author would also like to acknowledge Dr Lennox K. Archibald for his continuous support and is grateful to Shabneez Gangji and other staff members in Dar es Salaam for their assistance in the preparation of this chapter.

IMPORTANT FURTHER READING

International Diabetes Federation. IDF Diabetes Atlas, 6th edn. Brussels, Belgium: International Diabetes Federation, 2013. (http://www.idf.org/diabetesatlas

REFERENCES

Abbas ZG, Archibald LK. Epidemiology of the diabetic foot in Africa. Med Sci Monit 2005; 11:RA262–70.

Abbas ZG, Archibald LK. Challenges for management of the diabetic foot in Africa: doing more with less. Int Wound J 2007a; 4:305–313.

Abbas ZG, Archibald LK. The diabetic foot in Sub-Saharan Africa: a new management paradigm. Diab Foot J 2007b; 10:128–136.

Abbas ZG, Gill GV, Archibald LK. The epidemiology of diabetic limb sepsis: an African perspective. Diabet Med 2002a; 19:895–899.

Abbas ZG, Lutale JK, Bakker K, Baker N, Archibald LK. The 'Step-by-Step' Diabetic Foot Project in Tanzania: a model for improving patient outcomes in less-developed countries. Int Wound J 2011; 8:169–175.

Abbas ZG, Lutale JK, Morbach S, Archibald LK. Clinical outcome of diabetic patients hospitalized with foot ulcers, Dar es Salaam, Tanzania. Diabet Med 2002b; 19:575–579.

Abbas ZG, Viswanathan V. The diabetic foot in Africa and India. Int Diab Monitor 2007; 19:8–12.

Anichini R, Zecchini F, Cerretini I, et al. Improvement of diabetic foot care after the Implementation of the International Consensus on the Diabetic Foot (ICDF): results of a 5-year prospective study. Diabetes Res Clin Pract 2007; 75:153–158.

Apelqvist J, Larsson J. What is the most effective way to reduce incidence of amputation in the diabetic foot? Diabetes Metab Res Rev. 2000; 16:S75–S83.

Bakker K. The year of the diabetic foot and beyond. Diabetes Voice 2005; 50:43–45.

Bakker K, Abbas ZG, Pendsey S. Step-by-Step, improving diabetic foot care in the developing world. A pilot study for India, Bangladesh, The 'Step-by-Step' Diabetic Foot Project in Tanzania, 2004–2010 Sri Lanka and Tanzania. Pract Diab Intern 2006; 23:365–369.

Boulton AJM, Cavanagh PR, Rayman G (eds). The foot in diabetes, 4th edn. Chichester, UK: John Wiley & Sons, Ltd, 2006.

Ebskov B, Ebskov L. Major lower limb amputation in diabetic patients: development during 1982 to 1993. Diabetologia 1996; 39:1607–1610.

Faglia E, Favales F, Aldeghi A, et al. Change in major amputation rate in a center dedicated to diabetic foot care during the 1980s: prognostic determinants for major amputation. J Diabetes Complications 1998; 12:96–102.

Holstein P, Ellitsgaard N, Olsen BB, Ellitsgaard V. Decreasing incidence of major amputations in people with diabetes. Diabetologia 2000; 43:844–847.

Howard IM. The prevention of foot ulceration in diabetic patients. Phys Med Rehabil Clin N Am 2009; 20:595–609.

International Diabetes Federation. IDF Diabetes Atlas, 6th edn. Brussels, Belgium: International Diabetes Federation, 2013. http://www.idf.org/diabetesatlas

International Working Group on the Diabetic Foot (IWGDF). The development of global consensus guidelines on the management and prevention of the diabetic foot 2011. www.iwgdf.org

Larsson J, Apelqvist J, Agardh CD, Stenström A. Decreasing incidence of major amputation in diabetic patients: a consequence of a multidisciplinary foot care team approach? Diabet Med 1995; 12:770–776.

Leese GP, Stang D. Strategies for improving diabetic foot care: an example from Scotland. Diabetic Foot Canada 2014; 2:41–45.

Matwa P, Chabeli MM, Muller M, Levitt NS: Working Group of the National Diabetes Advisory Board: European IDDM Policy Group. Experiences and guidelines for footcare practices of patients with diabetes mellitus. Curationis 2003; 26:11–21.

Mayfield JA, Reiber GE, Sanders LJ, Janisse D, Pogach LM. Preventive foot care in people with diabetes. Diabetes Care 1998; 21:2161–2177.

Mayfield JA, Reiber GE, Sanders LJ, Janisse D, Pogach LM. American Diabetes Association. Preventive foot care in diabetes. Diabetes Care 2004; 27:S63–S64.

McGill M. Diabetic neuropathy: foot education. Diabetes education modules, Section 5 Part 4-III. 2006; International Diabetes Federation. www.idf.org/webdata/docs/Education%20modules%20Leaflet.pdf

Morbach S. Structures of diabetic foot care. European Endocrine Disease 2007; 2:56–58.

Müller E, Bergmann K, Brunk-Loch S, et al. Fubehandlungseinrichtung DDG - erste evaluation [in German]. Diabetologie 2006; 1:84.

Pendsey S, Abbas ZG. The step-by-step program for reducing diabetic foot problems: a model for the developing world. Curr Diab Rep 2007; 7:425–428.

Stang D. Target that risk: nationally agreed information and education leaflets for the diabetic. Diabet Foot J 2008; 11:156–160.

van Houtum WH, Rauwerda JA, Ruwaard D, Schaper NC, Bakker K. Reduction in diabetes-related lower-extremity amputations in The Netherlands: 1991-2000. Diabetes Care 2004; 27:1042–1046.

Van Rensburg GJ. Preventive foot care in people with diabetes: Quality patient education. JEMDSA 2009; 14:1–2.

Veves A, Uccioli L, Manes C, et al. Comparison of risk factors for foot problems in diabetic patients attending teaching hospital outpatient clinics in four different European states. Diabet Med 1994; 11:709–713.

Vileikyte L, Gonzalez JS, Leventhal H, et al. Patient Interpretation of Neuropathy Questionaire: an instrument for assessment of cognitive and emotional factors associated with foot ulceration. Diabetes Care 2006; 29:2617–2624.

Vileikyte L, Rubin RR, Leventhal H. Psychological aspects of diabetic neuropathic foot complications: an overview. Diabetes Metab Res Rev 2004; 20:13–18.

autonomic nerves 184–185
motor nerves 183–184
sensory nerves 184
pathological mechanisms for 187–189
aldose reductase and polyol pathway 188–189, *189*
hyperlipidemia 189
hypoxia 189
small fiber 183
testing for 185
Neuropathy and Foot Ulcer-specific Quality of Life (NeuroQoL) instrument 39, 40
Neuropeptide-specific peptidases (NEPs) 216
Neuropeptides (NPs), role of, in wound healing 216
Nicotinamide adenine dinucleotide phosphate (NADPH) 58, 188
Nitinol stents 164–165
Nitric oxide (NO) 103
role of, in diabetic ulcers 217
Nitric oxide synthase 3 (NOS-3) 246
Norfolk Quality of Life for Diabetic Neuropathy instrument (Norfolk QoL-DN) 40
NPWT *see* Negative pressure wound therapy (NPWT)
NSAIDs, for neuropathic pain 196
Nutrition, effect of, on wound healing 215

O

Obesity, effect of, on wound healing 215
Off-loading 345
devices 345–346, **346**
surgical 349–351, *350*
total contact cast 346–347
manufacture and application 347–349, *348, 349*
pros and cons of 347, **347**
Off-road system 161
Olive-type metal intraluminal occluders 145
Optical coherence tomography (OCT), in peripheral arterial disease 126
Optima Diab 306
OrthoWedge 347
Ostectomy **83**
Osteitis **58**
Osteomyelitis **58**
Osteoprotegerin (OPG) 297
Oxygen, for wound healing 213–214

P

PAD *see* Peripheral arterial disease (PAD)
'Painful painless feet' 193
Papaverine solution irrigation 143
Partial calcanectomy **83**
Patch angioplasty 145
Patient-reported outcome measures (PROMs) 39
PEDIS wound classification 16, **17**, 60
Percutaneous bone biopsy, in diagnosis of osteomyelitis 70–71, *71*
Percutaneous transluminal angioplasty (PTA) 153
see also Angioplasty
and anesthesia 156
antithrombotic therapy and 157
complications 155, **156**
effectiveness of 155
feasibility of 154–155, **155**, *155*
and hospital stay 156
indications for 153–154, **154**, *154*
and repeatability 156
and restenosis 156
revascularization after failed angioplasty 156–157

and stress 156
technological innovations in 157
vascular access for *157*, 157–158
Peripheral arterial disease (PAD) 95, 137, 171 *see also* Distal bypass techniques; Percutaneous transluminal angioplasty (PTA)
asymptomatic 98
atherosclerosis and 95, 111
cell-based therapy for 177
CO_2 angiography for 125
computed tomography angiography for
advantages and limitations of 121
optimizing contrast exposure 119
post-processing 120, *120*
radiation exposure 119, **120**
technology and principles 119
use of 120
and critical limb ischemia 98, 112
and diabetic foot ulcers 96, 171–172
diagnosis of 111
ankle brachial pressure index 113–114
clinical examination 112–113
pole test 114
symptoms of PAD 111–112, *112*
toe pressure measurement 114–115
transcutaneous oxygen tension measurements 115
treadmill test 114
digital subtraction angiography for 123–124, *124*
advantages and limitations of 124–125, *125*
contrast and contrast toxicity 122–123
contrast-induced nephrotoxicity 123, **124**
technology and principles 122
Fontaine and Rutherford classifications of **97**
gadolinium chelates for 122
imaging of 117 (see also Specific techniques)
insulin resistance and 111
intermittent claudication (IC) in 95, 98, 111–112
intravascular ultrasound for 126
lower limb 111
magnetic resonance angiography for 121
advantages and limitations of 121–122
technology and principles 121, *121*
molecular imaging for 126
natural history of *95*
in diabetes 98–99
in general population 97–98
optical coherence tomography for 126
pre-emptive revascularization 177–178
prevalence of
in diabetes 96–97
in general population 96
revascularization in diabetes with 172
amputation rate 174
angioplasty 176–177
distal disease and 175
limb salvage 174
outcomes of 173–175
patency rates 173, *173*, **174**
perioperative complications and mortality 173
surgical bypass 175–176
technical challenges 174
wound healing 173–174
risk factors for 95
rotational angiography/cone beam CT for 125–126
smoking and 96

ultrasonography for
advantages and limitations of *118*, 118–119
B-mode ultrasound 117
color Doppler 118
contrast-enhanced ultrasound 118
Doppler *117*, 117–118
volume–outcome relationship in surgery for 178
Peroneal artery 140, *140*
Phantom limb pain (PLP) 336, 340, 341
Photoplethysmography (PPG) 105, 114
Pioneer 161
Plantar hallux 12, *12*
Plantar neuropathic foot ulcers 5
Plantar ulcers with osteomyelitis 79
Plaster of Paris cast 348, *348*
PLP *see* Phantom limb pain (PLP)
Pneumatic postamputation mobility (PPAM) aid 336, *338*
Point-of-care test 238
Pole test 114
Polyhexamethylene biguanide (PHMB), in wound dressing 237
Polymorphonuclear (PMN) cell 57–58
Polytetrafluoroethylene (PTFE) graft 141
Polyurethane foam, as wound filler 245
Popliteal artery 138–139 *see also* Distal bypass techniques
occlusion of, treatment of 161–163, *162*
Postdebridement culture 323
Posterior tibial artery (PTA) 139, *140 see also* Distal bypass techniques
Probe-to-bone (PTB) test 69
Profunda femoris artery 138 *see also* Distal bypass techniques
Profundaplasty 145
Project LEAP 49
Propaten graft 141
Prostaglandin E1 therapy 147
Prosthetic graft failure 149
Prosthetic vascular grafts 141
Protease modulating dressings 238
Pseudomonas aeruginosa 61, **61**, 70
PTA *see* Percutaneous transluminal angioplasty (PTA)
Pulse volume recordings (PVR) 15

R

Removable cast walker (RCW) *305,* 305–306
Revascularization edema, after distal bypass 148
Risk classification 15, 16
PEDIS wound classification 16, 17
University of Texas (UT) ulcer classification system 15–16, 16
Wagner classification for foot ulcers 15
wound classification systems 15
RNA interference (RNAi) technology 220
Rotational angiography/cone beam CT 125–126
Rummel tourniquet 145

S

Sartorius flap 146
Semipermeable films 234, *235*
10-g Semmes–Weinstein monofilament 13
Sensory nerves 184
dysfunction of, consequences of 185, *186, 187*
Sequential bypass 146, *146*
Sesamoidectomy **83**
Short saphenous vein (SSV) 140, 142
Silver dressings 236

Skin and local tissue flaps 273
  external fixators, off-loading of 281
  local flaps 276, 276–277, 277
    bilobed flap 278
    local axial flaps 278–281, 280
    rhomboid flap 277, 278–279
    rotational flaps 277–278
    V-Y flap 278
  postoperative management 281
  preparation for 274, **274**, 275
  split-thickness skin grafts 276, **276**
  vascular and cutaneous anatomy of lower
    extremity 273–274
Skin perfusion pressure (SPP) 115
Skin substitutes, bioengineered 239
Smoking, effect of, on wound healing 215
Soft tissue infection **58**
Split-thickness skin graft (STSG) 273, 276 see also
  Skin and local tissue flaps
Spring ligament 261
Stabil-D device 306
Staphylococcus aureus 60, 70, 76
Staphylococcus epidermidis 69, 76
Statins, after distal bypass 147
Stenosis, on ultrasound 119
Step-by-Step Foot Project 51, 362, 363–365, **364**,
  364, **365**
Step-by-Step program xxi, 22, 25, 52
St Mary's boot 147, *147*
Stockinette 348
Supera stent 163
Superficial circumflex iliac artery perforator (SCIP)
  289–291, *290–291*
Superficial femoral artery (SFA) 138 see also Distal
  bypass techniques
Superoxide 58
Surgical debridement 267–272
  bone and 271
  callus 271
  in chronic wounds 271–272
  diabetic foot infection classification schemes
    268, 268–269
  fascia, muscle, and tendon 271
  skin 271
  subcutaneous tissue 271
  technique 269, *269*, *270*
    debridement tools 269
    tourniquet 269
  timing 267–269, **268**
  and wound closure 271
  and wound irrigation 271
Sutures, for vascular anastomosis 145

T
Tarsal tunnel syndrome 264
Taylor patch 147, *147*

TCC   *see* Total contact cast (TCC)
Telavancin 63
Thromboembolectomy 145
Tibial and foot arteries, calcification in 129
Tigecycline **61**, 63
TIMPs *see* Tissue inhibitors of metalloproteinases
  (TIMPs)
Tinel's sign, positive 202, 204
Tissue inhibitors of metalloproteinases (TIMPs)
  212, 213, 217, 238
Toe amputation, in osteomyelitis. *81,* 81–82
Toe–brachial index (TBI) 95, 114
Toe pressure measurements 114–115
Toll-like receptors (TLR) 210
Total contact cast (TCC) 303, *303,* 304–305, 316,
  346–349
Tourniquet, use of 145
Train the Foot Trainer program xxi–xxii, 51–52
Transcutaneous oxygen tension measurement
  105, 115, 285
Transfemoral amputation 335, *337* see also
  Amputation
Transtibial amputation 334–335, *335* see also
  Amputation
Transtibial prosthesis *336*
Treadmill test 114
TruePath device 160, *161*

U
Ulceration, diabetic foot **112**, 112–113 see also
  Diabetic foot ulcers (DFUs)
Ulcer recurrence, prevention of 353
  clinical guidelines 356
  conservative treatment 355
  footwear quality and adherence 356–357
  incidence and factors for ulcer recurrence 353,
    354
  methods of 353, 355
  surgical off-loading 355–356
Ultrasonic-assisted debridement 233
Ultrasonography, for peripheral arterial disease
  117, 117–119, *118*
University of Texas (UT) ulcer classification system
  15–16, **16**
Uridine diphosphate-*N*-acetylhexosamine
  (UDP-GlcNAc) 188

V
VACO ped-shoe 347
Vacuum-assisted closure (VAC) therapy system
  243–244
Vein graft, failure of 149 see also Distal bypass
  techniques
Vein patch adjuncts 176
Venlafaxine, in painful DSPN 197
Venoarteriolar reflex 103

Vessel loops 145
Viance Crossing Catheter Enteer Re-entry System
  160
Vibratory perception threshold monitor 13–14,
  14
Volcano s5i Imaging System console 161

W
Walking aid, use of 346
Western perspective of diabetic foot care
  365–366
Wildcat device 160, *161*
Windlass mechanism 263, *263*
World Diabetes Day (WDD) 2005 xx
Wound filler 245
Wound healing 209, 231, 251–252 see also
  Dressings; Free tissue transfer; Skin and local
  tissue flaps
  adjuncts to 243
    hyperbaric oxygen therapy 245–248
    negative pressure wound therapy
      243–245
  chronic wounds, development of 209, 213,
    213 (see also Diabetic foot ulcers (DFUs))
  normal process of 209–210, *210*
    angiogenesis 212
    extracellular matrix, formation of 212
    fibroblast migration 212
    growth factors and cytokines involved in
      211
    hemostasis 210
    inflammation 210–212
    proliferative phase 212
    re-epithelialization 212
    remodeling and scar maturation 212
    wound contraction 212
  outcome/end point of 252
    bias, avoidance of, in designing studies
      253–254
    cost and resource utilization studies,
      design of 254
    end point/outcome parameter 252
    European Wound Management
      Association (EWMA) survey document
      on 251–252
    recommendations for 254–255
    studies on, findings of 252–253
    surrogate end point/outcome parameter
      252
Wounds
  chronic 209, 213 (see also Wound healing)
  diabetic foot 3

X
X-ray, in diabetic foot osteomyelitis 71, *72*